Striking a Balance

HEALTH CARE SYSTEMS IN CANADA AND ELSEWHERE

CANADA HEALTH ACTION: BUILDING ON THE LEGACY
PAPERS COMMISSIONED BY THE NATIONAL FORUM ON HEALTH

Striking a Balance

HEALTH CARE SYSTEMS IN CANADA AND ELSEWHERE

ÉDITIONS
MULTIMONDES

FORUM NATIONAL
SUR LA SANTÉ

NATIONAL FORUM
ON HEALTH

Canadian Cataloguing in Publication Data

Main entry under title:

Canada Health Action: Building on the Legacy

Issued also in French under title: La santé au Canada: un héritage à faire fructifier
To be complete in 5 v.
Includes bibliographical references.
Contents: v. 1 Childen and Youth – v. 2. Adults and Seniors – v. 3. Settings
and Issues – v. 4. Health Care Systems in Canada and Elsewhere.
ISBN 2-921146-62-2 (set)
ISBN 2-921146-51-7 (v. 4)

1. Public health – Canada. 2. Medicine, Preventive – Canada. 3. Children – Health
and hygiene – Canada. 4. Adulthood – Health and hygiene – Canada. 5. Aged –
Health and hygiene – Canada. I. National Forum on Health (Canada).

RA449.C28 1998   362.1'0971   C97-941659-0

Linguistic Revision: Traduction Tandem
Proofreading: Traduction Tandem and Robert Paré
Cover Design: Gérard Beaudry
Graphics: Emmanuel Gagnon

Volume 4: Health Care Systems in Canada and Elsewhere
ISBN 2-921146-51-7   Cat. No.: H21-126/6-4-1997E
Legal Deposit– Bibliothèque nationale du Québec, 1998
Legal Deposit – National Library of Canada, 1998
© Her Majesty the Queen in Right of Canada, 1998

The series The National Forum on Health can be ordered at this address:
Éditions MultiMondes
930, rue Pouliot
Sainte-Foy (Québec)
G1V 3N9 CANADA
Telephone: (418) 651-3885; toll free in North America: 1 800 840-3029
Fax: (418) 651 6822; toll free in North America: 1 888 303-5931
E-mail: multimondes@multim.com
Internet: http://www.multim.com

Published by Éditions MultiMondes in co-operation with the National Forum on Health, Health
Canada, and Canadian Government Publishing, Public Works and Government Services Canada.

FOREWORD

In October 1994, the Prime Minister of Canada, The Right Honourable Jean Chrétien, launched the National Forum on Health to involve and inform Canadians and to advise the federal government on innovative ways to improve the health system and the health of Canada's people. The Forum was set up as an advisory body with the Prime Minister as Chair, the federal Minister of Health as Vice Chair, and 24 volunteer members who contributed a wide range of knowledge founded on involvement in the health system as professionals, consumers and volunteers.

To fulfil their mandate, the Forum focused on long-term and systemic issues. They saw their task as formulating advice appropriate to the development of national policies, and divided the work into four key areas – Values, Striking a Balance, Determinants of Health, and Evidence-Based Decision Making.

The complete report of the National Forum on Health consists of two volumes:

Canada Health Action: Building on the Legacy
    The Final Report of the National Forum on Health
and
    Canada Health Action: Building on the Legacy
    Synthesis Reports and Issues Papers

Copies available from: Publications Distribution Centre, Health Canada Communications, PL. 090124C, Brooke Claxton Building, Tunney's Pasture, Ottawa, Ontario K1A 0K9. Telephone: (613) 954-5995. Fax: (613) 941-5366. *(Aussi disponible en français.)*

The Forum based its recommendations on 42 research papers written by the most eminent specialists in the field. The papers are brought together in a five-volume series:

VOLUME 1 – CHILDREN AND YOUTH
VOLUME 2 – ADULTS AND SENIORS
VOLUME 3 – SETTINGS AND ISSUES
VOLUME 4 – HEALTH CARE SYSTEMS IN CANADA AND ELSEWHERE
VOLUME 5 – EVIDENCE AND INFORMATION

Individual volumes or the complete series can be ordered from: Editions MultiMondes, 930, rue Pouliot, Sainte-Foy (Québec) G1V 3N9. Telephone: 1 800 840-3029. Fax: 1 888 303-5931. *(Aussi disponible en français.)*

Values

The Values working group sought to understand the values and principles that Canadians hold about health and health care, so that the system continues to reflect and respond to these values. To explore Canadian core values that are connected to the health care system and to understand the implications for decision making, the group conducted some original public opinion research, using scenarios or short stories which addressed many of the issues being investigated by the other working groups of the Forum. The scenarios were tested in focus groups. Quantitative research supplemented the focus groups making the findings more generalizable. The group also contributed to a review of public opinion research on health and social policy. Finally, a review of Canadian and international experience with ethics bodies was commissioned to identify the contribution that such groups can make to continuing the discusssion of values in decision making.

Striking a Balance

The Striking a Balance working group considered how to allocate society's limited resources to best protect, restore and promote the health of Canadians. Attention was given to the balance of resources within the health sector and other sectors of the economy. The group commissioned a series of papers to assist in their deliberations. They conducted a thorough review of international trends in health expenditures, use of resources, and outcomes. They paid considerable attention to public and private financing issues, health system oganization and federal-provicial transfers. The group produced a separate discussion paper on public and private financing, and a position paper on the Canada Health and Social Transfer.

Determinants of Health

The Determinants of Health working group sought to answer the question: In these times of economic and social hardship, what actions must be taken to allow Canadians to continue to enjoy a long life and, if possible, to increase their health status? The group consulted specialists to assist in identifying appropriate actions on the non-medical determinants of health. Specialists were asked to prepare papers on issues of concern to the health of the population related to the macro-economic environment, the contexts in which people live (i.e. families, schools, work and communities), as well as on issues of concern to people's health at different life stages. Each paper presents a review of the literature, examples of success stories or failures, and relevant policy implications.

Evidence-Based Decision Making

The working group on Evidence-Based Decision Making considered how individually practioners and policy makers can have access to, and utilize the best available evidence in making decisions. The group held two workshops with leading authorities to discuss how health information can be used to support and encourage a culture of evicence-based decision making, and to consider what information Canadians need to be better health care consumers and how to get that information to them. The group commissioned papers to: examine the meaning and concepts of evidence and evidence-based decision making as well as cases that illustrate opportunities for improvement; identify the health information infrastructure needed to support evidence-based decision making; examine tools which support more effective health care decision making; and identify strategies for assisting and increasing the role of Canadians in decision making in health and health care.

Members

William R.C. Blundell, B.A.Sc. (Ont.)
Richard Cashin, LL.B. (Nfld.)
André-Pierre Contandriopoulos, Ph.D. (Que.)
Randy Dickinson (N.B.)
Madeleine Dion Stout, M.A. (Ont.)
Robert G. Evans, Ph.D. (B.C.)
Karen Gainer, LL.B. (Alta.)
Debbie L. Good, C.A. (PEI)
Nuala Kenny, M.D. (N.S.)
Richard Lessard, M.D. (Que.)
Steven Lewis (Sask.)
Gerry M. Lougheed Jr. (Ont.)

Margaret McDonald, R.N. (NWT)
Eric M. Maldoff, LL.B. (Que.)
Louise Nadeau, Ph.D. (Que.)
Tom W. Noseworthy, M.D. (Alta.)
Shanthi Radcliffe, M.A. (Ont.)
Marc Renaud, Ph.D. (Que.)
Judith A. Ritchie, Ph.D. (N.S.)
Noralou P. Roos, Ph.D. (Man.)
Duncan Sinclair, Ph.D. (Ont.)
Lynn Smith, LL.B., Q.C. (B.C.)
Mamoru Watanabe, M.D. (Alta.)
Roberta Way-Clark, M.A. (N.S.)

Secretary and Deputy Minister, Health Canada

Michèle S. Jean

Secretariat Staff

Executive Director
Marie E. Fortier

Joyce Adubofuor
Lori Alma
Rachel Bénard
Kathy Bunka
Barbara Campbell
Marlene Campeau
Carmen Connolly
Lise Corbett
John Dossetor
Kayla Estrin
Rhonda Ferderber
Annie Gauvin
Patricia Giesler
Sylvie Guilbault
Janice Hopkins

Lucie Lacombe
Johanne LeBel
Elizabeth Lynam
Krista Locke
John Marriott
Maryse Pesant
Marcel Saulnier
Liliane Sauvé
Linda St-Amour
Judith St-Pierre
Nancy Swainson
Catherine Swift
Josée Villeneuve
Tim Weir
Lynn Westaff

We extend our sincere thanks to all those who participated in the various production stages of this series of publications.

TABLE OF CONTENTS – VOLUME 4

HEALTH CARE FINANCING

INTERNATIONAL COMPARISON OF THE HOSPITAL SECTOR 3

Geoffroy Scott

Description of the Main Methods of Hospital Payment 7
Comparative Analysis of Acute Care Hospitals 7
Summary and Conclusion 22

CONTROLLING HEALTH EXPENDITURES: WHAT MATTERS 33

Astrid Brousselle

Introduction 39
Change in Expenditures in 13 OECD Countries 40
Explanation of the Deviation in Health Expenditures from the Average
of the Thirteen Countries Studied 43
Conclusion 51

MANAGING PHARMACEUTICAL EXPENDITURES:
HOW CANADA COMPARES 85

Wendy Kennedy

Methodology 90
Cross-Country Comparison of Per Capita Pharmaceutical Expenditures 91
Cross-Country Comparison of Drug Expenditures as a Percentage
of Total Health Expenditures 91
Cross-Country Comparison of Pharmaceutical Expenditures as
a Percentage of GDP 93
Cross-Country Comparison of the Relationship of Pharmaceutical
Expenditures to Wealth 94
Cross-Country Comparison of Drug Use 96
Cross-Country Comparison of Drug Sector Structures 97
Cross-Country Comparison of Health Indices 97
Discussion 98

HEALTH SPENDING AND HEALTH STATUS:
AN INTERNATIONAL COMPARISON 153

Centre for International Statistics

Health Care Spending among OECD Countries 157
The Relationship between Health Spending and Health Status 157
Other Forms of Social Spending that May Influence Health Status 162
Trends over Time 166
Conclusion 168

HOW CANADA'S HEALTH CARE SYSTEM COMPARES WITH
THAT OF OTHER COUNTRIES: AN OVERVIEW 173

Damien Contandriopoulos

Descriptive Analysis of the Various Health Care Systems 177
State of Health, Cost Control, and Performance of System 186
Conclusion 189

INTERNATIONAL COMPARISONS OF HEALTH EXPENDITURES 213

Delphine Arweiler

The Different Measurements of Health Expenditures 217
Prices and Quantities 225
Conclusion 236

THE IMPACT OF HEALTH CARE INFRASTRUCTURES AND
HUMAN RESOURCES ON HEALTH EXPENDITURES 253

Marc-André Fournier

Introduction 257
Breakdown of Expenditures and Resource Configurations 258
Configurations of Countries Successful and Unsuccessful
in Controlling Expenditures 275
Conclusion 282

HEALTH CARE EXPENDITURES AND THE AGING POPULATION
IN CANADA 285

Ellen Leibovich, Howard Bergman, and François Béland

Introduction 288
The Aging Population and the Cost of Health Care in Canada 288

System of Care for the Elderly in Sweden and the United Kingdom 296

Care of the Elderly in Canada 299

Strategy for the Development of a System of Care for the Frail
Elderly in Canada 300

Conclusion 302

PUZZLING ISSUES IN HEALTH CARE FINANCING 307

Raisa Deber and Bill Swan

Question One: Introduction and Summary 310

Overview of Data 310

Hypotheses 311

Discussion 329

Question Two (Supplementary Question): The Case of
the United Kingdom 331

Conclusions 335

*COMMENTARY ON HEALTH CARE EXPENDITURES, SOCIAL
SPENDING AND HEALTH STATUS* 343

Terrence Sullivan

Introduction 346

Overview of the Data 346

Hypotheses 347

Conclusions 352

INTERNATIONAL COMPARISONS

NATIONAL GOALS AND THE FEDERAL ROLE IN HEALTH CARE 367

Allan M. Maslove

Introduction 371

National and Provincial Goals in Health Care 372

Federal Levers in Health Care 380

National Goals and Federal Instruments: Options for Upholding
National Health Care Principles 384

Models of Financial Partnership 391

Conclusion 398

THE PUBLIC-PRIVATE MIX IN HEALTH CARE 423

**Raisa Deber, Lutchmie Narine, Pat Baranek, Natasha Sharpe,
Katya Masnyk Duvalko, Randi Zlotnik-Shaul, Peter Coyte,
George Pink, Paul Williams**

Objectives 431

Understanding the Basis for the Current Public-Private Mix of Services 431

Legislative and Regulatory Framework 457

The Case of Canada: Selected Data on the Extent of
the Public-Private Mix 469

Case studies of Some Experiences with Different Models 485

Evaluating the Models: Equity, Efficiency, Security and Liberty 503

Frameworks for Making Decisions about What Should and
What Should Not Be Insured 512

Policy Implications and Recommendations 531

*INTEGRATED MODELS. INTERNATIONAL TRENDS AND
IMPLICATIONS FOR CANADA* 547

John Marriott and Ann L. Mable

Introduction 551

Overviews of Systems in Selected Countries 558

Overview of the Canadian Health System and Models 609

Key Features of Integrated Models 626

Key Features of Integrated Models in the Canadian Context 640

Evaluation of Integrated Models 662

Conclusions and Observations 669

ISSUES FOR CANADIAN PHARMACEUTICAL POLICY 677

Steven G. Morgan

Introduction 681

The Economics and Politics of the Pharmaceutical Industry 688

Industry Trends and Corporate Strategies 699

Strategies for Managing Benefits 707

Conclusion 730

Health Care Financing

International Comparison of the Hospital Sector

GEOFFROY SCOTT

Doctorate Student in Public Health
University of Montreal

SUMMARY

The health care system, and more specifically, the hospital sector, is at a crossroads. Numerous budget cutbacks in recent years have raised questions about the optimum allocation of resources in this sector.

The National Forum on Health, through its "Striking a Balance" working group, is interested in this issue and believes that the public should be informed about the options. The primary purpose of international comparisons is to determine the relative ranking of the countries in order to provide an accurate and clear estimate of the resources invested in the sectors concerned. Using the most recent data available from the OECD, the comparative analysis presented in this report looks at some of the current trends in the hospital sector in the OECD countries studied.

It should be noted that there may be certain imperfections in the results of these international comparisons and consequently, they should be used with caution. The statistical data contains certain biases and it is imperative that the reader take note of them (this issue is addressed in the description of the methodology). This comparative analysis tries to answer four key questions:

- *Internationally, have acute care hospitals experienced a decrease in their share of total health expenditures?*
- *What components of the health sector have experienced an increase in their share of total health expenditures?*
- *Do the wealthier countries spend proportionately more on acute care hospitals than other countries?*

- *Does the quantity of physical resources have an impact on the use of acute care hospitals?*

  This report begins with a short description of the methods of hospital payment within OECD countries in order to help the reader better understand the various interactions between the utilization of hospital resources and hospital financing.

TABLE OF CONTENTS

Description of the Main Methods of Hospital Payment 7

Comparative Analysis of Acute Care Hospitals 7

Internationally, have acute care hospitals experienced a decrease
in their share of total health expenditures? 7

Which components of the health sector have experienced
an increase in their share of total health expenditures? 13

Do the wealthier countries spend relatively more on acute
care hospitals than other countries? 17

Does the quantity of physical resources have an impact
on the use of acute care hospitals? 19

Summary and Conclusion 22

Bibliography 24

APPENDICES

Appendix 1   Glossary 27

Appendix 2   Methodology 29

Appendix 3   Statistical Calculations 30

LIST OF FIGURES

Figure 1   Acute care hospital expenditures/Total health
expenditures 9

Figure 2   Acute care hospitals—Number of beds
per 1,000 inhabitants 10

Figure 3   Resources (personnel) available per occupied bed
(all hospitals except psychiatric hospitals) 11

Figure 4   Density (number of nurses) per 1,000 inhabitants 12

Figure 5   Hospital expenditures/Total health expenditures 14

Figure 6   Ambulatory care expenditures/Total health expenditures 15

Figure 7   Pharmaceutical goods expenditures/Total health
            expenditures 16

Figure 8   Other expenditures/Total health expenditures 16

Figure 9   Hospital expenditures/GDP 18

Figure 10   Acute care hospital expenditures/GDP 19

Figure 11   Correlation between admission rate and number of beds
            per 1,000 inhabitants 20

Figure 12   Correlation between length of stay and number of beds
            per 1,000 inhabitants 21

Figure 13   Correlation between occupancy rate and number of beds
            per 1,000 inhabitants 22

TABLE

Table 1   Main methods of hospital payment in OECD countries 8

DESCRIPTION OF THE MAIN METHODS OF HOSPITAL PAYMENT

It is crucial, in our view, to identify the main methods of payment to hospitals in order to give the reader a better understanding of the factors which have a major impact on the hospital sector. The incentives can vary widely from one payment model to another; even starting with the same amount, the various methods of payment will have different impacts on the realization of the objectives of equity, productivity, efficiency and cost control (Rhéault 1995). Furthermore, the methods of funding in the public sector are the result of a budget process, that is, a redistribution of public funds to the institutions.

Governments have five main methods of payment to finance *the activities of their institutions* (Rhéault 1995):

- *payment by global budget* by which the organization receives one payment to cover all of its activities;
- *per capita payment* by which the organization receives a payment based on the number of people to be served;
- *payment by episode of care* by which the organization receives a payment based on the complexity and intensity of anticipated services;
- *fee for service* which refers to the repayments made by a third party or by the government based on the number of services provided. More specifically, payment is made retroactively and the amount paid depends on the number of services provided, multiplied by the corresponding prices;
- *per diem payment* by which an amount (normally fixed) is paid to the organization under a contract for services.

Table 1 shows the main methods of payment used by OECD countries. Note that countries can use more than one method of payment but that for the vast majority the global budget is the one used most frequently.

COMPARATIVE ANALYSIS OF ACUTE CARE HOSPITALS

Internationally, have acute care hospitals experienced a decrease in their share of total health expenditures?

Expenditures for acute care hospitals account for approximately 80 percent of hospital expenditures. However, the budget constraints of recent years appear to have lead to a downsizing of the resources allocated to acute care hospitals in OECD countries.

To verify this trend, we will also examine a ratio with material resources and one with human resources.

Table 1

Main methods of hospital payment in OECD countries

	Payment by global budget	Per capita payment	Payment by episode of care	Fee-for-service payment	Per diem payment
Germany	X				
Australia	X				
Belgium	X				
Canada	X				
Denmark	X				
Spain	X				
United States		X	X		X
Finland	X				
France	X				
Greece					X
Ireland	X				
Italy	X				
Japan				X	
Luxembourg					X
New Zealand	X				
Norway	X		X		
Netherlands	X				
Portugal	X				
United Kingdom	X				X
Sweden	X				
Switzerland					X
Turkey	X				

Source: Contandriopoulos et al. 1993.

Acute Care Hospital Expenditures

First, it is necessary to determine the share of acute care hospital expenditures in total health expenditures. This ratio gives us the proportion of total health expenditures allocated to acute care hospitals since 1980. This first ratio was defined in two different ways (figure 1). First, based on OECD data, there has been a decrease in the share of total health expenditures allocated to acute care hospitals in Canada (falling from 40.9 percent in 1980 to 38.7 percent in 1992) and in the OECD countries as a whole (falling from 40.01 percent in 1980 to 34.8 percent in 1992). The reduction has been smaller in Canada compared to the OECD countries.

Figure 1

Acute care hospital expenditures/Total health expenditures

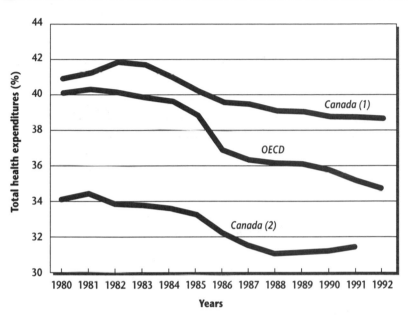

Second, based on the *Annual report of health institutions* (1995) which reports on the expenditures of Canadian hospitals, the proportion of total health expenditures allocated to acute care hospitals is lower than the average for the OECD countries by 4 percent to 5 percent. However, and this is the key point, the proportion of total health expenditures allocated to acute care hospitals in Canada is on the decline, dropping from 34.2 percent in 1980 to 31.5 percent in 1991.

Two observations need to be made concerning acute care hospital expenditures:

- In spite of a difference of almost 8 percent in results obtained from the two ratios, it is clear that the share of acute care hospital expenditures in total health expenditures is decreasing over time.
- Acute care hospitals continue to be the dominant component in health expenditures in all of the countries studied, regardless of the definition used for hospital care (OECD 1993).

However, the emphasis in such comparisons must be on the trends observed rather than on the absolute values.

Material Resources

The ratio of the number of beds per 1,000 inhabitants is an excellent indicator of the supply of beds in a country. Figure 2 shows a reduction in the number of beds per 1,000 inhabitants in Canada and in the OECD countries as a whole.[1] In Canada, the supply of acute care beds fell from 4.6 to 3.9 beds per 1,000 inhabitants between 1980 and 1991: the average supply of beds for the OECD countries as a whole fell from 5.4 to 4.6 beds per 1,000 inhabitants between 1980 and 1992.

Figure 2

Acute care hospitals—Number of beds per 1,000 inhabitants

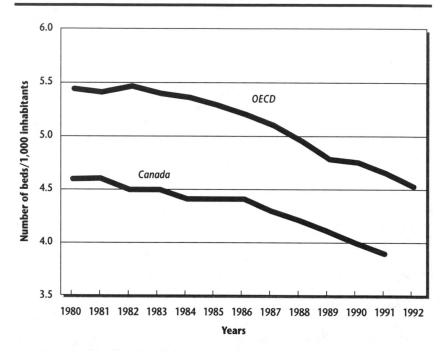

Canada therefore has fewer beds per 1,000 inhabitants than the average for the OECD countries. Medical technology and financial constraints are the main factors contributing to the drop in bed supply (OECD 1993).

---

1. The figures for 1980 to 1987 were supplied by the Canadian Institute for Health Information and not the OECD. They were adjusted based on the data for 1988 to 1991 since the most recent figures correspond to the number of beds approved in acute care units in all hospitals.

Human Resources

Two ratios are used to give us a good approximation of the level of human resources allocated per hospital bed. However, because there are many unoccupied beds (approximately 20 percent in Canada and 30 percent in the United States on average during the year), the ratio of personnel per occupied bed is a more significant figure (figure 3) and was retained for that reason. All types of institutions, except psychiatric facilities, were included in this ratio.

Figure 3

**Resources (personnel) available per occupied bed
(all hospitals except psychiatric hospitals)**

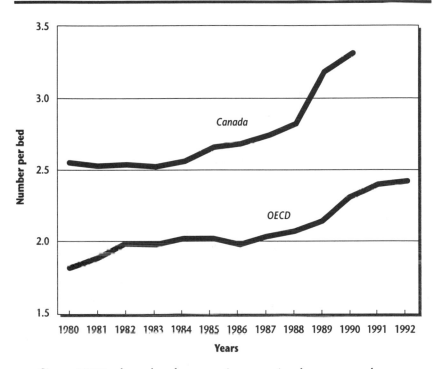

Since 1980, there has been an increase in the personnel resources allocated per occupied bed in Canada and in the OECD countries as a whole. In Canada, the rate increased from 2.56 in 1980 to 3.31 in 1990, compared to the average for the OECD countries which climbed from 1.8 in 1980 to 2.4 in 1992.

As for the second ratio, namely, the number of nurses per 1,000 inhabitants, figure 4 shows that it also increased in the OECD countries (from 5.3 in 1980 to 6.8 in 1991) and in Canada (9.6 in 1980 to 11.2 in 1991). These figures also reveal that the number of nurses in Canada is almost double the average for the OECD countries as a whole.

Figure 4

Density (number of nurses) per 1,000 inhabitants

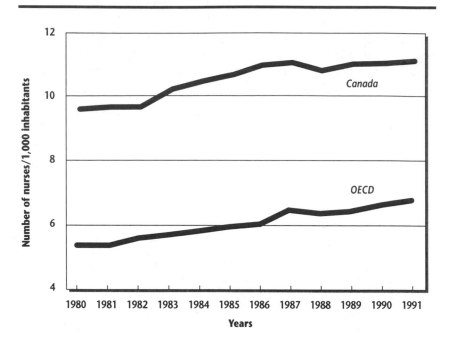

Canada appears to have more personnel per occupied bed than the average of the OECD countries. However, these figures must be interpreted with caution; a few clarifications will shed more light on the perceived gap. Hospital staff provide care to hospitalized patients and to outpatients. The increase in the number of personnel per bed reflects, at least in part, the growth in ambulatory care services (the numerator in the ratio covers all hospital personnel, while the denominator applies only to hospitalized patients). In addition, a drop in the length of stay in acute care hospitals, collective agreements, and the development of day surgery are all reasons for the higher number of human resources per bed. In short, a high ratio is not necessarily synonymous with a poor allocation of human resources in the hospital.

Conclusion

In short, although there has been an increase in human resources and nursing staff per bed, the proportion of acute care hospital expenditures in total health expenditures has decreased. The number of beds per 1,000 inhabitants has dropped, in absolute values, since 1980. It would appear that budget cutbacks imposed on acute care hospitals have led to a reduction in expenditures and in bed supply in this sector. However, it would be interesting to see the impact of these reductions on health performances.

Moreover, there appears to be a relationship between the number of acute care hospital beds per 1,000 inhabitants (figure 2) and the resources (personnel) available per occupied bed (figure 3). It appears that countries with a proportionately lower number of acute care hospital beds (such as Canada) use these beds more intensely and allocate more human resources to them. One hypothesis that might be drawn from these observations (it will have to be verified) is that the curative function of health care is greater when a country has proportionately fewer hospital beds.

Which components of the health sector have experienced an increase in their share of total health expenditures?

If the proportion of expenditures on acute care hospitals in the total health expenditures has decreased, then it is logical for there to have been increases among the other components of the health system. In order to verify this hypothesis and to determine the changes in the composition of expenditures, we have defined total health expenditures as follows:

Total health expenditures = hospital expenditures + ambulatory care expenditures + pharmaceutical goods expenditures + others

All of these components were examined to determine which ones had experienced growth since 1980. As with question 1 (see page 7), Canada was compared to the OECD countries as a whole.

Figure 5 clearly shows that hospital expenditures have dropped appreciably in Canada and the OECD countries as a whole. Indeed, Canada reduced the percentage of hospital expenditures[2] in the total expenditures from 53 percent in 1982 to 49 percent in 1991, while the OECD countries as a whole reduced the share of these expenditures from 51 percent in 1980 to 48 percent in 1991. This decrease was to be expected given the drop in acute care hospital expenditures noted in the previous section.

Canada spends proportionately slightly more than the OECD countries as a whole on hospital care but has followed the general trend which appears to be an appreciable reduction in this sector. Acute care, which accounts for almost 80 percent of hospital expenditures, has exercised strong downward pressure on this category of expenditures and surprisingly, there has been no increase in the share of total expenditures held by chronic care (except for home care).

---

2. Note that the category of hospital expenditures is more general than that of acute care hospital expenditures since it includes all types of institutions (see glossary).

Figure 5

Hospital expenditures/Total health expenditures

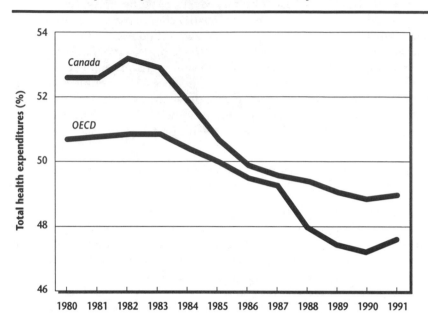

Figure 6, which deals with ambulatory care expenditures, reveals that there has been no increase in this sector in Canada since 1980, the percentage staying around 22 percent of total health expenditures. In the OECD countries as a whole, this sector has increased slightly, displaying a steady upward trend for about eight years. Canada appears to spend proportionately 5 percent less than the OECD countries as a whole. What is the reason for this? It is difficult to pinpoint but part of the reason may be that Canada is lagging behind in reform in this area.

Pharmaceutical goods expenditures (figure 7) have increased substantially in Canada, their proportion of total health expenditures climbing from 9 percent to 14 percent between 1989 and 1991. The proportion for OECD countries as a whole has remained stable at slightly less than 14 percent of total expenditures allocated to pharmaceutical goods. In spite of this sharp increase in just 10 years, Canada is now spending almost the same proportion of its total expenditures on pharmaceutical goods as the average for the OECD countries as a whole. The sharp rise in these expenditures over the past decade could be attributable to the predominance of private funding (Evans 1993).

Figure 6

Ambulatory care expenditures/Total health expenditures

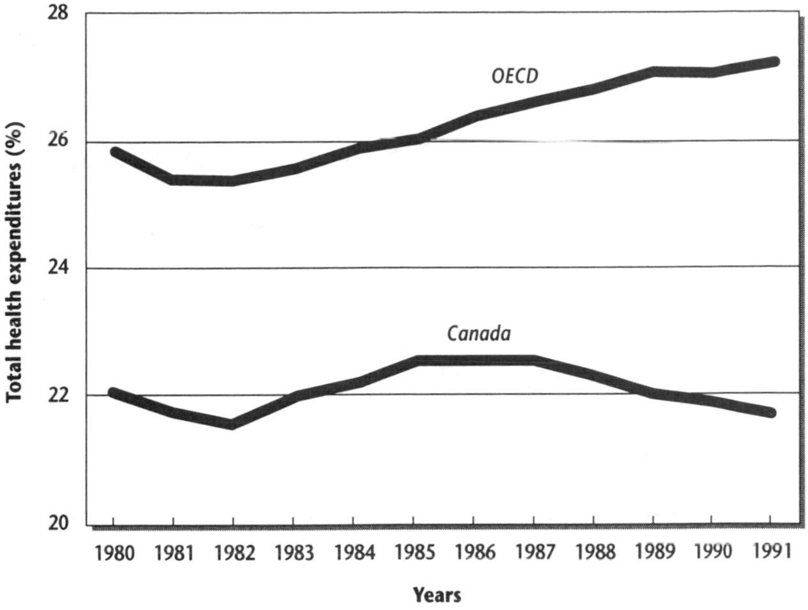

The last element of total health expenditures is the "other expenditures" sector (figure 8). This category includes, among other things, therapeutic devices, research and development, health administration, and medical investments. The OECD countries as a whole and Canada have experienced a decline in expenditures in this sector; between 1980 and 1989, they fell from 18.9 percent to 16.4 percent for the OECD countries as a whole, and from 16.4 percent to 15.4 percent for Canada. Note that the OECD countries as a whole experienced a greater drop in this category than Canada. This result would indicate that there has been a greater rationalization of these expenditures by OECD countries as a whole than by Canada.

Conclusion

There are several ways to define or categorize total health expenditures. The one used in this report highlights the major aggregates of total health expenditures. It is not exhaustive but it does provide a good overview of the issue.

Canada and the other OECD countries have a point in common: all have experienced an appreciable proportional decrease in their hospital expenditures. This would indicate that there has been a downsizing in this sector and that other avenues need to be explored in order to reform delivery mechanisms for health care.

Figure 7

Pharmaceutical goods expenditures/Total health expenditures

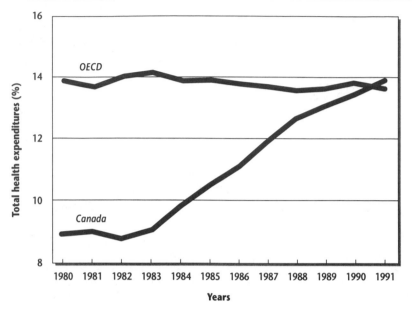

Years

Figure 8

Other expenditures/Total health expenditures

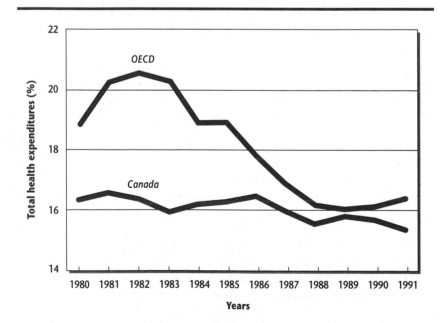

Years

Although ambulatory care expenditures have remained relatively stable for Canada and the OECD countries as a whole, there has been a marked increase in pharmaceutical goods expenditures in Canada. In fact, they have almost doubled in ten years and are now reaching the level of the average for the OECD countries.

What can be deduced from this information? Two conclusions can be drawn:

- In the OECD countries as a whole, the decrease in the proportion of total health expenditures allocated to the hospital care sector has been accompanied by an increase in the proportion of expenditures allocated to ambulatory care and to "other expenditures."
- In Canada, it appears that the pharmaceutical goods sector has absorbed all of the proportional reduction in expenditures in the hospital sector. It is somewhat difficult to determine the cause for this latter trend, but it is possible that the lack of a public national drug plan may have played a part (the other OECD countries have such a plan).

A brief review of the literature on health expenditures confirms these conclusions. The Conseil de la santé et du bien-être (1995) mentions that expenditures on pharmaceutical goods and medical services were the two areas that have experienced the greatest growth in Quebec in the past ten years.

Do the wealthier countries spend relatively more on acute care hospitals than other countries?

To verify this hypothesis, a simple linear regression was calculated for the variables being considered and then verified with a confidence interval of 99 percent. The index used for this comparison was the purchasing power parity per capita because it gives a good estimate of resource allocation. These correlations were determined using data from 1991 (figures 9 and 10).

The result obtained was significant[3] ($r^2 = 0.618425$), that is, there is a link between the wealth of a country and magnitude of its expenditures on acute care hospitals. For example, the United States has the highest per capita GDP ($21,574) and spends the most per capita on acute care ($935). At the other end of the scale, Spain has the lowest per capita GDP ($12,740) and spends the least, after the United Kingdom, on acute care ($392). Similarly, there is a link between the GDP of a country and the magnitude of all of its hospital expenditures. Although the latter correlation is weaker ($r^2 = 0.234265$) than that for acute care hospitals alone, it is still significant to a confidence interval of 95 percent.

This finding is corroborated indirectly by other studies. In fact, there is a strong correlation between a country's level of medical expenditures and the volume of resources it produces or which are available for consumption

---

3. A detailed description of the calculations is given in appendix 3.

Figure 9

Hospital expenditures/GDP

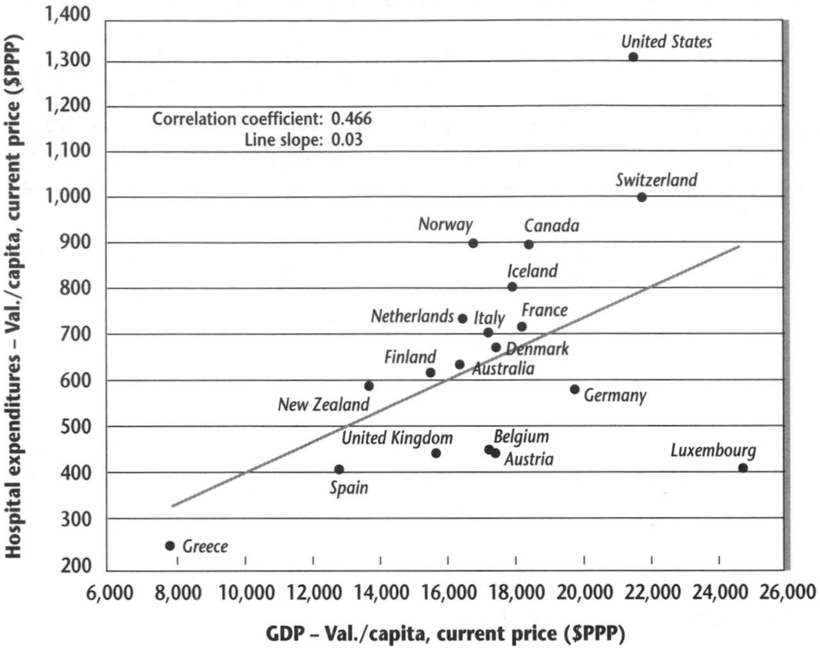

Source: OECD Health data 1995 (CREDES).

and investment (OECD 1993). This correlation even appears to have strengthened over the years. As a result, an upward trend in health care costs developed at a time when all new needs were met (Evans 1993).

Lastly, it is interesting to note in figures 9 and 10 that Canada's position above the line indicates a level of hospital spending higher than would be anticipated based on per capita GDP. The inverse is also true for other countries, such as the United Kingdom and Germany.

Conclusion

We can conclude from these findings that the wealthier countries (according to per capita GDP) very often have high hospital expenditures, especially in the acute care sector. Two observations are relevant:

- Expenditures on (and quantity of) hospital care and services increase as the per capita GDP increases;
- Hospital care and services (like health care) are becoming a luxury item because their consumption is higher in the wealthier countries.

Figure 10

Acute care hospital expenditures/GDP

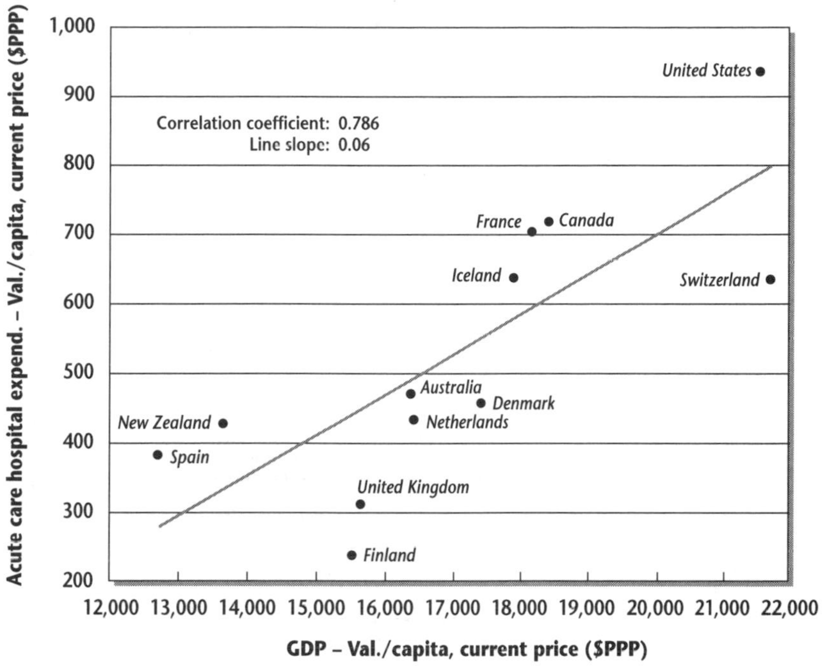

Correlation coefficient: 0.786
Line slope: 0.06

Source: OECD Health data 1995 (CREDES).

Does the quantity of physical resources have an impact on the use of acute care hospitals?

The use of acute care hospitals was examined in terms of three indicators: admission rate, length of stay, and occupancy rate. The same methodology was used as in question 3 (see page 17): simple linear regressions were calculated for the variables and verified with a confidence interval of at least 95 percent. Data from 1989 was used for the admission rate and occupancy rate calculations, while data from 1991 was used for the length of stay.

First, there appears to be a link between admission rates and bed supply (number of beds per 1,000 inhabitants) but this relationship is considered to be "weak" because it is significant only to 90 percent and not 95 percent ($r^2 = 0.150161$). We can conclude from this that the admission rate for acute care hospitals is influenced less by the supply of beds than the other indicators (figure 11). In actual fact, budget restrictions, the strive for excellence, technical progress, and aging populations with fixed resources are all factors which can have an impact on admission rates of acute care hospitals (OECD 1993).

Figure 11

**Correlation between admission rate and number of beds
per 1,000 inhabitants**

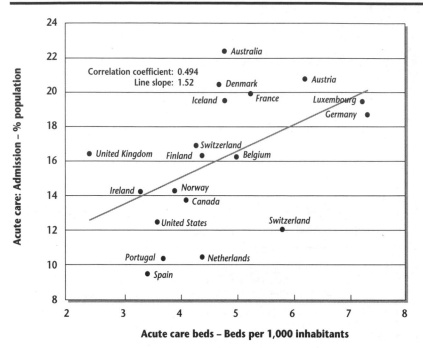

Source: OECD Health data 1995 (CREDES).

However, it was found that the length of stay in acute care hospitals was strongly influenced by bed supply (figure 12). Since $r^2 = 0.489$ and the variable is significant to a confidence interval of 99 percent, we can conclude that an increase in bed supply will result in an increase in length of stay. It is interesting to note, however, that countries with a short length of stay (United Kingdom, Denmark, and Japan) invest more in home care. One explanation for this phenomenon might be a better integration of resources allocated to chronic care. A study conducted by the Ministère de la Santé et des Services sociaux du Québec reached similar conclusions:

> … day surgery is much more developed in British Columbia than in Quebec; moreover, lengths of stay are shorter and the resources allocated to home care of the elderly are higher; the government also invests more than Quebec in social housing for the elderly (Turgeon 1995).

Figure 12

Correlation between length of stay and number of beds per 1,000 inhabitants

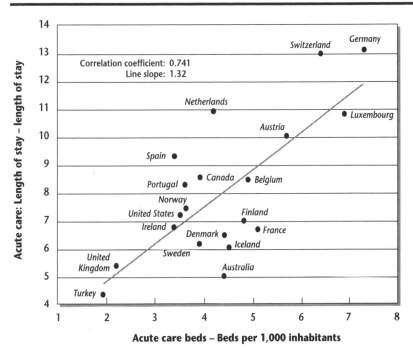

Source: OECD Health data 1995 (CREDES).

As for the occupancy rate, here again there appears to be a link with bed supply (figure 13). Although the correlation is weaker than with length of stay, it is still quite revealing (r^2 = 0.280 and the variable is significant to a confidence interval at 95 percent). A higher bed supply therefore tends to correlate to a higher occupancy rate. However, here again caution is warranted because higher rates may mask surplus capacity, as is the case when the length of hospitalization is longer than necessary or when it is motivated by deficiencies in social facilities (OECD 1993).

Overall, these observations support the hypothesis that a high bed supply leads to greater consumption of acute care. Similarly, the concept of induced demand, according to which the demand for health care and services is influenced primarily by the supply of care and services available on the market (Evans 1993), is also plausible in light of these findings.

Figure 13

Correlation between occupancy rate and number of beds per 1,000 inhabitants

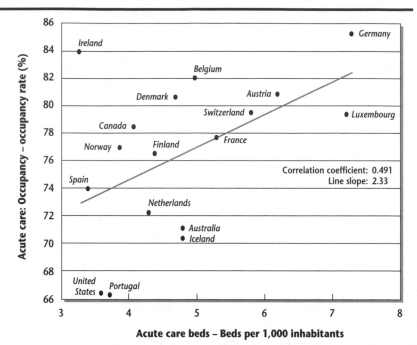

Source: OECD Health data 1995 (CREDES).

However, bed supply does not by itself determine the acute care consumption. Other factors also have a major impact on this consumption. For example, the payment of hospitals through a global budget gives hospitals the incentive to increase the length of stay and to reduce admission rates, while payment on an estimated case volume based on diagnosis-related groups (DRG) encourages hospitals to reduce the length of stay and increase admission rates (Schieber, Poullier, and Greenwald 1991). In the latter instance, the very nature of the budgetary process influences the productivity of hospital care and services in institutions.

SUMMARY AND CONCLUSION

The purpose of this comparative analysis was to identify the main trends for acute care hospitals in OECD countries. Given the scope and complexity of the subject, the study focused on expenditures and the consumption of care this component of the hospital system. The following trends were identified from the findings:

- Canada and the OECD countries as a whole have experienced a decline in the proportion of total health expenditures allocated to acute care hospital expenditures since 1980. The number of beds per 1,000 inhabitants has also fallen over the past decade. Budget cutbacks imposed on acute care hospitals appear to have reduced expenditures and bed supply.
- The number of personnel and the number of nurses per bed have risen since 1980. However, a high ratio does not necessarily mean a poor allocation of resources within hospitals.
- The decrease in the percentage of total health expenditures allocated to hospital care in Canada and the OECD countries as a whole necessarily translates into increases in the percentages of other categories of expenditures. For the OECD countries as a whole, the ambulatory care and "other expenditures" sectors experienced a proportional increase, while in Canada, it was the pharmaceutical goods sector which saw its share of expenditures rise.
- Hospital care and services expenditures (as well as the quantity of care and services) increase when the per capita GDP increases. The wealthier countries will therefore have to limit their hospital expenditures if they wish to bring them down to a reasonable percentage of their GDP.
- A high bed supply appears to produce a greater consumption of acute care.

However, these conclusions have limited scope since the variables examined reflect an incomplete view of reality. In actual fact, variables such as the methods of payment to hospitals, medical technologies, and budget cutbacks have a major impact on these trends. Consequently, it would be preferable to adopt a systemic perspective as much as possible.

Geoffroy Scott *is a doctoral candidate in public health at the University of Montreal. He holds a master's degree in public administration from the École nationale d'administration publique, and worked for the National Forum on Health as part of the "Striking a Balance" working group. His areas of interest include international comparisons, the use of oral services in developing countries, and the evaluation of health program.*

BIBLIOGRAPHY
(Sources cited and consulted)

ARWEILER, D., F. CHAMPAGNE, A.-P. CONTANDRIOPOULOS. 1994. *La privatisation du financement dans plusieurs pays de l'OCDE: convergence ou divergence?*, Montreal, GRIS, N94–01.

CHAPPELL, N. L. 1993. The Future of health care in Canada. *Journal of Social Policy* 22 (October).

CONSEIL DE LA SANTÉ ET DU BIEN-ÊTRE. 1995. *Un juste prix pour les services de santé.* Quebec, Government of Quebec.

CONTANDRIOPOULOS, A.-P., F. CHAMPAGNE, J. L. DENIS, A. LEMAY, S. DUCROT, M. A. FOURNIER, D. AVOKSOUMA. 1993. *Regulatory Mechanisms in the Health Care System of Canada and Other Industrialized Countries: Description and Assessment.* Queen's University–University of Ottawa Economics Projects.

EVANS, R. G. 1984. *Strained Mercy: The Economics of Canadian Health Care.* Toronto (ON): Butterworth.

———. 1993. Health care reform: The issue from hell. *Policy Options* July–August: 35–42.

GERDTHAM, G. 1992. Pooling international health care expenditure data. *Health Economics* 1: 217–231.

HEALTH CANADA. 1994. *National Health Expenditures in Canada 1975–1993.* Policy and Consultation Branch, Health Canada.

JEONG, H. S., and A. GUNJI. 1994. The influence of system factors upon the macro-economic efficiency of health care: Implications for the health policies of developing and developed countries. *Health Policy* 27: 113–140.

LAVIS, J. N., and G. M. ANDERSON. 1994. Can we have too much health care? *Daedalus* 123(fall): 43–60.

MAXWELL, J. 1995. *Sustainable Health Care for Canada.* Queen's University–University of Ottawa Economics Projects, University of Ottawa, Ottawa.

NAIR, C., and R. KARIM. 1993. An overview of health care systems: Canada and selected OECD countries. *Health Reports* 5(3). Statistics Canada.

NEWHOUSE, J. P., G. ANDERSON, L. L. ROOS. 1988. Hospital care in the United States and Canada: A comparison. *Health Affairs*, fall.

OECD. 1993. *OECD Health Systems: Facts and Trends 1960–1991.* Paris: Organization for Economic Cooperation and Development.

———1994. *The Reform of Health Care Systems: A Review of Seventeen OECD Countries.* Paris: Organization for Economic Cooperation and Development.

———. 1995. OECD Health data 1995 (CREDES).

PARÉ, I. 1995. L'hôpital, c'est fini! *Le Devoir*, Tuesday, April 4.

PORTER, B. (chairperson). 1991. *The Health Care System in Canada and Its Funding: No Easy Solutions.* First report of the Standing Committee on Health and Welfare, Social Affairs, Seniors and the Status of Women, Government of Canada, Ottawa.

RHÉAULT, S. 1995. *Évaluation des modalités de financement et de paiement dans le domaine sociosanitaire*, Collection Études et Analyses, no. 24, Direction générale de la planification et de l'évaluation, Ministère de la Santé et des Services sociaux, Government of Quebec.

SCHIEBER, G. J., and J. P. POULLIER. 1991. International health spendings: Issues and trends. *Health Affairs* spring: 106–116.

SCHIEBER, G. J., J. P. POULLIER, and L. M. GREENWALD. 1991. Health system performance in OECD countries, 1980–1992. *Health Affairs* fall: 100–112.

STATISTICS CANADA. 1995. *Annual Hospital Survey, Part 1.* Statistics Canada.

TURGEON, J. 1991. *Les soins hospitaliers de courte durée au Québec: une analyse comparative.* Direction générale de la planification et de l'évaluation, Ministère de la Santé et des Services sociaux, Bibliothèque nationale du Québec.

WORLD BANK. 1993. *World Development Report: Investing in Health.* New York (NY): Oxford University Press.

APPENDICES

APPENDIX 1

Glossary

Total health expenditures should include:
- final consumption by households of medical care and other health expenditures, including goods and services purchased by consumers of their own initiative, such as over-the-counter drugs, as well as the share of care financed or provided by the public sector that remains the responsibility of the patient;
- health services provided by the public sector, including health services at schools and in the armed forces;
- investment in consultation centres, laboratories, etc.;
- administrative costs;
- research and development, except for expenditures of pharmaceutical companies;
- occupational medicine (often treated as an intermediate consumption) is included when possible (such as expenditures of workers' compensation organizations);
- expenditures of volunteer organizations, medical equipment and therapeutic devices, and ambulance services.

Total Hospital Expenditures

Day-to-day expenditures, excluding investment expenditures for inpatient care hospitals, including public and private hospitals (acute and chronic care, convalescent). This definition covers all types of facilities: general hospitals; specialized hospitals (pediatric, orthopaedic, cancer, rehabilitation, extended care); psychiatric hospitals; sanatoriums.

Total Acute Care Hospital Expenditures

Day-to-day expenditures related to facilities which receive patients whose average length of stay is less than 30 days.

Number of Acute Care Beds per 1,000 Inhabitants

Average number of beds available in acute care facilities.

Admission Rate in Acute Care Hospitals

Number of admissions (or releases) in acute care hospitals, divided by the population and multiplied by 1,000   .

Average Length of Stay in Acute Care Hospitals

Number of bed-days in hospitals or acute care facilities, divided by the number of admissions (or releases).

Occupancy Rate for Acute Care Hospital Beds

Number of beds actually occupied in hospitals or acute care facilities, divided by the number of beds available and multiplied by 100.

Hospital Personnel Ratios

Workers, in full-time equivalents, employed in hospitals, and physicians, nursing staff and administrators (including contract personnel), paid on a full-time basis, divided by the number of beds available.

Nursing Staff Ratios

Level 1 and 2 nursing staff, in full-time equivalents, employed in hospital facilities, divided by the number of beds available.

Gross Domestic Product (GDP)

The GDP is the indicator used by the United Nations to measure a country's economic activity. Health expenditures are often expressed as a percentage of the GDP, which gives an approximate idea of the amount that is allocated to health in relation to society's ability to pay. The GDP and the GNP (gross national product) are similar measurements, but not identical. Canada's GDP is slightly higher than its GNP.

APPENDIX 2

Methodology

An international comparison can be both enriching and perilous: enriching because it makes it possible to determine the relative position of countries in various sectors, and perilous because there are a number of limitations in terms of methodology. Methodology limitations refer to the geographical, demographical, political, cultural, and economic differences which exist between countries, and to the differences in definitions from country to country. This is why the decision was made in this study to compare acute care hospitals because the definition of this concept is more uniform among countries. However, we are aware it would be preferable to have a systemic perspective. The ambiguity of definitions for alternative care and chronic care among OECD countries does not allow us, at present, to make an adequate comparison of these sectors.

All of the base data used was obtained from the *Health Data* database of the OECD. The OECD (Organization for Economic Cooperation and Development) is a worldwide organization which provides data in a variety of fields on its 24 member countries.[1] Although the data has some limitations, as discussed earlier, it nevertheless provides a good overview of the resources allocated by a country to its hospital sector. And that was the purpose of the exercise.

Lastly, the analysis was rounded off by a review of the literature which provided support for the initial findings. This study was also reviewed by individuals with the expertise to provide a constructive and valuable assessment.

---

1. Germany, Australia, Belgium, Canada, Denmark, Spain, the United States, Finland, France, Greece, Ireland, Italy, Japan, Luxembourg, New Zealand, Norway, the Netherlands, Portugal, the United Kingdom, Sweden, Switzerland, Turkey.

APPENDIX 3

Statistical Calculations

In the calculations given below and made using the Lotus 1-2-3 software, "p" has the following value:

$$\text{value of } p = \frac{\text{coefficient of X}}{\text{standard deviation of X}}$$

The value for p obtained from this calculation is compared to the table for t to determine whether p is significant to a confidence interval of $\geq$ 95 percent (t = 0.005). If it is, the variable is considered to be significant.

Question: Do the wealthier countries spend relatively more on acute care hospitals than other countries?

For acute care hospitals, the result is as follows:

$$\text{value of } p = \frac{0.056978}{0.014153} = 4.012$$

where p (4.012) is greater than 3.17 (t = 0.05).

*There is therefore a significant link between the GDP and the level of acute care expenditures.

For hospitals as a whole, the result is as follows:

$$\text{Value of } p = \frac{0.034789}{0.015255} = 2.2$$

Where p (2.2) is greater than 2.11 (t = 0.025).

*There is therefore a significant link between the GDP and the level of total hospital expenditures.

Question: Does the quantity of physical resources have an impact on the use of acute care hospitals?

For admission rate, the result is a follows:

$$\text{Value of } p = \frac{1.169333}{0.674681} = 1.74$$

where p (1.74) is less than 2.11 (t = 0.025), but equal to 1.74 (t = 0.05).

*There is therefore a link between admission rate and the supply of beds (number of beds per 1,000 inhabitants), but it is not retained because it is significant to 90 percent and not 95 percent.

For length of stay, the result is as follows:

$$\text{value of } p = \frac{1.286521}{0.318871} = 4.035$$

where p (4.035) is greater than 2.90 (t = 0.05).

*There is therefore a very significant link between length of stay and supply of beds (number of beds per 1,000 inhabitants).

For occupancy rate, the result is as follows:

value of p = $\dfrac{2.473295}{0.990699}$ = 2.4964848

where p (2.49) is greater than 2.12 (t = 0.025).

*There is therefore a significant link between occupancy rate and supply of beds (number of beds per 1,000 inhabitants).

Controlling Health Expenditures: What Matters

ASTRID BROUSSELLE

Doctoral Student in Public Health
Interdisciplinary Research Group on Health
Faculty of Medecine
University of Montreal

SUMMARY

Although the trend toward increasing costs is evident in all countries, there are significant differences from one country to another. The purpose of this project was to try to measure the differences in costs between the Canadian health system and that of 12 other OECD countries, and to identify the factors influencing these differences.

The first part of the project measured the differences in costs between the various countries between 1960 and 1993 using two indicators: per capita health expenditures and the percentage of GDP devoted to health expenditures. We also compared costs to the per capita GDP.

The second part of the project tried to explain the differences in relation to the average of the expenditures (regression curves). We tried to identify what aspects of financing, organization of the health system, and demand for health care in the various countries might explain these differences.

The analysis shows that health expenditures increase as a country develops. However, some countries control their health care costs much better than others. Moreover, the disparities in costs between the countries are not attributable to epidemiological or demographic differences; rather they are associated with the manner in which the health systems are organized, funded, and regulated.

Macroorganizational methods of regulation appear to be determinant. Micro-organizational methods are difficult to analyze, but the way in which physicians are paid seems to be a key factor. It also appears that controlling costs in the pharmaceutical sector is essential to controlling the total cost of the health system.

TABLE OF CONTENTS

Introduction 39

Change in Expenditures in Thirteen OECD Countries 40

Regressions 40
Linear Regressions 40
Logarithmic Regressions 40

Analysis 41
Change in per Capita Health Expenditures in Relation
to the per Capita GDP 41
Change in the Percentage of the GDP Allocated to Health in
Relation to the per Capita GDP 42

**Explanation of the Deviation in Health Expenditures
from the Average of the Thirteen Countries Studied** 43

Factors Associated with Health Demand 44
Population 65 Years and Older 44
Mortality Rate/1,000 Inhabitants 44

Macroorganizational Factors 45
Percentage of Public Financing 45
Number of Sources of Financing 46
Degree of Centralization 46

Microorganizational Factors 47
Hospital Sector 47
Ambulatory Sector 49
Medical Sector 49
Pharmaceutical Costs 51

Conclusion 51

Bibliography 53

Appendix 55

LIST OF FIGURES

Figure 1   Per capita health expenditures by per capita GDP
in 13 OECD countries, 1960 to 1993 57

Figure 2   Percentage of the GDP devoted to health by the
per capita GDP in 13 OECD countries, 1960 to 1993 57

Figure 3   Per capita health expenditures by per capita GDP,
Canada and Australia, 1960 to 1993 58

Figure 4   Per capita health expenditures by per capita GDP,
Canada and the United States, 1960 to 1993......................58

Figure 5   Per capita health expenditures by per capita GDP,
Canada and Germany, 1960 to 1993 59

Figure 6   Per capita health expenditures by per capita GDP,
Canada and France, 1960 to 1993 59

Figure 7   Per capita health expenditures by per capita GDP,
Canada and Japan, 1960 to 1993 60

Figure 8   Per capita health expenditures by per capita GDP,
Canada and the United Kingdom, 1960 to 1993................60

Figure 9   Per capita health expenditures by per capita GDP,
Canada and the Netherlands, 1960 to 1993 61

Figure 10   Per capita health expenditures by per capita GDP,
Canada and Sweden, 1960 to 1993 61

Figure 11   Per capita health expenditures by per capita GDP,
Canada and Denmark, 1960 to 1993 62

Figure 12   Per capita health expenditures by per capita GDP,
Canada and New Zealand, 1960 to 1993 62

Figure 13   Per capita health expenditures by per capita GDP,
Canada and Switzerland, 1960 to 1993 63

Figure 14   Per capita health expenditures by per capita GDP,
Canada and Italy, 1960 to 1993.......................................63

Figure 15   Percentage of the GDP devoted to health by the per
capita GDP, Canada and Australia, 1960 to 1993 64

Figure 16   Percentage of the GDP devoted to health by the per
capita GDP, Canada and the United States 1960 to 1993 ...64

Figure 17   Percentage of the GDP devoted to health by the per
capita GDP, Canada and Germany, 1960 to 1993 65

Figure 18 Percentage of the GDP devoted to health by the per capita GDP, Canada and France, 1960 to 1993 65

Figure 19 Percentage of the GDP devoted to health by the per capita GDP, Canada and Japan, 1960 to 1993 66

Figure 20 Percentage of the GDP devoted to health by the per capita GDP, Canada and the United Kingdom, 1960 to 1993 66

Figure 21 Percentage of the GDP devoted to health by the per capita GDP, Canada and the Netherlands, 1960 to 1993 67

Figure 22 Percentage of the GDP devoted to health by the per capita GDP, Canada and Sweden, 1960 to 1993 67

Figure 23 Percentage of the GDP devoted to health by the per capita GDP, Canada and Denmark, 1960 to 1993 68

Figure 24 Percentage of the GDP devoted to health by the per capita GDP, Canada and New Zealand, 1960 to 1993 68

Figure 25 Percentage of the GDP devoted to health by the per capita GDP, Canada and Switzerland, 1960 to 1993 69

Figure 26 Percentage of the GDP devoted to health by the per capita GDP, Canada and Italy, 1960 to 1993 69

Figure 27 Deviation e_i explained by the mortality rate/ 1,000 inhabitants 70

Figure 28 Deviation $e_{i'}$ explained by the mortality rate/ 1,000 inhabitants 71

Figure 29 Deviation e_i explained by the number of days of hospitalization per capita 72

Figure 30 Deviation $e_{i'}$ explained by the number of days of hospitalization per capita 73

Figure 31 Deviation e_i explained by hospital expenditures as a percentage of total expenditures 74

Figure 32 Deviation $e_{i'}$ explained by hospital expenditures as a percentage of total expenditures 75

Figure 33 Deviation e_i explained by hospital expenditures per capita 76

Figure 34 Deviation $e_{i'}$ explained by hospital expenditures per capita 77

Figure 35 Deviation e_i explained by per capita
ambulatory expenditures 78

Figure 36 Deviation $e_{i'}$ explained by per capita
ambulatory expenditures 79

Figure 37 Deviation e_i explained by the number of physicians/
1,000 inhabitants 80

Figure 38 Deviation $e_{i'}$ explained by the number of physicians/
1,000 inhabitants 81

Figure 39 Deviation e_i explained by the index of pharmaceutical
costs 82

Figure 40 Deviation $e_{i'}$ explained by the index of
pharmaceutical costs 83

LIST OF TABLES

Table 1   Scores for the different remuneration modalities
of physicians 50

Table 2   Results of regressions 84

INTRODUCTION

Faced with significant increases in expenditures in the health sector, the crisis in public finances and the importance which populations attribute to the health system, all countries are examining the future of their health system and the resources that will have to be devoted to it. They are right to be concerned. Between 1960 and 1993, the percentage of GDP which OECD countries spent on average on health rose from 3.88 percent to 8.32 percent. In 1993, average per capita expenditures expressed in $PPP[1] were more than 17 times what they were in 1960. In 1960, they were $87.14 PPP and in 1993, they were $1,536.91 PPP. While it is not possible to determine the optimum level of health spending, it is possible to draw some conclusions from the relative position of one OECD country compared to the others. Although the trend toward increasing costs is evident in all countries, there are significant differences from one country to another.

The purpose of this project was to try to measure the differences in costs between the Canadian health system and that of 12 other OECD countries, and to identify the factors influencing these differences.[2] To this end, the project is divided into two parts.

The first part measures the differences in costs between the various countries over the 33 years between 1960 and 1993 using two indicators: per capita health expenditures and the percentage of GDP devoted to health expenditures. To provide a better comparison of costs over time and between countries, we also compared them to the per capita GDP. In both cases, we calculated a logarithmic regression. The results are show graphically and analyzed.

The second part of the project tries to explain the differences in relation to the average of the expenditures (regression curves). This is done by calculating, for each country, each year and each of the two cost indicators, the difference between the observed value and the average: e_i (difference in per capita expenditures) and $e_{i'}$ (difference in health expenditures as a percentage of GDP). We then tried to identify what aspects of financing, organization of the health system, and demand for health care in the various countries might explain these differences.

The *Health Data* database was used.[3] All of the costs used in this study are in purchasing power parity dollars ($PPP).

---

1. Purchasing power parity.

2. The countries are Germany, Australia, Denmark, the United States, France, Italy, Japan, New Zealand, the Netherlands, the United Kingdom, Sweden, and Switzerland.

3. OECD. 1995. *Health Data*: Paris. Organization for Economic Cooperation and Development.

CHANGE IN EXPENDITURES IN THIRTEEN OECD COUNTRIES

In general, we found that, since 1960, strong economic growth in the developed countries has been parallelled by considerable development of their health care systems. We compared health expenditures to the GDP in order to better understand the change in spending in this field. In the first analysis, we explain per capita expenditures by per capita GDP and in the second, we explain the percentage of the GDP devoted to health by the per capita GDP. To see the trends in costs, we used data from 1960 to 1993 for the 13 countries selected.

Regressions

Linear Regressions

We began by trying to explain per capita costs and costs as a percentage of GDP using a linear regression.

We obtained the following results for the first regression which explains total per capita health expenditures ($PPP) by the per capita GDP ($PPP):

$$\text{TOT EXP/cap} = -144.006 + 0.094 \text{ GDP/cap} + e_i$$

DF = 434   t = (70.681) R^2 = 0.92 (p = 0.0001)

We obtained the following results for the second regression which explains health expenditures as a percentage of the GDP by the per capita GDP:

$$\text{TOT EXP/GDP} = 4.715 + 2.395 \times 10^{-4} \text{ GDP/cap} + e_i$$

DF = 434   t = (25.896) R^2 = 0.608 (p = 0.0001)

In both cases the results were significant. Total health costs, whether expressed in $PPP or as a percentage of GDP, had a positive relation to the per capita GDP. This means that the wealthier the country, the more it spends on its health system.

Logarithmic Regressions

We then used a logarithmic form for the two regressions so that we could obtain a direct estimate of the elasticity of expenditures to revenue.

The first regression, which explains per capita expenditures ($PPP) by the per capita GDP ($PPP), is expressed as follows:

$$\ln(\text{TOT EXP/cap}) = -5.219 + 1.284 \ln(\text{GDP/cap}) + e_i$$

DF = 434   t = (140.978) R^2 = 0.979 (p = 0.0001)

The second regression, which explains the percentage of GDP represented by health expenditures by the per capita GDP, is as follows:

$$\ln(\text{TOT EXP/GDP}) = -0.614 + 0.284 \ln(\text{GDP/cap}) + e_i$$

DF = 434   t = (31.123) $R^2 = 0.691$ (p = 0.0001)

Both regressions were significant. In both cases, the adjustment from the logarithm regression was higher than that from the linear regression. We therefore retained the logarithmic model to explain health expenditures.

Analysis

In both cases, the slope of the curve is positive; in other words, the countries with the higher GDPs are also those which spend the most in terms of dollar value and which devote a larger percentage of their GDP to health. However, the shape of the curves is not the same (figures 1 and 2).[4]

In the first instance, the elasticity of health expenditures in relation to the per capita GDP is greater than 1. Graphically, this gives a slightly convex curve. The rate of growth in per capita health expenditures increases with the increase in per capita GDP. Therefore, per capita health expenditures climb faster than the per capita GDP.

In the second case, the elasticity is less than 1. The share of the GDP devoted to health increases with the per capita GDP, but at a slower rate. The curve is concave and means that countries with a low GDP will decide, if their GDP rises, to increase the percentage of GDP allocated to health more than countries with a high GDP.

To be able to analyze the change in health spending by country, each figure shows the regression line and the real change in health expenditures in relation to the GDP for Canada and one of the other 12 countries (figures 3 to 26).

Change In per Capita Health Expenditures in Relation to the per Capita GDP

Among the countries above the average are the United States—which is significantly higher—and France and Canada, which have a similar pattern.

In general, Canada spends more per capita on health given its per capita GDP than the average of the 13 countries studied. It spent the same amount as the average in the early 1980s. Since then, health expenditures have risen faster than the average given the country's wealth. In 1989, Canada was above the average but was still close to it. Since then, per capita costs have risen more steeply. Expenditures jumped from $1,601 PPP per capita in 1989 to $1,971 PPP per capita in 1993. If Canada had had the same performance as the other OECD countries during this period, its

---

4. All of the graphs are appended.

expenditures would have risen from $1,601 PPP in 1989 to $1,763 PPP per capita in 1993.

In the United States, however, per capita expenditures have always increased faster in relation to per capita GDP. The trend in this country shows a widening of the gap between its expenditures and the average. In 1993, it spent per capita one-and-a-half times the average expenditures of the 13 countries studied.

Those countries which spend, per capita, less than the average on health are Japan, the United Kingdom, and Denmark since the end of the 1970s . Until the early 1980s, Japan's spending pattern was following the average, with its costs slightly less. Since the 1980s, its per capita health expenditures have fallen farther below the average. In 1993, Japan spent $1,495 PPP per capita on health. The trend in health costs in Denmark is almost the same as in Japan. Since the end of the 1970s, its per capita expenditures have fallen further below the average. The United Kingdom has spent less than the average of the 13 countries on health on a per capita basis since 1960. In 1993, its per capita health spending was $1,213 PPP.

Change in the Percentage of the GDP Allocated to Health in Relation to the per Capita GDP

The same countries are above the average for this comparison as are for the per capita expenditures, that is, the United States, Canada, and France. The United States shows the largest deviation. The percentage of the GDP it allocates to health increases constantly with the increase in the per capita GDP and continues to move farther from the average. In 1993, 14.12 percent of its GDP was allocated to health care. The change in Canada's expenditures is much less linear. Until the late 1970s, the percentage spent on health was higher than the average. There was a peak in 1971 when Canada spent 7.37 percent of its GDP on health. This figure was not reached again until 1980, when it was the same as the average. Since the early 1980s, the percentage of the GDP devoted to health in Canada has been higher than the average. In 1993, it was $10.22 percent. France's health spending pattern followed that of the average, although the share of its GDP allocated to this sector was higher than the average.

Japan, the United Kingdom, and Denmark are the countries which devote a smaller percentage of their GDP than the average to health. In 1993, Japan spent 7.2 percent of its GDP on health and the United Kingdom spent 7.07 percent. Between 1965 and the end of the 1970s, Denmark allocated a larger share of its GDP than the average to health care. Since the 1970s, Denmark's spending on health has fallen further and further below the average for the OECD countries. In 1993, it spent 6.67 percent of its GDP on health care.

Thus, there are two groups that are set apart both in terms of per capita health expenditures and the percentage of the GDP devoted to health. On the one hand, there are the countries which deviate the most from the average on the high side: the United States, Canada, and France. And then there are those which are the farthest below the average: Japan, the United Kingdom, and Denmark. Although expenditures were compared to the per capita GDP of each country, this does not appear to be a determinant in the change in expenditures (per capita and percentage of GDP) or the position of the country in relation to the average of the other countries. Although it is true that the country which spends the most in both cases is also the one with the highest per capita GDP ($23,358 in 1993), Denmark and Canada, which have almost the same per capita GDPs ($19,340 PPP and $19,271 PPP respectively in 1993), definitely do not have equivalent health expenditures. It would be interesting to know the reasons for these deviations from the average. This is what we will try to determine in the second part of this report.

EXPLANATION OF THE DEVIATION IN HEALTH EXPENDITURES FROM THE AVERAGE OF THE THIRTEEN COUNTRIES STUDIED

We used the two logarithmic regressions calculated in the first part of the study to calculate the e_i and $e_{i'}$ differences. "E_i" is the difference between the position of a country and the average value for the countries provided by the regression which compares per capita expenditures to per capita GDP. "E_i" is the difference between the estimated value of the percentage of per capita GDP devoted to health in relation to per capita GDP (second regression) and the real value of this percentage for the corresponding GDP. Deviations are positive for countries above the regression lines and negative for those below the lines. We tried to determine the factors which give rise to these deviations. They can be divided into three categories: factors related to demand for health care, macroorganizational variables and microorganizational variables. In the latter group, we are interested in four areas: the hospital sector, the ambulatory sector, the medical sector, and pharmaceutical expenditures.

In general, we made simple and polynomial regressions to explain e_i and $e_{i'}$ respectively, except in the case of the methods of payment for physicians in the ambulatory and hospital sectors. The regressions calculated test the degree to which the variables influence the results. Data for 1989 to 1993 inclusive was used for the microorganizational variables and the factors related to health care demand. In the case of the public financing, we used data from 1960 to 1993. Tests relating to the number of sources of financing, the degree of centralization, and the scores for payments to physicians were based on data for 1993.

The results are appended (table 2).

Factors Associated with Health Demand

Population 65 Years and Older

We often hear that high health costs are due to the fact that a significant percentage of the population is elderly. We tested this factor. The percentage of the population 65 years and older does not account for deviations in health expenditures. It therefore does not appear that the aging population, as a group, is responsible for high health expenditures.

Mortality Rate/1,000 Inhabitants

We also examined the mortality rate/1,000 inhabitants (figures 27 and 28). This variable is significant in both types of regression. However, it is more significant in the case of the polynomial regression:

$e_i = -20.205 + 4.615 \, (MORT/1,000 \, inhab.) - 0.259 \, (MORT/1,000 \, inhab.)^2 + z_i$

$DF = 61 \qquad t = 5.792 \qquad\qquad t = 6.053$

$R^2 = 0.439 \; (p = 0.0001)$

$e_{i'} = -20.171 + 4.608 \, (MORT/1,000 \, inhab.) - 0.259 \, (MORT/1,000 \, inhab.)^2 + z_i$

$DF = 61 \qquad t = 5.787 \qquad\qquad t = 6.049$

$R^2 = 0.439 \; (p = 0.0001)$

It would appear that there is a link between mortality and the level of health expenditures. The curve is concave. This means that there are countries in which mortality is low and health costs are low (Japan), countries in which the comparative mortality is average and expenditures are close to the relative average of the OECD countries, and countries where there is a high mortality rate and health expenditures are below what might be expected (United Kingdom, Denmark, Germany, and Sweden). The United States deviates significantly from the group because of its high expenditures. Canada also deviates from the regression curve. It appears that, given its mortality rate, it spends more than the average.

The findings clearly illustrate the difficulty involved in defining the causal relationship between the level of expenditures and the mortality rate. Two possible conclusions might be that health expenditures are low because the demand for care, expressed by the mortality rate, is low (Japan) or that the mortality rate is high because health expenditures are too low (United Kingdom, Denmark, etc.).

Macroorganizational Factors

We tested three types of variables in this area: percentage of public financing, number of sources of financing and degree of centralization. The first two variables were tested using linear and polynomial regressions. For the third variable, we compared the averages of the deviations for the various countries in each category.

Percentage of Public Financing

We explained the e_i and e_i' deviations by the percentage which public expenditures represent of the total expenditures using data for 1960 to 1993 inclusive. The results are as follows:

$e_i = 1.357 - 0.019$ (% PUBL EXP) $+ y_i$

$n = 426$ $t = 5.894$ $R^2 = 0.076$ $(p = 0.0001)$

$e_{i'} = 1.36 - 0.019$ (% PUBL EXP) $+ y_{i'}$

$n = 426$ $t = 5.914$ $R^2 = 0.076$ $(p = 0.0001)$

These regressions are significant. This means that the greater the percentage of public expenditures, the lower the health costs. Therefore, the greater the involvement of government in the financing of health expenditures, the lower the per capita costs and the lower the percentage of GDP allocated to health. However, this result is not borne out when the United States is excluded from the database:

$e_i = -0.18 + 4.799 \times 10^{-4}$ (% PUBL EXP) $+ y_i$

$DF = 392$ $t - 0.104$ $R^2 = 2.744 \times 10^{-5}$ $(p = 0.9176)$

$e_{i'} = -0.174 + 3.905 \times 10^{-4}$ (% PUBL EXP) $+ y_{i'}$

$DF = 392$ $t = 5.914$ $R^2 = 1.817 \times 10^{-5}$ $(p = 0.9329)$

If the United States is removed from the sample, public expenditures are no longer a significant factor in the deviation. This result may indicate that there is a threshold for private expenditures above which a country can no longer control its costs. The United States has apparently exceeded that threshold. It is actually the country with the smallest percentage of public health financing. Between 1989 and 1993, its average was 42.37 percent, while the average for the other countries, excluding the United States, was 77.3 percent of the total financing. Moreover, the United States is set apart from the other countries by the degree to which its costs deviate from the average.

For countries which have not reached this threshold, cost control may not depend on the percentage of private expenditures, but on other regulatory measures.

Number of Sources of Financing

We looked at the number of sources of financing of the health system, that is, whether the population participated only through paying taxes or whether it participated in some other way (insurance premiums, employer contributions, direct payment, etc.). Our purpose was to determine whether several sources of financing contributed to increased costs.

Number of sources of financing: Germany: 3; Australia: 3; Denmark: 3; United States: 5; France: 3; Italy: 4; Japan: 4; New Zealand: 2; Netherlands: 4; United Kingdom: 3; Sweden: 2; Switzerland: 3; Canada: 3.

However, this variable was not significant.

Degree of Centralization

Based on the descriptions of their health systems, we grouped the countries according to the way their systems were organized: centralized or decentralized. A system is considered to be centralized when funds are collected by only one level of government and when financing goes directly from the central level to the health care suppliers without regional intermediaries. There are two types of decentralization: administrative decentralization and political decentralization. Administrative decentralization occurs when funds are collected at only one level but are redistributed to various regional or local levels before being distributed to the health care suppliers. Political decentralization occurs when funds are collected at several levels (municipal, regional, national) and are also redistributed to regional and local levels. We used these groups to analyze the variances. The United States was not included in the analyzes as their organizational structure is that of the regulated market and is not a form of decentralization.

E_i variance test for centralization:

Categories	Countries	Average	F test
Centralized	3	– 0.250	0.102
Decentralized	9	– 0.445	prob. = 0.7558

$E_{i'}$ variance test for centralization:

Categories	Countries	Average	F test
Centralized	3	– 0.249	0.103
Decentralized	9	– 0.445	prob. = 0.7545

As can be seen, there is no significant difference between the centralized and decentralized systems for both e_i and $e_{i'}$.

E_i variance test for the type of decentralization:

Categories	Countries	Average	F test
D. Administrative	3	− 0.679	0.301
D. Political	6	− 0.328	prob. = 0.6005

$E_{i'}$ variance test for the type of decentralization:

Categories	Countries	Average	F test
D. Administrative	3	− 0.678	0.299
D. Political	6	− 0.329	prob. = 0.6014

Here again, there is no significant difference between the two types of decentralization for both e_i and $e_{i'}$. Therefore, no link can be established between expenditures control and the degree of centralization.

Microorganizational Factors

We are interested in three sectors: the hospital and medical sectors, and pharmaceutical expenditures. To the extent possible, we used variables which reflect quantities and others which reflect prices.

Hospital Sector

We looked at whether the number of beds/1,000 inhabitants and the number of days of hospitalization per capita might explain a wide deviation in health expenditures. Only the last variable—the number of days of hospitalization per capita—proved to be significant and only in the linear regression:

$e_i = 0.554 − 0.340 \text{ (DAYS HOSP/CAP)} + z_i$

DF = 62　　　　t = 2.129　　　　$R^2 = 0.069$ (p = 0.0373)

$e_{i'} = 0.55 − 0.340 \text{ (DAYS HOSP/CAP)} + z_{i'}$

DF = 62　　　　t = 2.131　　　　$R^2 = 0.069$ (p = 0.0372)

Thus, the higher the number of days of hospitalization, the lower the health expenditures. However, this result is no longer surprising when we look at the position of the United States. Here again, its results are totally different from those of the group. If it is removed from the sample, the linear regressions are no longer significant (for e_i, $R^2 = 0.006$, p = 0.5747; for $e_{i'}$, $R^2 = 0.006$, p = 0.5756). This phenomenon is explained by the fact that the United States has the lowest number of days of hospitalization and the highest costs for its health care system. Its position biases the regressions.

The polynomial regressions are significant only when the United States is excluded:

$$e_i = -6.817 + 4.901 \text{ (DAYS HOSP/CAP)} - 0.87 \text{ (DAYS HOSP/CAP)}^2 + z_i$$

DF = 57   t = 5.1   t = 5.055

$R^2 = 0.321$ (p = 0.0001)

$$e_{i'} = -6.806 + 4.893 \text{ (DAYS HOSP/CAP)} - 0.868 \text{ (DAYS HOSP/CAP)}^2 + z_{i'}$$

DF = 57   t = 5.095   t = 5.051

$R^2 = 0.321$ (p = 0.0001)

There would therefore appear to be a link between the number of days of hospitalization per capita and the level of expenditures. The countries at the two extremes for days of hospitalization (maximum: Japan, and minimum: United Kingdom, Denmark) are the also the ones with the lowest expenditures. The countries located around the average of the 13 countries are the ones which have the highest expenditures (figures 29 and 30).

In terms of expenditures, we tested the percentage which hospital expenditures represented of total expenditures, as well as hospital expenditures per capita.

In the first case, only the polynomial regressions were significant (figures 31 and 32):

$$e_i = -17.427 + 0.783 \text{ (HOSP EXP/TOT EXP)} - 0.009 \text{ (HOSP EXP/TOT EXP)}^2 + z_i$$

DF = 54   t = 4.903   t = 5.011

$R^2 = 0.33$ (p = 0.0001)

$$e_{i'} = -17.402 + 0.782 \text{ (HOSP EXP/TOT EXP)} - 0.009 \text{ (HOSP EXP/TOT EXP)}^2 + z_{i'}$$

DF = 54   t = 4.899   t = 5.006

$R^2 = 0.329$ (p = 0.0001)

These curves are concave. Japan (low percentage of total expenditures allocated to hospital expenditures and negative deviations) and Denmark (high percentage of total expenditures allocated to hospital expenditures and slight deviations) are at the two extremes. In general, the countries seem to align themselves along the regression curve. The United States and the United Kingdom are the only two which stray from the norm: the United States with very high expenditures and the United Kingdom with low expenditures.

In the case of per capita hospital expenditures, both types of regression were significant.

However, the polynomial regressions appeared to have a slightly better adjustment. We therefore chose to use them (figures 33 and 34):

$e_i = -2.909 + 0.003 \, (\text{HOSP EXP/CAP}) + 4.909 \times 10^{-7} \, (\text{HOSP EXP/CAP})^2 + z_i$

DF = 54   t = 1.824   t = 0.485

$R^2 = 0.71 \ (p = 0.0001)$

$e_{i'} = -2.906 + 0.003 \, (\text{HOSP EXP/CAP}) + 4.917 \times 10^{-7} \, (\text{HOSP EXP/CAP})^2 + z_{i'}$

DF = 54   t = 1.822   t = 0.487

$R^2 = 0.71 \ (p = 0.0001)$

Thus, the greater the hospital expenditures, the higher the overall expenditures. Moreover, the growth is almost linear. Only one country deviates significantly from this finding and that is Denmark (low expenditures). The United States is at right angles to the figure, above the curve.

Ambulatory Sector

We explained the ei and ei' deviations on the basis of per capita ambulatory expenditures. Both the linear and polynomial regressions were significant. However, the polynomial regressions gave a better adjustment and we therefore chose to use them (figures 35 and 36).

$e_i = -0.138 - 0.003 \, (\text{AMB EXP/CAP}) + 5.489 \times 10^{-6} \, (\text{AMB EXP/CAP})^2 + z_i$

DF = 50   t = 1.504   t = 3.137

$R^2 = 0.449 \ (p = 0.0001)$

$e_{i'} = -0.137 - 0.003 \, (\text{AMB EXP/CAP}) + 5.486 \times 10^{-6} \, (\text{AMB EXP/CAP})^2 + z_{i'}$

DF = 50   t = 1.506   t = 3.138

$R^2 = 0.449 \ (p = 0.0001)$

The United States deviated from the group. It is likely that it biases the results. However, if we include the United States, our results clearly indicate that the higher the ambulatory care expenditures, the higher the e_i and $e_{i'}$ deviations.

Medical Sector

We looked first at the number of care staff and more specifically, the number of nurses/1,000 inhabitants, which did not prove significant, and then at the number of physicians/1,000 inhabitants, which was significant in the case of the polynomial regressions (figures 37 and 38):

$e_i = -11.447 + 9.938\,(\text{NO PHYS}/1{,}000\,\text{INHAB}) - 2.087\,(\text{NO PHYS}/1{,}000\,\text{INHAB})^2 + z_i$

DF = 47   t = 4.532   t = 4.532

$R^2 = 0.334$ (p = 0.0001)

$e_{i'} = -11.44 + 9.932\,(\text{NO PHYS}/1{,}000\,\text{INHAB}) - 2.086\,(\text{NO PHYS}/1{,}000\,\text{INHAB})^2 + z_{i'}$

DF = 47   t = 4.533   t = 4.363

$R^2 = 0.334$ (p = 0.0001)

The curve is therefore concave. However, the United States appears to draw the curve upwards. Moreover, it is important to place this variable in context since it does not take into consideration the percentage of health expenditures attributable to physicians' salaries. Consequently, it is difficult to draw conclusions about the impact of the number of physicians on health expenditures, since remuneration varies widely from country to country. It was not possible to acquire data on the remuneration of physicians.

We also developed variables which might measure the degree of control over health expenditures. The scores were assessed using the following model (9 would be the score which would allow the greatest control over costs associated with payments to physicians).

Table 1

Scores for the different remuneration modalities of physicians

Determination of price		Payment mechanism		Method of remuneration		Score
Physician	1	Individual	1	Fee for service	1	3
Physician	1	Third party	2	Fee for service	1	4
Negotiation	2	Individual	1	Fee for service	1	4
Negotiation	2	Third party	2	Fee for service	1	5
Negotiation	2	Third party	2	Salary	2	6
Administrative decision	3	Third party	2	Fee for service	2	7
Negotiation	2	Third party	2	Per capita	3	7
Negotiation	2	Organization	3	Salary	2	7
Administrative decision	3	Third party	2	Salary	2	7
Administrative decision	3	Organization	3	Salary	2	8
Administrative decision	3	Organization	3	Per capita	3	9

Source: Based on the model of Contandriopoulos et al. 1993.

Scores were calculated for each country for generalists and specialists working in the public hospital sector (HOSP PAY) and the ambulatory care sector (AMB PAY). We used these scores to calculate the regressions in order to explain the e_i and $e_{i'}$ deviations.

The variable "score for hospital sector payment" was not significant. However, the "score for ambulatory care sector" was significant in the linear regression:

$e_i = 3.078 - 0.606$ (AMB PAY) $+ y_i$

DF = 11   t = 3.015 $R^2 = 0.476$ (p = 0.013)

$e_{i'} = 3.075 - 0.605$ (AMB PAY) $+ y_{i'}$

DF = 11   t = 3.015 $R^2 = 0.476$ (p = 0.013)

Consequently, it would appear that the greater the control, the lower the expenditures on health. This regression confirms what many studies show: that fee for service is not the remuneration system which allows the greatest reduction in costs and that, on the contrary, it creates inflationary pressures.

Pharmaceutical Costs

We calculated a cost index as follows:

PE index = (z (pharma exp/GDP) + 2 × z (pharma exp per capita))/3

This index explains the ei and ei' disparities. The linear regressions were more definitive than the polynomial regressions (figures 39 and 40).

$e_i = -0.298 + 0.494$ (PE) $+ y_i$

DF = 58   t = 4.216 $R^2 = 0.238$ (p = 0.0001)

$e_{i'} = -0.298 + 0.493$ (PE) $+ y_{i'}$

DF = 58   t = 4.215 $R^2 = 0.238$ (p = 0.0001)

Thus, the higher the index, the higher the ei and ei' deviations. Once again, the results for the United States deviated from those for the group (higher expenditures). The United Kingdom and Denmark stand out below the line.

CONCLUSION

We can draw a few broad conclusions from our analyses. Health expenditures increase as a country develops, at a faster rate along a convex trajectory in the case of per capita expenditures, and along a concave trajectory for the percentage of GDP allocated to health. There are, however, considerable vaiations from country to country and some countries control their health costs much better than others. The comparison between Denmark and Canada is striking in this regard. Although they have had similar per capita GDP growth, the percentage of the GDP allocated to health is 3 percent lower in Denmark than in Canada.

Our analysis of the e_i and $e_{i'}$ variations showed that the disparities in costs between the countries were not attributable to any epidemiological or demographic differences in populations. Rather, the factors which explain a country's position relative to the average trajectory of change are associated with the manner in which its health system is organized, funded, and regulated.

Macroorganizational methods of regulation appear to be determinant. Public financing of the system is a powerful cost control mechanism. When the direct contribution from government is only a relatively small proportion of the total cost—as in the United States—there is very little capacity to control costs. That does not mean to say that as long as the government finances a large proportion of the expenditures, it will control expenditures effectively. The capacity to control and the implementation of that control are two different things.

It was difficult to analyze the microorganizational methods of regulation individually and without taking into consideration the macroregulation of the system. Nevertheless, the results did reveal a few patterns. The data on the hospital and ambulatory care sectors were difficult to analyze without taking into consideration the organizational context of each country. However, our results appear to indicate that the way in which physicians are paid is a key factor and particularly, the way in which front-line physicians are paid. Better cost control of the system can be achieved if payment is not made on a fee-for-service basis. It also appears that controlling costs in the pharmaceutical sector is essential to controlling the total cost of the health system.

Astrid Brousselle *is a doctoral student in public health at the University of Montreal. She also holds a master's degree in health administration from the University of Montreal. The subject of her doctoral thesis is the "model building of condom use in the prevention of AIDS in prostitutes in Sub-Saharan Africa." She has also studied economics and is particularly interested in health economics.*

BIBLIOGRAPHY
(Sources cited and consulted)

BEFORT, A.-F. 1990. *Le système de soins et la maîtrise des dépenses de santé en RFA (The Health Care System and Controlling Health Expenditures in the FRG).* Paris: Les cahiers Institut La Boétie.

CONTANDRIOPOULOS, A.-P. et al. 1993. *Regulatory Mechanisms in the Health Systems of Canada and Other Industrialized Countries: Description and Assessment.* Ottawa (ON): University of Ottawa, Faculty of Medicine, Health Sciences.

GRIS, UNIVERSITÉ DE MONTRÉAL/GROUPE SECOR. 1996. *Financial Incentives/Disincentives in Canada's Health System.* GRIS. Université de Montréal.

MAYNARD, A. et al. 1990. *La réforme du système de santé britannique (Reform of the British Health System).* Paris: Les cahiers Institut La Boétie.

OECD. 1994. *Health Policy Studies No 5. Reform of Health Care Systems: A Review of Seventeen OECD Countries.* Paris: Organization for Economic Cooperation and Development.

_____. 1995. *Health Data.* Paris: Organization for Economic Cooperation and Development.

OMS. Groupe spécial de l'OMS sur le développement sanitaire des pays d'Europe centrale et orientale. 1991. *Organisation, financement et réforme des systèmes de soins dans les pays d'Europe Centrale et Orientale, Compte rendu de la réunion qui s'est tenue à l'Organisation Mondiale de la Santé à Genève, du 22 au 26 avril 1991.* (WHO. Special working group of the WHO on health development in the countries of Central and Eastern Europe. 1991. *Organization, Financing and Reform of Health Systems in the Countries of Central and Eastern Europe, Minutes of the meeting held at the World Health Organization in Geneva, April 22 to 26, 1991).*

POMEY, M.-P. 1993. *La réforme du système de santé aux Pays-Bas (Reform of the Health System in the Netherlands).* Paris: Les cahiers Institut La Boétie.

APPENDIX

Figure 1

**Per capita health expenditures by per capita GDP
in 13 OECD countries, 1960 to 1993**

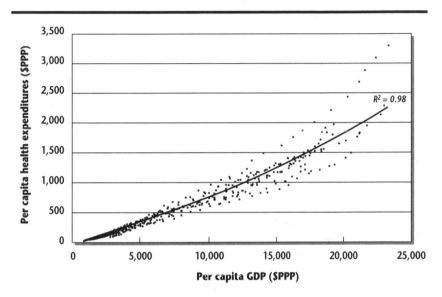

Figure 2

**Percentage of the GDP devoted to health by the per capita GDP
in 13 OECD countries, 1960 to 1993**

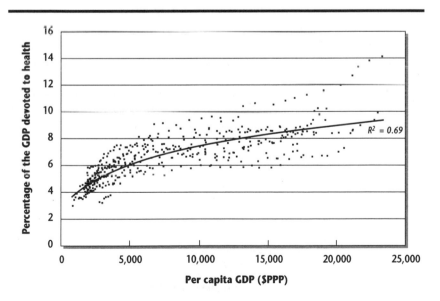

Figure 3

**Per capita health expenditures by per capita GDP,
Canada and Australia, 1960 to 1993**

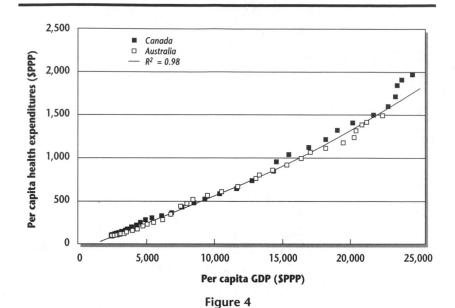

Figure 4

**Per capita health expenditures by per capita GDP,
Canada and the United States, 1960 to 1993**

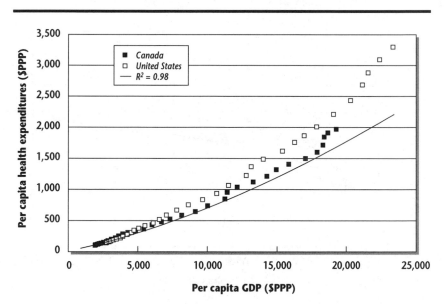

Figure 5

**Per capita health expenditures by per capita GDP,
Canada and Germany, 1960 to 1993**

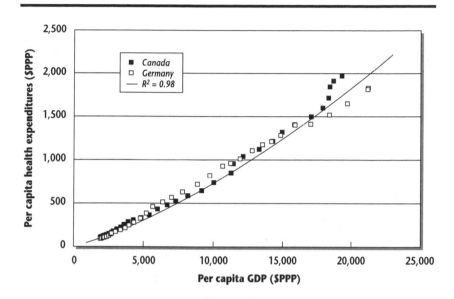

Figure 6

**Per capita health expenditures by per capita GDP,
Canada and France, 1960 to 1993**

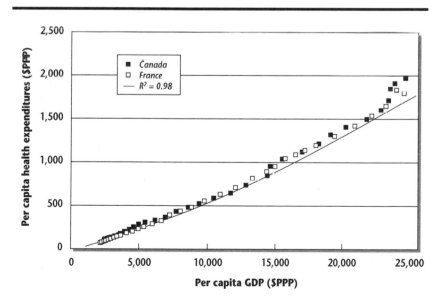

Figure 7

**Per capita health expenditures by per capita GDP,
Canada and Japan, 1960 to 1993**

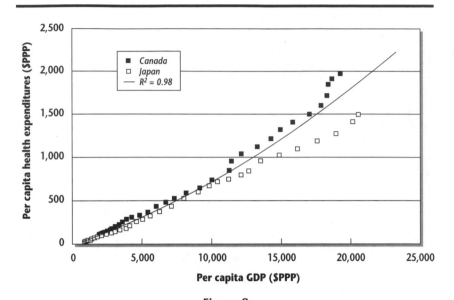

Figure 8

**Per capita health expenditures by per capita GDP,
Canada and the United Kingdom, 1960 to 1993**

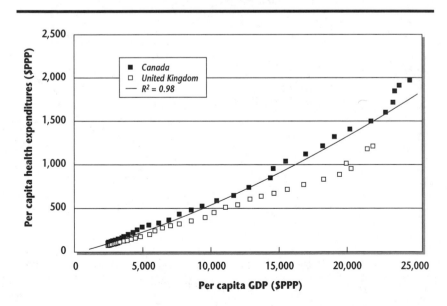

Figure 9

**Per capita health expenditures by per capita GDP,
Canada and the Netherlands, 1960 to 1993**

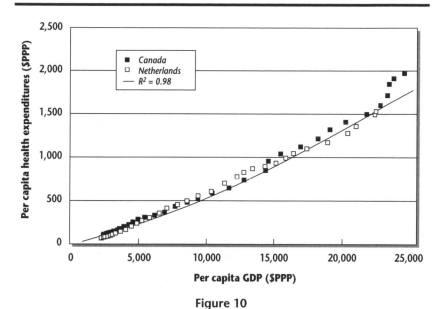

Figure 10

**Per capita health expenditures by per capita GDP,
Canada and Sweden, 1960 to 1993**

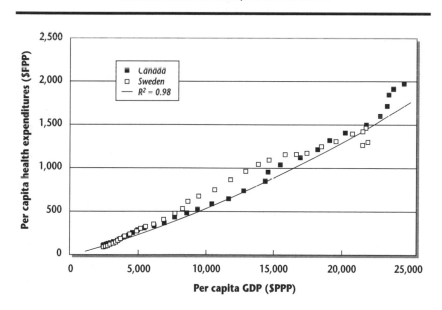

Figure 11

**Per capita health expenditures by per capita GDP,
Canada and Denmark, 1960 to 1993**

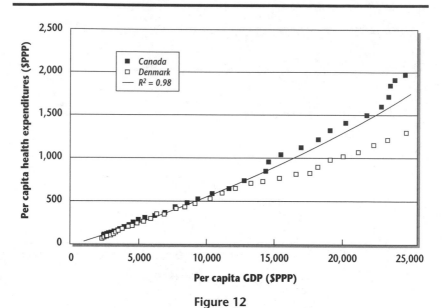

Figure 12

**Per capita health expenditures by per capita GDP,
Canada and New Zealand, 1960 to 1993**

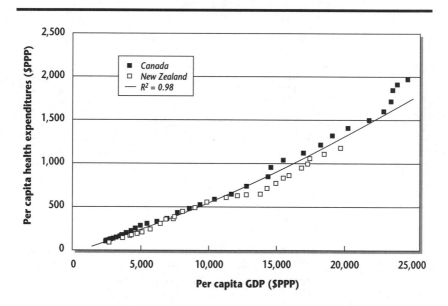

Figure 13

**Per capita health expenditures by per capita GDP,
Canada and Switzerland, 1960 to 1993**

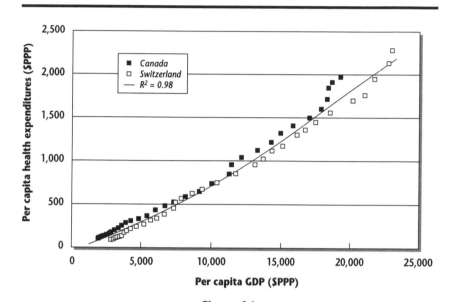

Figure 14

**Per capita health expenditures by per capita GDP,
Canada and Italy, 1960 to 1993**

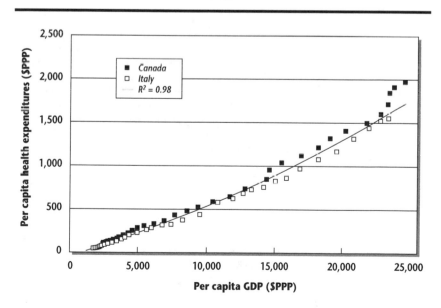

Figure 15

Percentage of the GDP devoted to health by the per capita GDP, Canada and Australia, 1960 to 1993

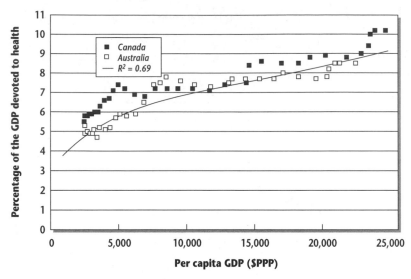

Per capita GDP ($PPP)

Figure 16

Percentage of the GDP devoted to health by the per capita GDP, Canada and the United States, 1960 to 1993

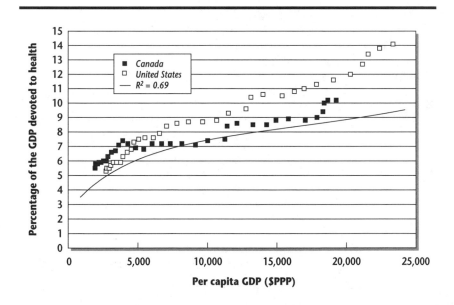

Per capita GDP ($PPP)

Figure 17

**Percentage of the GDP devoted to health by the per capita GDP,
Canada and Germany, 1960 to 1993**

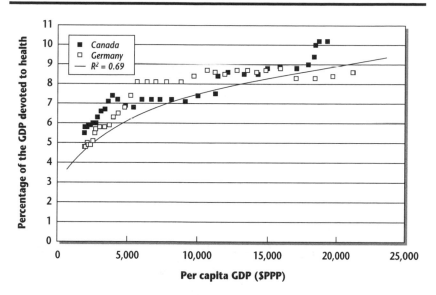

Figure 18

**Percentage of the GDP devoted to health by the per capita GDP,
Canada and France, 1960 to 1993**

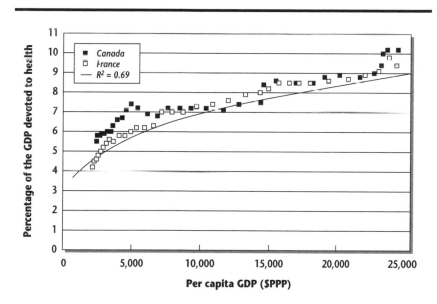

Figure 19

Percentage of the GDP devoted to health by the per capita GDP, Canada and Japan, 1960 to 1993

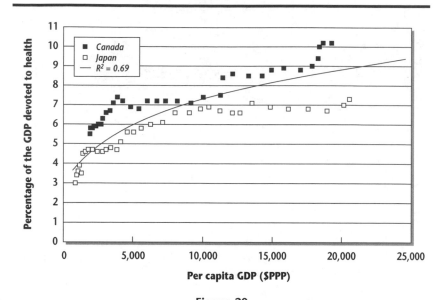

Figure 20

Percentage of the GDP devoted to health by the per capita GDP, Canada and the United Kingdom, 1960 to 1993

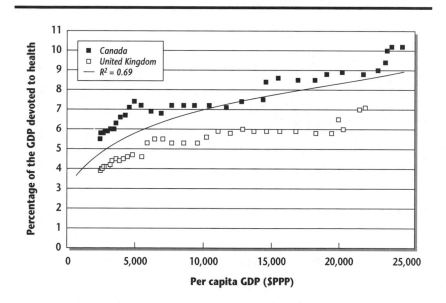

Figure 21

Percentage of the GDP devoted to health by the per capita GDP, Canada and the Netherlands, 1960 to 1993

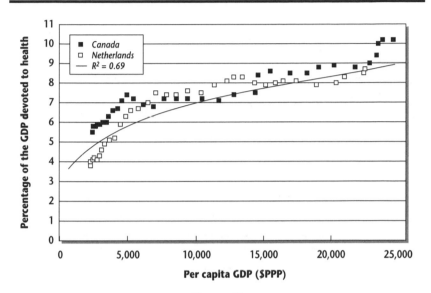

Figure 22

Percentage of the GDP devoted to health by the per capita GDP, Canada and Sweden, 1960 to 1993

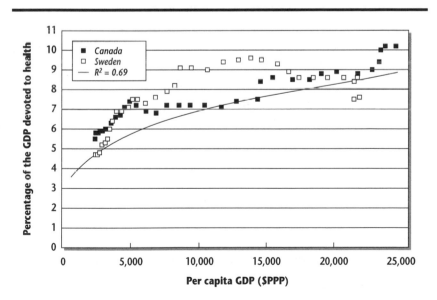

Figure 23

Percentage of the GDP devoted to health by the per capita GDP, Canada and Denmark, 1960 to 1993

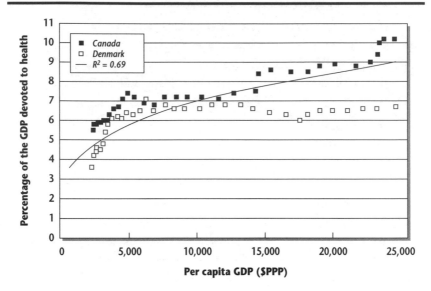

Figure 24

Percentage of the GDP devoted to health by the per capita GDP, Canada and New Zealand, 1960 to 1993

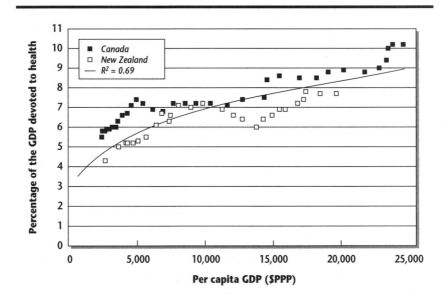

Figure 25

Percentage of the GDP devoted to health by the per capita GDP, Canada and Switzerland, 1960 to 1993

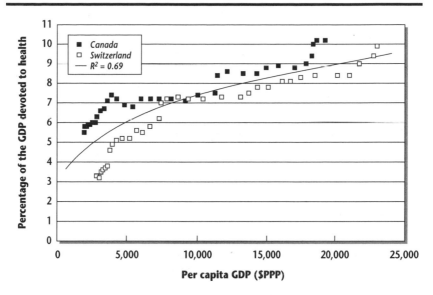

Figure 26

Percentage of the GDP devoted to health by the per capita GDP, Canada and Italy, 1960 to 1993

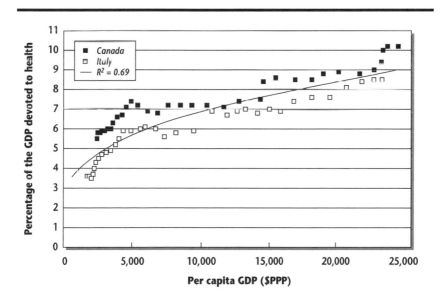

Figure 27

Deviation e$_i$ explained by the mortality rate/1,000 inhabitants

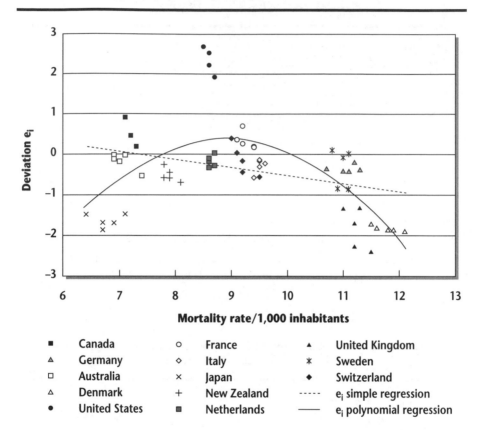

■	Canada	○	France	▲	United Kingdom
▵	Germany	◇	Italy	*	Sweden
□	Australia	×	Japan	◆	Switzerland
△	Denmark	+	New Zealand	-----	e$_i$ simple regression
●	United States	▣	Netherlands	——	e$_i$ polynomial regression

Figure 28
Deviation $e_{i'}$ explained by the mortality rate/1,000 inhabitants

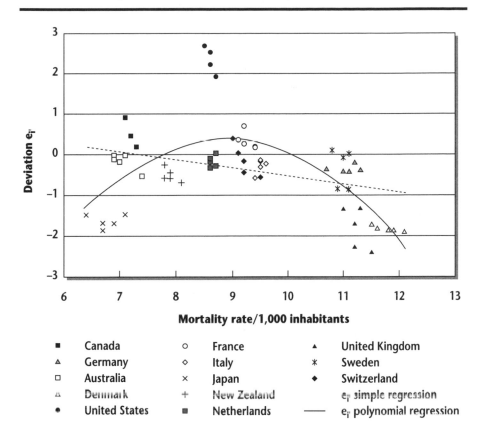

■	Canada	○	France	▲	United Kingdom
▵	Germany	◇	Italy	*	Sweden
□	Australia	×	Japan	◆	Switzerland
▵	Denmark	+	New Zealand		$e_{i'}$ simple regression
●	United States	▪	Netherlands	——	$e_{i'}$ polynomial regression

Figure 29

Deviation e_i explained by the number of days of hospitalization per capita

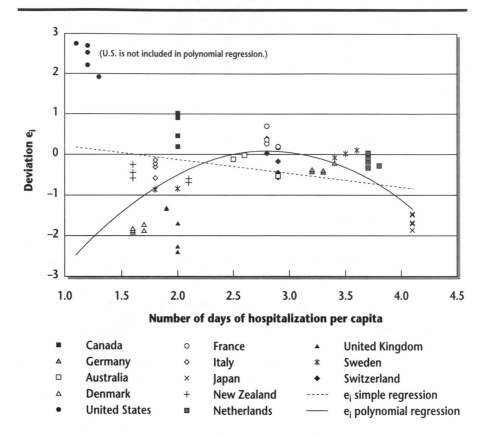

Number of days of hospitalization per capita

■	Canada	○	France	▲	United Kingdom
▲	Germany	◇	Italy	*	Sweden
□	Australia	×	Japan	◆	Switzerland
△	Denmark	+	New Zealand	-----	e_i simple regression
●	United States	▣	Netherlands	——	e_i polynomial regression

Figure 30

Deviation $e_{i'}$ explained by the number of days of hospitalization per capita

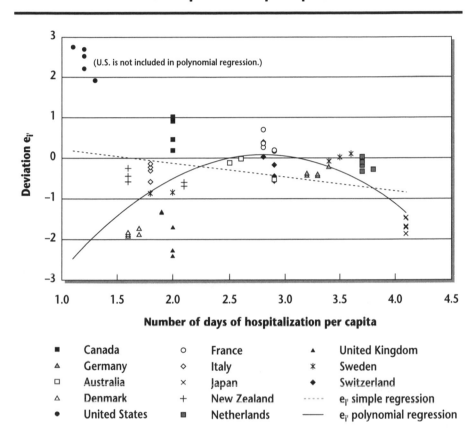

Number of days of hospitalization per capita

■	Canada	○	France	▲	United Kingdom
▲	Germany	◇	Italy	*	Sweden
□	Australia	×	Japan	◆	Switzerland
△	Denmark	+	New Zealand	-----	$e_{i'}$ simple regression
●	United States	▣	Netherlands	——	$e_{i'}$ polynomial regression

Figure 31

Deviation e$_i$ explained by hospital expenditures as a percentage of total expenditures

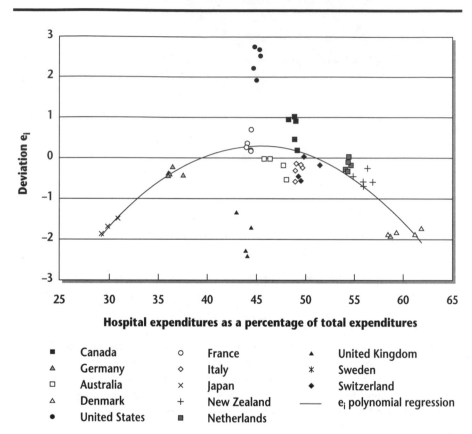

Hospital expenditures as a percentage of total expenditures

■	Canada	○	France	▲	United Kingdom
▲	Germany	◇	Italy	✳	Sweden
□	Australia	×	Japan	◆	Switzerland
△	Denmark	+	New Zealand	——	e$_i$ polynomial regression
●	United States	▥	Netherlands		

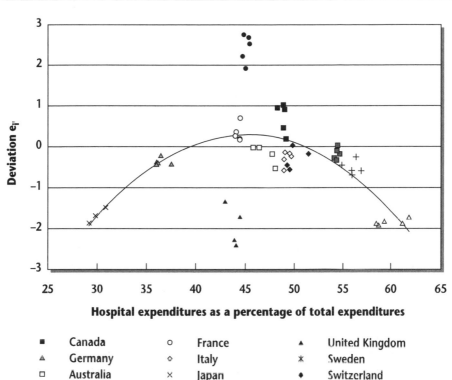

Figure 32

**Deviation $e_{i'}$ explained by hospital expenditures
as a percentage of total expenditures**

■	Canada	○ France	▲ United Kingdom
▲	Germany	◇ Italy	✳ Sweden
□	Australia	✕ Japan	◆ Switzerland
△	Denmark	+ New Zealand	—— $e_{i'}$ polynomial regression
●	United States	▣ Netherlands	

Figure 33

Deviation e_i explained by hospital expenditures per capita

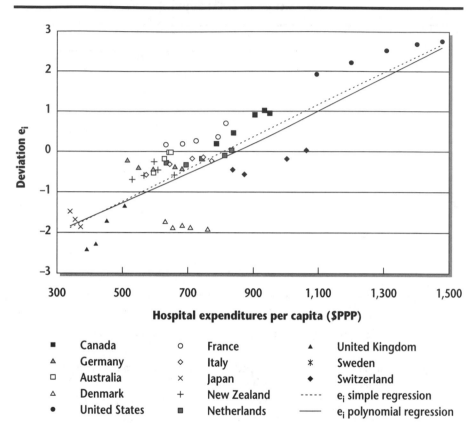

Figure 34

Deviation $e_{i'}$ explained by hospital expenditures per capita

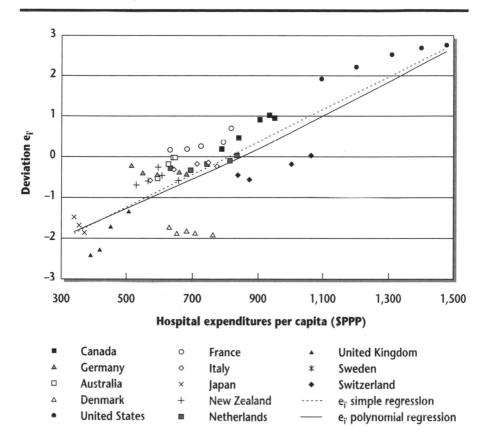

Hospital expenditures per capita ($PPP)

▪	Canada	○	France	▲	United Kingdom
▲	Germany	◇	Italy	*	Sweden
◻	Australia	×	Japan	◆	Switzerland
△	Denmark	+	New Zealand	-----	$e_{i'}$ simple regression
●	United States	▪	Netherlands	——	$e_{i'}$ polynomial regression

Figure 35

Deviation e_i explained by per capita ambulatory expenditures

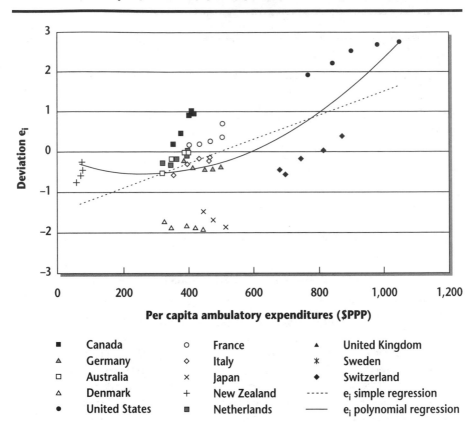

■	Canada	○	France	▲	United Kingdom
▲	Germany	◇	Italy	✳	Sweden
□	Australia	✕	Japan	◆	Switzerland
△	Denmark	+	New Zealand	-----	e_i simple regression
●	United States	▣	Netherlands	———	e_i polynomial regression

Figure 36

Deviation e_i explained by per capita ambulatory expenditures

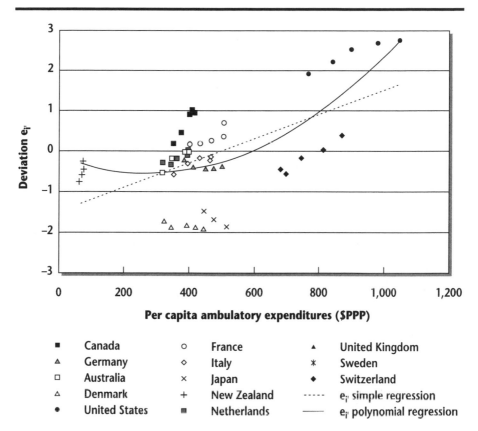

Figure 37

Deviation e$_i$ explained by the number of physicians/1,000 inhabitants

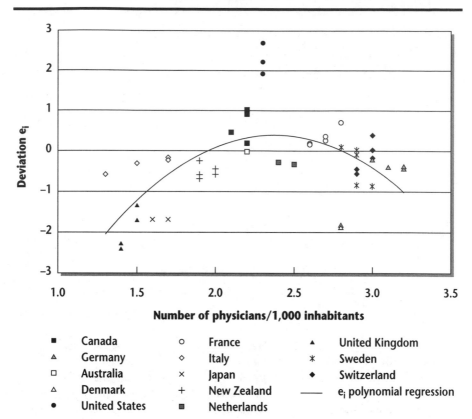

Number of physicians/1,000 inhabitants

■	Canada	○	France	▲	United Kingdom
▲	Germany	◇	Italy	*	Sweden
□	Australia	×	Japan	◆	Switzerland
△	Denmark	+	New Zealand	——	e$_i$ polynomial regression
●	United States	▣	Netherlands		

Figure 38

Deviation e_i explained by the number of physicians/1,000 inhabitants

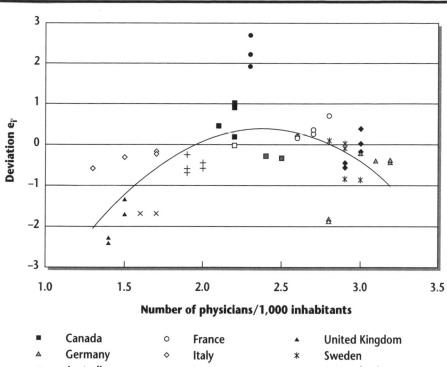

■	Canada	○ France	▲ United Kingdom
▲	Germany	◇ Italy	* Sweden
□	Australia	× Japan	◆ Switzerland
△	Denmark	+ New Zealand	— e_i polynomial regression
●	United States	▣ Netherlands	

Figure 39

Deviation e_i explained by the index of pharmaceutical costs

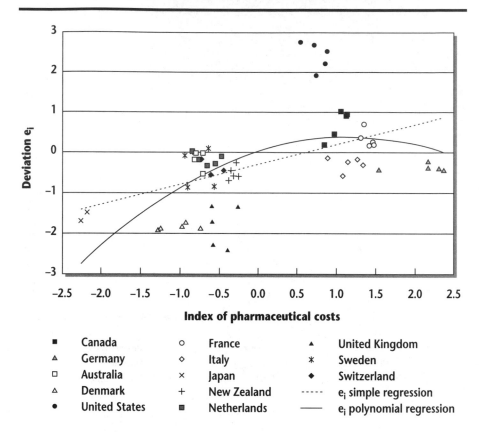

■	Canada	○ France	▲ United Kingdom
▲	Germany	◇ Italy	* Sweden
□	Australia	× Japan	◆ Switzerland
△	Denmark	+ New Zealand	----- e_i simple regression
●	United States	▣ Netherlands	—— e_i polynomial regression

Figure 40

Deviation $e_{i'}$ explained by the index of pharmaceutical costs

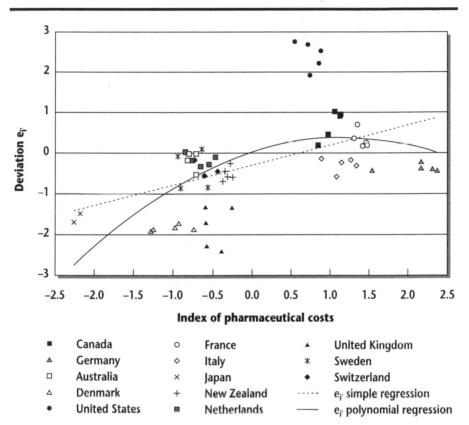

■	Canada	○	France	▲	United Kingdom
▲	Germany	◇	Italy	✳	Sweden
□	Australia	×	Japan	◆	Switzerland
△	Denmark	+	New Zealand	-----	$e_{i'}$ simple regression
●	United States	▣	Netherlands	——	$e_{i'}$ polynomial regression

Table 2

Results of regressions

	Simple regressions				Polynominal regressions			
	e_i		$e_{i'}$		e_i		$e_{i'}$	
	R^2	p	R^2	p	R^2	p	R^2	p
Factors associated with health demand								
Population 65 years and older	0.098	0.0756	0.099	0.0748	0.123	0.1396	0.123	0.1385
Mortality rate/1,000 inhabitants	0.090	0.0176	0.091	0.0175	0.439	0.0001	0.439	0.0001
Macroorganizational factors								
Percentage of public financing	0.076	0.0001	0.076	0.0001				
Number of sources of financing	0.232	0.0955	0.232	0.0953	0.36	0.1071	0.361	0.1067
Microorganizational factors								
Hospital sector								
Number of beds /1,000 inhabitants	0.030	0.2233	0.030	0.228	0.030	0.4799	0.030	0.4792
Number of days of hospitalization per capita	0.069	0.0373	0.069	0.0372	0.567	0.0001	0.566	0.0001
Hospital expenditures/total expenditures	0.006	0.5658	0.006	0.5665	0.330	0.0001	0.329	0.0001
Hospital expenditures per capita	0.709	0.0001	0.709	0.0001	0.710	0.0001	0.710	0.0001
Ambulatory sector								
Per capita ambulatory expenditures	0.336	0.0001	0.336	0.0001	0.449	0.0001	0.449	0.0001
Medical sector								
Number of physicians/1,000 inhabitants	0.052	0.1197	0.052	0.1200	0.334	0.0001	0.334	0.0001
Number of nurses/1,000 inhabitants	0.005	0.6828	0.005	0.6825	0.008	0.8834	0.008	0.8835
Score for ambulatory care sector	0.476	0.013	0.476	0.013				
Score for hospital sector payment	0.186	0.1858	0.186	0.185				
Pharmaceutical costs								
Pharmaceutical costs index	0.238	0.0001	0.238	0.0001	0.332	0.0001	0.332	0.0001

Managing Pharmaceutical Expenditures: How Canada Compares

WENDY KENNEDY, L.L.B., M.B.A.

Interdisciplinary Research Group on Health
University of Montreal

SUMMARY

To show how Canada compares internationally in the way it manages pharmaceutical expenditures, we used variables related to pharmaceutical expenditure and use, health outcome and economic status indices and compared them across all OECD member countries using OECD health data.

Member countries were compared for each year from 1989 to 1993. Expenditure and income variables are expressed in purchasing power parities (PPP) per capita, in order to eliminate the effect of population and currency exchange differences.

We selected 11 OECD member countries with socioeconomic characteristics similar to Canada's that all have a health care and drug reimbursement program. Expenditures on pharmaceuticals in these countries over the past fifteen years were then compared. We also used the least squares regression to compare per capita pharmaceutical expenditures against per capita GDP for the OECD countries for the years 1981 to 1991.

Comparisons were also made between the structure of the pharmaceutical distribution systems of the countries examined. Finally, we tried to explain the differences observed between the pharmaceutical reimbursement programs in several countries, as well as their relative performance.

Some countries have succeeded in controlling their expenditures on pharmaceuticals through price control measures. By comparison, Canada was the poorest performer in terms of cost control for the years 1981 to 1991. Canada has only limited centralized control over the prices of pharmaceuticals under patent protection.

TABLE OF CONTENTS

Methodology 90

Cross-Country Comparison of per Capita Pharmaceutical
Expenditures 91

Cross-Country Comparison of Drug Expenditures
as a Percentage of Total Health Expenditures 91

Cross-Country Comparison of Pharmaceutical Expenditures
as a Percentage of GDP 93

Cross-Country Comparison of the Relationship of Pharmaceutical
Expenditures to Wealth 94

Cross-Country Comparison of Drug Use 96

Cross-Country Comparison of Drug Sector Structures 97

Cross-Country Comparison of Health Indices 97

Discussion 98

Bibliography 101

Appendix 105

LIST OF FIGURES

Figure 1.1 Total pharmaceutical expenditures per capita ($PPP),
1989 128

Figure 1.2 Total pharmaceutical expenditures per capita ($PPP),
1990 129

Figure 1.3 Total pharmaceutical expenditures per capita ($PPP),
1991 130

Figure 1.4 Total pharmaceutical expenditures per capita ($PPP),
1992 131

Figure 1.5 Total pharmaceutical expenditures per capita ($PPP),
1993 132

Figure 2 Total pharmaceutical expenditures in $U.S. purchasing
power parities per capita, 1980–1994 133

Figure 3.1 Total pharmaceutical expenditures as a percentage
of total health care expenditures, 1989 134

Figure 3.2 Total pharmaceutical expenditures as a percentage
of total health care expenditures, 1990 135

Figure 3.3 Total pharmaceutical expenditures as a percentage
of total health care expenditures, 1991 136

Figure 3.4 Total pharmaceutical expenditures as a percentage
of total health care expenditures, 1992 137

Figure 3.5 Total pharmaceutical expenditures as a percentage
of total health care expenditures, 1993 138

Figure 4   Total pharmaceutical expenditures as a percentage
of total health care expenditures in $U.S. purchasing
power parities per capita, 1980–1994 139

Figure 5.1 Total pharmaceutical expenditures as a percentage
of gross domestic product, 1989 140

Figure 5.2 Total pharmaceutical expenditures as a percentage
of gross domestic product, 1990 141

Figure 5.3 Total pharmaceutical expenditures as a percentage
of gross domestic product, 1991 142

Figure 5.4 Total pharmaceutical expenditures as a percentage
of gross domestic product, 1992 143

Figure 5.5 Total pharmaceutical expenditures as a percentage
of gross domestic product, 1993 144

Figure 5.6 Global pharmaceutical expenditures index (total
pharmaceutical expenditures as a percentage of GDP + 2
pharmaceutical expenditures per capita /3, 1989–1993 145

Figure 6   Pharmaceutical expenditures as a percentage of gross
domestic product in $U.S. purchasing power parities
per capita, 1980–1984 146

Figure 7   Regression: Total expenditures on pharmaceuticals
and GDP, 21 countries, 1981 147

Figure 8   Regression: Total expenditures on pharmaceuticals
and GDP, 21 countries, 1991 147

Figure 9   Consumption of medications measured by the number
of boxes per capita, 1981 and 1989 148

Figure 10   Number of pharmacists per thousand population, 1981
and 1991 149

Figure 11   Percentage of public and private expenditures
on pharmacy as a percentage of total expenditures
on pharmacy, 1989 150

Figure 12   Global health index of OECD countries, 1989 to 1993 ... 151

LIST OF TABLES

Table A   Position of expenditures on pharmaceuticals with respect
to regression of pharmaceutical expenditures
against GDP 95

Table 1.1   OECD member country data (except Iceland) for 1980 ... 107

Table 1.2   OECD member country data (except Iceland) for 1981 ... 108

Table 1.3   OECD member country data (except Iceland) for 1982 ... 109

Table 1.4   OECD member country data (except Iceland) for 1983 ... 110

Table 1.5   OECD member country data (except Iceland) for 1984 ... 111

Table 1.6   OECD member country data (except Iceland) for 1985 ... 112

Table 1.7   OECD member country data (except Iceland) for 1986 ... 113

Table 1.8   OECD member country data (except Iceland) for 1987 ... 114

Table 1.9   OECD member country data (except Iceland) for 1988 ... 115

Table 1.10 OECD member country data (except Iceland) for 1989 ... 116

Table 1.11 OECD member country data (except Iceland) for 1990 ... 117

Table 1.12 OECD member country data (except Iceland) for 1991 ... 118

Table 1.13 OECD member country data (except Iceland) for 1992 ... 119

Table 1.14 OECD member country data (except Iceland) for 1993 ... 120

Table 1.15 OECD member country data (except Iceland) for 1994 ... 121

Table 2   Confidence intervals for regressions, 1981 and 1991 122

Table 3   Number of pharmacists 124

Table 4   Program performance 125

METHODOLOGY

To show how Canada compares internationally in the way it manages pharmaceutical expenditures, we used variables related to pharmaceutical expenditure and use, health outcome and economic status indices and compared them across all OECD member countries using OECD health data. Member countries were compared for each year from 1989 to 1993. Expenditure and income variables are expressed in purchasing power parities (PPP) per capita, in order to eliminate the effect of population and currency exchange differences in so far as this is possible. Because the OECD PPP is based on the cost of a similar basket of goods in each country, the inflation factor should be constant across all countries over time, but this has not been eliminated from the analysis.

In addition, we selected 11 OECD member countries with socioeconomic characteristics similar to Canada's that all have a health care and drug reimbursement program—Australia, Denmark, France, Germany, Italy, the Netherlands, New Zealand, Sweden, Switzerland, the United Kingdom, and the United States (comparator countries).[1] We then compared expenditures on pharmaceuticals in these countries over the past fifteen years.

We also used the least squares regression of per capita pharmaceutical expenditures against per capita gross domestic product (GDP) for the OECD group of countries (minus Iceland) for the years 1981 and 1991 to see the changes that had occurred over the decade.

A comparison of the relative consumption of pharmaceuticals, expressed in boxes per inhabitant, was made between countries. Unfortunately, this information is not available for Canada.

The number of pharmacists per 1,000 inhabitants as well as the proportion of pharmaceutical expenditures from public funding sources gave us some information with which to compare the structure of the pharmaceutical distribution systems of the countries examined. These variables were measured and compared for the years 1981 and 1991.

Finally, the main characteristics of the pharmaceutical reimbursement programs in several countries were outlined and compared, and some explanation was sought for the differences that were observed and relative performance as demonstrated by pharmaceutical expenditure levels of the comparator countries.

All tables and figures referred to in the report may be found at the end of the document. Tables 1.1 to 1.17 contain the data from which all the figures were drawn.

---

1. Originally, Japan was included in the list but problems with the OECD information on its total sources of pharmaceutical expenditures required us to drop this country from the analysis.

CROSS-COUNTRY COMPARISON OF PER CAPITA PHARMACEUTICAL EXPENDITURES

Figures 1.1 to 1.5 illustrate the total pharmaceutical expenditures[2] for OECD countries from 1989 to 1993 and include the mean of all the countries in question. Canada is consistently above the mean in each of the years. In 1989, Canada had the sixth highest total expenditure per capita on pharmaceuticals; in 1990, it was in fifth place (having surpassed Luxembourg); in 1991, it came fourth (along with the United States); in 1992, it was still fourth (the United States having dropped into fifth place); and in 1993, it was third (Italy having dropped from third to fifth place). Over the period, Germany and France were consistently in first and second place respectively.

Figure 2 (A and B) compares Canada with the comparator countries, and illustrates the development of pharmaceutical expenditures in PPPs per capita for the period 1980 to 1993 (1994 for Canada and Italy). There are two basic country groups: the higher level includes Germany, Italy, France, Canada, and the United States, and the balance (Australia, the United Kingdom, Switzerland, the Netherlands, Sweden, Denmark, and New Zealand) fall in the lower range.

Germany, as expected, occupies the highest position in each year of the period. Canada can be seen to be least successful in controlling expenditure increase over that time period. Switzerland saw a dramatic decrease in 1985, after which expenditures increased at a slower rate. New Zealand saw a temporary decrease in 1989. Germany, although showing the steepest increases until 1992, showed a marked decrease from 1992 to 1993 as a result of pharmaceutical budget controls that considerably reduced prescriptions. Italy, whose expenditure pattern closely resembled Canada's until 1992, showed a marked decline from 1992 to 1993 and an even stronger drop in 1993 to 1994. The decline reflects the effect of penalties that physicians incur for improper prescribing.[3]

CROSS-COUNTRY COMPARISON OF DRUG EXPENDITURES AS A PERCENTAGE OF TOTAL HEALTH EXPENDITURES

Decisions about the categories to which health care expenditures should be allocated will differ from one country to another. The proportion of total health care expenditures allocated to pharmaceuticals is compared by country to determine whether there is an impact on the control of drug costs. It is

---

2. This includes expenditures from public and private sources.
3. The national health service has drawn up a list of drugs with appropriate indications and manner of prescribing. The service pays for drugs so prescribed, and penalties can be incurred by physicians who prescribe outside these rules (Simini 1995).

reasonable to assume that certain trade-offs can be made in types of expenditures; a lower level of pharmaceutical expenditures might be explained by higher levels of expenditures in other areas. A comparison was made, therefore, of total pharmaceutical expenditures as a proportion of total health care expenditures.

Figures 3.1 to 3.5 illustrate total pharmaceutical expenditures expressed as a percentage of total health care expenditures for OECD countries from 1989 to 1993 and include the mean for all the countries under consideration. These figures present quite an interesting picture. Canada's position from 1989 to 1992 is at or just above the mean. Many countries spend proportionately more of their total health care expenditures on pharmaceuticals, including those with total drug expenditures well above the Canadian level (such as Germany and France) and well below (such as Greece, Spain, and the United Kingdom). The mean percentage can also be seen to be increasing gradually over the period, from just under 13 percent in 1989 to 14 percent in 1993.[4] High relative percentages are the result of two factors: the relative size of total overall health expenditures (and the majority of OECD countries[5] are below the Canadian level), and the relative size of total pharmaceutical expenditures.

Figure 4 (A and B) shows the development of total pharmaceutical expenditures for the comparator countries as a percentage of total health care expenditures (all sources) for the years 1980 to 1993. Once again, countries could be divided into two groups, although this time the demarcation between the higher and lower groups is less obvious. What should be noted here is that Canada has the steepest overall increase in proportionate expenditures on pharmaceuticals. Sweden also shows a substantial rise, although at a consistently lower proportionate spending level than Canada. Despite temporary decreases in 1989 and 1990, New Zealand also shows an overall increase, to a level above that of Canada's in 1993.

Of the group of countries consistently occupying a position higher than Canada, most display a pattern of relatively flat proportionate spending, and Germany again showed a decrease from 1992 to 1993. Italy saw an increase until about 1987, while the trend in proportionate spending flattened thereafter. Switzerland is the only country which showed an overall, and quite dramatic, decrease in proportionate spending over the period examined, although we have no results after 1991.

---

4. The value for 1993 is based on considerably fewer countries than that of the previous years, and may be not representative of the true median; however, the value is well within the expected range for the time period.

5. With the exception of the United States and Switzerland; and Luxembourg in 1993.

These results underline the previous message: Canada clearly has problems in controlling its pharmaceutical expenditures, both absolutely and in proportion to overall health expenditures.

CROSS-COUNTRY COMPARISON OF PHARMACEUTICAL EXPENDITURES AS A PERCENTAGE OF GDP

Although a relatively clear picture emerges from the previous comparisons, differences in wealth of the countries under review have not been taken into consideration. Expenditures on pharmaceuticals may also be measured by how well countries can afford them. As it is known that increases in wealth are generally accompanied by increases in health expenditures (Contandriopoulos et al. 1993), spending levels should be analyzed relative to each country's wealth. Gross pharmaceutical expenditure data may therefore be refined using the ratio of pharmaceutical expenditures to per capita GDP.

Figures 5.1 to 5.5 illustrate total pharmaceutical expenditures expressed as a percentage of GDP for OECD countries from 1989 to 1993 and include the mean of all the countries under consideration. As was the case for total pharmaceutical expenditures expressed as a proportion of GDP, Canada was consistently above the mean in each of the years. In 1989, Canada was seventh highest in proportionate per capita expenditure on pharmaceuticals, tied with Spain; in 1990, it was fifth (having passed Iceland and Belgium); in 1991, fourth (passing Greece); in 1992, it was fourth again; and in 1993, it was third (Italy having fallen from third to fifth place). Germany and France were consistently first and second during the period.

For a more complete comparative picture, a proportion of pharmaceutical expenditures to GDP, combined with total pharmaceutical expenditures, were indexed to the average of OECD member countries (figure 5.6). This clearly shows the relative positions internationally over the five-year period under review. Canada is in fourth position overall, after Germany, France and Italy, and ahead of the United States, Belgium, Iceland, and Luxembourg, all of which are above the OECD member country mean.[6]

Figure 6 (A and B) shows the development in total pharmaceutical expenditures as a percentage of gross domestic product for comparator countries from 1980 to 1994. The chart shows that Italy and Canada differ from the other countries over the period because of the increase in their spending relative to their economic wealth. For most of the period under consideration, Germany had the highest ratio of pharmaceutical spending

---

6. Total pharmaceutical expenditures as a percentage of GDP were added to twice the total pharmaceutical expenditures per capita and the sum was divided by three.

per capita relative to its per capita wealth. The slight but steady increase in France's relative expenditures over the period reached the German level only in 1993 when a sharp decrease was again noted in relative German spending on pharmaceuticals. Italy's relative spending, which had consistently exceeded Canada's, fell below the Canadian level in 1993, both because of the greater relative increase in Canada's expenditure pattern and because of a sharp drop in Italian spending from 1993 to 1994.

Once again, Canada compares poorly to other countries with respect to its management of pharmaceutical expenditures. This third intercountry comparison reveals that relative to economic wealth, Canada had the steepest and most consistent increase over the period.

CROSS-COUNTRY COMPARISON OF THE RELATIONSHIP OF PHARMACEUTICAL EXPENDITURES TO WEALTH

We reviewed per capita expenditures on pharmaceuticals as a function of the expenditures that might be expected from the least squares regression of per capita expenditures on pharmaceuticals against per capita GDP, using the values for OECD member countries for the years 1981 and 1991. Information for the years after 1991 was too incomplete to allow reasonable comparisons. Results of the analyses and the regression coefficients for the years 1981 and 1991 are given in figures 7 and 8 respectively.

The least squares regression for 1981 produces the following formula:

$$\$Rx = 3D\ .009GDP + 1.02$$

where $Rx is total per capita expenditures on pharmaceuticals, expressed in PPPs, and GDP is per capita gross domestic product, expressed in PPPs. The correlation coefficient of per capita pharmaceutical expenses to per capita GDP for the year 1981 is a respectable 0.6, with an r^2 of 0.4; the ANOVA of the variable is seen to be significant ($p = .001$).[7]

The least squares regression for 1991 produces the following formula:

$$\$Rx = .011GDP - 1.86$$

The correlation coefficient for 1991 is again 0.6, with an r^2 of 0.4; the ANOVA of the variable is seen to be significant ($p = .005$).[8] Not surprisingly, the relationship of pharmaceutical expenditures to GDP is not as strong as

7. Results of a simple regression of 21 OECD member countries in Statview® Student: missing are Iceland, Ireland, Mexico, and Japan.

8. Results of a simple regression of 21 OECD member countries in Statview® Student: missing are Mexico, Japan, Portugal, and Turkey.

that of total health care expenditures to GDP.[9] Pharmaceutical expenditures will reflect the interplay of many factors that together influence how total health care dollars are allocated among health sectors, including the kind of treatment health professionals choose and the controls exercised over the type, price, and quantity of pharmaceuticals.

We have measured the positions of the comparator countries for both 1981 and 1991 above and below the regression line within the 90 percent and the 95 percent confidence intervals. Table 2 provides the expected value and confidence information data from which table A was created.

Table A

Position of expenditures on pharmaceuticals with respect to regression of pharmaceutical expenditures against GDP

Country	Position in 1981	Position in 1991
Australia	–	–
Canada	–	+
Denmark	–	–
France	+	+
Germany	+++	++
Italy	+	+
Netherlands	–	–
New Zealand	–	+–*
Sweden	–	–
Switzerland	+	–
United Kinqdom	–	–
United States	–	+

Note: + indicates a position above the regression line and wlthIn the 90 percent confidence interval (CI) , ++ above and within the 95 percent CI, and +++ above the 95 percent CI, and the converse for – and – –. For example, a notation of +++ indicates extremely poor control of pharmaceutical expenditures relative to the expected value given the least squares regression against GDP, and – indicates rather good relative control.

* New Zealand was almost on the regression line.

From 1981 to 1991, the relative positions of most countries remained more or less the same. This gauge shows that the relative control of pharmaceuticals costs improved since only Switzerland, Germany, and three other

9. For 1981, total health care expenditures as a function of GDP resulting from a simple least squares regression yields a correlation coefficient of .9 with an r^2 of .867; the ANOVA of the variable is seen to be significant (p = .0001). The same analysis for 1991 yields a correlation coefficient of .9 with an r^2 of .732; the ANOVA of the variable is significant (p = .0001).

countries (Canada, the United States and, to a lesser extent, New Zealand) showed a deterioration in cost control.

CROSS-COUNTRY COMPARISON OF DRUG USE

Figure 9 illustrates the difference in average consumption of pharmaceuticals among the comparator countries for the years 1981 and 1989 on the basis of the average number of boxes per person. Unfortunately, the OECD data does not provide any information on the consumption of pharmaceuticals for Canada. France shows the highest per capita consumption by a wide margin, with Italy and Switzerland tied for second but only about half that of France for 1989. From the information available, only France shows any great change in consumption over the decade with an increased per capita consumption of almost 25 percent.

Information about per capita consumption, however, varies according to the source. For 1989, Rigter (1994) reports consumption of almost 50 boxes per capita in France, between 20 and 30 for Germany and Italy, between 10 and 20 for the United Kingdom, Sweden and Switzerland, and less than 10 for the Netherlands.

The lack of information on Canadian consumption levels makes it difficult to position Canada with respect to the comparator countries. However, we took liberties by using some crude price comparison information to indirectly estimate a very rough range of per capita consumption.[10] The calculation produces a result of between 8 and 30 boxes per capita, too wide a margin to be of much use.

The number of prescriptions per capita in Canada is difficult to ascertain, as coverage for prescription costs is extremely variable with much of the population not covered at all. However, partial information is available from a variety of sources. Saskatchewan's drug plan covers nearly 100 percent of its population. It reported an average of 5.4 prescriptions per capita in 1989. Drug plan users have a much higher rate prescription rate: on average there were 8.2 prescriptions per user in Saskatchewan,[11] 16.16 per user for the income security beneficiary drug reimbursement program for Quebec,

---

10. Prices of the top-selling products in Canada in 1993 were compared to various countries, and the ratio of Canadian prices to those of some of the other comparator countries are as follows: France 1.36, Germany 0.96, Italy 1.31, Sweden 1.20, Switzerland 0.98, United Kingdom 1.16, and the United States 0.72. We calculated the average cost (in PPP) per unit of consumption in 1989 for these countries. Using the price ratio of a given country to that of Canada, we calculated the expected Canadian consumption level, given that the per capita expenditures on pharmaceuticals in Canada in 1991 was $256 PPP.

11. Quinn 1992.

and 31.58 for the over-65 drug reimbursement program for Quebec.[12] Comparing this to per-packet information is extremely problematic, because prescriptions may cover time periods that would require the dispensing of the equivalent of two or more "packets."

CROSS-COUNTRY COMPARISON OF DRUG SECTOR STRUCTURES

Except for Italy and Switzerland, for which no information was available, the number of pharmacists per 1,000 population varies for the comparator countries from the Netherlands, with the lowest ratio, to Belgium, with the highest. Although the change in ratio of individual countries between 1981 and 1991 is usually fairly minor, we see a rather large increase for Belgium. Australia, Denmark, and New Zealand reported decreases. It is not clear that these figures bear any relationship to differences in managing pharmaceutical expenditures (table 3 and figure 10).

For countries for which information is available, the percentage of total drug expenditures from public funding sources has remained more or less unchanged from 1989 to 1993. Because of this stability and the increasing scantiness of more recent information, we will focus on 1989 (figure 11). The average percentage of total drug expenditures covered by public funding sources for OECD member countries is just under 60 percent. When we examine comparator countries, only the United States' public sources funding level is lower than Canada's. At 25 percent, Canada's public funding proportion is well below that of most comparator countries, with only Denmark, Australia, and the United States below the OECD average. The level of public funding does not seem to be directly related to cost control: for example, Italy and the United Kingdom, although they have very different cost control profiles, fund pharmaceuticals at an almost identical level (66 percent) of public financing.

CROSS-COUNTRY COMPARISON OF HEALTH INDICES

The comparator countries were reviewed relative to their respective positions in terms of population health status (figure 12). In terms of the Global Health Index and relative to the OECD mean index of zero, Canada is behind Sweden and Switzerland but ahead of Germany, Australia, France, Italy, and the Netherlands, which are all above the mean for most of the period from 1989 to 1993. It is well ahead of Denmark, New Zealand, the United Kingdom and the United States, which are at or below the mean for the majority of the period. On the basis of this information, it is difficult to relate the level of pharmaceutical expenditures, however measured, to the

---

12. Simard 1991.

health of the population. The country that spends most (Germany) has a health index not much higher than the mean, while the one that spends least (the United Kingdom) falls on the mean, higher than countries that spend more, like New Zealand. An attempt at regression of these two variables yields no obvious relationship.[13]

DISCUSSION

Characteristics of the drug reimbursement programs of some comparator countries, namely, Australia, Denmark, New Zealand, the United Kingdom, the Netherlands, France, and Germany are found in table 3.

There is no easy correlation to be drawn between effective control over medication costs and measures taken to curb increases in these costs. When contrasted with inflationary cost increases in Canada, the countries we examined have controlled their increased expenditures on pharmaceuticals relatively well.

Because expenditures are the result of the product of two factors, price and quantity, countries that have succeeded in controlling pharmaceutical costs should, in theory, have implemented both quantity control and price regulation. In fact, strong quantity control measures appear to have been adopted only relatively recently, if at all. More often, expenditures on pharmaceuticals were regulated through price controls, with some very limited control over quantity.

Australia imposed a measure of quantity control in 1987 by requiring authorization to prescribe certain products; Denmark, by restricting the type of physician allowed to prescribe certain items; and the United Kingdom in 1991, by controls on the average number of prescriptions, with notices to overprescribers. The Netherlands continues to control increases in pharmaceutical expenditures quite well without major quantity controls. However, the Netherlands has been able to reach some consensus on the need to reduce pharmaceutical costs. To some extent, manufacturers, wholesalers, and pharmacists have voluntarily reduced their revenue. This is an indication of the responsible attitude that Dutch health care professionals have adopted towards achieving the objectives of the system, and hence the need to assure financial resources for the whole sector. Limits on quantity in the United States are due in large part to the lack of a universal publicly funded drug program, which is also the case in most Canadian provinces.[14]

Prices can be regulated either directly, as in Australia, or indirectly, as in the United Kingdom. All the countries reviewed here have introduced

---

13. A simple least squares regression yields a $p > 0.9$.

14. Universal in terms of the population covered, not in terms of the benefits available.

price controls by way of positive, negative and/or restrictive lists which have necessitated the negotiation of prices by the pharmaceutical industry and the program payers to a level seen as appropriate by reimbursement programs.

New Zealand, which was subject to serious economic and political turmoil during the decade, seems to have brought pharmaceutical expenditures under control for a brief time through a mix of quantity control (prescription of certain items limited to specialists, and/or to the permission of a specialist) and price control (positive list and reference pricing). It seems to have been unable to sustain that control.

Countries that failed to control the increase of pharmaceutical expenditures in the 1980s also lacked any effective mechanism to control the quantities of prescriptions. This problem was recognized in Germany and led the government in its 1993 health care reform to make doctors responsible for the level of drugs prescribed. Any prescription levels above regional medication budget caps will be matched by decreases in doctors' revenue. The effect can be seen in the 1993 figures. Interestingly, the 1993 reform follows an unsuccessful 1989 attempt to curb pharmaceutical costs. In the 1989 reform, a reference-pricing system was introduced, fixing the reimbursement limit above which patients had to pay the difference. Although initially successful, the effect did not last, as less than a third of the drugs available could be reference priced and manufacturers simply compensated for the loss in revenue by raising the prices of drugs not found on the list.

Italy's recent decrease results from a reduced number of available products. This measure has been recently combined with legislation incorporating stiff penalties aimed at problematic physician prescribing. France has implemented recent reforms to curb excessive physician prescribing practices, although the available data do not yet reflect the effect of these 1994 reforms.

Over the ten-year period studied, Canada was clearly the poorest performer in terms of cost control. From a position of relatively good control, its performance declined. There have been some Canadian efforts to control drug prices,[15] and recent increases in mechanisms to control the quantities of prescriptions, in particular, an increased need for special authorization for physicians to prescribe certain products. Because of different provincial programs, it is difficult to comment on Canada-wide cost controls.

Finally, in the United Kingdom, where cost increases were already well under control, fund holding has been introduced recently as an additional and apparently effective incentive to reduce prescribing levels.

---

15. The Patented Medicines Prices Review Board controls the prices of drugs still under patent protection.

Price controls seem to have worked in a limited fashion. There are many examples of price control mechanisms in the countries we examined: Australia negotiates the pricing of all products; and Great Britain controls prices indirectly by regulating promotional costs and profits. Canada has limited centralized control over the prices of pharmaceuticals still under patent protection. Certain parts of the Canadian market are subject to some price control pressures, resulting, for example, from the negotiation of provincial formulary prices and the tender-purchasing practices of many hospitals and hospital groups.

From the point of view of overall efficiency in controlling pharmaceutical costs, the option of global budgets, with financial responsibility (as in the United Kingdom) or financial incentives (as in Germany), show the most promise. In addition, a shift away from a fee-for-service reimbursement of physician practitioners toward a system of either salary or capitation would allow some measure of control over the use of health services. A fee-for- service system, by its very nature, encourages an increase in the use of health services by offsetting price controls with changes in volume and types of service.

What remains largely unknown is the effect of these programs on the overall efficiency of the health care system. Controls on pharmaceutical use are very likely to affect the system as a whole both positively and negatively, but to what extent we do not know. Problems associated with the under-use of necessary medication will no doubt arise, along with long-term implications for the health of the individuals affected and consequences in terms of increased demands on the system as a whole. These increased demands will either be dealt with at the expense of other services, or by means of an increase in total costs. Whatever happens, the system's efficiency should increase as resources are reallocated from less efficient purposes to patients deemed most in need, and treatments considered most effective. An evaluation of the extent of these consequences would be of interest for future study.

Wendy Kennedy *is a research assistant with GRIS (Interdisciplinary Research Group on Health) and the Faculty of Pharmacy at the University of Montreal, and with the Quebec Centres for Excellence in Respiratory Disease at Sacré-Coeur Hospital. With an LL.B. and an M.B.A., Ms. Kennedy has worked in university, industry, and government. Her research interests are in the areas of pharmacoeconomics, pharmacoepidemiology, and pharmaceutical policy. She is finishing a doctorate in public health at the University of Montreal.*

BIBLIOGRAPHY

(Sources cited and consulted)

ANDERSON, G. M., and J. N. LAVIS. 1994. *Prescription Drug Use in the Elderly: Expenditures and Patterns of Use under Ontario and British Columbia Provincial Drug Benefit Programs*. Queen's–University of Ottawa Economic Projects, Ottawa.

ANGUS, D. E., A. LUDWIG, J. E. CLOUTIER, and T. ALBERT. 1995. *Sustainable Health Care for Canada*. Ottawa (ON): Queen's–University of Ottawa Economic Projects.

ARISTIDES, M., and A. MITCHELL. 1994. Applying the Australian guidelines for the reimbursement of pharmaceuticals. *Pharmacoeconomics* 6(3): 196–201.

BARIS, E., A.-P. CONTANDRIOPOULOS, and F. CHAMPAGNE. 1992. *Cost Containment in Health Care: A Review of Policy Options, Strategies and Tools in Selected OECD Countries*. GRIS, University of Montreal, Montreal, R92–07.

BEFORT, A.-F. 1990. *Le système de soins et la maîtrise des dépenses de santé en RFA*. Paris: Institut La Boétie.

BOYD, G. R. 1994. Manager. Therapeutics Section, Ministry of Health of New Zealand. December, Personal communication. December .

CADE, J. 1992. New Zealand. In *International Pharmaceutical Services: The Drug Industry and Pharmacy Practice in Twenty-Three Major Countries of the World*, eds. R. N. SPIVEY, A. I. WERTHEIMER, and T. D. RUCKERS. New York (NY): Pharmaceutical Products Press.

COMMONWEALTH DEPARTMENT OF HUMAN SERVICES AND HEALTH. 1994. *Schedule of Pharmaceutical Benefits*. Canberra: Australian Government Publishing Service.

CONTANDRIOPOULOS A.P., F. CHAMPAGNE F., J. L. DENIS, A. LEMAY, S. DUCROT, M. A. FOURNIER, and A. DJONA. 1993. *Regulatory Mechanisms in the Health Care Systems of Canada and Other Industrialized Countries: Description and Assessment*. Ottawa (ON): Queen's–University of Ottawa Economic Projects.

CUMMING, J. 1995. Health Services Research Centre, Victoria University of Wellington. Personal communication. January.

DAVIES, R., and M. TATCHELL. 1992. Australia: The national health care system. In *International Pharmaceutical Services: The Drug Industry and Pharmacy Practice in Twenty-Three Major Countries of the World*, eds. R. N. SPIVEY, A. I. WERTHEIMER, and T. D. RUCKERS. New York (NY): Pharmaceutical Products Press.

EUROPEAN TRANSPLANT AND DIALYSIS ASSOCIATION. 1991. Combined report on regular dialysis and transplantation in Europe, XXI. *Nephrol Dial Trans* 6(suppl. 4): 5–29.

FURNISS, S. J. 1995. Head. Pharmaceutical Industry Branch, Department of Health. Personal communication. February.

GENERAL ACCOUNTING OFFICE. 1993. *German Health Reforms: New Cost Control Initiatives. Report to the Chairman, Committee on Governmental Affairs, U.S. Senate*. GAO/HRD–93–103.

GREEN, D. G. 1994. The national health service pharmaceuticals market. Recent and prospective reforms. *Pharmacoeconomics* 6(suppl. 1): 11–14.

GRIFFIN, J. P. 1993. Is therapeutic conservatism cost effective? Presentation to EFPIA General Assembly, Salzburg. IMS International. p. 1.

GUNNAR G. Bundesministerium für Gesundheit (Federal Ministry of Health). Personal communication.

HARTMANN-BESCHE. Bundesministerium für Gesundheit (Federal Ministry of Health). Personal communication.

KEMP, R. and J. WLODARCZYK. 1994. Australian pharmaceutical pricing guidelines: Preliminary practical experience. *Pharmacoeconomics* 5(6): 465–471.

KIELGAST, P., and J. POVELSEN. 1992. Denmark. In *International Pharmaceutical Services: The Drug Industry and Pharmacy Practice in Twenty-Three Major Countries of the World*, eds. R. N. SPIVEY, A. I. WERTHEIMER, and T. D. RUCKERS. New York (NY): Pharmaceutical Products Press.

KLETCHKO S. L., D. E. MOORE, and K. L. JONES. 1995. *Targeting Medicines Rationalising Resources in New Zealand.* Wellington (NZ): Pharmac, June.

KNOX, R. *Germany's Health System.* 1993. Washington: Faulkner & Gray, Inc.

LEUFKENS, H. G., and A. BAKKER. 1992. Netherlands. In *International Pharmaceutical Services: The Drug Industry and Pharmacy Practice in Twenty-Three Major Countries of the World*, eds. R. N. SPIVEY, A. I. WERTHEIMER, and T. D. RUCKERS. New York (NY): Pharmaceutical Products Press.

MALING, T. J. B. 1994. The New Zealand preferred medicines concept. *Pharmacoeconomics* 6: 5–14.

MEDICINES CONTROL AGENCY. *Annual report and account 1993/1994.* London: HMSO.

MINISTÈRE DE LA SANTÉ ET DES SERVICES SOCIAUX, Direction de l'Evaluation. 1995. *Recension des options en matière de financement, de partage et de contrôle des coûts d'un programme universel de médicaments et évaluation sommaire de ces options.* Quebec, August .

MITCHELL, A. November 1994 and March 1995. Personal communication.

MÜNNICH, F. E., and K. SULLIVAN. 1994. The impact of recent legislative change in Germany. *Pharmacoeconomics* 6(suppl. 1): 22–27.

NATIONAL ECONOMIC RESEARCH ASSOCIATES (NERA). 1993. The health care system of Germany. In *Financing Health Care with Particular Reference to Medicines, Volume 5.* NERA, May.

NOYCE, P. R., and J. A. HOWE. 1992. United Kingdom. In *International Pharmaceutical Services: The Drug Industry and Pharmacy Practice in Twenty-Three Major Countries of the World*, eds. R. N. SPIVEY, A. I. WERTHEIMER, and T. D. RUCKERS. New York (NY): Pharmaceutical Products Press.

OECD. 1993. *OECD Health System Facts and Trends 1960–1991.* Paris: OECD.

_____. 1995. *OECD Comparative Analysis of Health Systems (Statistical Publications on Diskettes).* Paris: CREDES, OECD.

OFFICE OF HEALTH ECONOMICS. 1992. *Compendium of Health Statistics.* 8th ed. Box 4.17, p. 49.

_____. 1992. *Compendium of Health Statistics.* 8th ed. Table 4.26, p. 64.

PARRY, T. G. 1994. Costing and funding of health care in Australia: Pharmaceuticals in context. *Pharmacoeconomics* 5(3): 180–187.

PBS. 1994. *The Pharmaceutical Benefits Scheme.* June.

PHARMACEUTICAL BENEFITS PRICING AUTHORITY. 1993. *Annual Report for the Year Ending 30 June 1993.* Canberra: Australian Government Publishing Service.

POLICY AND CONSULTATION BRANCH, HEALTH CANADA. 1994. *National Health Expenditures in Canada 1975–1993.* Ottawa (ON): Ministry of Supply and Services Canada.

QUINN, K., M. J. BAKER et al. 1992. A population-wide profile of prescription drug use in Saskatchewan, 1989. *Canadian Medical Association Journal* 146(12): 2177–2186.

REDWOOD, H. 1994. Public policy trends in drug pricing and reimbursement in the European community. *Pharmacoeconomics* 6(suppl. 1): 3–10.

REICHELT, H. 1990. Implementation and consequences of the "Reference Price System" in Germany. Paper of the 4th DPHM-INSERM conference, Paris, November.

RIETVELD, 1995. Ad. Senior Economist. Ministry of Health of the Netherlands. Personal communication. January.

RIGTER, H. 1994. Recent public policies in the Netherlands to control pharmaceutical pricing and reimbursement. *Pharmacoeconomics* 6(suppl. 1):15–21.

Scrip World Pharmaceutical News, no. 1944, July 29, 1994. PJB Publications, London, U.K. p. 20.

Scrip World Pharmaceutical News, no. 1946, August 5, 1994. PJB Publications, London, U.K. p. 19.

Scrip World Pharmaceutical News, no. 1952, August 26, 1994. PJB Publications, London, U.K. p. 13.

Scrip World Pharmaceutical News, no. 1954/55, September 2–6, 1994. PJB Publications, London, U.K. p. 23.

Scrip World Pharmaceutical News, no. 1957, September 13, 1994. PJB Publications, London, U.K. p. 20.

Scrip World Pharmaceutical News, no. 1961, September 27, 1994. PJB Publications, London, U.K. p. 3

Scrip World Pharmaceutical News, no. 1965, October 11, 1994. PJB Publications, London, U.K. p. 21–22.

Scrip World Pharmaceutical News, no. 1979, November 29, 1994. PJB Publications, London, U.K. p. 3, 20.

SERMEUS, G., and G. ADRIAENSSENS. 1989. *Drug Prices and Drug Legislation in Europe.* Brussels: BEUC, March.

SIMARD, R. 1991. Les principales causes de variation de coûts dans le programme de médicaments 1983–1989. Quebec (QC): Conseil consultatif de pharmacologie.

SIMINI, B. 1995. Prescribing in Italy—letter to the editor. *Lancet* 345: 1630.

SITZIUS-ZEHENDER, H., B. DERVENILCH, F. DIENER, and G. FOH. 1992. Federal Republic of Germany. In *International Pharmaceutical Services: The Drug Industry and Pharmacy Practice in Twenty-Three Major Countries of the World*, eds. R. N. SPIVEY, A. I. WERTHEIMER, and T. D. RUCKERS. New York (NY): Pharmaceutical Products Press.

THOMSEN, E. 1995. Medicines Division, National Board of Health, Denmark. Personal communication. May.

APPENDIX

Table 1.1

OECD member country data (except Iceland) for 1980

Country	Total exp. on health	Med. goods expenditure	Macroecon. references	Med. goods expenditure
	Total exp. on health val./capita $PPP	Total exp. pharm. goods val./capita $PPP	GDP val./capita $PPP	Public exp. pharm. goods val./capita $PPP
Australia	671	53	9,206	23
Austria	697	84	8,849	50
Belgium	586	102	8,827	58
Canada	739	66	10,018	15
Denmark	595	54	8,746	25
Finland	521	56	8,004	26
France	711	113	9,415	73
Germany	819	154	9,731	107
Greece	187	65	4,325	9
Ireland	451	50	5,169	24
Italy	581	81	8,460	57
Japan	526	12	8,011	6
Luxembourg	693	101	11,044	87
Mexico	–	–	3,503	–
Netherlands	702	55	8,880	37
New Zealand	556	–	7,723	49
Norway	558	56	8,392	24
Portugal	263	52	4,526	36
Spain	332	70	5,868	45
Sweden	867	56	9,250	41
Switzerland	851	129	11,721	56
Turkey	76	–	2,259	–
United Kingdom	452	58	8,020	37
United States	1,067	92	11,512	7

Source: OECD Health Data 1995 (CREDES).

Table 1.2
OECD member country data (except Iceland) for 1981

Country	Total exp. on health	Med. goods expenditure	Macroecon. references	Med. goods expenditure
	Total exp. on health val./capita $PPP	Total exp. pharm. goods val./capita $PPP	GDP val./capita $PPP	Public exp. pharm. goods val./capita $PPP
Australia	764	62	10,247	29
Austria	794	92	9,658	54
Belgium	687	110	9,584	61
Canada	849	77	11,257	18
Denmark	649	59	9,513	26
Finland	594	61	8,906	29
France	817	134	10,391	–
Germany	928	175	10,662	122
Greece	211	69	4,704	12
Ireland	484	–	5,793	–
Italy	625	90	9,321	63
Japan	600	13	9,036	7
Luxembourg	783	113	12,014	98
Mexico	–	–	4,045	–
Netherlands	776	61	9,608	41
Norway	609	61	9,255	26
New Zealand	608	69	8,848	56
Portugal	312	57	5,028	24
Spain	372	77	6,394	49
Sweden	963	63	10,134	42
Switzerland	956	141	13,104	64
Turkey	93	9	2,554	8
United Kingdom	513	65	8,673	43
United States	1,226	103	12,779	8

Source: OECD Health Data 1995 (CREDES).

Table 1.3

OECD member country data (except Iceland) for 1982

Country	Total exp. on health	Med. goods expenditure	Macroecon. references	Med. goods expenditure
	Total exp. on health val./capita $PPP	Total exp. pharm. goods val./capita $PPP	GDP val./capita $PPP	Public exp. pharm. goods val./capita $PPP
Australia	804	64	10,441	29
Austria	831	97	10,348	55
Belgium	762	117	10,323	62
Canada	956	84	11,419	21
Denmark	709	64	10,408	28
Finland	661	65	9,704	30
France	894	144	11,220	–
Germany	960	181	11,222	125
Greece	220	62	4,981	12
Ireland	496	49	6,217	29
Italy	685	109	9,912	78
Japan	671	13	9,826	9
Luxembourg	819	114	12,895	103
Mexico	–	–	4,209	–
Netherlands	826	67	10,005	45
Norway	664	67	9,818	29
New Zealand	629	–	9,494	59
Portugal	335	61	5,436	43
Spain	404	86	6,820	55
Sweden	1,045	71	10,857	50
Switzerland	1,022	148	13,696	67
Turkey	81	9	2,754	8
United Kingdom	541	74	9,372	48
United States	1,367	115	13,136	8

Source: OECD Health Data 1995 (CREDES).

Table 1.4

OECD member country data (except Iceland) for 1983

Country	Total exp. on health	Med. goods expenditure	Macroecon. references	Med. goods expenditure
	Total exp. on health val./capita $PPP	Total exp. pharm. goods val./capita $PPP	GDP val./capita $PPP	Public exp. pharm. goods val./capita $PPP
Australia	860	70	11,204	31
Austria	880	103	10,979	56
Belgium	814	127	10,779	68
Canada	1,040	94	12,127	25
Denmark	729	68	11,095	30
Finland	714	71	10,297	32
France	954	150	11,700	–
Germany	1,012	194	11,904	132
Greece	239	70	5,168	13
Ireland	516	49	6,400	31
Italy	729	118	10,392	84
Japan	719	14	10,416	11
Luxembourg	859	119	13,802	102
Mexico	–	–	4,125	–
Netherlands	869	69	10,504	43
Norway	726	74	10,645	31
New Zealand	641	80	10,008	63
Portugal	328	63	5,630	39
Spain	433	86	7,208	57
Sweden	1,094	75	11,475	54
Switzerland	1,116	159	14,319	72
Turkey	89	10	2,936	8
United Kingdom	605	82	10,082	53
United States	1,489	127	14,005	9

Source: OECD Health Data 1995 (CREDES).

Table 1.5

OECD member country data (except Iceland) for 1984

Country	Total exp. on health	Med. goods expenditure	Macroecon. references	Med. goods expenditure
	Total exp. on health val./capita $PPP	Total exp. pharm. goods val./capita $PPP	GDP val./capita $PPP	Public exp. pharm. goods val./capita $PPP
Australia	920	73	12,018	35
Austria	919	107	11,562	58
Belgium	849	127	11,451	69
Canada	1,122	110	13,279	28
Denmark	767	72	12,048	32
Finland	761	76	10,967	34
France	1,045	161	12,294	–
Germany	1,107	214	12,777	147
Greece	249	74	5,492	14
Ireland	539	53	6,897	33
Italy	757	122	11,091	85
Japan	748	13	11,218	11
Luxembourg	929	132	15,234	114
Mexico	–	–	4,333	–
Netherlands	895	77	11,222	48
Norway	760	78	11,665	33
New Zealand	649	86	10,813	69
Portugal	338	67	5,734	38
Spain	437	81	7,570	54
Sweden	1,157	77	12,400	54
Switzerland	1,172	166	15,093	77
Turkey	93	10	3,202	8
United Kingdom	638	91	10,729	57
United States	1,618	138	15,380	10

Source: OECD Health Data 1995 (CREDES).

Table 1.6

OECD member country data (except Iceland) for 1985

Country	Total exp. on health Total exp. on health val./capita $PPP	Med. goods expenditure Total exp. pharm. goods val./capita $PPP	Macroecon. references GDP val./capita $PPP	Med. goods expenditure Public exp. pharm. goods val./capita $PPP
Australia	995	80	12,848	37
Austria	992	116	12,246	63
Belgium	887	139	11,943	71
Canada	1,215	127	14,263	33
Denmark	815	78	12,997	35
Finland	852	83	11,682	37
France	1,090	176	12,898	116
Germany	1,175	232	13,519	159
Greece	284	82	5,838	15
Ireland	569	57	7,331	34
Italy	827	148	11,770	101
Japan	796	13	12,112	12
Luxembourg	1,008	149	16,179	128
Mexico	–	–	4,509	–
Netherlands	934	84	11,859	53
Norway	816	83	12,669	36
New Zealand	714	104	11,201	85
Portugal	386	68	6,102	42
Spain	455	92	8,007	58
Sweden	1,159	82	13,056	58
Switzerland	1,300	115	16,124	61
Turkey	73	10	3,356	8
United Kingdom	671	95	11,459	61
United States	1,759	151	16,259	12

Source: OECD Health Data 1995 (CREDES).

Table 1.7

OECD member country data (except Iceland) for 1986

Country	Total exp. on health	Med. goods expenditure	Macroecon. references	Med. goods expenditure
	Total exp. on health val./capita $PPP	Total exp. pharm. goods val./capita $PPP	GDP val./capita $PPP	Public exp. pharm. goods val./capita $PPP
Australia	1,067	86	13,371	42
Austria	1,051	118	12,681	67
Belgium	939	148	12,402	81
Canada	1,321	146	14,938	39
Denmark	825	84	13,786	37
Finland	906	87	12,216	39
France	1,140	186	13,445	123
Germany	1,212	243	14,170	169
Greece	325	93	6,060	20
Ireland	579	60	7,479	37
Italy	862	158	12,414	99
Japan	842	15	12,662	13
Luxembourg	1,043	159	17,232	137
Mexico	–	–	4,341	–
Netherlands	991	92	12,421	56
Norway	952	95	13,474	40
New Zealand	773	117	11,709	95
Portugal	456	69	6,514	48
Spain	474	90	8,440	56
Sweden	1,173	86	13,655	61
Switzerland	1,359	121	16,730	63
Turkey	96	11	3,605	10
United Kingdom	716	101	12,221	65
United States	1,867	166	16,950	15

Source: OECD Health Data 1995 (CREDES).

Table 1.8

OECD member country data (except Iceland) for 1987

Country	Total exp. on health	Med. goods expenditure	Macroecon. references	Med. goods expenditure
	Total exp. on health val./capita $PPP	Total exp. pharm. goods val./capita $PPP	GDP val./capita $PPP	Public exp. pharm. goods val./capita $PPP
Australia	1,113	89	14,262	49
Austria	1,114	125	13,274	71
Belgium	999	159	13,031	90
Canada	1,408	167	15,830	43
Denmark	897	84	14,238	39
Finland	979	94	13,073	43
France	1,197	194	14,094	117
Germany	1,283	262	14,827	184
Greece	322	89	6,208	18
Ireland	597	72	8,073	39
Italy	971	182	13,202	121
Japan	959	17	13,524	15
Luxembourg	1,195	182	18,240	157
Mexico	–	–	4,460	–
Netherlands	1,045	102	12,872	62
Norway	1,045	101	14,108	42
New Zealand	834	123	12,133	100
Portugal	481	–	7,091	58
Spain	523	98	9,166	62
Sweden	1,249	95	14,474	67
Switzerland	1,449	120	17,482	71
Turkey	110	14	3,929	12
United Kingdom	771	107	13,163	70
United States	2,009	180	17,844	17

Source: OECD Health Data 1995 (CREDES).

Table 1.9

OECD member country data (except Iceland) for 1988

Country	Total exp. on health	Med. goods expenditure	Macroecon. references	Med. goods expenditure
	Total exp. on health val./capita $PPP	Total exp. pharm. goods val./capita $PPP	GDP val./capita $PPP	Public exp. pharm. goods val./capita $PPP
Australia	1,176	98	15,282	50
Austria	1,198	138	14,313	79
Belgium	1,087	179	14,150	101
Canada	1,499	190	17,041	47
Denmark	979	94	14,950	44
Finland	1,044	100	14,203	46
France	1,301	217	15,179	131
Germany	1,403	293	15,872	205
Greece	336	88	6,720	20
Ireland	620	79	8,748	44
Italy	1,079	195	14,265	131
Japan	1,025	18	14,854	17
Luxembourg	1,363	199	19,918	–
Mexico	–	–	4,593	–
Netherlands	1,100	108	13,634	66
Norway	1,114	113	14,502	44
New Zealand	863	124	12,465	99
Portugal	558		7,798	63
Spain	633	113	9,986	85
Sweden	1,309	93	15,300	61
Switzerland	1,558	129	18,530	74
Turkey	119	–	4,077	–
United Kingdom	832	116	14,317	78
United States	2,210	192	19,073	19

Source: OECD Health Data 1995 (CREDES).

Table 1.10

OECD member country data (except Iceland) for 1989

Country	Total exp. on health	Med. goods expenditure	Macroecon. references	Med. goods expenditure
	Total exp. on health val./capita $PPP	Total exp. pharm. goods val./capita $PPP	GDP val./capita $PPP	Public exp. pharm. goods val./capita $PPP
Australia	1,238	108	15,912	54
Austria	1,316	147	15,423	85
Belgium	1,160	188	15,228	106
Canada	1,601	210	17,878	53
Denmark	1,019	94	15,685	42
Finland	1,151	108	15,610	51
France	1,423	239	16,350	149
Germany	1,413	289	17,003	195
Greece	371	88	7,238	21
Ireland	652	91	9,869	52
Italy	1,170	213	15,317	141
Japan	1,098	19	16,168	20
Luxembourg	1,442	214	21,939	181
Mexico	–	–	4,860	–
Netherlands	1,172	114	14,804	71
Norway	1,128	118	15,161	44
New Zealand	949	119	13,172	110
Portugal	573	–	8,702	60
Spain	711	128	10,895	93
Sweden	1,396	113	16,239	80
Switzerland	1,698	134	20,168	80
Turkey	120	–	4,180	–
United Kingdom	887	125	15,228	83
United States	2,433	212	20,299	21

Source: OECD Health Data 1995 (CREDES).

Table 1.11

OECD member country data (except Iceland) for 1990

Country	Total exp. on health	Med. goods expenditure	Macroecon. references	Med. goods expenditure
	Total exp. on health val./capita $PPP	Total exp. pharm. goods val./capita $PPP	GDP val./capita $PPP	Public exp. pharm. goods val./capita $PPP
Australia	1,315	118	16,023	53
Austria	1,395	154	16,600	91
Belgium	1,247	194	16,333	118
Canada	1,716	231	18,304	61
Denmark	1,068	95	16,548	37
Finland	1,291	121	16,193	58
France	1,538	256	17,347	156
Germany	1,520	312	18,369	211
Greece	395	95	7,424	23
Ireland	749	101	11,209	58
Italy	1,317	242	16,286	161
Japan	1,188	–	17,596	22
Luxembourg	1,532	225	23,398	190
Mexico	–	–	5,211	–
Netherlands	1,279	127	15,948	85
Norway	1,202	125	16,006	46
New Zealand	996	140	13,518	96
Portugal	616	94	9,380	68
Spain	813	145	11,755	103
Sweden	1,464	120	17,018	86
Switzerland	1,761	144	21,020	80
Turkey	133	35	4,668	–
United Kingdom	955	132	15,896	88
United States	2,685	236	21,162	25

Source: OECD Health Data 1995 (CREDES).

Table 1.12

OECD member country data (except Iceland) for 1991

Country	Total exp. on health	Med. goods expenditure	Macroecon. references	Med. goods expenditure
	Total exp. on health val./capita $PPP	Total exp. pharm. goods val./capita $PPP	GDP val./capita $PPP	Public exp. pharm. goods val./capita $PPP
Australia	1,384	133	16,369	56
Austria	1,490	161	17,364	97
Belgium	1,377	213	17,162	135
Canada	1,846	256	18,400	68
Denmark	1,151	126	17,440	59
Finland	1,416	140	15,508	67
France	1,649	275	18,156	169
Germany	1,650	341	19,677	233
Greece	414	94	7,764	23
Ireland	846	110	11,975	64
Italy	1,440	258	17,170	163
Japan	1,273	–	18,951	26
Luxembourg	1,616	236	24,695	200
Mexico	–	–	5,487	–
Netherlands	1,358	135	16,429	90
Norway	1,339	144	16,764	57
New Zealand	1,059	151	13,643	102
Portugal	730	–	10,421	80
Spain	907	162	12,740	–
Sweden	1,423	126	16,840	90
Switzerland	1,949	152	21,729	86
Turkey	164	–	4,809	–
United Kingdom	1,016	142	15,619	92
United States	2,882	256	21,574	29

Source: OECD Health Data 1995 (CREDES).

Table 1.13

OECD member country data (except Iceland) for 1992

Country	Total exp. on health	Med. goods expenditure	Macroecon. references	Med. goods expenditure
	Total exp. on health val./capita $PPP	Total exp. pharm. goods val./capita $PPP	GDP val./capita $PPP	Public exp. pharm. goods val./capita $PPP
Australia	1,415	135	16,642	66
Austria	1,672	176	18,674	110
Belgium	1,532	250	18,889	155
Canada	1,912	276	18,661	76
Denmark	1,211	138	18,249	66
Finland	1,406	151	15,017	69
France	1,798	299	19,190	185
Germany	1,831	378	21,196	260
Greece	469	110	8,545	27
Ireland	906	128	13,377	76
Italy	1,553	281	18,343	160
Japan	1,411	24	20,150	31
Luxembourg	1,817	–	27,048	233
Mexico	340	–	6,962	–
Netherlands	1,494	156	17,534	147
Norway	1,531	–	18,555	–
New Zealand	1,109	153	14,471	108
Portugal	815	139	11,497	87
Spain	963	175	13,305	–
Sweden	1,300	148	17,138	104
Switzerland	2,133	–	22,779	–
Turkey	148	–	5,003	–
United Kingdom	1,181	169	16,824	108
United States	3,094	267	22,396	31

Source: OECD Health Data 1995 (CREDES).

Table 1.14

OECD member country data (except Iceland) for 1993

Country	Total exp. on health	Med. goods expenditure	Macroecon. references	Med. goods expenditure
	Total exp. on health val./capita $PPP	Total exp. pharm. goods val./capita $PPP	GDP val./capita $PPP	Public exp. pharm. goods val./capita $PPP
Australia	1,493	–	17,555	–
Austria	1,777	191	19,126	120
Belgium	1,601	267	19,373	160
Canada	1,971	298	19,271	81
Denmark	1,296	147	19,340	71
Finland	1,363	–	15,530	–
France	1,835	309	18,764	191
Germany	1,815	335	21,163	205
Greece	500	–	8,782	–
Ireland	922	129	13,847	81
Italy	1,523	275	17,865	135
Japan	1,495	–	20,550	–
Luxembourg	1,993	–	28,741	–
Mexico	–	–	7,019	–
Netherlands	1,531	168	17,602	158
Norway	1,592	–	19,467	–
New Zealand	1,179	189	15,409	125
Portugal	866	–	11,800	80
Spain	972	–	13,330	–
Sweden	1,266	161	16,828	111
Switzerland	2,283	–	23,033	–
Turkey	146	–	5,376	–
United Kingdom	1,213	181	17,152	114
United States	3,299	280	23,358	34

Source: OECD Health Data 1995 (CREDES).

Table 1.15

OECD member country data (except Iceland) for 1994

Country	Total exp. on health	Med. goods expenditure	Macroecon. references	Med. goods expenditure
	Total exp. on health val./capita $PPP	Total exp. pharm. goods val./capita $PPP	GDP val./capita $PPP	Public exp. pharm. goods val./capita $PPP
Australia	–	–	18,511	–
Belgium	–	–	–	–
Canada	–	323	20,312	–
Denmark	–	–	–	–
Finland	–	–	165,017	–
France	–	–	–	–
Germany	–	–	–	–
Greece	–	–	–	–
Ireland	–	–	–	–
Italy	–	249	18,573	–
Japan	–	–	–	–
Luxembourg	–	–	–	–
Mexico	–	–	–	–
Netherlands	–	–	–	–
Norway	–	–	–	–
New Zealand	–	–	–	–
Austria	–	–	–	–
Portugal	–	–	–	–
Spain	–	–	–	–
Sweden	–	–	–	–
Switzerland	–	–	–	–
Turkey	–	–	2,792	–
United Kingdom	–	–	–	–
United States	–	–	–	–

Source: OECD Health Data 1995 (CREDES).

Table 2

Confidence intervals for regressions, 1981 and 1991

Confidence intervals for regressions, 1981

Drugs from GNP	GDP per cap.	Drugs per cap.	Expected value	Difference	90% conf. interval Lower	Upper	95% conf. interval Lower	Upper
Australia	10,247	62	93,043	−31,043	41,808	144,278	31,561	154,525
Canada	11,257	77	102,133	−25,133	45,848	158,418	34,591	169,675
Denmark	9,513	59	86,437	−27,437	38,872	134,002	29,359	143,515
France	10,391	134	94,339	39,661	42,384	146,294	31,993	156,685
Germany	10,662	175	96,778	78,222	43,468	150,088	32,806	160,750
Italy	9,321	90	84,709	5,291	38,104	131,314	28,783	140,635
Netherlands	9,608	61	87,292	−26,292	39,252	135,332	29,644	144,940
New Zealand	8,848	69	80,452	−11,452	36,212	124,692	27,364	133,540
Sweden	10,134	63	92,026	−29,026	41,356	142,696	31,222	152,830
Switzerland	13,104	141	118,756	22,244	53,236	184,276	40,132	197,380
United Kingdom	8,673	65	78,877	−13,877	35,512	122,242	26,839	130,915
United States	12,779	103	115,831	−12,831	51,936	179,726	39,157	192,505

Table 2 (cont.)

Confidence intervals for regressions, 1991

Drugs from GNP	GDP per cap.	Drugs per cap.	Expected value	Difference	90% conf. interval		95% conf. interval	
					Lower	Upper	Lower	Upper
Australia	16,369	133	178,199	−45,199	79,985	276,413	63,616	292,782
Canada	18,400	256	200,540	55,460	90,140	310,940	71,740	329,340
Denmark	17,440	126	189,980	−63,980	85,340	294,620	67,900	312,060
France	18,156	275	197,856	77,144	88,920	306,792	70,764	324,948
Germany	19,677	341	214,587	126,413	96,525	332,649	76,848	352,326
Italy	17,170	258	187,010	70,990	83,990	290,030	66,820	307,200
Netherlands	16,429	135	178,859	−43,859	80,285	277,433	63,856	293,862
New Zealand	13,643	151	148,213	2,787	66,355	230,071	52,712	243,714
Sweden	16,840	126	183,380	−57,380	82,340	284,420	65,500	301,260
Switzerland	21,729	152	237,159	−85,159	106,785	367,533	85,056	389,262
United Kingdom	15,619	142	169,949	−27,949	76,235	263,663	60,616	279,282
United States	21,574	256	235,454	20,546	106,010	364,898	84,436	386,472

Source: OECD 1995 Health Data (CREDES).

124

Table 3

Number of pharmacists

Country	Number of pharmacists 1981	Population (in thousands) 1981	Pharmacists per thousand	Number of pharmacists 1991	Population (in thousands) 1991	Pharmacists per thousand
Austrialia	10,189	14,923	0.68	10,880	17,284	0.63
Belgium	9,942	9,853	1.01	12,490	10,004	1.25
Canada	–	24,900		17,296	28,118	0.62
Denmark	1,344	5,122	0.26	990	5,154	0.19
France	39,533	54,182	0.73	51,277	57,050	0.90
Germany	29,454	61,682	0.48	37,550	64,074	0.59
Italy	–	56,516		–	56,748	
Netherlands	1,601	14,247	0.11	2,287	15,070	0.15
New Zealand	2,290	3,147	0.73	2,223	3,406	0.65
Sweden	3,875	8,320	0.47	5,285	8,617	0.61
Switzerland	–	6,354		–	6,808	
United Kingdom	–	56,379		32,913	57,649	0.57
United States	–	237,568		182,000	262,200	0.69

Source: OECD 1995 Health Data (CREDES).

Table 4

Program performance

Country	Liberty	Equity	Efficiency score*
Australia	• List of medications • Control on certain medication prescriptions • Economic criteria for listing of medication	• The Pharmaceutical Benefits Scheme covers all residents for all drugs listed in the Schedule • Varying copayment: lower for some pensioners, invalids and socio-economically underpriviledged	Med./GDP 1981: – Med./GDP 1991: –
Canada	• Most provinces have a list of medications eligible for government subsidy	• Coverage generally for seniors, the poor and chronically ill • Copayment generally minimal for the poor and chronically ill	Med./GDP 1981: – Med./GDP 1991: +
Denmark	• Two positive lists • One negative list • Some prescriptions limited to specialists • Subsidies for medications depending on the type of list	• No copayment: certain groups of patients, residents of homes for the elderly and handicapped • Subsidy of medications is universal (for residents of Denmark)	Med./GDP 1981: – Med./GDP 1991: –
France	• Lists of medications eligible for different levels of subsidy (3 types) • Copayment related to classification of drug • Penalties for overprescribers	• Universal coverage • Copayment minimal for the poor, chronically ill, and handicapped	Med./GDP 1981: + Med./GDP 1991: +

Table 4 (cont.)

Country	Liberty	Equity	Efficiency score*
Germany	• Cap on pharmaceutical budget: overruns are matched by reductions in physicians' fees • Control of physicians exceeding standards (based on their speciality, patient mix, use of technology, and regional location) • Reference price system: limit under which SFs reimburse medications • Negative list for SFs reimbursement	• 92 percent of the population covered by a statutory Sickness Fund. Eight percent covered by private insurance • Copayment related to the quantity of drug purchased • Upper limit of copayment based on income, marital status, and family size • No copayment for low-income persons and chronically ill	Med./GDP 1981: +++ Med./GDP 1991: ++
Netherlands	• Negative list (with the public insurance plan) • Copayment related to classification of drug	• 60 percent of the population covered by the compulsory public health insurance plan; 40 percent by private insurance	Med./GDP 1981: – Med./GDP 1991: –
New Zealand	• List of medications eligible for government subsidy. For drugs within therapeutic subgroups, subsidy is based upon the lowest-priced drug in that subgroup • Some products available only if prescribed by a specialist, others through hospital pharmacies. For some products, GPs are required to consult a specialist	• Universal coverage (all residents) • Copayment minimal for the poor, children, chronically ill, and accident cases • Maximized for others with a ceiling per family per year	Med./GDP 1991: +/- Med./GDP 1981: –

Table 4 (cont.)

Country	Liberty	Equity	Efficiency score*
United Kingdom	• Restrictive list for some therapeutic groups • Information on level of individual prescribing habits sent to overprescribing physicians	• Copayment: fixed amount by item. Forty-eight percent of the population is exempt from copayment.	Med./GDP 1981: – Med./GDP 1991: –

Source: Adapted and reproduced with permission from Kennedy et al., *Selected National Drug Programs: Description and Review of Performance.* Report of the Pharmaceuticals Policy Division, Drugs Directorate, Health Canada, Ottawa, October 1995.

* Below the line (relative underexpenditure) but within the 90 percent confidence interval (CI) range is designated by –, within the 95 percent CI is designated by – –, outside by – – –. Above the line (relative overexpenditure) but within the 90 percent CI is designated by +, within the 95 percent CI is designated by ++, outside by +++. For example, a notation of +++ indicates extremely poor control of pharmaceutical expenditures relative to the expected value given the least squares regression against GDP, and – indicates rather good relative control.

Figure 1.1

Total pharmaceutical expenditures per capita ($PPP), 1989

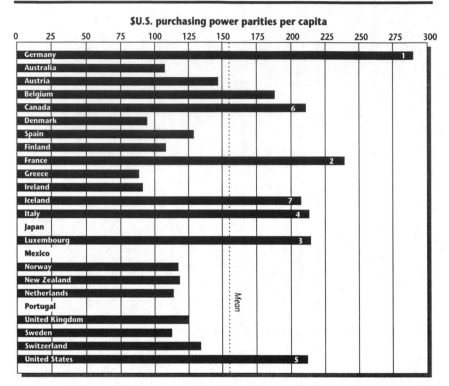

$U.S. purchasing power parities per capita

Source: OECD Health Data 1995 (CREDES).

Figure 1.2

Total pharmaceutical expenditures per capita ($PPP), 1990

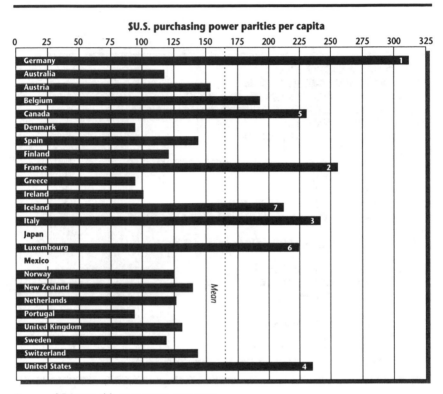

Source: OECD Health Data 1995 (CREDES).

Figure 1.3

Total pharmaceutical expenditures per capita ($PPP), 1991

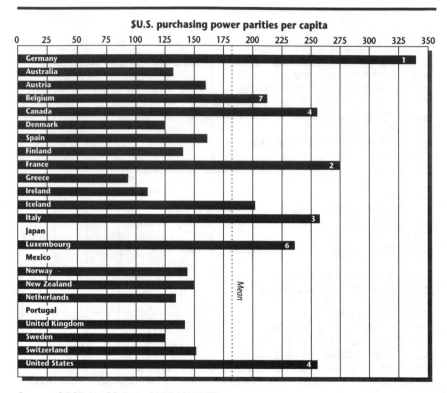

Source: OECD Health Data 1995 (CREDES).

Figure 1.4

Total pharmaceutical expenditures per capita ($PPP), 1992

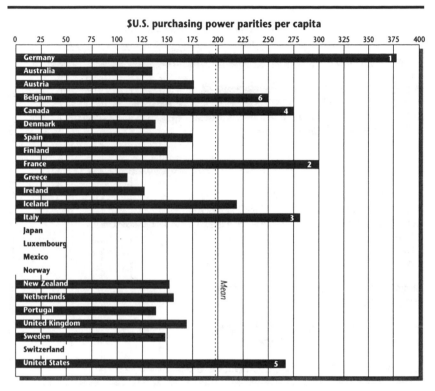

Source: OECD Health Data 1995 (CREDES).

Figure 1.5

Total pharmaceutical expenditures per capita ($PPP), 1993

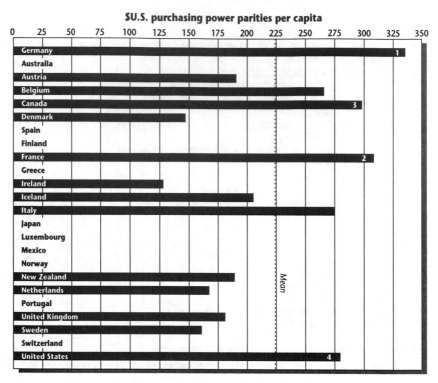

$U.S. purchasing power parities per capita

Source: OECD Health Data 1995 (CREDES).

Figure 2A

Total pharmaceutical expenditures in $U.S. purchasing power parities per capita, 1980–1994

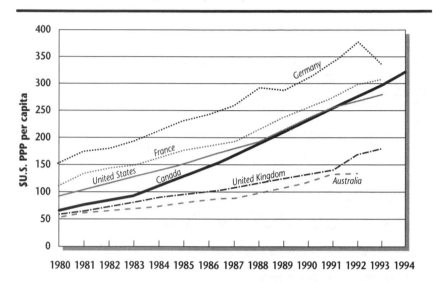

Figure 2B

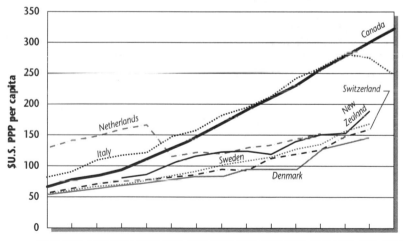

Source: OECD Health Data 1995 (CREDES).

Figure 3.1

Total pharmaceutical expenditures as a percentage of total health care expenditures, 1989

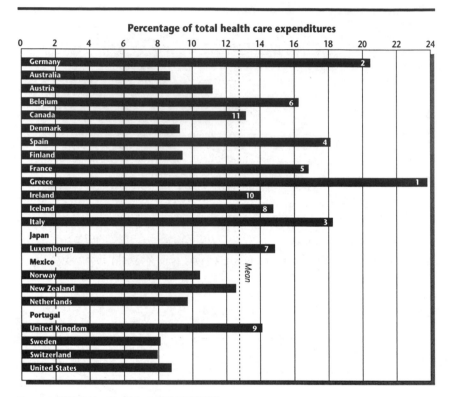

Source: OECD Health Data 1995 (CREDES).

Figure 3.2

Total pharmaceutical expenditures as a percentage
of total health care expenditures, 1990

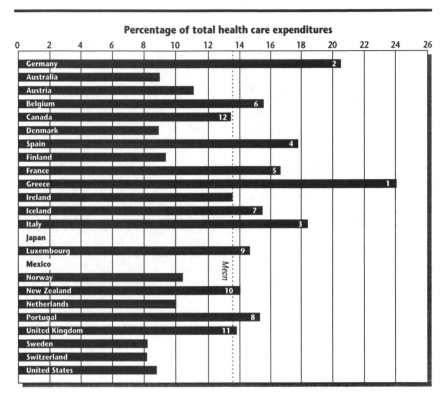

Source: OECD Health Data 1995 (CREDES).

Figure 3.3

Total pharmaceutical expenditures as a percentage of total health care expenditures, 1991

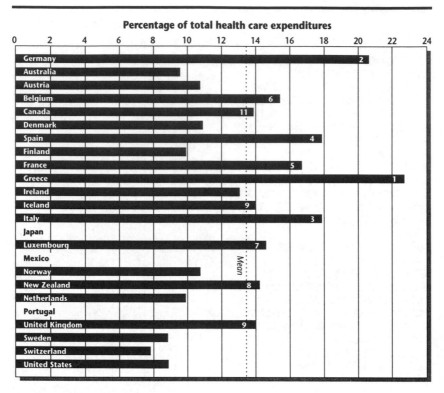

Source: OECD Health Data 1995 (CREDES).

Figure 3.4

Total pharmaceutical expenditures as a percentage of total health care expenditures, 1992

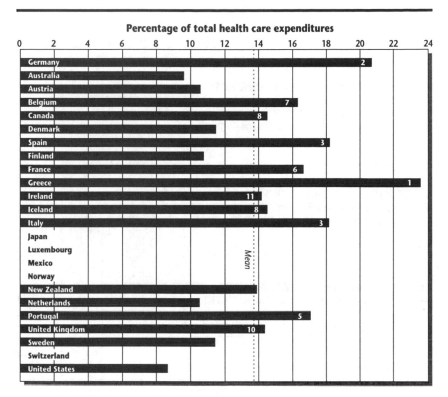

Source: OECD Health Data 1995 (CREDES).

Figure 3.5

Total pharmaceutical expenditures as a percentage of total health care expenditures, 1993

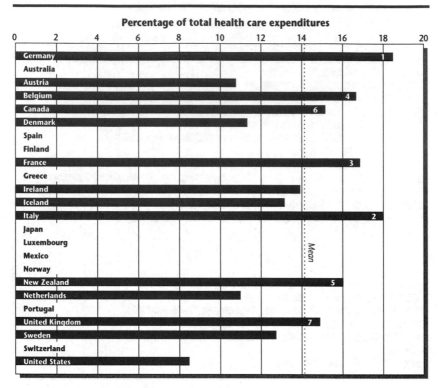

Source: OECD Health Data 1995 (CREDES).

Figure 4A

Total pharmaceutical expenditures as a percentage of total healthcare expenditures in $U.S. purchasing power parities per capita, 1980–1994

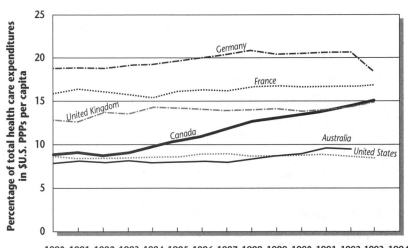

Figure 4B

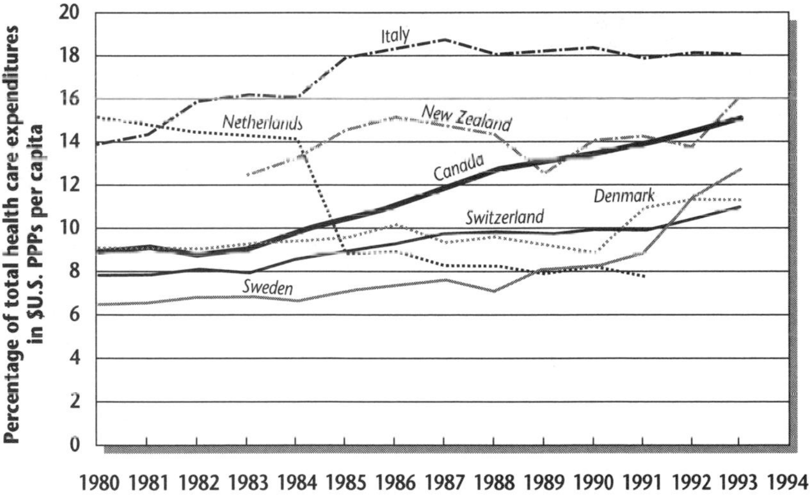

Source: OECD Health Data 1995 (CREDES).

Figure 5.1

Total pharmaceutical expenditures as a percentage of gross domestic product, 1989

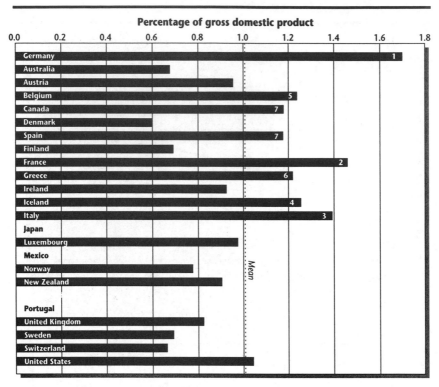

Source: OECD Health Data 1995 (CREDES).

Figure 5.2

Total pharmaceutical expenditures as a percentage of gross domestic product, 1990

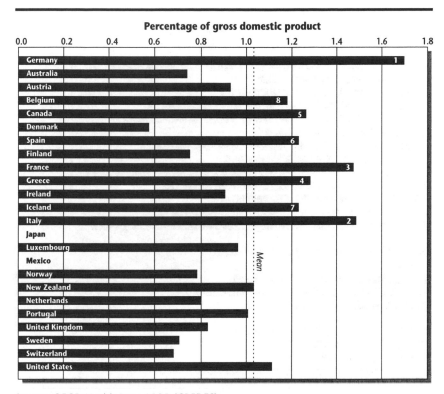

Source: OECD Health Data 1995 (CREDES).

Figure 5.3

Total pharmaceutical expenditures as a percentage of gross domestic product, 1991

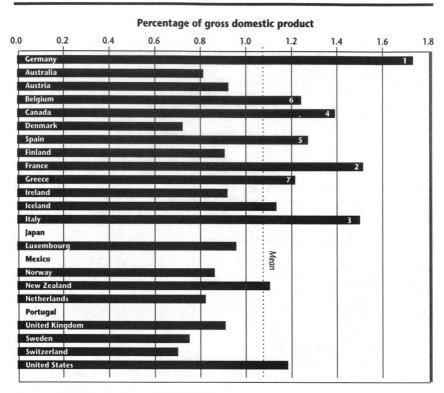

Source: OECD Health Data 1995 (CREDES).

Figure 5.4

Total pharmaceutical expenditures as a percentage
of gross domestic product, 1992

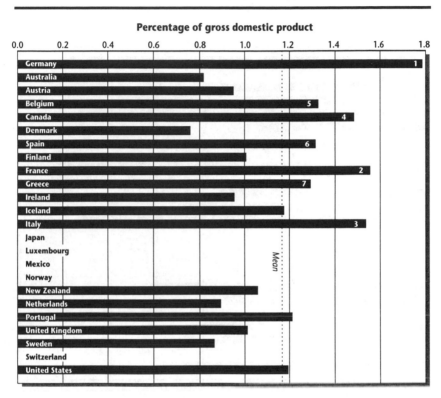

Source: OECD Health Data 1995 (CREDES).

Figure 5.5

Total pharmaceutical expenditures as a percentage of gross domestic product, 1993

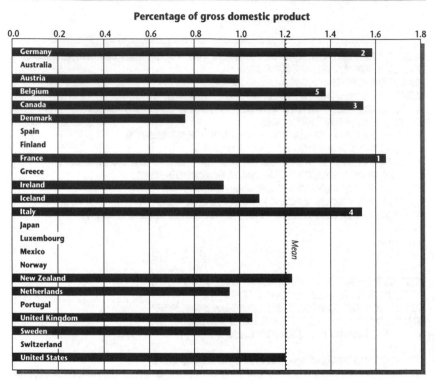

Source: OECD Health Data 1995 (CREDES).

Figure 5.6

Global pharmaceutical expenditures index
(total pharmaceutical expenditures as a percentage
of GDP + 2 pharmaceutical expenditures per capita /3, 1989–1993)

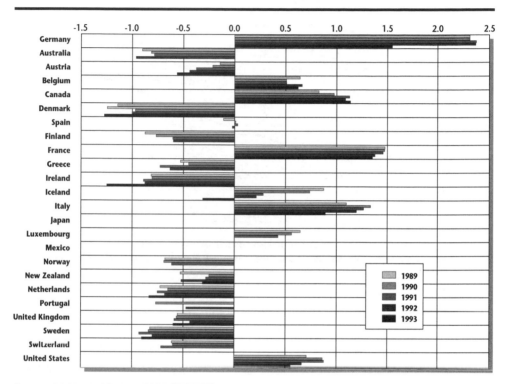

Source: OECD Health Data 1995 (CREDES).

Figure 6

Pharmaceutical expenditures as a percentage of gross domestic product in $U.S. purchasing power parities per capita, 1980–1984

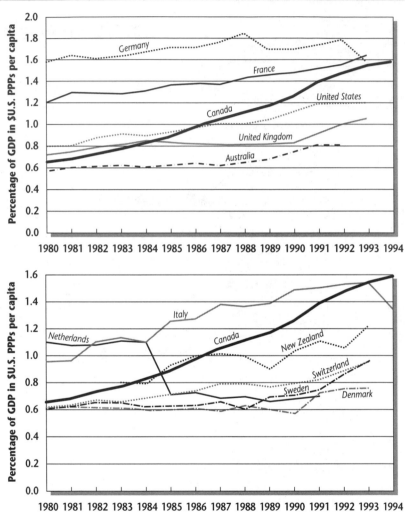

Source: OECD Health Data 1995 (CREDES).

Figure 7

Regression: Total expenditures on pharmaceuticals and gross domestic product, 21 countries, 1981

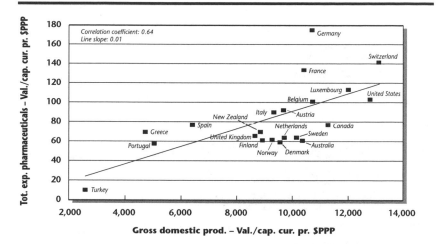

Source: 1995 OECD Health Data (CREDES).

Figure 8

Regression: Total expenditures on pharmaceuticals and gross domestic product, 21 countries, 1991

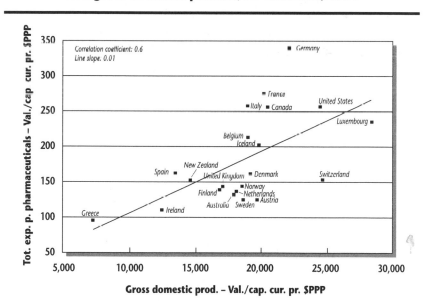

Source: OECD Health Data 1995 (CREDES).

Figure 9

Consumption of medications measured by the number of boxes per capita, 1981 and 1989

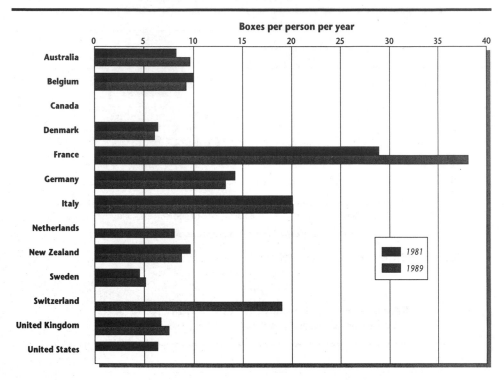

Source: OECD Health Data 1995 (CREDES).

Figure 10

Number of pharmacists per thousand population, 1981 and 1991

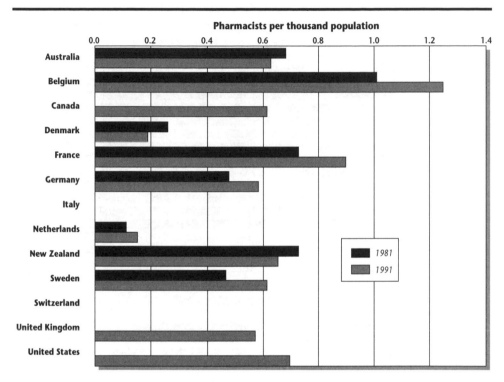

Source: OECD Health Data 1995 (CREDES).

Figure 11

Percentage of public and private expenditures on pharmacy as a percentage of total expenditures on pharmacy, 1989

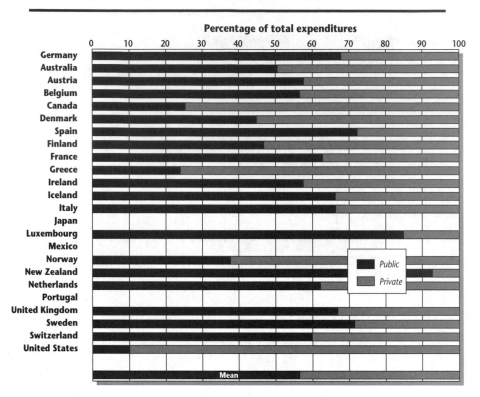

Source: OECD Health Data 1995 (CREDES).

Figure 12

Global health index of OECD countries, 1989 to 1993

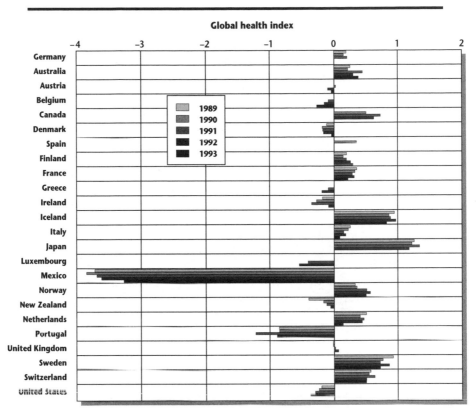

Source: OECD Health Data 1995 (CREDES).

Health Spending and Health Status: An International Comparison

CENTRE FOR INTERNATIONAL STATISTICS

Ottawa

SUMMARY

This paper presents an international comparison of public health care expenditures and other selected types of social spending. The objective of the paper is to comparatively examine the relationship between various forms and levels of public expenditure and the health status of the population in each of the member countries of the OECD. Two indicators of national health status are used: life expectancy at birth, and infant mortality rate. The paper addresses several questions:

- *How does Canada's level of health care spending compare with that of other industrialized countries?*
- *Do countries that spend more on health care have higher life expectancies and lower infant mortality rates than other countries?*
- *What impact do other social and economic factors such as income inequality, poverty levels, and GDP per capita have on health status?*

The findings show that relative to other industrialized nations, Canada's spending on health care is high. And while the health status of Canada's population, as measured by life expectancy and infant mortality, compares favourably with other countries, the relationship between health care spending and health outcomes is ambiguous. In several countries, high life expectancy and low infant mortality are obtained with lower health care expenditures than in Canada. In other words, international comparisons show that higher levels of national health spending are not unequivocally linked with better health status. The findings also show an ambiguous relationship between health status and other forms of social spending such as expenditures on income security and education. It would appear that among industrialized nations, simple measures of the amount of spending are poor predictors of a country's ranking on life expectancy and infant mortality.

A word of caution is warranted. This paper is limited to an exploratory overview of the relationship between public spending and health status of the populations in industrialized nations. No attempt has been made to control for the complexity of social, demographic, environmental, and biological factors that may influence the health status of a given population. Accordingly, all results should be read with caution. Further in-depth research is required.

TABLE OF CONTENTS

Health Care Spending among OECD Countries 157

Does Canada Spend More on Health than Other Industrialized
Countries? 157

Public versus Private Health Care Expenditures 157

Are Canada's Public Health Care Expenditures Higher than
Other Countries? 157

The Relationship between Health Spending and Health Status 157

Do Countries that Spend More on Health Care Have Better
Health Status? 157

Health Spending and Life Expectancy 159

**Other Forms of Social Spending That May Influence
Health Status** 162

Income Security Spending and Health Status 162

Income Inequality, Poverty, and Health Status 164

Trends over Time 166

Conclusion 168

Bibliography 171

LIST OF FIGURES

Figure 1   Total public and private health expenditure as
a percentage of GDP, OECD countries, 1993 158

Figure 2   Public health expenditure as a percentage of GDP,
OECD countries, 1993 159

Figure 3   Total health spending and infant mortality, selected
OECD countries, 1993 160

Figure 4   Total health expenditure and life expectancy,
selected OECD countries 161

Figure 5   Total health spending and life expectancy of women,
1993 161

Figure 6   Income security expenditure (1990) and infant
             mortality (1993), selected OECD countries 164

Figure 7   Family poverty and infant mortality, selected OECD
             countries 166

Figure 8   Change in infant mortality (1980–1993) and change
             in health care expenditure as a percentage of GDP
             (1983–1993), OECD countries 169

Figure 9   Change in infant mortality and change in inequality
             over time 169

LIST OF TABLES

Table 1   Public expenditure (as a percentage of GDP) on income
             security, education, and labour market programs:
             Selected OECD countries, various years 163

Table 2   Rank order correlations, selected expenditure,
             and health status variables, OECD countries 165

Table 3   Changes in selected indicators over time, OECD 167

HEALTH CARE SPENDING AMONG OECD COUNTRIES

Does Canada Spend More on Health than Other Industrialized Countries?

Compared with the 25 member countries of the Organization for Economic Cooperation and Development (OECD), Canada ranks second in its total health care spending as a percentage of GDP (figure 1). Total health care expenditures include those financed through the public purse, as well as private spending, such as insurance premiums and out-of-pocket expenditures. Total health care spending amounts to 10.2 percent of GDP in Canada, second only to the United States at 14.1 percent. On average, OECD countries spend 8 percent of GDP on health care.

Public versus Private Health Care Expenditures

In almost all industrialized countries, the majority of health care spending is financed through the public purse. In Canada, 73 percent of total health care expenditures are financed publicly, which is consistent with the average among all OECD countries. The United States stands out as being the *only* OECD country to spend more privately on health care than publicly, with only 44 percent of total health spending coming from public sources. At the other extreme is Norway, where 93 percent of total health expenditures are financed publicly.

Are Canada's Public Health Care Expenditures Higher than Other Countries?

Compared with other OECD countries, Canada has the second highest public health expenditure measured as a percentage of GDP (figure 2). In 1993, public health expenditures in Canada amounted to 7.4 percent of GDP ($40.4 billion). Despite its high ranking, Canada's level of public health expenditure is similar to several other European countries, including Norway, Belgium, and France.

THE RELATIONSHIP BETWEEN HEALTH SPENDING AND HEALTH STATUS

Do Countries that Spend More on Health Care Have Better Health Status?

From an international perspective, there is no clear relationship between levels of health care expenditure and health status of the population. One commonly used indicator of a population's health status is the infant mortality rate, which refers to the number of deaths before the age of one per 100 live births. The

Figure 1

Total public and private health expenditure as a percentage of GDP, OECD countries, 1993

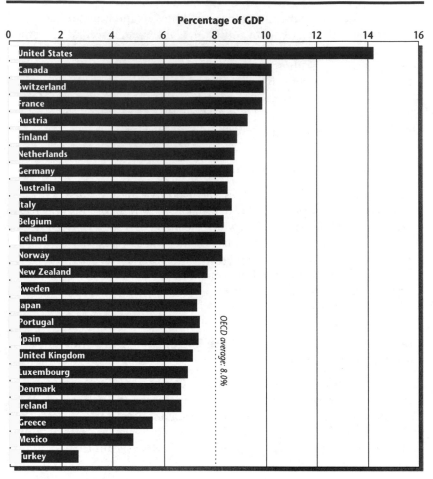

Source: *OECD in Figures*, 1995.

relationship between total health spending and infant mortality rates is presented in figure 3 (see table 2 for rank order correlation coefficients). The figure shows that higher spending on health care does not necessarily result in lower infant mortality. The United States, for example, spends 38 percent more than Canada on health, and has an infant mortality rate that is 25 percent greater than in Canada. On the other hand, the infant mortality rate in Norway and Sweden is considerably lower than in Canada, and yet these countries spend considerably less on health care.

Figure 2

Public health expenditure as a percentage of GDP, OECD countries, 1993

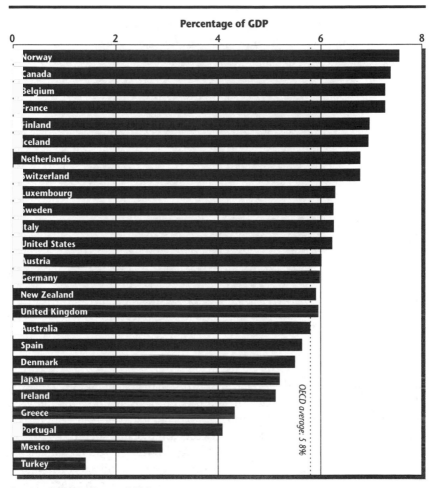

Source: *OECD in Figures*, 1995.

Health Spending and Life Expectancy

Another indicator used to assess the health status of a nation's population is life expectancy at birth, which refers to the number of years a newborn would live if the prevailing patterns of mortality at birth remain constant throughout the child's life. Among OECD countries, Canada has the ninth highest life expectancy at birth. Of the 10 OECD countries with the highest life expectancies, Canada has the highest expenditure on health care. In other words, several other industrialized countries have relatively high life

Figure 3

**Total health spending and infant mortality,
selected OECD countries, 1993**

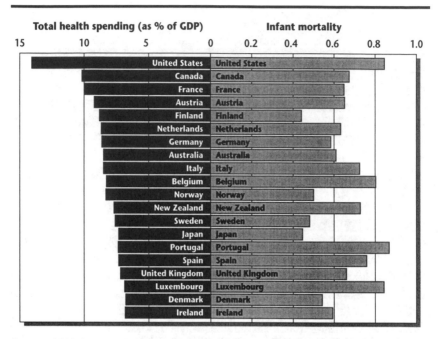

Source: *OECD in Figures*, 1995.

expectancy but lower health care expenditures than Canada. From a comparative international perspective, there is no significant relationship between
level of health care spending and life expectancy (figure 4).There is a
statistically significant correlation between total health spending and the
life expectancy of *women*. That is, the life expectancy of women tends to be
higher in those countries with higher health care expenditures (figure 5).
An examination of the reasons why this relationship exists for women, and
not for men, is beyond the scope of this paper. It is worth noting however,
that despite this positive association, there are several exceptions. The United
States, for example, has the highest level of spending on health care and a
relatively low female life expectancy. Sweden, on the other hand, has
comparably low spending on health care and high life expectancy for women.

Figure 4

Total health expenditure and life expectancy, selected OECD countries

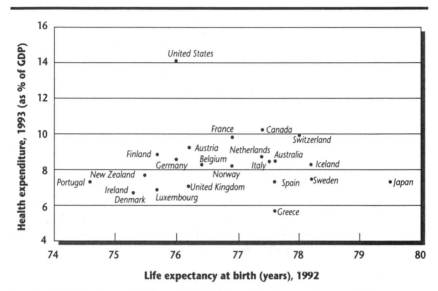

Sources: *OECD in Figures*, 1995; and UNDP, *Human Development Report*, 1995.

Figure 5

Total health spending and life expectancy of women, 1993

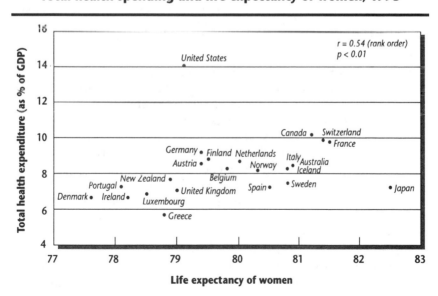

Source: *OECD in Figures*, 1995.

OTHER FORMS OF SOCIAL SPENDING THAT MAY INFLUENCE HEALTH STATUS

Direct public expenditures on health care are not the only form of spending that may influence the health status of a nation's population. Public spending on income security, education, and labour market programs, for example, can promote and enhance quality of life, and consequently the health and well-being of the population. These forms of spending are not typically thought of as health spending, but there is evidence of a relationship between socioeconomic status and health (see, for example, Wilkinson 1994; the Canadian Institute of Child Health 1994; and Wilkins, Adams, and Brancker 1989).

Income Security Spending and Health Status

While Canada's health care spending is among the highest in the industrialized world, its level of public spending on income security programs is more modest. Expenditures on income security refers to the provision of social welfare, public pensions, unemployment benefits and other income support schemes, and amounts to 11.9 percent of GDP, placing Canada below the OECD average, and well below the level of other OECD countries such as Sweden and Denmark (table 1).

While the objectives and design of income security programs can vary considerably within and between countries, in most (if not all) industrialized nations, these programs have the common purpose of supporting, supplementing, and stabilizing the incomes generated by private market economies. Examples include income support and supplementation for the poor, replacement income for the unemployed, public assistance for the disabled and the sick, and retirement pensions for the elderly, to name only a few. To the extent that income security spending leads to improvements in socioeconomic status, particularly among the more vulnerable groups in society, it may have a positive (if indirect) impact on health status.

Figure 6 compares the level of public spending on income security with the infant mortality rate in each of 20 OECD countries for which data is available. Based on these 20 countries, there is no statistically significant association between infant mortality and income security spending as a percentage of GDP (see rank order correlation coefficients in table 2). As seen from figure 6, however, three countries—Luxembourg, Japan, and Australia—appear as "outliers" in what would otherwise seem to be a linear relationship. In fact, when these three countries are removed from the analysis, there is a strong and significant rank order correlation between income security spending and infant mortality ($r = -.73$, $p < .001$). In other words, those countries with higher levels of income security spending tend to have lower infant mortality rates. If we focus on the 15 countries that have higher income security spending than Canada, five of them have a higher infant mortality rate and ten have a lower infant mortality rate.

Table 1

Public expenditure (as a percentage of GDP) on income security, education and labour market programs: Selected OECD countries, various years

			Labour market programs	
	Income security	Education	Unemp. comp.	Other
Sweden	26.3	7.5	2.7	3.1
Denmark	23.1	7.6	3.6	3.2
Netherlands	23.0	5.6	2.2	1.2
Luxembourg	22.7	–	0.3	0.8
Norway	21.6	–	1.6	1.3
Finland	20.8	8.3	4.6	2.3
France	20.5	5.5	1.6	1.4
Austria	19.0	5.8	1.4	0.4
Italy	18.5	5.1	0.6	1.2
United Kingdom	18.5	5.1	1.2	0.5
Belgium	18.4	6.0	2.2	1.8
Germany	16.8	4.1	2.0	2.2
Ireland	15.2	5.6	2.8	1.5
Spain	14.5	4.6	3.5	0.5
New Zealand	12.9	6.5	2.0	0.7
Canada	11.9	7.1	2.3	0.6
Portugal	11.3	–	0.9	1.0
United States	9.4	5.3	0.6	0.3
Australia	7.4	5.5	1.9	0.8
Japan	6.8	3.6	0.3	0.1
Average	16.9	5.5	1.9	1.2

Notes:

1. Income security expenditures refer to social welfare spending in the areas of pensions, unemployment benefits, and other income schemes in 1990.

2. Education expenditure is from the OECD, and refers to public expenditure on all levels of education as a pecentage of GDP in 1991–1992.

3. Labour market expenditure is from the *OECD Employment Outlook,* 1994, and is expressed as a percentage of GDP in 1992–1993.

The relationship between other forms of social spending and various indicators of health status is summarized in table 2. As seen from the table, there is a statistically significant correlation between infant mortality and labour market expenditure. The latter refers to a wide range of program spending including unemployment compensation as well as labour market

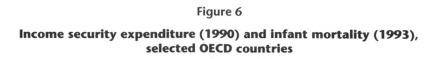

Figure 6

**Income security expenditure (1990) and infant mortality (1993),
selected OECD countries**

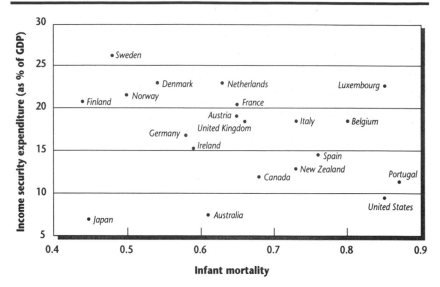

Sources: OECD, *OECD in Figures*, 1995, and *New Orientations for Social Policy*, 1994.

training, youth employment programs, measures for the disabled, and employment subsidies. The correlation coefficient between labour market expenditure and infant mortality is negative, indicating that higher levels of spending are associated with lower infant mortality rates.

There is no significant correlation between education spending and infant mortality or life expectancy.

Income Inequality, Poverty, and Health Status

There is a substantial amount of research showing that measures of health within countries are related to income. In Canada, for example, a Statistics Canada Health Report presents evidence to suggest a relationship between infant mortality, low birthweight and income (Wilkins, Adams, and Brancker 1989). It may thus be reasonable to expect that countries with a large degree of income inequality or high levels of relative poverty may have comparably lower standards of national health. As shown in table 2, there is some evidence to support this. There is a significant association between the share of income held by the bottom 40 percent of households and life expectancy. That is, those countries with a larger share held by the bottom 40 percent tend to have higher life expectancy. In addition, there is a strong correlation

Table 2

Rank order correlations, selected expenditure, and health status variables, OECD countries[1]

	Life expectancy at birth (all)	Life expectancy at birth (men)	Life expectancy at birth (women)	Infant mortality
Health expenditure (total) as a % of GDP	0.16	0.10	0.54**	– 0.10
Health expenditure (public) as a % of GDP	0.18	0.16	0.48**	– 0.21
Income security expenditure as a % of GDP[2]	– 0.08	– 0.14	– 0.14	– 0.31
Education expenditure as a % of GDP[3]	– 0.32	– 0.22	– 0.26	– 0.23
Labour market expenditure (total) as a % of GDP[4,5]	– 0.14	– 0.11	– 0.11	– 0.46**
Labour market compensation expenditure as a % of GDP[4,6]	– 0.09	– 0.04	– 0.09	– 0.39*
Labour market program expenditure as a % of GDP[4,7]	– 0.24	– 0.19	– 0.17	– 0.41*
Per capita GDP	0.12	0.06	0.28	– 0.14
Ratio of top income quintile to bottom income quintile[8]	– 0.38	– 0.17	– 0.22	0.27
Income share of bottom 40%[8]	0.41*	0.19	0.28	– 0.17
Family poverty[9]	0.13	0.18	0.24	0.71**

Sources: OECD, *OECD in Figures*, 1995, and *OECD Employment Outlook*, 1994; UNDP, *Human Development Report*, 1995; and the Luxembourg Income Study.

* p < .10; ** p < .05.

1. All correlations based on 23 OECD countries. Mexico and Turkey have been excluded on the basis that they did not receive a high human development rank on the United Nations Human Development Report (1995), and appear as outliers on much of the analysis. Additional notes refer to other countries excluded due to data limitations. 2. Excludes Iceland and Switzerland. Income security expenditures refer to the provision of social welfare, public pensions, unemployment benefits, and other income support programs. 3. Excludes Greece, Iceland, Luxembourg, Norway, and Portugal. 4. Excludes Greece, Iceland, and Switzerland. 5. Includes early retirement provisions as labour force adjustment programs, plus labour market compensation and programs. 6. Includes labour market training, youth employment programs, measures for the disabled, employment subsidies. 7. Includes labour market compensation for the unemployed. 8. Excludes Austria, Greece, Iceland, Ireland, Luxembourg, and Portugal. 9. Includes only Sweden, Finland, Denmark, Belgium, Norway, the Netherlands, Canada, Australia, and the United States.

between family poverty and infant mortality: countries with higher rates of family poverty tend to have a higher rate of infant mortality (figure 7). It should be noted that the relationship between family poverty and infant mortality is based on only nine countries (due to availability of data). Results should therefore be used with caution.

TRENDS OVER TIME

This section of the paper examines the relationship between changes in infant mortality over time and a number of selected items: average annual change in GDP; change in total health care expenditure; change in spending on income security programs; and change in the degree of income inequality.

As table 3 shows, in all OECD countries for which data is available, infant mortality was lower in 1993 than in 1980. In Canada, for example, infant mortality (percentage of live births) decreased from 1.04 in 1980 to 0.68 in 1993. During roughly the same period, OECD countries demonstrated considerable variation in level of economic growth, health spending, income security spending, and income inequality. For example, in Canada, total health care expenditure as a percentage of GDP increased by 1.6 percentage points between 1983 and 1993 (from 8.6 percent to 10.2 percent), while in Sweden, total health expenditure decreased by 2.0 percentage points (from 9.5 percent to 7.5 percent).

Figure 7
Family poverty and infant mortality, selected OECD countries

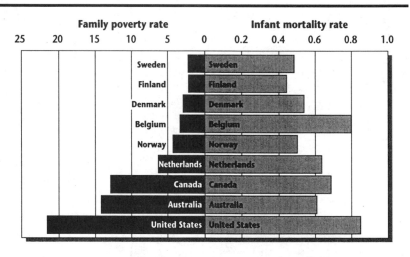

Sources: The Luxembourg Income Study; and OECD, *OECD in Figures*, 1995.

Table 3

Changes in selected indicators over time, OECD

Country	[1] infant mortality 1980–1993	[2] % average annual change in GDP 1983–1993	[3] % point change in health care expenditure as % of GDP 1983–1993	[4] % point change in spending on income security 1980–1990	[5] inequality: % point change in Gini coefficient	[6] inequality: % point change in Gini coefficient (adjusted)*
Australia	− 0.46	3.3	0.8	1.0	0.8	0.02
Austria	− 0.78	2.3	1.2	1.0	–	–
Belgium	− 0.30	2.0	0.7	− 1.5	0.7	0.23
Canada	− 0.36	2.6	1.6	3.0	0.3	0.05
Denmark	− 0.30	1.9	0.1	2.9	–	–
Finland	− 0.32	1.0	1.9	4.5	0.8	0.27
France	− 0.36	1.9	1.6	2.6	0.0	0.00
Germany	− 0.69	2.8	0.1	− 2.3	–	–
Greece	− 0.94	1.7	1.1	–	–	–
Iceland	− 0.29	2.2	1.0	–	–	–
Ireland	− 0.52	4.4	− 1.4	2.2	–	–
Italy	− 0.70	2.2	1.5	4.3	–	–
Japan	− 0.30	3.7	0.4	1.0	–	–
Luxembourg	− 0.30	3.7	0.7	3.0	–	–
Mexico	–	2.0	–	–	–	–
Netherlands	− 0.23	2.5	0.4	1.7	2.1	0.53
New Zealand	− 0.56	1.6	1.3	3.7	–	–
Norway	− 0.31	2.7	1.4	6.7	1.2	0.17
Portugal	− 1.73	2.8	1.5	1.9	–	–
Spain	− 0.35	2.8	1.3	2.3	–	–
Sweden	− 0.21	1.2	− 2.0	2.6	2.1	0.35
Switzerland	− 0.30	1.8	2.1	–	–	–
Turkey	–	5.3	− 0.3	–	–	–
United Kingdom	− 0.55	2.2	1.1	2.4	3.4	0.49
United States	− 0.41	2.8	3.5	− 0.8	3.2	0.46

Sources: Columns 1,2,3: 1993 data from OECD, OECD in Figures, 1995; 1980 data from OECD, Measuring Health Care 1960–1983, 1985. Column 4: OECD, New Orientations for Social Policy, 1994. Columns 5,6: OECD, Income Distribution in OECD Countries, 1995 (based on data from the Luxembourg Income Study, 1995).

* Measures the difference in Gini coefficients at 2 points (late 1970s to mid-1980s). Differences are divided by the number of years between observation points.

Is there a relationship between trends in economic growth, health spending, income security spending, or income inequality and changes in infant mortality? Are countries that have increased their health expenditures also those that have had the greatest decline in infant mortality? Have infant mortality rates decreased more rapidly in those countries that have moved toward greater income equality? The analysis of rank order correlations shows no significant relationship between change in infant mortality and any of the items identified in table 3 (see plots in figures 8 and 9).

CONCLUSION

Compared with other industrialized nations, Canada's health care expenditures (measured as a percentage of GDP) are high. Total health care spending (public and private combined) amounts to 10.2 percent of GDP, second only to the United States. Public health care expenditures amount to 7.4 percent of GDP, second only to Norway.

Countries that spend more on health care do not necessarily have higher life expectancy or lower infant mortality than countries spending less. The simple measure of health care spending as a percentage of GDP appears to be a poor predictor of a country's ranking on these two measures of population health status. There is a statistically significant association between health spending and the life expectancy of women—a relationship that is not found for men. Further research is required to better understand this relationship.

The relationship between other forms of spending—income security, education, and labour market programs—and health status is also ambiguous. Neither income security spending nor education spending is significantly correlated with health status. The statistically significant correlation found between labour market expenditures and infant mortality also requires further research and explanation.

In short, the examination of rank order correlations between measures of the amount of spending and health status (life expectancy and infant mortality) do not yield any consistent patterns. While further in-depth research is required to better understand these relationships, the findings presented here suggest that a country's ranking on health status is not a function of spending per se.

There is some limited evidence suggesting a relationship between health status and income inequality. Countries with a relatively high rate of family poverty, for example, tend to have comparably high infant mortality. A number of factors could account for this relationship, including access to health care, nutrition, and lifestyle. Again, further research is warranted.

Perhaps the only conclusion that can be made with any degree of confidence is that international differences in life expectancy and infant mortality are unlikely to be explained with reference to a single factor.

Figure 8

Change in infant mortality (1980–1993) and change in health care expenditure as a percentage of GDP (1983–1993), OECD countries

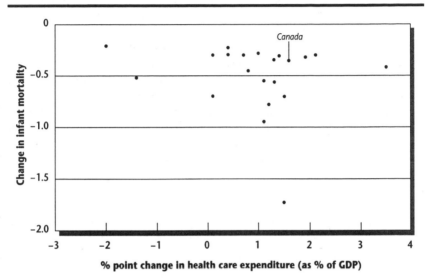

See data table for sources and explanatory notes.

Figure 9

Change in infant mortality and change in inequality over time

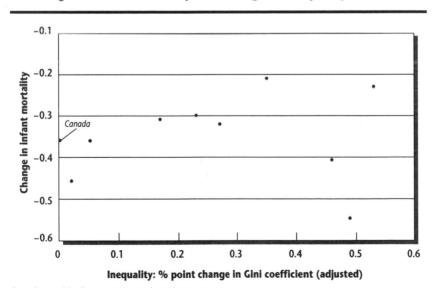

See data table for sources and explanatory notes.

Throughout this paper, the analysis has included all OECD countries for which data was available. It is worth noting that in many instances, statistically significant correlations between otherwise unrelated variables could be obtained by selectively excluding a few countries from the analysis. This was the case in terms of the relationship between spending on income security and infant mortality. While no significant correlation was found based on the analysis of 20 OECD countries for which data was available, the exclusion of three countries resulted in a strong and significant association. Data selectivity is therefore a critical issue in international comparisons, and must be a key consideration in future research.

Finally, this report has drawn upon secondary data sources for its measures of health status and spending levels. These data have been drawn from standard international data sources, and no attempt has been made to evaluate the comparability of these measures across nations.

BIBLIOGRAPHY

CANADIAN INSTITUTE OF CHILD HEALTH. 1994. *The Health of Canada's Children.* 2nd edition.

Luxembourg Income Study. 1995. Special Tabulations by the Centre for International Statistics, circa, 1991.

ORGANIZATION FOR ECONOMIC COOPERATION AND DEVELOPMENT (OECD). 1995. *Income Distribution in OECD Countries.*

_____. 1985 *Measuring Health Care 1960–1983.* Paris: OECD.

_____. 1994. *New Directions in Social Policy.* Paris: OECD.

_____. 1994. *OECD Employment Outlook.* Paris: OECD.

_____. 1995. *OECD in Figures.* Paris: OECD.

UNITED NATIONS DEVELOPMENT PROGRAM (UNDP). 1995. *Human Development Report.*

WILKINS, R., O. ADAMS, and A. BRANCKER. 1989. Changes in mortality by income in urban Canada from 1971 to 1986. Ottawa (ON): Industry, Science and Technology. *Health Reports* 3(1): 7–31.

WILKINSON, R. G. 1994. *Unfair Shares.* Essex: Barnardo's.

How Canada's Health Care System Compares with That of Other Countries: An Overview

DAMIEN CONTANDRIOPOULOS

Doctoral Student in Public Health
Interdisciplinary Research Group on Health
Faculty of Medecine
University of Montreal

SUMMARY

The purpose of this document is to describe the performance of Canada's health care system and compare it to the situation in 23 other OECD countries during the past 5 years for which data is available, that is, from 1989 to 1993. All of the data used has been drawn from the OECD Health Data database. The report has been divided into two parts.*

In the first part, we will present various graphs of raw data on health or the health care system in the 24 countries studied and we will analyze that data. We will then compare the health expenditures of these countries based on each one's wealth.

In the second part, we will use the raw data to calculate three composite indices of the costs of the system, the health of the population, and the system's performance. We will then examine Canada's position in relation to the other countries based on these indices.

---

* Germany, Australia, Austria, Belgium, Denmark, Spain, the United States, Finland, France, Greece, Ireland, Iceland, Italy, Japan, Luxembourg, Mexico, Norway, New Zealand, the Netherlands, Portugal, the United Kingdom, Sweden, and Switzerland.

Lastly, in appendix, we will present a table describing the main features of the various systems in each country.

From these comparisons, we will be able to determine where Canada's health care system stands in relation to those of the other OECD countries, and to identify which countries have a situation comparable to that of Canada.

TABLE OF CONTENTS

Descriptive Analysis of the Various Health Care Systems 177

Epidemiological and Demographic Data 177

Combined Life Expectancy (Men and Women) 177

Infant Mortality (Rate for 100 Births) 178

Percentage of Persons Older than 65 Years 179

Capacity of Service Supply 180

Number of Beds per 1,000 Inhabitants 180

Number of Physicians per 1,000 Inhabitants 180

Health Expenditures 181

Health Expenditures Expressed as a Percentage of GDP and
in $PPP 181

Percentage of Public and Private Expenditures on Health 184

Regressions on Health Expenditures in Relation to GDP 185

State of Health, Cost Control, and Performance of System 186

Composite Index of the Costs of the System 186

Presentation of the Index 186

Analysis of the Results 186

Composite Index of the State of Health of the Population 187

Presentation of the Index 187

Analysis of the Results 188

Composite Index of the System's Performance 188

Presentation of the Index 188

Analysis of the Results 189

Conclusion 189

Bibliography 191

Appendix 193

LIST OF FIGURES

Figure 1   Combined life expectancy (men and women) at birth 199

Figure 2   Infant mortality (rate for 100 births) 200

Figure 3   Percentage of the population older than 65 years 201

Figure 4   Number of hospital beds per 1,000 inhabitants 202

Figure 5   Number of physicians per 1,000 inhabitants 203

Figure 6   Health expenditures as a percentage of GDP 204

Figure 7   Per capita health expenditures in $PPP 205

Figure 8   Percentage of private health expenditures......................... 206

Figure 9   Per capita health expenditures in relation to per capita
             GDP in 1989 207

Figure 10   Per capita health expenditures in relation to per capita
             GDP in 1990 207

Figure 11   Per capita health expenditures in relation to per capita
             GDP in 1991 208

Figure 12   Per capita health expenditures in relation to per capita
             GDP in 1992 208

Figure 13   Per capita health expenditures in relation to per capita
             GDP in 1993 209

Figure 14   Global health expenditures index from 1989 to 1993 210

Figure 15   Global index of the state of health of the population
             from 1989 to 1993 211

Figure 16   Global index of the performance of the health care system
             from 1989 to 1993 212

LIST OF TABLES

Table 1   Ranking of countries (average 1989–1993)....................... 182

Table 2   Descriptive tables of the various health systems 195

DESCRIPTIVE ANALYSIS OF THE VARIOUS HEALTH CARE SYSTEMS

In all of our raw data analyses, we analyzed the average data from the five years of the study: this is why the figures we mention cannot be found directly on the graphs appended to the report. However, whenever a trend is visible in the changes over the five-year period, it is explicitly noted.

The raw data used can be divided into three categories. First, there are descriptive measurements of the population (percentage of people over 65 years of age) and measurements of the state of the population's health (life expectancy at birth and infant mortality). Second, there are indicators of the capacity to offer health services (number of beds per 1,000 inhabitants and number of physicians per 1,000 inhabitants). And lastly, there are cost indicators (per capita health expenditures, health expenditures as a percentage of GDP, and percentage of private and public expenditures).

Epidemiological and Demographic Data

Combined Life Expectancy (Men and Women)

In this report, we have analyzed the combined life expectancy of men and women because we are interested in the overall state of health of the population. However, it must be remembered that, in relation to this global life expectancy index, the life expectancy of women is always higher and the life expectancy of men is always lower. This phenomenon arises from the fact that the life expectancy of women in all of the countries studied is higher than that of men (on average, for all of the countries combined, between 6.2 and 6.4 years depending on the year). However, this gap tends be narrowing on a global basis over time.

The second general comment that should be made is that life expectancy is increasing in all of the countries studied (except in certain countries where it is impossible to determine the change in this variable due to missing data). On average, the combined life expectancy increased by 1.13 years between 1989 and 1993, as is shown in figure 1[1].

From the 1930s to the 1950s, life expectancy increased dramatically, in part because of a drop in infant mortality rates. Today, gains are attributable more to a decline in mortality rates among the middle aged and elderly. However, these additional years of life are not necessarily spent in good health. "Various studies have determined that a not insignificant part of these additional years were spent incapacitated and with a loss of functional autonomy" (Government of Quebec 1995, 25).

Canada (77.63 years) is among the five countries with the longest life expectancy, behind Japan (79.08), Iceland (78.13), Sweden (77.85), and

---

1. All of the graphs are appended.

Switzerland (77.64). The countries with the shortest life expectancies are Mexico (71.11), Portugal (74.14), Ireland (74.78), Denmark (74.94), and Finland (75.30).

The life expectancy in some countries is different from what one might expect at first glance. In Greece, for example, which is close to Mexico for many variables, the life expectancy is quite high (76.70), less than a year short of the life expectancy in Canada. Conversely, Luxembourg (75.38) and the United States (75.30), which are wealthy countries, have relatively short life expectancies.

Infant Mortality (Rate for 100 Births)

Before analyzing this variable, it is important to clarify two points. First, this variable is acknowledged as a good indicator of the quality of health care because very significant gains have been made in these rates as a result of improved medical techniques. Second, there is a not insignificant possibility of bias when making international comparisons of infant mortality rates. In developed countries, infant mortality is concentrated primarily during the first hours or days after birth and involves primarily premature and low-birthweight babies. However, regulations vary from country to country on how to distinguish between stillbirths and borderline cases of infant mortality.[2] There are also differences in the efforts made to resuscitate premature and low-birthweight children.

> The unofficial degree of latitude, which is smaller but varies widely from country to country, is a factor which must be added to that of the heterogeneity of the official regulations. In some countries, it is easier not to report as live births babies who do not live more than a few hours. There may also be systemic trends in the reporting of certain "borderline" cases: depending on the country, they may be registered as a live birth, as a stillbirth, or not registered at all, depending on the habits, customs and values of the societies concerned, or on the specific laws and regulations with respect to the advantages or disadvantages associated with a live birth (funeral costs or disposal of the body, special allowance at the time of birth, etc.). Japan is often cited as one country in which underreporting may be significant (Governement of Quebec 1995, 117).

---

2. Infant mortality refers to all deaths which occur in live births between the time of their birth and the age of one year. Stillbirths are deaths which occur between the presumption of viability of the fetus and birth. However, the distinction is not always clear cut since, in some instances, death occurs very shortly before or after birth. Moreover, depending on the country, infants less than 28 weeks gestation or less than 1,000 g at birth are not considered to be cases of infant mortality but of stillbirths, regardless of their status at birth (Chevalier et al. 1995, 144).

In analyzing the data, it is evident that infant mortality rates (figure 2) are declining in all of the countries studied, falling from an overall average of 0.87 to 0.70 for 100 births. Although this decrease is no longer the key factor in the increase in life expectancy, it definitely plays a role.

In this area, Canada is not among the countries with the lowest rates, ranking ninth of 24 with a rate of 0.67. However, Canada is acknowledged as a country which reports infant mortality cases relatively systematically, a practice which may increase its mortality rate compared to certain other countries. Japan (0.45), Iceland (0.53), Finland (0.54), Sweden (0.56), and Norway (0.64) had the lowest rates. In the case of Japan, it is often noted that the level of nonreporting may be significant and could bias the comparison.

Among the countries with the highest rates, Mexico is in a class of its own with a rate of 2.16, followed by Portugal (1.04), the United States (0.91), Greece (0.91), and Luxembourg (0.88). Here again, some countries do not rank where they might be expected to. The United States and Luxembourg, for example, which are among the wealthiest countries in our study, ranked with the poorest countries of Mexico, Greece, and Portugal. In the United States, the great disparity in the redistribution of wealth— which produces highly disadvantaged groups—may explain the abnormally high infant mortality rate.

Percentage of Persons Older than 65 Years

The number of elderly persons is often given as one of the factors which influence the level of health expenditures. However, using the data available to us, it was not possible to establish a statistical link between the health expenditures of a country and the percentage of persons over 65 years of age, even though this percentage varies quite significantly among the countries studied. This finding means that, contrary to popular opinion, the percentage of people older than 65 years does not seem to be a real factor influencing the costs of the health care systems in the countries in our sample.

Based on the increase in the average between 1989 and 1993, the number of people over 65 years of age (figure 3) is on the rise overall in the OECD countries (more than 1.05 percent in five years). This increase is evident in some of the countries, such as Canada, Australia, Finland, Greece, and the Netherlands. However, in those countries which already have very high rates, such as Sweden, Norway, and Austria, there has been no increase. Moreover, there is a great deal of missing data for this variable and two of the countries, Germany and Mexico, were not included at all.

The countries with the highest percentage of people over 65 years of age are Sweden (17.72), Norway (16.26), the United Kingdom (15.65), Denmark (15.56), and Austria (15.08). Those countries with the lowest percentage are Iceland (10.63), New Zealand (10.91), Canada (10.99), Australia (11.32), and Ireland (11.33). Canada's ranking in terms of the percentage of people over 65 years, shows that it still has a very young population in relation to other OECD countries.

Capacity of Service Supply

Number of Beds per 1,000 Inhabitants

The number of beds per 1,000 inhabitants (figure 4) is a variable with a very high standard deviation (4.00), which means that there are significant differences between the countries. For example, the difference between the highest (Switzerland with 20.7 beds per 1,000 inhabitants) and lowest number of beds (Mexico with 0.78 beds per 1,000 inhabitants) is 19.92 beds.

Overall, the number of beds is declining in the 24 countries studied, the average in 1989 (8.95) being 2.27 beds higher than in 1993 (6.68). In some countries, such as Canada, the decrease is only slight, while in others—and Sweden in particular—it is considerable.

For this variable, Canada is not among the countries at the extremes; it ranks sixteenth of 24 in the list of countries with the most beds per inhabitants. Those with the greatest number of beds per 1,000 inhabitants are Switzerland (20.70 beds), Iceland (16.54), Japan (15.78), Norway (14.50), and Finland (11.95). The countries with the fewest number of beds are Mexico (in a class of its own with 0.78), Spain (4.27), Portugal (4.54), the United States (4.63), and Greece (5.05).

The fact that there are many countries in which the number of hospital beds is far fewer than in Canada, combined with the rapid decrease in beds, appears to indicate that there may be an opportunity for Canada to downsize.

Number of Physicians per 1,000 Inhabitants

In contrast to the number of beds, the number of physicians per 1,000 inhabitants (figure 5) is on the increase in OECD countries. For all of the countries combined, the 1993 average (2.63) is 0.20 physicians higher than in 1989 (2.43). The rate of increase varies from country to country: in Canada, for example, the situation is stable, while in Spain and Greece, the number is increasing rapidly. It is also evident that the countries in which the ratio is increasing the fastest are often those which already have the highest number of physicians.

Here again, Canada was not among the countries at the extremes, ranking seventeenth of 24 countries with the highest number of physicians per 1,000 inhabitants. The countries ranking the highest were Spain (3.90), Greece (3.55), Belgium (3.48), Norway (3.15), and Germany (3.13). The lowest scores were obtained by Mexico (0.96), the United Kingdom (1.45), Italy (1.55), Japan (1.65), and Ireland (1.70). In the case of Italy, there are a number of indications[3] that, because of special criteria used in the survey of physicians, the rate may be considerably underestimated.

The results produced some surprises in this case as well, since it was not the richest countries which had the most physicians. Greece and Spain had the highest scores, followed by a series of much richer countries. Similarly, Japan, Italy, and the United Kingdom ranked much closer to Mexico among the countries with the smallest number of physicians per 1,000 inhabitants.

Health Expenditures

Health Expenditures Expressed as a Percentage of GDP and in $PPP

Analysis of the Differences between the Two Measurements of Expenditures

In this report, we analyze two different measurements of health expenditures. Health expenditures expressed as a percentage of GDP (figure 6) is a measurement of the proportion of a country's wealth that is devoted to the health of its population. Health expenditures per capita expressed in purchasing power parity dollars (figure 7) is a measurement of the average amount in PPP dollars that is spent on health for each person in a country.[4]

A review of the ranking of average expenditures by OECD countries during the five years of the study (1989 to 1993) for the two indicators shows that they measure related variables since the order of the two rankings is similar (table 1). For example, Mexico and Greece are the two countries which spend the least, both as a proportion of GDP and in $PPP per capita. Similarly, Canada and the United States are among the three countries which spend the most based on both indicators.

However, there are disparities between the indicators for several of the countries, and the gaps are sometimes considerable. For example, Luxembourg spends little in terms of percentage of its GDP, but a great deal in $PPP. These findings may result from the fact that Luxembourg has an extremely

---

3. The OECD publications (OECD. 1994. *Health Policy Studies No. 5. Reform of Health Care Systems: A Review of Seventeen OECD Countries*. Paris: Organization for Economic Cooperation and Development) give contradictory information on this subject. On page 45, the number of physicians per 1,000 inhabitants is estimated at 1.3, while on page 196 of the same report, it gives an estimate of 4.6 physicians per 1,000 inhabitants....

4. Dollars adjusted by the purchasing power parity make it possible to compare the prices of identical products in various countries. Purchasing power parity is not, therefore, simply a monetary conversion but an equivalence which takes into consideration a real value assigned to a basket of goods and services.

Table 1

**Ranking of countries
(average 1989–1993)**

Percentage of GDP devoted to health (%)		Amount in $PPP spent per capita on health ($PPP)		Difference between standardized scores for per capita expenditures and expenditures as % of GDP	
Mexico	4.89	Mexico	340	Portugal	– 0.59
Greece	5.39	Greece	430	Finland	– 0.41
United Kingdom	6.49	Portugal	720	Spain	– 0.35
Denmark	6.58	Ireland	815	New Zealand	– 0.31
Luxembourg	6.66	Spain	873	Ireland	– 0.30
Ireland	6.76	United Kingdom	1,050	United States	– 0.29
Japan	6.91	New Zealand	1,058	Canada	– 0.24
Portugal	6.92	Denmark	1,149	Greece	– 0.20
Spain	7.02	Japan	1,293	Netherlands	– 0.18
New Zealand	7.53	Finland	1,325	Australia	– 0.18
Norway	7.87	Norway	1,359	France	– 0.18
Belgium	7.93	Netherlands	1,367	Austria	– 0.16
Sweden	8.15	Australia	1,369	Sweden	– 0.09
Iceland	8.19	Sweden	1,370	Italy	– 0.08
Italy	8.22	Belgium	1,383	Mexico	– 0.07
Netherlands	8.28	Italy	1,401	Norway	0.05
Australia	8.29	Iceland	1,460	Iceland	0.06
Germany	8.44	Austria	1,530	Belgium	0.07
Finland	8.52	Germany	1,646	Germany	0.26
Austria	8.75	France	1,648	United Kingdom	0.31
Switzerland	9.01	Luxembourg	1,680	Denmark	0.45
France	9.16	Canada	1,809	Japan	0.52
Canada	9.77	Switzerland	1,965	Switzerland	0.52
United States	13.20	United States	2,879	Luxembourg	1.41

high per capita GDP and can therefore spend a great deal per inhabitant without it accounting for a large percentage of its wealth. The inverse is true for Portugal which, in spite of the fact that its per capita expenditures are among the three lowest, spends quite a high percentage of its GDP on health because it has a relatively low GDP.

In order to measure the gap between the two indicators, we determined the difference between the standardized score of per capita expenditures and the standardized score of expenditures as a percentage of GDP. The greater the positive value of the difference, the more a country spends less per capita than would be expected based on the country's GDP. The greater the negative value of the difference, the more a country spends more per capita than its wealth would indicate.

The main interest in comparing the two measurements of health expenditures is the fact that, depending on what we wish to study—and the results that we wish to obtain—either of the measurements can be used. In the second part of our study, we use a cost index calculated from both of the measurements but with different weighting. It should therefore be remembered that the farther the score a country obtains in the difference between the two standardized indices is from zero, the greater is the possibility that a bias exists as a result of the methods of measurement used.

Analysis of Health Costs in the Various Countries

In terms of the costs themselves, it is apparent that Canada, regardless of the measurement used, is one of the countries which spends the most on health. It is surpassed only by the United States and Switzerland (Switzerland surpasses Canada only for per capita expenditures).

The United States' position, in terms of health expenditures, places it almost in a class of its own since it spent on average (1989 to 1993) 13.2 percent of its GDP on health, which is 5.46 percent higher than the average of the other countries for the same period, and 3.43 percent of GDP higher than Canada which ranked second on the list. The situation is similar with per capita expenditures. The United States spent almost one thousand dollars more per capita than Switzerland (second on the list) and Canada (third on the list), while its per capita expenditures were more than twice as high as those of Japan.

Although Canada's costs are high, they are not out of proportion compared to those of several other countries, and while Canada can be considered one of the countries which spends the most, it is in a group with France, Switzerland, Luxembourg, Austria, and Germany.

At the other extreme, the countries which spend the least can be divided into two groups. First, there are Mexico and Greece which have health expenditures significantly below those of the other OECD countries. Then there is another group—consisting of Ireland, Spain, Portugal, and the United Kingdom—which spends less than the majority of countries but which is not far off the average.

In terms of the trend in health expenditures over the five years of the study, it is clear that, based on the two indicators, health spending increased in absolute terms. From the two graphs on health expenditures, it is clear that the 1989 average is considerably lower than the 1993 average. The graphs also show that, for a majority of the countries including Canada, health expenditures rose in absolute terms between 1989 and 1993. Indeed, expenditures rose in all of the countries studied with the notable exception of Sweden, where expenditures fell steadily and significantly over the five years, from $1,396 PPP to $1,213 PPP (less $130 PPP) per capita: this represents a drop of 1.07 percent of GDP spent on health.

Percentage of Public and Private Expenditures on Health

Although this study is interested in the proportion of public and private total expenditures, in order to make the discussion more understandable, we will talk only of the percentage of private expenditures, public expenditures in this case being equal to 100 less the private expenditures.

Overall, there has been a very slight increase among OECD countries in private health expenditures (figure 8), which rose from 23.89 percent to 24.58 percent. However, the country-by-country analysis shows that there have been quite different trends. Ireland, Japan, the Netherlands, and the United States, for example, have seen a decline in private sector health expenditures. On the other hand, Germany, Greece, Iceland, Italy, New Zealand, and Sweden experienced a slight increase in the privatization of their health care systems.

Canada was not among the countries at either extreme, and ranked ninth of 24 among countries with the most private health systems. The United States (57.6 percent), Portugal (45.6 percent), Mexico (42.0 percent), Austria (34.1 percent), and Australia (32.1 percent) are the countries with systems with the highest proportion of private expenditures. The systems with the smallest private expenditures are found in Norway (5.5 percent), Luxembourg (9.1 percent), Belgium (11.3 percent), Sweden (12.9 percent), and Iceland (14.0 percent).

Before moving on to the next section, we can briefly summarize Canada's situation in terms of the raw variables we have identified. The health status of the population in Canada is very good—low infant mortality and long life expectancy—although some countries, such as Iceland and Japan, are doing better. Moreover, although the Canadian population is aging, it is still very young. In terms of health resources, Canada is again doing well. Both the number of physicians and the number of beds have been kept under control and Canada remains slightly below the average of OECD countries for these variables. However, in terms of expenditures, the situation is less promising. Canada is one of the three OECD countries which spends the most on health in proportion to its wealth, along with Switzerland and the United States. In terms of expenditures in $PPP, Canada is closer to the average but continues to be among the three countries with the highest expenditures. Lastly, in terms of the level of privatization, Canada's system is relatively public but is close to the OECD average.

Regressions on Health Expenditures in Relation to GDP

In analyzing the measurements of health expenditures, and particularly the difference between the two measurements (health expenditures expressed as a percentage of GDP, and per capita health expenditures in $PPP), it was clear that a country's spending on health was related to its wealth.

To measure the relationship which exists between a country's wealth (measured here by per capita GDP in $PPP) and its health expenditures (in $PPP per capita), we placed the countries on a graph with per capita GDP on the abscissa and per capita health expenditures on the ordinate. This gives us a graph (figures 9 to 13) for each year from 1989 to 1993 on which the countries are distributed approximately along an axis which places the poorest countries, and consequently those with the lowest health expenditures, below and to the left and the richest countries, with the highest health expenditures, above and to the right.

To verify whether this placement along a rich/poor axis could really be used to partly explain health expenditures, we calculated a regression between these two variables. We used a logarithmic regression which not only gives a very good adjustment, but also gives a direct estimate of the elasticity of health expenditures in relation to GDP. Our regression equations were as follows:

$$Ln(\text{per capita health expenditures}) = [a(Ln(\text{per capita GDP})) + b + e_i]$$

Where "a" is the estimate of elasticity of health expenditures to GDP, "b" is a constant, and "e_i" is the difference between a country's health expenditures "i" and the average for OECD countries. This e_i difference is used later as an indication of the level of a country's spending in relation to the OECD average based on its national wealth.

All of the regressions were highly significant (probability $\alpha < 0.0001$) and the R^2 varied from 0.82 to 0.89 depending on the year. This means that a country's wealth can be used to predict, to a certain degree, its spending on health and that these two variables are closely related.

The graphs show that the closer a country is to the curve, the closer the amount it spends on health is proportional to its national wealth; the farther above the curve a country is, the more its expenditures on health are greater than would be anticipated based on its wealth. The inverse is also true. If we look at whether a country spends a great deal, not in relation to the average of the other countries, but in relation to the other countries, while also taking into account the wealth of the country, it is possible to make an even more precise adjustment. A complete analysis of this type of regression and the significance of the e_i error is presented in *Controlling Health Care Costs: What Matters* (Brousselle 1998).

STATE OF HEALTH, COST CONTROL, AND PERFORMANCE OF SYSTEM

In the previous section, we analyzed raw data. We will now use this raw data to build composite indices. Each raw variable measures a very specific aspect of the health of the population or of the health care system. What we are trying to do is bring together in a single index several standardized raw variables in order to compare certain complex factors such as the health of the population, the costs of the system, or the system's performance. The composite indices developed from the standardized scores of the variables pinpoint the position of each country in relation to the average of the OECD countries.

Composite Index of the Costs of the System

Presentation of the Index

To examine the global costs of health care systems, we used two cost measurements:
  a. total health expenditures expressed as a percentage of gross domestic product (GDP);
  b. total per capita health expenditures in dollars adjusted by the purchasing power parity ($PPP).

The composite index of costs is determined by averaging these two standardized measurements after applying a weighting of two to per capita expenditures and a weighting of one to expenditures as a percentage of GDP ($[(1z(a)+2z(b))/3]$). In table 1 given earlier, we determined the difference between the two health expenditure measurements. The greater the gap between these two measurements for a given country, the greater the theoretical risk of bias for that country due to the weighting used in this study. For example, because of Luxembourg's very high per capita GDP, its ranking may have been slightly biased. Nevertheless, this weighting, which attributes more weight to per capita health expenditures, makes it possible to rank the countries on the basis of the value of services available per capita, that is, on the basis of a measurement of access to health care services. The measurement of expenditures in PPP dollars is more relevant, however, because it is a more direct measurement of the accessibility of health services and is less biased by the relative wealth of the country. In any event, changing the weighting to test the sensitivity of the index produced no significant changes in the results.

Analysis of the Results

Figure 14 shows that, in general, over the past five years, Canada was one of the countries with the highest cost index. On average during this period, it ranked third with a score of 0.97, behind Switzerland (1.12) and particularly the United States (3.13). These three countries had relatively stable cost indices over the past five years, although Canada shows a slight decrease in overall expenditures beginning in 1993. The other countries with cost indices markedly higher than the average over this period were, in descending order, France (0.63), Germany (0.48), and Austria (0.38).

The countries with the lowest levels of spending were Mexico (– 1.90), Greece (– 1.80), Portugal (– 1.10), Ireland (– 1.00), Spain (– 0.87), the United Kingdom (– 0.75), Denmark (– 0.58), New Zealand (– 0.50), and Japan (– 0.38).

The remaining countries had cost indices close to the average (which is 0). Lastly, it should be noted that Iceland (0.19) and Sweden (0.08) had average levels of spending close to zero but their costs decreased steadily in relation to the OECD average during the five-year period. The drop was 0.52 and 1.09 respectively.

Composite Index of the State of Health of the Population

Presentation of the Index

We used three raw measurements to create the composite index of the state of health of the population:
   a. life expectancy of women at birth;
   b. life expectancy of men at birth;
   c. infant mortality rate for 100 births.

The composite index of the state of health of the population is calculated by averaging these three standardized measurements after attributing a weighting of one to each of the life expectancies and a weighting of minus three to the infant mortality rate which gives: ($[(1z(a)+1z(b) - 3z(c))/5]$). The infant mortality rate is given a strong weighting because it is generally recognized as the indicator of the population's state of health that is most sensitive to the performance of the health care system. The weighting is negative because it is important that a high infant mortality rate decrease the state of health index and not the opposite.

It is important to reiterate at this point the warnings given earlier about international comparisons of infant mortality rates and the potential biases associated with them, particularly in view of the strong weighting given to this variable. It should also be borne in mind that, while this index provides a general idea of the health status of the population, it is not a true measure of that status, which would be very difficult to do accurately. Lastly, remember that, for developed countries where health care systems have achieved a certain level of performance—as is the case in the OECD countries being studied in this report (except perhaps for Mexico)—there is no direct relationship between the care provided by the system and our index of the population's state of health.

Analysis of the Results

Here again, it is easy to see (figure 15) that the index of the state of health of the population for Canada is high. More specifically, Canada's average score for the five years of the study was 0.57, which places it behind Japan (1.29), Iceland (0.88), and Sweden (0.76). In terms of health, Canada's score is almost the same as Switzerland's (0.56). They are followed by Norway, the Netherlands, Australia, Spain, France, Finland, Germany, and Italy, all of which have indices of the population's state of health that are above the average.

The countries with the lowest state of health indices are Mexico (– 3.67), Portugal (– 0.95), Luxembourg (– 0.48), and the United States (– 0.37). Mexico's score improved by 0.37 over the five years of the study, but it continues to lag well behind. It is surprising to find two countries as rich as the United States and Luxembourg joining Mexico and Portugal as the countries with the worst indices of the state of health of the population. In the case of the United States, the reason may lie in the country's vast social heterogeneity caused by such factors as the distribution of wealth and education.

Composite Index of the System's Performance

Presentation of the Index

The composite index of the system's performance is calculated from the two indices described earlier. This performance index combines the population's state of health with the funds invested in the health care system. Thus, a country which invests little in its health system and whose population's state of health is poor, and a country which invests a great deal and whose population's state of health is good will have a performance index near zero. In contrast, a country which invests a great deal in its health system and whose population is in poor health will have a negative performance index. Lastly, a country which invests little in health care but whose population is in good health will have a positive health index.

To obtain a performance index which shifts in the direction indicated, the normalized cost index must be subtracted from the standardized state of health index.

A word of caution is important at this point. As we mentioned earlier, the care provided by a health care system is not directly related to the state of health index. This relationship would be relatively direct in a country where the health system is still being developed, such as in third world countries. However, once a certain level of care has been surpassed, there is a sort of levelling off and the infant mortality rate ceases to decline, just as life expectancy ceases to rise. It is not a total plateauing and gains continue to be made, but at a much slower pace. In addition, certain variables, such as life expectancy, are very closely tied to factors outside the health system and which have not been fully identified. Under these circumstances, it is important to remember when analyzing this performance index that there may be considerable biases.

Analysis of the Results

The countries with the highest performance indices (figure16) are, in order, Greece (0.84), Japan (0.84), Spain (0.60), the United Kingdom (0.41), Ireland (0.38), Iceland (0.35), Sweden (0.34), Norway (0.23), and Denmark (0.23); the United States (– 1.77), Mexico (– 0.94), Luxembourg (– 0.29), Switzerland (– 0.24), Canada (– 0.22), Austria (– 0.21), and France (– 0.17) had the lowest scores.

One feature of this index is that countries which invest little in their health systems, like Greece, Spain, and the United Kingdom, but whose population's state of health is close to the average obtain a very good performance index for their health systems. In such instances, it is important to bear in mind that the population's state of health is not the direct result of the health system and that several other factors come into play.

The opposite is also true: countries such as Canada and France, which have an index of the population's state of health significantly higher than the average, but which also spend much more than the average, obtain a negative performance index. The record in this area is held by the United States: its population's state of health is poor and it has exorbitant costs which result in an extremely low performance index.

Figure 16 also shows that Iceland and Sweden have performance indices which are increasing. This improvement is the result of the cutbacks they have made in health system costs over the last five years. The change is particularly evident in Sweden's case.

Although the absolute value of the performance index is difficult to interpret, its change over time for a given country provides interesting information on the position of that country relative to the average for OECD countries. Indeed, over a relatively short period of time, it can be said that the determining factors of state of health have remained stable and, as a result, changes in the performance index can be attributed to changes in the health care systems. From this perspective, we can see that Canada's relative position has improved over the three years for which data is available.

CONCLUSION

We were therefore able to compare Canada's situation with that of 24 other OECD countries. We were able to draw three conclusions from the raw data analyzed. First, the state of health of the population in Canada is among the best in the world. Second, there are fewer medical resources—number of beds and physicians—than the average for the OECD countries. This is not an indication of insufficient resources but rather a sign of efficient management. Lastly, Canada is in a less enviable position with respect to health expenditures since it is one of the three OECD countries which spends the most on health. Since, as we recently noted, the quantity of medical resources is under control, it can be concluded that the price of these resources is much higher than in other countries, with the exception of the United States.

A more detailed analysis can be made of Canada's expenditures by looking at health expenditures in relation to the country's wealth, which we did using regressions. Figures 9 to 13 show that Canada, while remaining among the wealthiest OECD countries, saw its relative position decline between 1989 and 1990. During the same time, Canada's health expenditures rose rapidly. The consequences of this change can be seen in looking at the three composite indices on the state of the health care system.

Canada's state of health index is among the highest in the world. However, because of the volume of its health expenditures, its health system performance index is very mediocre. Canada is not alone in this situation, France, Switzerland and Germany being in comparable positions. Some countries—the United States in particular—are in an even worse position in terms of the performance of their health care systems. However, it must be remembered that, while the Canadian system is often compared to that of Nordic countries, such as Sweden, Denmark, and Norway, these countries are well ahead of Canada in terms of the performance of their systems.

Finally, the observation from these analyses is that, by bringing Canada's health expenditures closer to the average of OECD countries, it may be possible to improve its performance index significantly. Another way to achieve this result would be to maintain the current level of medical resources but to reduce their price. Indeed, the only explanation for why Canada's performance index is so low compared to other OECD countries is the price of its medical resources. However, given the proximity of the United States, it may be difficult to implement such a policy.

Damien Contandriopoulos *is a doctoral student in public health at the University of Montreal. He obtained a master's degree in anthropology in 1997 and a major in biology in 1994, both from the University of Montreal. He has worked as a research assistant with GRIS (Interdisciplinary Research Group on Health) at the University of Montreal since 1993.*

BIBLIOGRAPHY

BROUSSELLE, A. 1998. Controlling health expenditures: What matters. International Comparison
   Series Paper. Papers commissioned by the National Forum on Health. Ottawa (ON). Published
   in this volume.

CHEVALIER, S. et al. 1995. Groupe de travail pour les systèmes d'information sur la santé communautaire.
   Indicateurs sociosanitaires: Définitions et interprétations. (Working group on community health
   information systems. *Socio-health indicators: Definitions and interpretations*). Quebec (QC):
   Publisher I.C.I.S.

CONTANDRIOPOULOS, A.-P. et al. 1993. *Regulatory Mechanisms in the Health Care Systems of Canada
   and Other Industrialized Countries: Description and Assessment.* University of Ottawa (ON): Faculty
   of Medicine, Health Sciences.

EVANS, G. R. et al. 1994. *Why Are Some People Healthy and Others Not? The Determinants of Health of
   Populations.* New York (NY): Aldine de Gruyter.

GOVERNMENT OF QUEBEC. 1995. Department of Health and Social Services, Planning and Evaluation
   Branch. *Quebec: A Comparative Study of Health, Demographic and Socioeconomic Indicators. The
   Changing Situation in Quebec, Canada and Internationally.*

OECD. 1994. *Health Policy Studies No. 5. Reform of Health Care Systems: A Review of Seventeen OECD
   Countries.* Paris: Organization for Economic Cooperation and Development.

_____. 1995. *Health Data.* Paris: Organization for Economic Cooperation and Development.

APPENDIX

Table 2

Descriptive tables of the various health systems

Country	Percentage of public coverage	National health system	Type of financing	Description
Germany	*93*	*NO*	*Social and private insurance*	*Health insurance fund; mandatory below an income threshold set by the state; optional otherwise; (0.3% of population not covered)*
Australia	100	NO	Public financing (1984), social insurance	Medicare system; universal coverage; financing through a system of federal taxation
Austria		NO	Public financing, social insurance, and private insurance	Mandatory membership in a social insurance fund; 99% of population covered, the remaining 1% are members of a liberal profession or inmates; 38% of population have complementary private insurance
Belgium	*100*	*NO*	*Social insurance*	*Social security system; mandatory membership in a mutual insurance company; unlimited choice of specific company; additional coverage and private hospitalization coverage available*
Canada	100	NO	Public financing	Universal coverage; federal and provincial financing through an income tax system
Denmark	100	YES (1973)	Public financing	Insured choose between 2 groups; group 1 (96.4% of pop.) free care (except for dental care); group 2 (3.6% of pop.) contribution to costs (choice of physician, free access to specialists)

Table 2 (cont.)

Country	Percentage of public coverage	National health system	Type of financing	Description
Spain	96.7	YES (1986)	Social insurance	Services financed through social security (INSALUD); financing by government, business, and households; objective to ultimately have financing through taxes only
Finland	100	Public organization	Public financing and private insurance	Salary and fee-for-service payment; private insurance less and less common
France	99	NO	Social insurance	Social security system; mandatory membership; funds: CNAMTS, MSA, self-employed workers
Greece	100	YES (1983)	Social insurance, public financing	IKA social insurance fund (39%), OGA (35%), and TEVE (9.5%)
Ireland	100	YES (1970)	Social insurance, public financing	Several categories of insured groups; category 1: low income (38%); category 2: middle income (47%); category 3: high income (15%)
Iceland	100	YES	Public financing	Universal access and patient contribution
Italy	100	YES (1978)	Social insurance	Uniform coverage for entire population; national health service receives contributions from employers, employees, and self-employed workers, and redistributes money to the regions
Japan		NO	Social insurance	A system for salaried workers (health insurance for private sector, the navy, and mutual companies [65% of pop.]); a national health insurance system for nonsalaried workers; special payment system for the elderly

Table 2 (cont.)

Country	Percentage of public coverage	National health system	Type of financing	Description
Luxembourg	99	NO	Social insurance	Several insurance funds (depending on profession); membership in a fund
Mexico				
Norway	100	NO	Social insurance	National insurance system; mandatory membership
New Zealand		YES (1938)	Public financing	Universal coverage for basic care; patient contribution
Netherlands	70	NO	Social insurance and private insurance	ZFW covers all individuals with an income below a certain threshold; AWBZ covers entire population for certain risks (long-term hospitalization, psychiatric internment, etc.)
Portugal	100	YES (1979)	Social insurance, public financing	Universal coverage by national health care system but certain funds still exist (ex.: for government employees) and cover 24% of population
United Kingdom	100	YES (1948)	Public financing and contributions	Financing primarily through taxes; National Solidarity Fund to which employers and households contribute
Sweden	100	YES	Social insurance, public financing	National health insurance system covers fee-for-service payments and salaries

Table 2 (cont.)

Country	Percentage of public coverage	National health system	Type of financing	Description
Switzerland		NO	Social insurance, private insurance	Mandatory or optional insurance depending on place of residence (99% of population insured)
United States	15	NO	Private insurance and public financing	Medicare for the elderly (federal) and Medicaid for the poorest (state and federal); 14% of population has no coverage

Sources: Information in italics is from: Contandriopoulos et al. 1993. All other information is from: OECD 1994.

Figure 1

Combined life expectancy (men and women) at birth

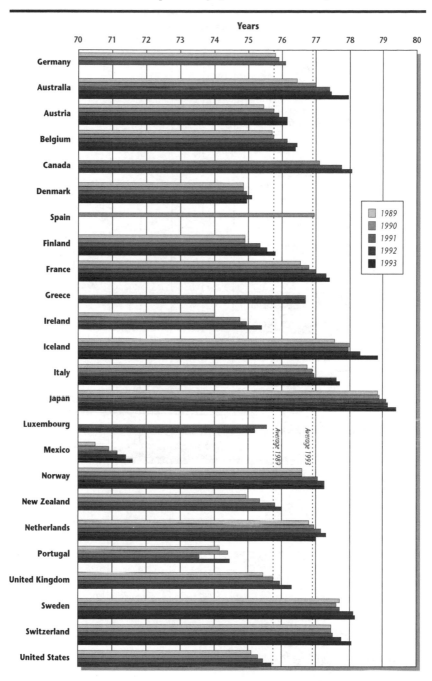

Figure 2

Infant mortality (rate for 100 births)

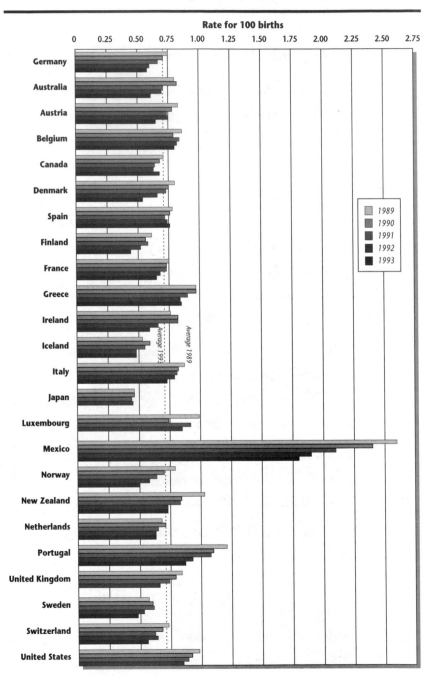

Figure 3

Percentage of the population older than 65 years

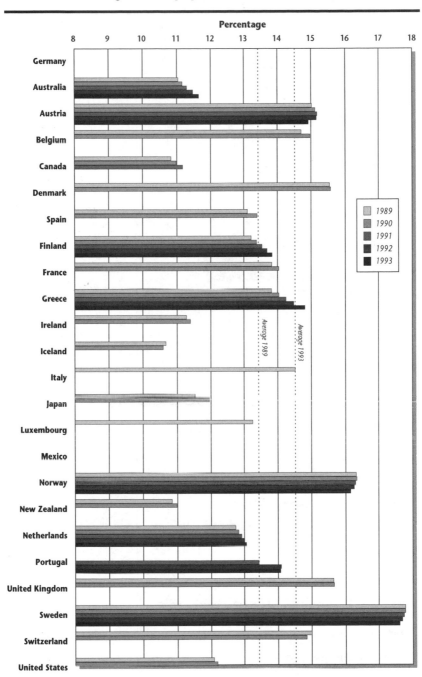

Figure 4

Number of hospital beds per 1,000 inhabitants

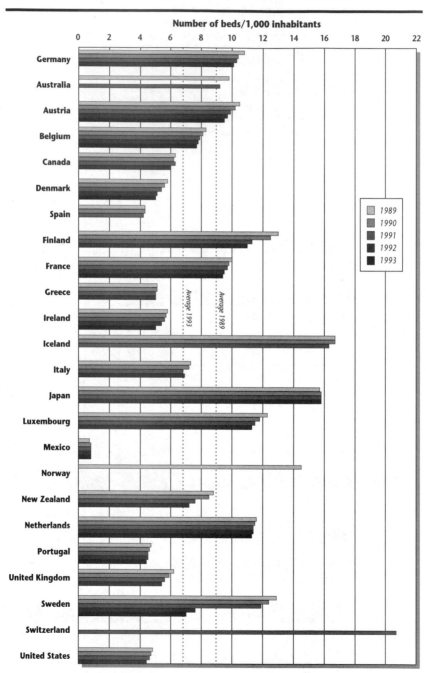

Number of beds/1,000 inhabitants

Figure 5

Number of physicians per 1,000 inhabitants

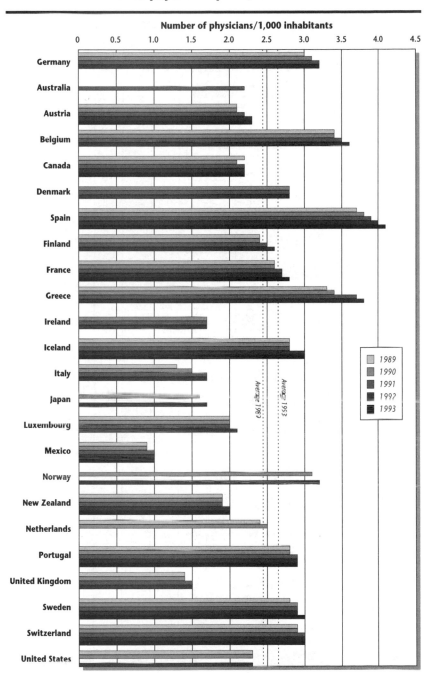

Figure 6

Health expenditures as a percentage of GDP

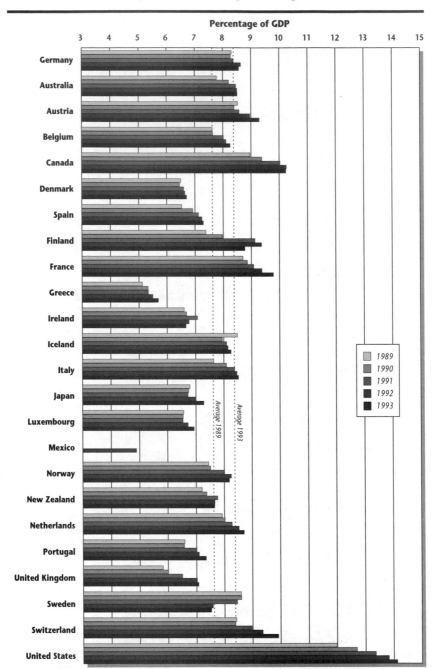

Figure 7

Per capita health expenditures in $PPP

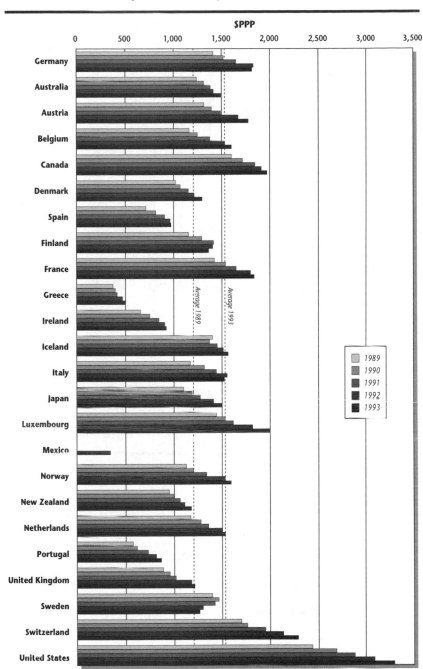

Figure 8

Percentage of private health expenditures

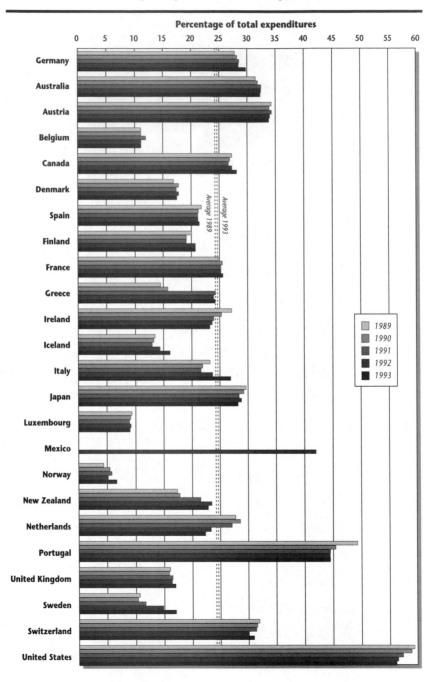

Figure 9

Per capita health expenditures in relation to per capita GDP in 1989

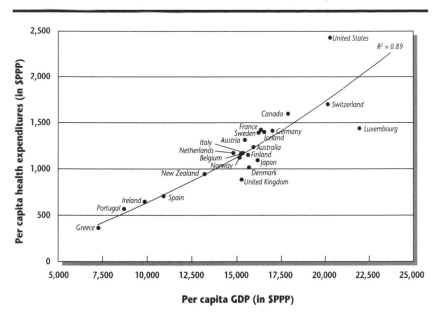

Per capita GDP (in $PPP)

Figure 10

Per capita health expenditures in relation to per capita GDP in 1990

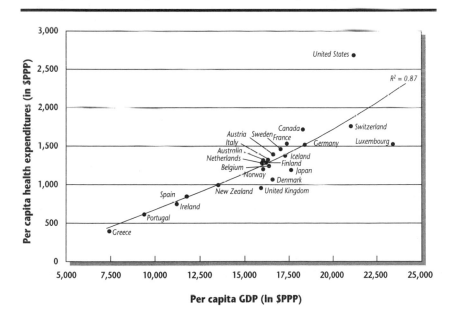

Per capita GDP (In $PPP)

Figure 11

Per capita health expenditures in relation to per capita GDP in 1991

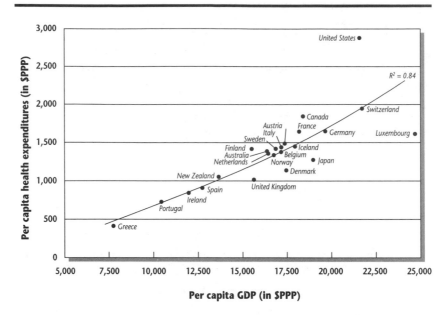

Figure 12

Per capita health expenditures in relation to per capita GDP in 1992

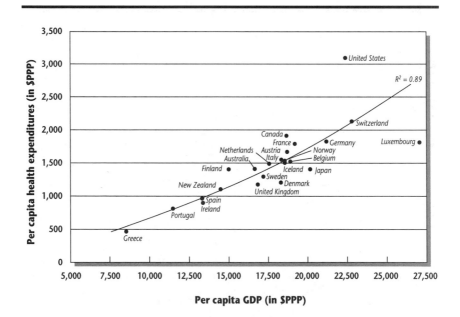

Figure 13

Per capita health expenditures in relation to per capita GDP in 1993

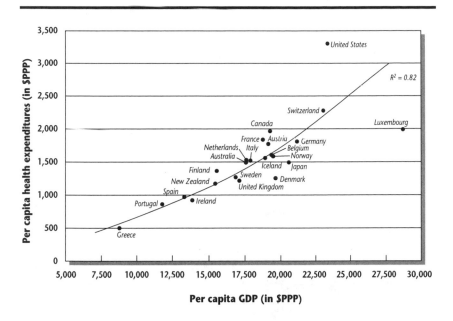

Per capita GDP (in $PPP)

Figure 14

Global health expenditures index from 1989 to 1993

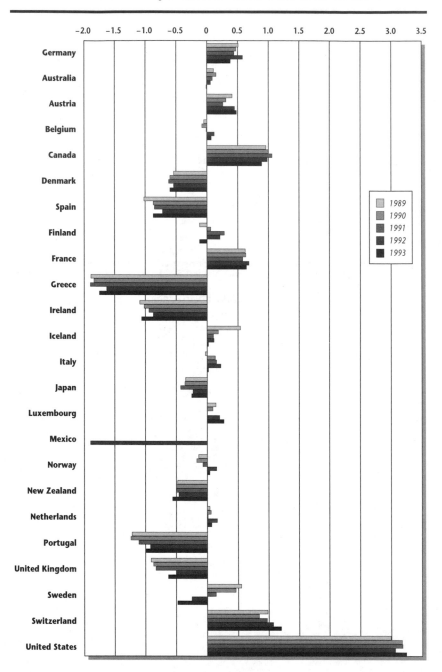

Figure 15

Global index of the state of health of the population
from 1989 to 1993

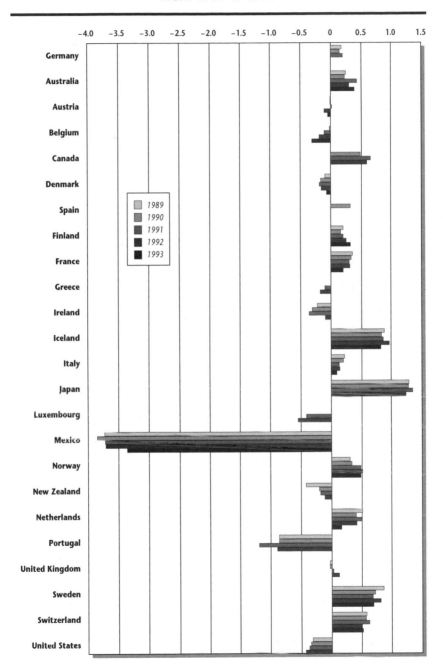

Figure 16

Global index of the performance of the health care system from 1989 to 1993

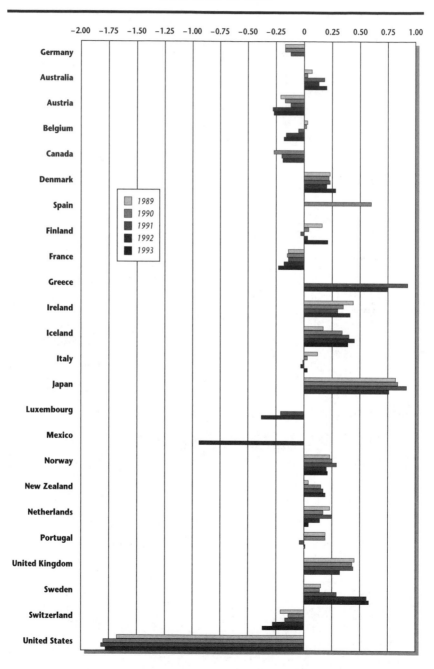

International Comparisons of Health Expenditures

DELPHINE ARWEILER

Doctoral Student in Public Health
Interdisciplinary Research Group on Health
University of Montreal

SUMMARY

International comparisons are a good way of getting to know the health system of one's own country and of examining alternative configurations of this system without having to conduct costly social experiments (Parkin, McGuire, and Yule 1989). International comparisons of health expenditures are essential (McGuire et al 1993) when debating the optimum size of the health sector, both from the point of view of the volume of expenditures and the factors which cause them to increase. However, as with all comparisons of indicators, the aggregates selected must be comparable and carefully defined.

In the first part of this report, we examine the problem of comparing monetary indicators. After ensuring the comparability of health expenditure indicators, we give a more precise interpretation of what is measured by each of these indicators. In the second part, we try to identify the possible causes of an increase in health expenditures based on their relationship to the wealth of the country, prices, and the quantity of care consumed.

TABLE OF CONTENTS

The Different Measurements of Health Expenditures 217

   Diversity of Monetary Conversions 217

      Exchange Rate and Nominal Health Expenditures 217

      Purchasing Power Parity (GDP) and Real Health
      Expenditures 217

      Purchasing Power Parity (Health) and Quantities of
      Care Consumed 218

   Health Expenditures and GDP 224

      The Health Expenditures/GDP Ratio 224

      Change in Health Expenditures and the GDP 225

Prices and Quantities 225

   Impact of Prices and Quantities 225

      Real GDP 225

      Expenditures 230

      Quantities 230

      Prices 230

   Results of Other Studies 230

   Methods 231

   Results 231

   A Look at the Method 235

Conclusion 236

Bibliography 237

APPENDICES

   Appendix 1   The Variables 241

   Appendix 2   Price and Income Elasticities 244

   Appendix 3   Figures and Bar Graphs 245

LIST OF FIGURES

Figure 1   Change in GDP 1979–93 245

Figure 2   Change in health expenditures 1979–93 245

Figure 3   Growth rate of GDP and health expenditures
in Canada 1986–93 246

Figure 4   Price and GDP/cap. 1993 246

Figure 5   Relative price of care and GDP 247

Figure 6   Health expenditures and GDP/cap. (1993) 247

Figure 7   Health quantities and GDP/cap. (1993) 248

LIST OF BAR GRAPHS

Bar graph 1   GDP/cap. 1993 ($PPP) 248

Bar graph 2   Price level (GDP) 1993 249

Bar graph 3   Relative price of care 1993 249

Bar graph 4   Health expenditures 1993 ($U.S.) 250

Bar graph 5   Health expenditures 1993 ($PPP) 250

Bar graph 6   Health expenditures 1993 ($PPP health) 251

Bar graph 7   Health expenditures/GDP 1993 (%) 251

LIST OF TABLES

Table 1   GDP and price 219

Table 2   Quantities 221

Table 3   Expenditures 222

Table 4   Health expenditures/GDP (%) 224

Table 5a   Change in GDP (curr. price val. (M$PPP)) 226

Table 5b   GDP growth rate (%) 227

Table 6a   Health expenditures (curr. price val. (M$PPP)) 228

Table 6b   Growth rate in expenditures (%) 229

Table 7   Quantity forecasts 234

THE DIFFERENT MEASUREMENTS OF HEALTH EXPENDITURES

The problem with international comparisons is to decide on the unit in which health expenditures will be expressed and consequently, the indicator selected. Three monetary conversions are used: the exchange rate and purchasing power parity calculated for all goods and services produced or only for health care. Four indicators can be deduced from these conversions: nominal expenditures, real expenditures, quantities, and the expenditures/GDP ratio.

Diversity of Monetary Conversions

Exchange Rate and Nominal Health Expenditures

The exchange rate is the price of the national monetary unit in foreign currency. This price is set on the currency market based on supply and demand and the interventions of monetary authorities (OECD 1995). This is why the levels of prices set on goods and services markets are different from the levels of exchange rates (Gilbert and Kravis 1954).

When health expenditures are converted using the exchange rate, we obtain their nominal value (Ward 1985) because in this instance the currency is a unit of account. The American dollar is the unit of account used most often. In nominal value, the United States ($3,299), Switzerland ($3,294), Japan ($2,463) and Germany ($2,308) have the highest expenditures/capita. Canada ($1,943) ranks sixteenth in ascending order of expenditures converted using exchange rates (table 3). It is not possible to draw any conclusions with respect to volume of care because it is difficult to determine the impact of monetary operations on the indicators. However, the countries with the highest expenditures are also those whose national currency is considered to be "strong." Moreover, the nominal expenditures reflect both differences in quantities of goods and services in each country and differences in the level of prices (Ward 1985).

Purchasing Power Parity (GDP) and Real Health Expenditures

Purchasing power parity is an international price index calculated by comparing the prices of identical products in various countries (Ward 1985). It indicates the rate at which one currency should be converted into another to be able to purchase an equivalent basket of goods and services in the two countries (Ward 1985). The PPPs therefore eliminate price disparities between countries (appendix 1). The OECD chose the American dollar as its legal tender and the reader will note the use of $PPP throughout this study. Expenditures made in each country will consequently be expressed in the same unit, $PPP. For example, in 1993, it was possible to purchase the same quantity of a good with $1 in the United States, $1.27 in Canada, and $183.16 in Japan (table 1). The PPP is a good basis for comparing standards of living, estimating the allocation of resources between various producing sectors, and examining levels of productivity (Ward 1985). Since expenditures in PPP (GDP) are expressed in relation to a basket of goods representative of the GDPs of all of the OECD countries, they provide a measure of the opportunity cost of care (Saez and Murillo 1994) in relation to the utilization that might have been made of the resources mobilized in other producing sectors. In terms of the real value per capita, the United States ($3,299 PPP), Switzerland ($2,283 PPP), Luxembourg ($1,993 PPP), and Canada ($1,971 PPP) have the highest expenditures, Japan being far behind (table 3). Real expenditures are by nature comparable. However, it is difficult to determine from them whether the countries which have high expenditures are in this position because their medical professionals are highly paid, the relative global costs of care are high, the quantities of care consumed are high, or a combination of these elements.

Purchasing Power Parity (Health) and Quantities of Care Consumed

The PPP(health) indicates the rate at which one currency should be converted to another to be able to purchase an equivalent basket of health goods and services in the two countries. For example, in 1993, it was possible to purchase the same quantity of care with $1 in the United States, $0.83 in Canada, and $71 in Japan (table 1). By using the PPP (health), we are measuring the volume of resources allocated to the care sector, which is expressed in this study as the quantity of care per capita (Saez and Murillo 1994). If national health expenditures calculated from various monetary conversions are compared, the same countries do not come up with the highest levels of expenditures/capita (table 3). In terms of quantities (table 2), France ($4,128), Japan ($3,258) and Switzerland ($3,801) consume the most, while Canada ($3,020) ranks fifteenth in ascending order of expenditures in $PPP (health). Since France's real expenditures are not among the highest, but its quantity of care consumed is relatively high, we can conclude that the relative prices of care are lower than in the United States or Switzerland. Since Canada has high real health expenditures and average quantities of care consumed close to the average for OECD countries, it can be concluded that Canada's relative prices of care appear to be higher than the average for OECD countries. These conclusions lead us to ask whether the quantities consumed, the relative prices of care, and the per capita national income of the country have a significant effect on the level of health expenditures. This question will be discussed in the following section.

Table 1

GDP and price

Country	Macroeconomic references	Monetary conversion	Monetary conversion	Monetary conversion	Price	Relative
	Gross domestic product Val./cap. $PPP	Purch. power parity (GDP) NMU/$PPP	Exchange rate NMU/$U.S.	Purch. power parity (health) NMU/$PPP	level (GDP)	price of care
Turkey	5,376	5,943.99	10,966.00	2,606.000	0.54	0.44
Greece	8,782	184.27	229.10	87.000	0.80	0.47
Portugal	11,800	116.88	160.70	74.000	0.73	0.63
Spain	13,330	118.90	127.70	59.000	0.92	0.50
Ireland	13,847	0.66	0.68	0.410	0.96	0.63
New Zealand	15,409	1.51	1.85	0.850	0.82	0.56
Finland	15,530	6.08	5.72	3.520	1.06	0.58
Sweden	16,828	9.83	7.79	5.770	1.26	0.59
United Kingdom	17,152	0.64	0.67	0.332	0.95	0.52
Australia	17,555	1.37	1.47	0.750	0.93	0.55
Netherlands	17,602	2.13	1.86	1.150	1.15	0.54
Italy	17,865	1,533.16	1,572.00	776.000	0.98	0.51
France	18,764	6.57	5.66	2.920	1.16	0.44
Iceland	18,931	82.23	67.64	41.500	1.22	0.50
Austria	19,126	13.86	11.63	7.800	1.19	0.56
Canada	19,271	1.27	1.29	0.830	0.99	0.65

Table 1 (cont.)

Country	Macroeconomic references	Monetary conversion	Monetary conversion	Monetary conversion	Price level (GDP)	Relative price of care
	Gross domestic product Val./cap. $PPP	Purch. power parity (GDP) NMU/$PPP	Exchange rate NMU/$U.S.	Purch. power parity (health) NMU/$PPP		
Denmark	19,340	8.79	6.48	5.43	1.36	0.62
Belgium	19,373	37.29	34.56	19.50	1.08	0.52
Norway	19,467	8.74	7.09	5.15	1.23	0.59
Japan	20,550	183.16	111.20	71.00	1,65	0.39
Germany	21,163	2.10	1.65	1.24	1.27	0.59
Switzerland	23,033	2.13	1.48	1.28	1.44	0.60
United States	23,358	1.00	1.00	1.00	1.00	1.00
Luxembourg	28,741	39.61	34.56	20.9	1.15	0.53

Source: OECD Health Data 1995 (CREDES).

Table 2

Quantities

Country	Monetary conversion	Total health expenditures	Total health expenditures
	Purch. power parity (health) NMU/$PPP	Total health expenditures Val./cap. NMU	Val./cap. PPP (health)
Turkey	2,606.00	868,563	333
Greece	87.00	92,110	1,059
Portugal	74.00	101,221	1,368
Spain	59.00	113,604	1,925
Ireland	0.41	604	1,473
New Zealand	0.85	1,778	2,092
Finland	3.52	8,291	2,355
Sweden	5.77	12,444	2,157
United Kingdom	0.33	773	2,328
Australia	0.75	2,050	2,733
Netherlands	1.15	3268	2,842
Italy	776.00	2,334,322	3,008
France	2.92	12,054	4,128
Iceland	41.50	128,644	3,100
Austria	7.80	24,621	3,157
Canada	0.83	2,507	3,020
Denmark	5.43	11,385	2,097
Belgium	19.50	59,699	3,061
Norway	5.15	13,915	2,702
Japan	71.00	273,896	3,858
Germany	1.24	3,814	3,076
Switzerland	1.28	4,865	3,801
United States	1.00	3,299	3,299
Luxembourg	20.90	78,947	3,777

Source: OECD Health Data 1995 (CREDES).

Table 3

Expenditures

Country	Macroeconomic references Gross domestic product Val./cap. $PPP	Total health expenditures Total health expenditures Val./cap. $(change)	Rank	Total health expenditures Total health expenditures Val./cap. $PPP	Rank	Total health expenditures Val./cap. $PPP (health)	Rank
Turkey	5,376	79	1	146	1	333	1
Greece	8,782	402	2	500	2	1,059	2
Portugal	11,800	630	3	866	3	1,368	3
Spain	13,330	890	5	972	5	1,925	5
Ireland	13,847	884	4	922	4	1,473	4
New Zealand	15,409	961	6	1,179	6	2,092	6
Finland	15,530	1,449	9	1,363	10	2,355	10
Sweden	16,828	1,598	11	1,266	8	2,157	8
United Kingdom	17,152	1,161	7	1,213	7	2,328	9
Australia	17,555	1,392	8	1,493	11	2,733	12
Netherlands	17,602	1,760	14	1,531	14	2,842	13
Italy	17,865	1,485	10	1,523	13	3,008	14
France	18,764	2,129	19	1,835	20	4,128	24
Iceland	18,931	1,902	15	1,564	15	3,100	18
Austria	19,126	2,117	18	1,777	18	3,157	19
Canada	19,271	1,943	16	1,971	21	3,020	15

Table 3 (Cont.)

Country	Macroeconomic references Gross domestic product Val./cap. $PPP	Total health expenditures Total health expenditures Val./cap. $(change)	Rank	Total health expenditures Total health expenditures Val./cap. $PPP	Rank	Total health expenditures Val./cap. $PPP (health)	Rank
Denmark	19,340	17,56	13	1,296	9	2,097	7
Belgium	19,373	17,27	12	1,601	17	3,061	16
Norway	19,467	19,62	17	1,592	16	2,702	11
Japan	20,550	24,63	22	1,495	12	3,858	23
Germany	21,163	23,08	21	1,815	19	3,076	17
Switzerland	23,033	32,94	23	2,283	23	3,801	22
United States	23,358	32,99	24	3,299	24	3,299	20
Luxembourg	28,741	22,84	20	1,993	22	3,777	21

Health Expenditures and GDP

The Health Expenditures/GDP Ratio (Table 4)

In 1979, Sweden (9 percent), the United States (8.8 percent), and Germany (8.1 percent) had the highest ratios, the ratios for the other countries being between 5 percent and 8 percent: Canada's ratio was 7.1 percent. Between 1979 and 1993, while Sweden and Germany—with ratios of 8.6 percent and 7.5 percent respectively—maintained relatively stable ratios (Sweden even experienced a decrease of 1.5 percent), the United States saw a strong increase in its ratio. In 1993, with the ratios for most countries between 6 percent and 9 percent, three countries stood out: the United States (14.1 percent), Canada (10.1 percent), and Switzerland (9.9 percent). However, an increase in health expenditures greater than the growth in the GDP can be interpreted either as an acceleration in the growth in expenditures or a slowdown in the growth of the GDP.

Table 4

Health expenditures/GDP (%)

Country	1979	1981	1983	1985	1987	1989	1991	1993
Australia	7.4	7.5	7.7	7.7	7.8	7.8	8.5	8.5
Austria	7.9	8.2	8.0	8.1	8.4	8.5	8.6	9.3
Belgium	6.8	7.2	7.6	7.4	7.7	7.6	8.0	8.3
Canada	7.1	7.5	8.6	8.5	8.9	9.0	10.0	10.2
Denmark	6.6	6.8	6.6	6.3	6.3	6.5	6.6	6.7
Finland	6.6	6.7	6.9	7.3	7.5	7.4	9.1	8.8
France	7.4	7.9	8.2	8.5	8.5	8.7	9.1	9.8
Germany	8.1	8.7	8.5	8.7	8.7	8.3	8.4	8.6
Greece	4.4	4.5	4.6	4.9	5.2	5.1	5.3	5.7
Iceland	6.2	6.4	7.3	7.3	7.9	8.5	8.1	8.3
Ireland	7.8	8.4	8.1	7.8	7.4	6.6	7.1	6.7
Italy	5.9	6.7	7.0	7.0	7.4	7.6	8.4	8.5
Japan	6.1	6.6	6.9	6.6	7.1	6.8	6.7	7.3
Luxembourg	6.1	6.5	6.2	6.2	6.6	6.6	6.5	6.9
Netherlands	7.5	8.1	8.3	7.9	8.1	7.9	8.3	8.7
New Zealand	7.0	6.9	6.4	6.4	6.9	7.2	7.8	7.7
Norway	6.9	6.6	6.8	6.4	7.4	7.4	8.0	8.2
Portugal	5.0	6.2	5.8	6.3	6.8	6.6	7.0	7.3
Spain	5.5	5.8	6.0	5.7	5.7	6.5	7.1	7.3
Sweden	9.0	9.5	9.5	8.9	8.6	8.6	8.4	7.5
Switzerland	7.2	7.3	7.8	8.1	8.3	8.4	9.0	9.9
Turkey	3.3	3.6	3.0	2.2	2.8	2.9	3.4	2.7
United Kingdom	5.3	5.9	6.0	5.9	5.9	5.8	6.5	7.1
United States	8.8	9.6	10.6	10.8	11.3	12.0	13.4	14.1

Source: OECD Health Data 1995 (CREDES).

Change in Health Expenditures and the GDP

All of the countries experienced an upward trend in their GDP between 1979 and 1993, although there were marked slowdowns in certain years, such as 1990–1991 and 1992–1993 (table 5a). In 1993, certain countries had negative GDP growth rates: Sweden (–1.23 percent), Germany (–1.26 percent), France (–2 percent), and Italy (–2.26 percent) (table 5b). The same trend is obvious in total health expenditures (table 6a). It should be noted, however, that 1992–1993 saw the smallest growth rates ever in health expenditures, below 8 percent for the countries as a whole (table 6b). The growth rates for health expenditures and the GDP in Canada have been asymmetrical since 1986–1987 (graph 3). This makes it difficult to interpret and compare its expenditures/GDP ratio year to year. Since 1991, health expenditures and the GDP have risen less quickly; in 1992–1993, the GDP growth rate was 4.42 percent, while that of expenditures was 4.19 percent. At the least, this phenomenon might indicate that, in Canada, the increase in the expenditures/GDP ratio is not the result of an acceleration in the growth of health expenditures.

PRICES AND QUANTITIES

Impact of Prices and Quantities

In this section we update Gerdtham and Jönsson's (1991) research for 1985 to 1993. We try to identify the relationships between health expenditures, prices, quantities of health care consumed, and national income (GDP) for the 24 OECD countries included in the study.

Real GDP

When the PPP is used to convert the GDP, it gives the real value of the GDP (Ward 1985) which can be used to make international comparisons of volume (table 1). In 1993, Canada, with a per capita GDP of $19,271 PPP had the ninth highest per capita GDP. Luxembourg had the highest GDP ($28,741 PPP) and Turkey, the lowest ($5,376 PPP).

Table 5a

Change in GDP (curr. price val. (M$PPP))

Country	1979	1981	1983	1985	1987	1989	1991	1993
Australia	120,222.9	152,909.2	172,460.2	202,848.7	231,958.1	26,747.7	282,925.5	309,953.4
Austria	59,348.5	73,062.5	83,077.5	92,796.4	100,857.0	118,126.0	135,663.0	152,835.5
Belgium	76,186.7	94,434.2	106,230.5	117,736.4	128,611.7	151,333.8	171,684.6	195,360.9
Canada	221,936.8	280,296.6	308,694.6	369,999.2	420,275.2	489,489.4	517,375.2	554,110.8
Denmark	41,164.5	48,726.3	56,759.7	66,465.5	72,998.3	80,508.9	89,883.7	100,352.9
Finland	33,209.6	42,750.6	50,001.3	57,266.1	64,475.8	77,485.8	77,755.1	78,674.6
France	457,429.4	563,032.2	640,322.5	711,603.8	786,768.7	922,522.1	1,035,826.8	1,078,935.2
Germany	54,239.4	657,656.4	731,174.4	824,968.3	905,586.9	1,055,237.2	1,260,761.9	1,357,611.8
Greece	37,473.6	45,769.4	50,886.3	57,993.8	61,982.4	72,658.3	79,190.1	91,046.7
Iceland	1,873.4	2,476.1	2,729.8	3,158.2	3,848.4	4,180.7	4,622.3	4,997.9
Ireland	15,593.1	19,944.7	22,430.4	26,951.3	28,595.3	34,690.4	42,199.4	49,296.2
Italy	418,955.0	526,787.8	587,925.8	666,231.6	747,230.0	867,713.0	974,376.4	1,017,580.7
Japan	825,499.9	1,063,028.5	1,242,260.3	1,462,579.5	1,651,092.0	1,990,559.6	2,348,438.1	2,558,534.8
Luxembourg	3,654.8	4,397.0	5,051.4	5,937.7	6,767.0	8,270.9	9,532.2	10,921.8
Netherlands	113,923.1	136,879.9	150,914.9	171,858.6	188,766.1	219,805.0	247,589.0	269,133.1
New Zealand	22,066.9	27,932.2	32,244.7	36,650.9	40,086.5	43,864.3	46,468.5	53,624.0
Norway	30,089.4	37,947.2	43,941.8	52,613.8	59,072.1	64,086.5	71,448.0	83,943.4
Portugal	38,849.6	49,534.0	55,705.4	60,439.0	70,189.8	85,118.7	102,603.9	117,854.9
Spain	198,015.5	240,218.4	275,080.0	308,055.1	354,860.9	423,693.2	495,798.9	520,977.0
Sweden	69,133.5	84,314.4	95,573.6	109,020.1	121,553.5	137,921.2	145,110.0	146,727.1
Switzerland	65,406.4	83,260.5	91,913.9	104,324.9	115,713.3	134,053.6	147,933.4	160,978.4
Turkey	93,971.5	116,740.8	140,797.6	170,031.3	208,674.7	231,590.4	275,699.5	321,862.9
United Kingdom	421,803.8	488,986.5	568,387.6	648,765.0	749,362.3	871,594.9	900,401.9	985,401.9
United States	2,465,969.0	3,035,796.0	3,394,298.0	4,016,649.0	4,496,574.0	5,204,600.0	5,656,600.0	6,259,900.0

Source: OECD Health Data 1995 (CREDES).

Table 5b

GDP growth rate (%)

Country	1986–87	1987–88	1988–89	1989–90	1990–91	1991–92	1992–93
Australia	8.30	8.92	5.90	2.20	3.47	4.87	6.53
Austria	4.81	8.07	8.33	8.61	5.74	6.85	3.42
Belgium	5.16	8.94	8.01	7.57	5.46	6.57	2.96
Canada	7.37	9.05	6.60	3.92	1.71	10.66	4.42
Denmark	3.40	5.06	4.97	5.67	5.65	11.31	6.36
Finland	7.32	8.95	10.30	4.20	– 3.69	7.53	3.91
France	5.35	8.26	8.30	6.69	5.25	10.48	– 2.00
Germany	4.66	7.70	8.19	10.11	8.51	12.44	– 1.26
Greece	2.63	8.47	8.07	3.09	5.73	8.37	3.31
Iceland	11.97	3.80	4.66	5.32	4.98	2.84	3.11
Ireland	7.98	8.24	12.08	13.19	7.47	9.05	3.89
Italy	6.33	8.08	7.44	6.41	5.53	8.94	– 2.26
Japan	7.33	10.30	9.30	9.20	8.04	10.51	2.23
Luxembourg	6.13	9.79	11.32	7.50	7.21	2.56	3.53
Netherlands	4.29	6.61	9.23	8.49	3.83	– 2.62	1.09
New Zealand	4.47	3.14	6.09	3.61	2.25	4.68	7.66
Norway	5.16	3.33	4.99	5.92	5.25	4.97	5.55
Portugal	8.81	9.87	10.38	8.64	10.95	6.29	3.96
Spain	8.92	9.22	9.32	8.08	8.27	7.19	0.38
Sweden	6.35	6.18	6.86	5.61	– 0.38	2.37	– 1.23
Switzerland	5.23	6.85	8.43	6.56	3.56	6.91	1.79
Turkey	11.52	6.06	4.64	13.83	4.58	6.31	9.81
United Kingdom	8.02	9.02	6.69	4.70	– 1.34	11.29	0.99
United States	6.28	7.95	7.22	5.47	3.04	4.96	5.43

Source: OECD Health Data 1995 (CREDES).

Table 6a

Health expenditures (curr. price val. (M$PPP))

Country	1979	1981	1983	1985	1987	1989	1991	1993
Australia	8,873.9	11,399.0	13,237.2	15,710.9	18,097.8	20,819.4	23,928.4	26,365.6
Austria	4,666.2	6,005.0	6,662.6	7,520.0	8,462.3	10,078.0	11,642.2	14,198.4
Belgium	5,213.0	6,765.9	8,022.2	8,746.3	9,856.9	11,532.1	13,776.2	16,143.3
Canada	15,714.2	21,128.5	26,480.4	31,512.5	37,388.2	43,839.9	51,913.2	56,660.4
Denmark	2,704.5	3,326.1	3,727.0	4,170.0	4,599.1	5,232.5	5,932.6	6,723.5
Finland	2,189.0	2,851.6	3,465.2	4,176.0	4,829.8	5,715.4	7,102.0	6,903.4
France	33,911.1	44,292.5	52,197.5	60,160.2	66,839.0	80,275.6	94,053.0	105,492.8
Germany	44,168.0	57,223.7	62,147.2	71,696.8	78,348.5	87,704.0	105,714.3	116,412.9
Greece	1,632.5	2,053.0	2,350.0	2,819.8	3,219.5	3,719.6	4,221.0	5,182.7
Iceland	116.9	158.0	199.2	229.2	303.9	354.8	374.2	413.0
Ireland	1,219.1	1,667.8	1,809.5	2,015.3	2,115.3	2,291.0	2,982.0	3,282.4
Italy	24,806.0	35,322.0	41,262.9	46,821.5	54,949.1	66,286.4	81,731.7	86,724.8
Japan	50,458.7	70,625.7	85,707.5	96,090.9	117,064.0	135,224.1	157,754.9	186,180.1
Luxembourg	221.9	286.6	314.2	369.8	443.4	543.7	623.8	757.4
Netherlands	8,513.3	11,059.9	12,487.9	13,537.8	15,320.1	17,403.2	204,64.4	23,414.7
New Zealand	1,450.7	1,919.2	2,064.4	2,337.1	2,756.4	3,161.5	3,607.4	4,103.4
Norway	2,077.7	2,495.4	2,998.6	3,390.2	4,373.4	4,769.3	5,707.9	6,865.0
Portugal	1,941.1	3,077.8	3,243.6	3,825.9	4,756.2	5,606.9	7,191.5	8,649.8
Spain	10,921.7	13,971.6	16,506.9	17,491.5	20,245.6	27,660.5	35,310.5	37,979.9
Sweden	6,221.5	8,010.1	9,111.4	9,680.3	10,491.3	11,852.7	12,259.0	11,038.8
Switzerland	4,706.3	6,075.7	7,165.5	8,413.3	9,592.5	11,286.7	13,268.1	15,954.0
Turkey	3,091.9	4,234.5	4,252.8	3,710.9	5,866.0	6,667.7	9,390.9	8,748.3
United Kingdom	22,194.0	28,925.0	34,116.1	37,994.5	43,897.0	50,769.5	58,549.5	69,714.3
United States	218,272.0	291,369.0	360,782.0	434,498.0	506,178.0	623,914.0	755,551.0	884,205.0

Source: OECD Health Data 1995 (CREDES).

Table 6b

Growth rate in expenditures (%)

Country	1986–87	1987–88	1988–89	1989–90	1990–91	1991–92	1992–93
Australia	5.85	7.45	7.07	7.81	6.61	3.39	6.57
Austria	6.08	7.83	10.45	6.97	7.99	13.68	7.28
Belgium	6.41	9.17	7.17	7.79	10.82	11.69	4.92
Canada	8.04	7.80	8.77	8.81	8.83	4.76	4.19
Denmark	8.83	9.19	4.20	4.97	8.02	5.55	7.37
Finland	8.38	6.90	10.7	12.62	10.33	-0.19	-2.61
France	5.54	9.19	9.99	8.68	7.80	9.66	2.28
Germany	5.84	10.04	1.72	9.64	9.94	12.35	-1.98
Greece	-0.52	4.43	10.63	7.11	5.94	14.61	7.13
Iceland	14.87	11.28	4.91	4.91	6.94	5.52	4.6
Ireland	3.20	3.72	4.42	4.42	13.68	7.71	2.19
Italy	12.59	11.19	8.49	8.49	9.42	7.84	-1.61
Japan	14.49	7.34	7.61	7.61	7.47	11.08	6.25
Luxembourg	14.93	14.67	6.93	6.93	7.15	13.63	6.86
Netherlands	6.09	5.93	7.23	7.23	7.03	10.84	3.22
New Zealand	8.80	3.91	10.39	10.39	7.75	5.80	7.51
Norway	10.15	7.18	1.75	1.75	11.93	14.96	4.62
Portugal	5.34	16.08	1.55	1.55	18.37	11.75	7.63
Spain	10.58	21.36	12.58	14.49	11.5	6.37	1.12
Sweden	6.88	5.27	7.33	5.69	-2.14	-8.09	-2.02
Switzerland	7.36	8.33	8.61	6.05	10.85	11.61	7.74
Turkey	17.53	10.39	2.97	13.06	24.57	-7.94	1.19
United Kingdom	8.02	8.22	6.87	6.87	6.81	16.96	1.80
United States	3.63	11.09	10.95	11.64	8.47	8.58	7.78

Source: OECD Health Data 1995 (CREDES).

Expenditures

Given the heterogeneity of units of quantity of care (it is not possible to add medical interventions and boxes of drugs) and their lack of comparability between countries (for example, for nursing care), it is necessary to find a common unit that facilitates comparisons. We therefore chose currency as the unit of account—the American dollar for the OECD—and health expenditures as the indicators—specifically, the product of quantities of care and their prices. The study was conducted at an aggregate level; expenditures are given by the OECD in $U.S. PPP (GDP) in order to provide more reliable international comparisons (Gilbert and Kravis 1954; Kravis, Heston, and Summers 1978).

Quantities

The relative quantities of goods and services purchased in two countries can vary because of (1) differences in tastes and needs, (2) disparities in income levels, and (3) differences in relative prices (Gilbert and Kravis 1954). This study looks at the latter two aspects: quantities are expressed by care expenditures in PPP (health) described earlier (Kravis, Heston, and Summers 1978), and income is expressed in terms of per capita GDP (appendix 1).

Prices

Disparities in the relative prices of care can be explained by differences in the availability of natural resources or manpower relative to capital, differences in the relative efficiency of producing various types of goods and services, or even differences in demand profiles which might influence production efficiency (Gilbert and Kravis 1954). In this study, we refer to two relative prices: the GDP, calculated on the basis of a basket of various goods, and the more specific price of care (appendix 1). Canada, like all of the OECD countries, has a relative price of care (0.65) that is a great deal less than that of the United States (1.00), although it still ranks second behind the United States (table 1).

Results of Other Studies

In a brief review of the literature, Murillo, Piatecki and Saez (1993) point out the contradictory results found in empirical studies of the relationship between health expenditures and per capita GDP. In the article from which we have taken our methodology (Gerdtham and Jönsson 1991), health expenditures increased with the per capita GDP, but were not higher in the countries with high relative prices. The relative price of care had a counter-balancing effect on the quantity of care consumed.

Methods

Estimates of the impact of prices and quantities were determined using linear regressions, with a logarithmic transformation of the variables: the latter has proven to be the most effective method in international comparisons of health expenditures (Gerdtham and Jönsson 1991). The betas were interpreted in economic terms of elasticity (appendix 2). The confidence interval of the elasticity was 95 percent.

- Definitions of all of the variables and of the main concepts are given in appendix 1.
- All of the data were taken from *Health Data* (OECD 1995), except for the PPP (health) which were provided directly by the OECD and will be incorporated in the *Health Data* in 1996.
- All of the OECD countries were used, except for Mexico (24 countries). To avoid overloading the charts, only 13 countries are displayed: Germany, Australia, Canada, Denmark, France, Italy, Japan, New Zealand, the Netherlands, the United Kingdom, Sweden, Switzerland, and the United States.

Results

• Do wealthy countries have higher relative prices of care?

Is price level a function of the GDP/cap.?

$$\ln(\text{price level}) = -5.39 + 0.56 \ln(\text{GDP/cap.}) + e_i$$

t (-6.20) (6.26) $N = 24$ $R^2 = 64\%$

The per capita GDP explains significantly 64 percent of the variance in the level of price, which is 20 percent lower than in 1985. When the per capita GDP increases 1 percent, the price level increases 0.56 percent. With a confidence interval of $(-1.2; 2.32)$, the elasticity is not significantly different from 0.

Is the relative price of care a function of GDP/cap.?

$$\ln(\text{relative price of care}) = -2.24 + 0.17 \ln(\text{GDP/cap.}) = e_i$$

t (1.60) (-2.17) $N = 24$ $R^2 = 10.4\%$

The relationship is not significant.

Conclusion – Wealthy countries have a higher overall level of price but the relative prices of care are not significantly higher in these countries. As for Gerdtham and Jönsson (1991), *Health Data* did not contain data on the remuneration of physicians for 1993 from a sufficient number of countries to be able to determine whether this element contributes to the higher relative price of care for the OECD countries as a whole.

• **Do wealthy countries have higher expenditures and quantities of care?**

Are care expenditures per capita a function of GDP/cap.?

ln(care expenditures per cap.) = $- 9.03 + 1.67$ ln(GDP/cap.) + e_i

t $(- 8.03)$ (14.89) N = 24 $R^2 = 90\%$

    Per capita GDP explains significantly 90 percent of the variance in care expenditures. With a confidence interval of (1.45; 1.89), the income elasticity is significantly higher than 0. When per capita income increases 1 percent, care expenditures increase 1.67 percent.

Are per capita quantities of care a function of GDP/cap.?

ln (quantities of care/cap.) = $- 6.81 + 1.50$ ln(GDP/cap.) + e_i

t $(- 6.48)$ (13.88) N = 24 $R^2 = 90\%$

    The per capita GDP explains significantly 90 percent of the variance in per capita quantities of care. With a confidence interval of (1.28; 1.72), the income elasticity is significantly higher than 0. When per capita income increases 1 percent, the quantity of care increases 1.50 percent.

    Conclusion – Wealthy countries have higher care expenditures and also consume greater quantities of care. The income elasticity is weaker for quantities of care than for expenditures but both elements are elastic with respect to income. Health care therefore becomes a luxury item with the wealthiest consuming the most care. We can conclude that care is rationed according to level of income.

• **Are care expenditures higher in countries with higher relative care prices?**

Are care expenditures per capita a function of the relative price of care and GDP/cap.?

ln(care expenditures/cap.) = $- 7.86 + 2.56$ ln(GDP/cap.) + 0.52 ln (relative price of care) + e_i

t (7.37) (15.02) (2.62)

                                             N = 24 $R^2 = 93.2\%$

    The per capita GDP combined with the relative price of care explains significantly 93.2 percent of the variance in care expenditures per capita.

With a confidence interval of (1.36; 1.8), the income elasticity is significantly higher than 0. When per capita income rises 1 percent, quantity of care increases 1.58 percent. With a confidence interval of (0.13; 0.91), the price elasticity is significantly higher than –1. When relative price of care increases 1 percent, care expenditures per capita increase 0.52 percent.

Is the quantity of care consumed per capita a function of the relative price of care and GDP/cap.?

ln (quantity of care/cap.) = – 7.87 + 1.58 ln(GDP/cap.) – 0.47 ln(relative price of care) + e_i

t   (– 7.50) (15.28)   (– 2.40)

$N = 24$ $R^2 = 92\%$

The per capita GDP combined with the relative price of care explains significantly 92 percent of the variance in the quantity of care consumed. With a confidence interval of (1.38; 1.78), the income elasticity is significantly higher than 0. When per capita income increases 1 percent, quantity of care per capita increases 1.58 percent. The price elasticity is significantly different from –1 with a confidence interval of (– 0.86; – 0.08). When relative price of care increases 1 percent, quantity of care per capita decreases 0.47 percent.

Conclusion – The income elasticity of care in terms of expenditures or quantities is higher than the price elasticity. Although Gerdtham and Jönsson (1991) found a price elasticity for expenditures that was not significant in relation to – 1 in 1985, it was significant in this study for 1993. This means that a 1 percent increase in the relative price of care will not be offset by a 1 percent drop in quantity. Disparities in expenditures between countries can be explained either in terms of price or quantity; in 1985, disparities in expenditures on care between countries could be explained only in relation to weighted quantities of care. It can therefore be concluded that countries with a higher relative price of care have higher expenditures, everything else being equal. The same reasoning applies to quantity. Everything else being equal, countries consuming higher quantities of care have higher health expenditures.

• **Which countries consume the greatest quantities of care after correcting for differences in GDP/cap. and relative price of care?**

After correcting for differences in per capita GDP and relative price of care, two countries stand apart in terms of the disparity between the real quantities of care they consumed and the quantities they would be expected to consume (table 7). Luxembourg's consumption was 34 percent less than expected. This disparity is significant because the real quantity is outside the confidence interval calculated at 95 percent. At the other extreme, France consumed a quantity of care 31 percent higher than predicted, but this value remains within the confidence interval. In Gerdtham and Jönsson's study of OECD countries in 1995, France, Ireland, the Netherlands, Portugal, Austria, and Sweden consumed significantly greater quantities than expected. Denmark, Norway, and Luxembourg had significantly smaller quantities of care consumed than expected. As for Canada, in 1993, its real quantity of care was 11 percent higher than the quantity predicted, but it remained within the limits of the confidence interval.

Table 7

Quantity forecasts

| Country | Real | Confidence interval 95 percent | | | |
		Predicted quantities	Difference quantities	Ci: Lower limit	Ci: Upper limit
Turkey	333	437	−104	290	659
Greece	1,059	919	140	638	1,323
Portugal	1,368	1,275	93	894	1,819
Spain	1,925	1,725	200	1,223	2,431
Ireland	1,473	1,642	−169	1,159	2,324
New Zealand	2,092	2,055	37	1,463	2,886
Finland	2,355	2,046	309	1,456	2,876
Sweden	2,157	2,304	−147	1,639	3,237
United Kingdom	2,328	2,520	−192	1,793	3,542
Australia	2,733	2,546	187	1,813	3,574
Netherlands	2,842	2,579	263	1,836	3,622
Italy	3,008	2,712	296	1,928	3,817
France	4,128	3,143	985	2,204	4,482
Iceland	3,100	3,000	100	2,128	4,231
Austria	3,157	2,890	267	2,056	4,061
Canada	3,020	2,725	295	1,930	3,848
Denmark	2,097	2,803	−706	1,990	3,947
Belgium	3,061	3,054	7	2,169	4,301
Norway	2,702	2,899	−197	2,062	4,077
Japan	3,858	3,842	16	2,637	5,596
Germany	3,076	3,308	−232	2,348	4,659
Switzerland	3,801	3,751	50	2,655	5,298
United States	3,299	3,010	289	1,999	4,533
Luxembourg	3,777	5,641	−1,864	3,934	8,090

A Look at the Method

International comparisons of health expenditures present the same inherent problems as any international comparison (Schieber and Poullier 1990): the data is not comparable, health systems are difficult to assess, especially health outputs or access to care. It is also difficult to allow for the socio-cultural, economic, and medical characteristics of each country. Such differences are certainly not reflected in the calculation of price indices which are then used with caution in the analyses (Gerdtham and Jönsson 1991). For all of these reasons, the transposition of health policies from one country to another is problematic. Other problems and constraints arise with econometric analyses of health expenditures, particularly in relation to per capita GDP. Some of these problems are mentioned below.

First, the relationship between health expenditures and per capita GDP does not reflect care and health needs. Consequently, considerations of efficiency and equity are not included in the analysis (McGuire et al. 1993).

All of the variables in these analyses are economic aggregates. Moreover, health economics has not yet developed macroeconomic theories which could be used specifically to analyze health expenditures (McGuire et al. 1993). This is why the conclusions made in these studies are dependent on the validity of theoretical hypotheses, that are highly restrictive, to the extent that these empirical studies explain macroeconomic variables by micro-economic behaviours (Parkin, McGuire, and Yule 1987; McGuire et al. 1993). For example, care expenditures are presented as a reflection of global demand for care expressed in terms of global income (GDP). At the macroeconomic level, care expenditures are determined by a market through the adjustment of global supply of and demand for care and not solely by the consumer's willingness to pay.

Furthermore, with respect to interpretation, these studies concentrate on the effects of individual income (and no longer global income) on global expenditures (income elasticity of expenditures) or on quantities of care (income elasticity of demand). As a result, any attempt to explain global expenditures by individual behaviour presents significant aggregation problems that can only be resolved by making assumptions about the properties of the taste structures of consumers as a whole, such as additivity. Numerous studies have also shown that, in terms of microeconomics, individual income has a limited ability to explain the level of care expenditures, notably by the existence of health insurance. Moreover, this elasticity is calculated in relation to per capita GDP, an indicator which assumed an equal distribution of income between members of a country's population since it is calculated from an average (Parkin, McGuire, and Yule 1987).

The use of cross-sectional studies—and particularly those dealing with groups of countries—to determine income elasticity has proven inappropriate unless the health systems are homogeneous (Murillo, Piatecki, and

Saez 1993). In effect, since the definitions of care expenditures vary from country to country, as do the variables, the same relationships are not being measured in all of the countries.

CONCLUSION

It would appear at first glance to be difficult to measure on a comparable basis both the level of health expenditures and the change in such expenditures. In Canada, the ratio of health expenditures to GDP varies widely from year to year. In 1993, this ratio was among the highest (10.1 percent). However, the increases noted do not appear to have come about as a result of an acceleration in the growth of health expenditures.

The study showed that wealthier countries have higher care expenditures and consume more in terms of quantity of care. For Canada, which had a per capita GDP of $19,271 PPP (ranking ninth) in 1993, real health expenditures per capita were $1,971 PPP (ranking fourth), while quantities of care consumed were $3,020 PPP (health)(ranking tenth).

Canada has the highest price of care (0.65) behind the United States. Statistical analyses conducted in 1993 on all OECD countries revealed that the countries consuming large quantities of care had high expenditures on care and that countries with a high relative price of care, care expenditures were also high. The counterbalancing effect of prices no longer applies: an increase in prices will not be entirely offset by a decrease in the quantity of care consumed. In Canada, the high relative price of care is not entirely offset by a decrease in the quantity of care consumed, which explains the country's relatively high real care expenditures.

After correcting for differences in per capita GDP and relative prices of care, Canada is not far off the other OECD countries in terms of quantity of care consumed. Among all of the countries, Luxembourg is the only one in which the quantities of care consumed are significantly below the expected levels.

Caution is warranted in interpreting these results. Major problems in the area of methodology (such as calculating price indices) and theory (particularly in terms of the level of aggregation of the analysis) must be taken into consideration when using the results.

Delphine Arweiler *is a doctoral student in public health at the University of Montreal. The subject of her thesis is the conceptualization of health in economics. She is also working on the ethical aspects of economic theories, and on the funding and organization of the health care system.*

BIBLIOGRAPHY

GERDTHAM, U. G., and B. JÖNSSON. 1991. Price and quantity in international comparisons of health care expenditures. *Applied Economics* 23: 1519–1528.

GILBERT, M., and I. B. KRAVIS. 1954. *An International Comparison of National Products and the Purchasing Power Parities of Currencies.* Paris: OECD.

HENDERSON, J. M., and R. C. QUANDT. 1972. *Microéconomie. Formulation mathématique élémentaire.* Paris: Dunod.

KRAVIS, I. B., A. W. HESTON, and R. SUMMERS. 1982. *World Product and Income. International Comparisons of Real Gross Product.* Baltimore (MD): Johns Hopkins University Press.

McGUIRE, A., D. PARKIN, D. HUGHES, and K. GERARD. 1993. Econometric analysis of national health expenditures: Can positive economics help answer normative questions? *Health Economics* 2: 113–126.

MURILLO, C., C. PIATECKI, and M. SAEZ. 1993. Health care expenditure and income in Europe. *Health Economics* 2: 127–138.

OECD. 1995. *Health Data.* Paris: Organization for Economic Cooperation and Development.

PARKIN, D., A. McGUIRE, and B. YULE. 1987. Aggregate health care expenditure and national income: Is health care a luxury good? *Journal of Health Economics* 6: 109–127.

SAEZ, M., and C. MURILLO. 1994. Shared features in prices: Income and price elasticities for health care expenditure. *Health Economics* 3: 267–279.

SCHIEBER, G. J., and J. P. POULLIER. 1990. Comparaisons internationales des dépenses de santé: un survol. *OECD: Les systèmes de santé à la recherche d'efficacité* (International comparisons of health expenditures: An overview. In *OECD: Health care systems and efficiency*). Paris: OECD. pp. 9–16.

WARD, M. 1985. *Parités de pouvoir d'achat et dépenses réelles dans les pays de l'OCDE (Purchasing power parities and real expenditures in OECD countries).* Paris: OECD.

APPENDICES

APPENDIX 1

The Variables

Per Capita Gross Domestic Product (GDP/Cap.) in $

$$\text{GDP/cap. \$} = \frac{\text{GDP/cap. in national currency}}{\text{rate of exchange (national currency/\$1)}}$$

The gross domestic product is defined as the sum of the final consumption of households, investments (gross aggregate of fixed capital plus stock fluctuations) and exports, from which imports are subtracted (OECD 1995). The GDP includes all economic activity within a country, while the GNP includes all economic activity relating to the country.

Purchasing Power Parity (PPP)

Purchasing power parity is an international price index calculated by comparing the prices of identical goods in various countries (Ward 1985). It indicates the rate at which one currency must be converted into another currency to be able to purchase an equivalent basket of goods and services in the two countries (Ward 1985).

The PPP in currency j in the unit of account chosen is equal to:

$$\text{PPP}_j = \frac{\Sigma\, P_{ij}\, Q_{ij}}{\Sigma\, \pi i\, Q_{ij}}$$

where π_i = average international price of good i in the unit of account chosen;

Q_{ij} = quantity of goods sold in the currency of country j;

P_{ij} = price of good i sold in the currency of country j (Ward 1985).

Per Capita Gross Domestic Product (GDP/Cap.) in Real Value (Purchasing Power Parity of GDP)

$$\text{GDP/cap.} \atop \text{(real value)} = \frac{\text{GDP/cap. in national currency}}{\text{PPP in national currency/\$1}}$$

In this case, the GDP is expressed in terms of volume, estimated at market prices, the effects of inflation and monetary fluctuations in general having been neutralized by dividing the GDP by an international price index.

Comparative Price Level of the Dollar for Final Expenditures Attributed to the GDP

$$\text{Price level} = \frac{\text{PPP}}{\text{exchange rate}} * 100$$

The price level of each country is a comparative price for a basket of goods and services representative of the GDPs of all of the OECD countries.

Relative Prices of Health Expenditures Attributed to the GDP

$$\text{Relative price of care} = \frac{\text{PPP(health)}}{\text{PPP(GDP)}}$$

This gives the price of care in relation to the price of a representative basket of goods of national consumption. If the relative price is greater than 1, the price of health is higher than that of a representative basket of goods.

Health Expenditures

Total health expenditures (HE) can be defined as:

$$HE_{ik} = Q_{ik} * P_{ik} = N_{jk} * Y_{ik}$$

where P_{ik} = average price per unit of type i care offered;

Q_{ik} = quantities of various types of care i offered;

N_{jk} = number of people earning various types j of income by supplying care;

Y_{ik} = average level of income earned by supplying care (Evans 1984).

In *Health Data*, total health expenditures are composed of (OECD 1995):
– final consumption of medical care by households;
– health care supplied by the public sector including expenditures for communities and special public health programs;
– investments in hospitals, clinics, and consultation centres;
– administrative costs;
– financing of research and development programs;
– company physicians;
– expenditures by volunteer organizations, private insurance and rehabilitation institutions.

Health Expenditures in Real Value or in PPP (GDP)

$$\text{Health expenditures (real value GDP)} = \frac{\text{health expenditures in national currency}}{\text{PPP in national currency}/\$1}$$

Real health expenditures or expenditures by volume estimated at market prices measures the opportunity cost of care, the effects of inflation and monetary fluctuations in general having been neutralized by dividing the expenditures by an international price index, in this case the PPP(GDP).

Health Expenditures in PPP (Health) or Weighted Quantity of Care

$$\text{Weighted quantity of care} = \frac{\text{health expenditures in national currency}}{\text{PPP(health)}}$$

By using health expenditures in PPP(health), we are always measuring the volume of resources allocated to the health sector but in terms of quantity of care per capita.

APPENDIX 2

Price and Income Elasticities

The income elasticity of demand is used to measure the variation in quantities demanded of a good l when the consumer's income increases one unit:

$$\mu_l = \frac{\partial \log q_l}{\partial \log y} \quad \text{(for a good 1, q: quantity and y: income)}$$

$\mu_l > 0$, the expenditure for q_1 increases with an increase in individual income.

$\mu_l = 0$, the expenditure for q_1 does not change with respect to individual income.

$\mu_l < 0$, the expenditure for q_1 decreases with an increase in individual income.

The price elasticity of demand is used to measure the variation in the quantity demanded of a good l by the consumer when the price increases by a unit.

$$e_{11} = \frac{\partial (\log q_1)}{\partial (\log p_1)} = \frac{p_1}{q_1} * \frac{\partial q_1}{\partial p_1} \quad \text{(for a good 1, p: price and q: quantity)}$$

$e_{11} > -1$, consumer spending for good q_1 increases with the price p_1.

$e_{11} = -1$, spending is constant regardless of p_1.

$e_{11} < -1$, consumer spending decreases with an increase in p_1 (Henderson and Quandt 1972).

The elasticities with respect to expenditure are also used. Expenditures substitute for quantities in the elasticity formulae.

APPENDIX 3

Figures and Bar graphs

Figure 1

Change in GDP 1979–93

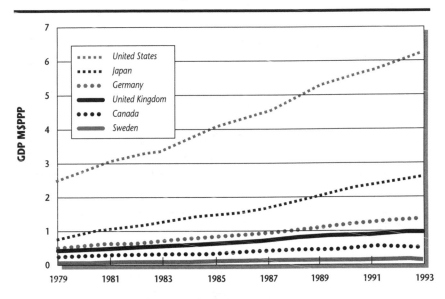

Figure 2

Change in health expenditures 1979–93

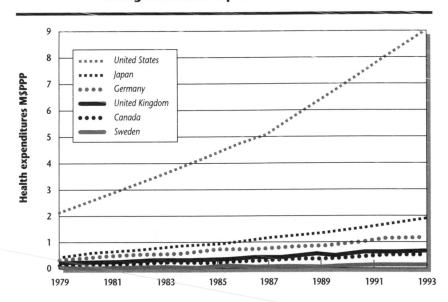

Figure 3

Growth rate of GDP and health expenditures in Canada 1986–93

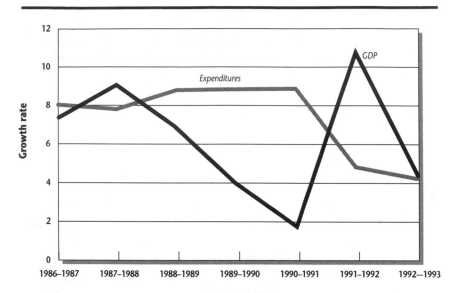

Figure 4

Price and GDP/cap. 1993

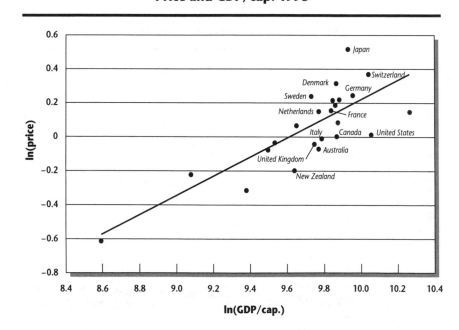

Figure 5

Relative price of care and GDP

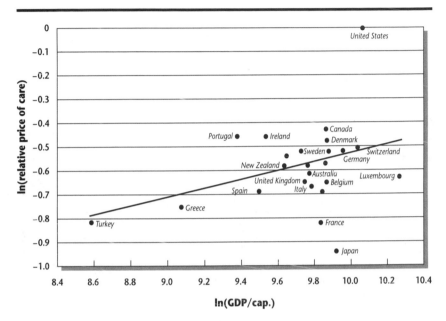

Figure 6

Health expenditures and GDP/cap. 1993

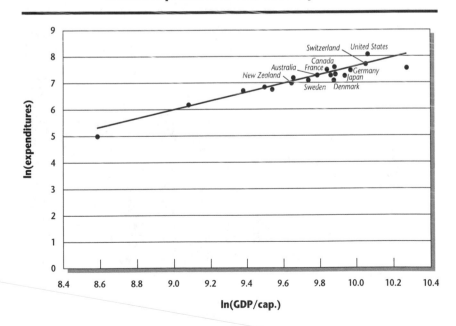

Figure 7

Health quantities and GDP/cap. 1993

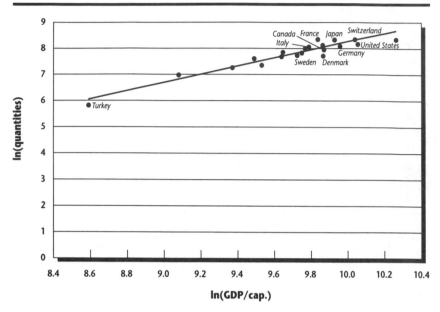

Bar graph 1

GDP/cap. 1993 ($PPP)

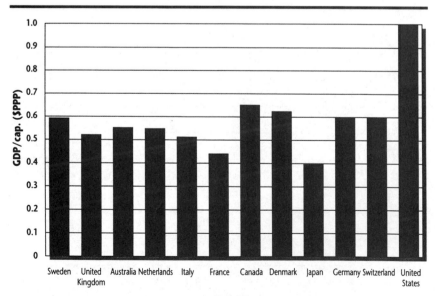

Bar graph 2

Price level (GDP) 1993

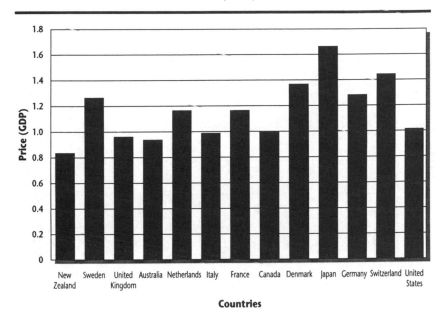

Countries

Bar graph 3

Relative price of care 1993

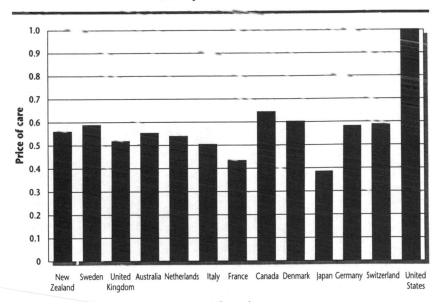

Countries

Bar graph 4

Health expenditures 1993 ($U.S.)

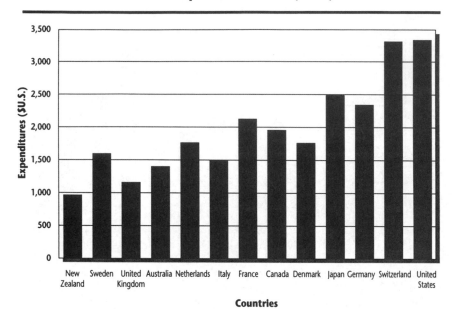

Bar graph 5

Health expenditures 1993 ($PPP)

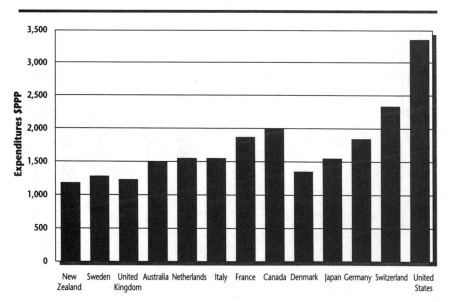

Bar graph 6

Health expenditures 1993 ($PPP health)

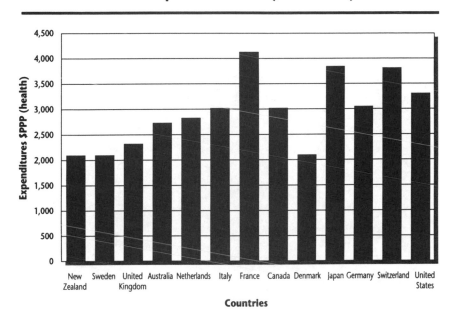

Bar graph 7

Health expenditures/GDP 1993 (%)

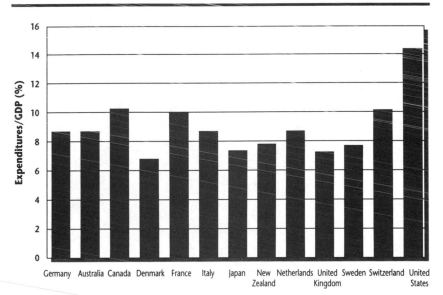

The Impact of Health Care Infrastructures and Human Resources on Health Expenditures

MARC-ANDRÉ FOURNIER

Doctoral Student in Public Health
Interdisciplinary Research Group on Health
Faculty of Medicine
University of Montreal

PUZZLING ISSUE NO. 1

Canada does not have a significantly greater supply of physicians and hospital beds than other industrialized countries, yet Canada's health expenditures are among the highest in the developed world. A more complete picture of human resource and infrastructure configurations is needed to shed light on the mix and intensity of health system resources, including comparisons of GP/specialist ratios, supply of nurses, and acute care vs. other institutional care and their relationship with costs.

TABLE OF CONTENTS

Introduction 257

Breakdown of Expenditures and Resource Configurations 258

Breakdown of Expenditures between the Main Sectors 258

Hospital Services 263

Human Resources 268

    Personnel 268

    Level of Remuneration 268

**Configurations of Countries Successful and Unsuccessful
in Controlling Expenditures** 275

Comparisons between the Two Groups of Countries 275

Organizational Strategies Relating to Physicians 278

Conclusion 282

Bibliography 284

LIST OF TABLES

Table 1   Comparative breakdown of health expenditures
(% of total spending). Selected OECD countries.
Last year available (1988–1993) 259

Table 2   Health expenditures per capita ($PPP) selected
OECD countries, by type of expenditure, 1988 261

Table 3   Funding and characteristics of hospital sector
(all hospitals) 264

Table 4   Resources and performance of acute care hospitals (AC) ... 265

Table 5   Ambulatory physicians: Costs, level of activity,
and utilization 267

Table 6   Human resources in health. Selected OECD countries.
Last year available (1988–1993) 269

Table 7   Income levels ($PPP) of physicians, nurses, and health
            workers compared with the average income of workers
            in the country as a whole. Last year available. Data
            adjusted for 1991 273

Table 8   Relative position (country/mean) of selected countries
            in which health expenditures/GDP are the highest
            or the lowest; selected indicators 276

Table 9   Characteristics of the most and the least successful
            countries in terms of control of entry in system
            and method of payment of physicians (in early '90s) 279

Table 10   Current health expenditures ($PPP), selected OECD
            countries, by type of expenditure, 1988 280

INTRODUCTION

A number of studies, including some conducted for the Forum, show that Canada ranks second among OECD countries in terms of health expenditures as a percentage of the GDP, but that the number of beds and physicians per 1,000 inhabitants compares with the average of the other countries (Arweiler 1998; Brousselle 1998). Considerable differences in the regulation, organization, and funding of health systems have also been mentioned as factors explaining the variations in costs and performance. These differences also make it difficult to make comparisons between countries in order to understand the key factors contributing to these variations.

In spite of these problems, we must determine whether the infrastructure configurations of the health system (mix, intensity, and cost of human and material resources) can explain the differences in health expenditures from country to country. We must also try to identify the regulatory mechanisms that would ensure greater control of the system's costs and performance.

This study examines these issues by comparing the hospital and human resource allocations of various OECD countries. The first part of the study is descriptive. Data is presented on (1) the breakdown of health expenditures between the various sectors of activity, (2) the resources and use of hospital sector services, (3) the importance of human resources (physicians, nurses, and health workers as a whole), and (4) the income levels of these three categories of personnel. The main purpose of this part is to compare Canada with the average of certain OECD countries in the study. The second part of the study analyzes the data by identifying, from among the countries in the study, the four with the highest levels of expenditures in relation to the GDP, and the four with the lowest levels of expenditures. The results will then be considered from the perspective that the dynamics of the health system depend, to a large extent, on the organizational and regulatory mechanisms controlling the practice of medicine and especially, access to the profession and physician payment configurations.

The data is taken from the *Health Data* database, version 3.6 (1995). A number of other sources have been used to offset the shortcomings of the *Health Data* database (Health Canada 1995,1996).

In general, the data applies to 1993. When data for that year was unavailable, the previous year's data was used and, if necessary, adjusted to ensure its comparability with that of the other countries.

Data from 17countries was included in the study. We excluded those countries in which the health expenditures' portion of the GDP is low or for which there was little data available in *Health Data.*

BREAKDOWN OF EXPENDITURES AND RESOURCE CONFIGURATIONS

Breakdown of Expenditures between the Main Sectors

It is difficult to make international comparisons because of the differences in the way in which health systems are organized and expenditures are accounted for, and in the availability of data. As many authors have indicated, this data must be used with caution.

The *Health Data* database has certain major limitations in terms of the distribution of health expenditures (table 1). For example, the "acute care or short-term care hospitals" category should include only those costs for patients hospitalized in this type of facility. However, several countries (Australia, Canada, Sweden, and the United Kingdom) include expenditures for outpatients in this category. In Austria and Belgium, a significant proportion of the public funding is not included. In the case of Canada, the acute/short-term care hospitals category (38 percent of expenditures) includes the expenditures of all hospitals (long-term care hospitals, psychiatric hospitals, etc.); the "nursing homes" category (10.2 percent of expenditures) covers this type of facility and others (rehabilitation, substance abuse, etc.); the "all hospitals" category (48.2 percent of expenditures) is the sum of the previous two categories. The definition of the "nursing homes" category varies from country to country. In virtually all countries, the "acute care" category includes expenditures for chronic care patients hospitalized in these hospitals, and this proportion can vary considerably from one country to another. Lastly, the remuneration of physicians is often included in hospital expenditures when the physicians who work in these facilities are employees, but not when they are paid on a fee-for-service basis (as in Canada and the United States). For these two countries, accepted national statistics would show that the expenditures allocated to medical services for ambulatory care correspond, in fact, to the total remuneration of physicians (Health Canada 1996; Rublee and Schneider 1991).

In light of these problems, Rublee and Schneider (1991) validated and harmonized the various categories of expenditures for several OECD countries using 1988 data. Even this data, which appears more coherent, reveals still significant spreads in health expenditures in the various sectors of activity (table 2). The breakdown of expenditures in the Canadian system is virtually the same as the average for the countries as a whole, except for the proportion of expenditures allocated to acute care given to hospitalized patients (all types of hospitals, including physician remuneration) and to medical services for ambulatory care (nonhospitalized patients and visits to private clinics). Hospital expenditures are higher (48.5 percent compared to 43.8 percent), while those for ambulatory care are lower (10.6 percent compared to 15.5 percent).

Table 1

Comparative breakdown of health expenditures (% of total spending)
Selected OECD countries. Last year available (1988-1993)

	% exp./ GDP	Hospitals		Ambulatory	Ambulatory physicians	Nursing homes	Home	Drugs
		Total	Acute care					
United States	14.10	44.80	32.50	31.70	19.40	7.9	2.40	8.50
Canada	10.20	48.20	38.00	21.10	14.20	10.2	1.00	12.70
Switzerland	9.90	51.40	33.10	38.10	16.80	13.4	–	7.80
France	9.80	44.40	43.40	27.50	11.90	1.1	1.30	16.80
Austria	9.30	29.90	–	21.30	16.20	–	–	10.70
Finland	8.80	43.60	17.20	34.90	–	–	0.70	10.70
Netherlands	8.70	54.40	32.40	25.90	9.70	10.2	–	10.90
Germany	8.60	37.60	–	26.10	16.90	8.7	1.20	18.50
Australia	8.50	45.80	34.60	28.20	19.20	7.7	0.50	9.60
Italy	8.50	49.00	–	30.60	20.30	–	1.20	18.00
Belgium	8.30	35.20	–	37.00	–	–	–	16.70
Norway	8.20	69.90	36.60	23.60	12.20	19.4	–	10.80
New Zealand	7.70	55.90	38.10	6.90	11.20	3.2	–	16.00
Sweden	7.50	–	–	–	13.50	–	–	12.70
Japan	7.30	29.20	–	40.50	33.50	3.3	1.90	1.70
United Kingdom	7.10	43.00	29.80	–	–	–	3.00	14.90
Denmark	6.70	58.70	40.90	34.30	–	–	2.70	11.30
Mean	7.95	43.51	31.28	26.40	15.05	7.72	1.35	11.75
Standard deviation	0.99	10.61	6.91	8.44	6.05	5.37	0.81	4.19

Table 1 (cont.)

	% exp./GDP	Hospitals		Ambulatory	Ambulatory physicians	Nursing homes	Home	Drugs
		Total	Acute care					
				Relative index (country/mean)				
United States	1.28	1.11	1.21	0.80	0.94	1.32	0.74	1.08
Canada	1.28	1.11	1.21	0.80	0.94	1.32	0.74	1.08
Switzerland	1.25	1.18	1.06	1.44	1.12	1.74	–	0.66
France	1.23	1.02	1.39	1.04	0.79	0.14	0.96	1.43
Austria	1.17	0.69	–	0.81	1.08	–	–	0.91
Finland	1.11	1.00	0.55	1.32	0.00	–	0.52	0.91
Netherlands	1.09	1.25	1.04	0.98	0.64	1.32	–	0.93
Germany	1.08	0.86	–	0.99	1.12	1.13	0.89	1.57
Australia	1.07	1.05	1.11	1.07	1.28	1.00	0.37	0.82
Italy	1.07	1.13	–	1.16	1.35	–	0.89	1.53
Belgium	1.04	0.81	–	1.40	0.00	–	–	1.42
Norway	1.03	1.61	1.17	0.89	0.81	2.51	–	0.92
New Zealand	0.97	1.28	1.22	0.26	0.74	0.41	–	1.36
Sweden	0.94	–	–	–	0.90	–	–	1.08
Japan	0.92	0.67	–	1.53	2.23	0.43	1.41	0.14
United Kingdom	0.89	0.99	0.95	–	0.00	–	2.22	1.27
Denmark	0.84	1.35	1.31	1.30	0.00	–	2.00	0.96
Mean	1.00	1.00	1.00	1.00	1.00	1.00	1.00	1.00
Standard deviation	0.13	0.24	0.21	0.32	0.57	0.66	0.58	0.35

Note: Expenditures cannot be added up by sector since, in some cases, expenditures related to one sector could be accounted for in another (e.g., nursing homes and hospitals).

Table 2

**Health expenditures per capita ($PPP)[a],
selected OECD countries, by type of expenditure, 1988**

	% exp./GDP	Total	Hospitals[b]	Ambulatory physicians	Drugs[c]	Long-term care	Dental services	Medical aids and appliances	Other services
United States	14.1	2,007	868	419	170	193	119	82	156
Canada	10.2	1,495	725	159	183	184	86	59	99
Switzerland	9.9	1,385	679	232	145	117	121	49	42
France	9.8	1,158	531	186	201	57	75	48	60
Austria	9.3	999	460	175	93	125	93	29	24
Netherlands	8.7	1,062	461	108	98	197	54	52	92
Germany	8.6	1,201	408	194	198	93	156	87	65
Italy[d]	8.5	997	425	242	180	73	–	45	32
Belgium	8.3	918	324	194	148	78	32	47	95
Sweden	7.5	1,330	623	137	90	213	77	52	138
Japan	7.3	989	326	156	173	108	55	46	125
United Kingdom	7.1	856	406	117	116	111	36	19	51
Denmark	6.7	1,091	552	80	83	212	51	36	77
Mean	**8.92**	**1,191.38**	**522**	**185**	**144**	**135**	**73**	**50**	**81**

Table 2 (cont.)

	% exp./ GDP	Total	Hospitals[b]	Ambulatory physicians	Drugs[c]	Long-term care	Dental services	Medical aids and appliances	Other services
			Breakdown of expenditures (%)						
United States	99.95	43.20	20.88	8.47	9.62	5.93	4.09	7.77
Canada	**100.01**	**48.50**	**10.64**	**12.24**	**12.31**	**5.75**	**3.95**	**6.62**
Switzerland	99.97	49.00	16.75	10.47	8.45	8.74	3.54	3.03
France	99.95	45.80	16.06	17.36	4.92	6.48	4.15	5.18
Austria	99.95	46.00	17.52	9.31	12.51	9.31	2.90	2.40
Netherlands	99.99	43.40	10.17	9.23	18.55	5.08	4.90	8.66
Germany	100.00	33.97	16.15	16.49	7.74	12.99	7.24	5.41
Italy[d]	100.00	42.63	24.27	18.05	7.32	–	4.51	3.21
Belgium	100.00	35.29	21.13	16.12	8.50	3.49	5.12	10.35
Sweden	100.00	46.84	10.30	6.77	16.02	5.79	3.91	10.38
Japan	100.00	32.96	15.77	17.49	10.92	5.56	4.65	12.64
United Kingdom	100.00	47.43	13.67	13.55	12.97	4.21	2.22	5.96
Denmark	100.00	50.60	7.33	7.61	19.43	4.67	3.30	7.06
Mean	**100.00**	**43.83**	**15.49**	**12.13**	**11.37**	**6.17**	**4.20**	**6.82**
Standard deviation	0.02	5.64	4.75	4.00	4.24	2.53	1.17	2.98

Source: Beratungsgesellschaft für angewandte Systemforschung (BASYS) Ltd.; Rublee and Schneider 1991.

[a] Purchasing Power Parity (PPP) is an international index which express the rate at which one currency should be converted to purchase the same set of good and services in different countries.

[b] Includes physician services provided in hospitals.

[c] Excludes drugs prescribed in hospitals.

[d] Ambulatory physician services included dental services.

Hospital Services[1]

Canada has the fewest number of private hospitals after the United Kingdom: the percentage of private beds is 3.6 percent compared to the average of 3.9 percent (table 3). On the other hand, private funding is relatively high. Although the proportion of private funding for hospitals is lower than the average (14.4 percent compared to 22.4 percent), Canada still ranks eighth of 16.

Table 4 shows that, in relation to the average for the countries as a whole, the proportion of acute care beds in hospitals in Canada is slightly higher than the average (63.1 percent of all beds compared to 57.1 percent), but the number of beds per 1,000 inhabitants in these acute care hospitals is lower than the average (3.9 compared to 4.7). However, the length of stay and bed occupancy rate are higher.

As for the use of hospital services, in Canada, the percentage of the population hospitalized (in theory, including acute care) is lower than the average (13.8 percent compared to 16.9 percent). This lower use of hospital services does not appear to be explained by the use of ambulatory care services since, as we saw in tables 1 and 2, the percentage of ambulatory care expenditures is lower in Canada. Furthermore, table 5 shows that the number of contacts per person with a physician is close to the average. However, these results are difficult to interpret because of differences in data collection methods in the various countries and the reservations that must be exercised with respect to the comparability of the data. Physician performance is also difficult to interpret because of the vast differences in how services are accounted for from one country to another.

These statistics would therefore indicate that, compared to the average of the other developed countries, Canada has a relatively large hospital system which belongs almost exclusively to the public sector, with a measurable share of private funding, a relatively low number of acute care beds but a slightly high length of stay, and an underdeveloped ambulatory care sector. Some of these differences can be explained by demographics (Canada's population is younger than that of most of these countries).[2]

---

1. The *Health Data* data on hospital resources (number of beds and staff) and on certain features of performance and use of hospital services is more reliable than that on costs. This is because such factual data is easier to identify and is often required for administrative purposes. The data on acute care (or short-term care) hospitals covers hospitals which deliver mainly acute care but includes, in most countries, chronic care patients hospitalized in such facilities. The percentage of these patients varies significantly from one country to another. In some instances, it has not been included in the statistics.

2. For example, in a study of medical services, Contandriopoulos et al. (1989) showed that by standardizing the costs of medical services for age and gender, and by using the level of use by age and gender in Quebec in 1986, the number of physicians required in most European countries would be 7 percent to 11 percent higher than in Quebec and Canada.

Table 3

Funding and characteristics of hospital sector (all hospitals)

	% exp./ GDP	% private beds	% private funding	Hosp. exp.: % AC/ total
United States	14.10	81.60	42.80	72.50
Canada	**10.20**	**3.60**	**14.40**	**78.80**
Switzerland	9.90	–	28.70	64.50
France	9.80	36.00	9.40	97.60
Austria	9.30	30.00	64.50	–
Finland	8.80	4.90	7.70	39.50
Netherlands	8.70	–	15.50	59.50
Germany	8.60	47.80	14.90	–
Australia	8.50	39.10	24.30	75.60
Italy	8.50	20.50	14.60	–
Belgium	8.30	61.80	31.60	–
Norway	8.20	–	0.00	52.30
New Zealand	7.70	35.50	5.00	68.10
Sweden	7.50	8.50	–	–
Japan	7.30	67.30	7.40	–
United Kingdom	7.10	3.50	9.80	69.40
Denmark	6.70	–	0.00	70.00
Mean	**8.78**	**33.85**	**22.35**	**67.98**
Standard deviation	1.64	24.68	16.46	14.21
Relative index (country/mean)				
United States	1.61	2.41	1.91	1.07
Canada	**1.16**	**0.11**	**0.64**	**1.16**
Switzerland	1.13	–	1.28	0.95
France	1.12	1.06	0.42	1.44
Austria	1.06	0.89	2.89	–
Finland	1.00	0.14	0.34	0.58
Netherlands	0.99	–	0.69	0.88
Germany	0.98	1.41	0.67	0.00
Australia	0.97	1.16	1.09	–
Italy	0.97	0.61	0.65	–
Belgium	0.95	1.83	1.41	–
Norway	0.93	–	0.00	0.77
New Zealand	0.88	1.05	0.22	1.00
Sweden	0.85	0.25	–	–
Japan	0.83	1.99	0.33	–
United Kingdom	0.81	0.10	0.44	1.02
Denmark	0.76	–	0.00	1.03
Mean	**1.00**	**1.00**	**1.00**	**1.00**
Standard deviation	0.19	0.73	0.74	0.35

Table 4

Resources and performance of acute care hospitals (AC)

	% exp./ GDP	% AC hosp./ tot. exp.	% beds/ total beds	# beds/ 1,000 pop.	Length of stay	Occupancy rate	% hosp. pop.	# hosp. days p.c.
United States	14.10	32.50	78.40	3.50	7.10	66.20	13.00	0.80
Canada	**10.20**	**38.00**	**63.10**	**3.90**	**8.60**	**78.60**	**13.80**	**1.40**
Switzerland	9.90	33.10	30.80	6.20	12.10	78.70	14.90	1.80
France	9.80	43.40	52.70	5.00	6.50	76.50	21.10	1.40
Austria	9.30	–	57.00	5.40	9.20	78.50	24.00	2.10
Finland	8.80	17.20	42.20	4.60	5.70	70.10	19.10	1.10
Netherlands	8.70	32.40	36.00	4.10	10.40	72.00	10.30	1.10
Germany	8.60	–	70.70	7.20	12.40	85.90	18.50	2.20
Australia	8.50	34.60	48.00	4.40	5.00	75.40	17.40	0.90
Italy	8.50	–	80.20	5.50	–	–	14.90	1.00
Belgium	8.30	–	62.10	4.80	8.00	81.10	17.70	1.40
Norway	8.20	36.60	26.90	3.50	6.80	77.10	13.30	1.10
New Zealand	7.70	38.10	94.00	7.10	–	–	–	–
Sweden	7.50	–	48.50	3.40	5.50	76.20	17.20	0.90
Japan	7.30	–	–	–	–	–	–	–
United Kingdom	7.10	29.80	40.60	2.10	5.10	–	19.10	0.90
Denmark	6.70	40.90	82.20	4.10	6.30	82.80	19.80	1.30
Mean	**8.78**	**34.24**	**57.09**	**4.68**	**7.76**	**76.85**	**16.94**	**1.29**
Standard deviation	1.64	6.61	19.27	1.33	2.38	5.04	3.45	0.42

Table 4 (cont.)

	% exp./ GDP	% AC hosp./ tot. exp.	% beds/ total beds	# beds/ 1,000 pop.	Length of stay	Occupancy rate	% hosp. pop.	# hosp. days p.c.
		Relative index (country/mean)						
United States	1.61	0.95	1.37	0.75	0.91	0.86	0.77	0.62
Canada	1.16	1.11	1.11	0.83	1.11	1.02	0.81	1.08
Switzerland	1.13	0.97	0.54	1.33	1.56	1.02	0.88	1.39
France	1.12	1.27	0.92	1.07	0.84	1.00	1.25	1.08
Austria	1.06	–	1.00	1.16	1.18	1.02	1.42	1.62
Finland	1.00	0.50	0.74	0.98	0.73	0.91	1.13	0.85
Netherlands	0.99	0.95	0.63	0.88	1.34	0.94	0.61	0.85
Germany	0.98	–	1.24	1.54	1.60	1.12	1.09	1.70
Australia	0.97	1.01	0.84	0.94	0.64	0.98	1.03	0.70
Italy	0.97	–	1.40	1.18	–	–	0.88	0.77
Belgium	0.95	–	1.09	1.03	1.03	1.06	1.04	1.08
Norway	0.93	1.07	0.47	0.75	0.88	1.00	0.79	0.85
New Zealand	0.88	1.11	1.65	1.52	–	–	–	0.00
Sweden	0.85	–	0.85	0.73	0.71	0.99	1.02	0.70
Japan	0.83	–	–	–	–	–	–	0.00
United Kingdom	0.81	0.87	0.71	0.45	0.66	–	1.13	0.70
Denmark	0.76	1.19	1.44	0.88	0.81	1.08	1.17	1.01
Mean	1.00	1.00	1.00	1.00	1.00	1.00	1.00	1.00
Standard deviation	0.19	0.19	0.34	0.28	0.31	0.07	0.20	0.44

Table 5

Ambulatory physicians: Costs, level of activity, and utilization

	% exp./ GDP	Phys. exp./ total exp.	# serv./ phys.	# contacts/ person
United States	14.10	19.40	6,735	5.90
Canada	**10.20**	**14.20**	**3,858**	**6.90**
Switzerland	9.90	16.80	–	11.00
France	9.80	11.90	4,748	6.30
Austria	9.30	16.20	3,996	5.10
Finland	8.80	–	1,862	3.30
Netherlands	8.70	9.70	8,551	5.70
Germany	8.60	16.90	–	12.80
Australia	8.50	19.20	4,055	10.60
Italy	8.50	20.30	–	11.00
Belgium	8.30	–	3,210	8.00
Norway	8.20	12.20	–	3.80
New Zealand	7.70	11.20	–	–
Sweden	7.50	13.50	–	3.00
Japan	7.30	33.50	9,100	12.90
United Kingdom	7.10	–	7,089	5.80
Denmark	6.70	–	–	4.40
Mean	**8.78**	**16.54**	**5,320**	**7.28**
Relative index (country/mean)				
United States	1.61	1.17	1.27	0.81
Canada	**1.16**	**0.86**	**0.73**	**0.95**
Switzerland	1.13	1.02	–	1.51
France	1.12	0.72	0.89	0.87
Austria	1.06	0.98	0.75	0.70
Finland	1.00	–	0.35	0.45
Netherlands	0.99	0.59	1.61	0.78
Germany	0.98	1.02	–	1.76
Australia	0.97	1.16	0.76	1.46
Italy	0.97	1.23	–	1.51
Belgium	0.95	–	0.60	1.10
Norway	0.93	0.74	–	0.52
New Zealand	0.88	0.68	–	–
Sweden	0.85	0.82	–	0.41
Japan	0.83	2.03	1.71	1.77
United Kingdom	0.81	–	1.33	0.80
Denmark	0.76	–	–	0.60
Mean	**1.00**	**1.00**	**1.00**	**1.00**
Standard deviation	0.19	0.35	0.43	0.45

Human Resources

Personnel

The data on health personnel must also be interpreted with caution. In some countries, the figures correspond to the number of people, while in others they correspond to full-time equivalents. Also, in certain countries, especially those with a high percentage of private clinics, the number of personnel other than physicians and nurses has been underestimated. Canada, for example, is currently reevaluating its data to include the staff of physicians' private offices (secretary, accountant, etc.). We should point out that we have corrected the data on nurses in Canada and removed assistant nurses from the original *Health Data* data.

Canada is close to the average in terms of the number of physicians, nurses, and other health personnel (table 6) per 1,000 inhabitants. However, nurses represent a higher percentage of health personnel as a whole (38.8 percent compared to 29.2 percent). Canada also has a higher nurses to physicians ratio (3.8 compared to 3.2). On the other hand, in hospitals (acute and chronic care), the ratio of nurses to beds is slightly below the average (0.82 compared to 0.9), while the ratio of the other categories of personnel is higher. As to the breakdown between general practitioners and specialists, this is a more difficult comparison to make with certain countries, especially the Nordic countries, because of differences in how physicians qualify as specialists or "consultants" (Contandriopoulos 1989). Based on these data, however, Canada would appear to have fewer generalists than specialists (1.14 compared to 1.41). If Norway and Denmark are excluded, this difference disappears. In light of these results and given the quality of the data, it is not possible to identify key configurations of intensity and mix of manpower which would set Canada apart from the other countries.

Level of Remuneration

In an effort to compare the cost of labour in the health system and to evaluate the impact of income level on the percentage of the GDP allocated to health, we compared the average income (in $PPP) of physicians, nurses, and health workers as a whole to the average income of workers in the country as a whole.

Table 6

Human resources in health
Selected OECD countries. Last year available (1988–1993)

	% GDP	#/1,000 pop.				Ratio		% health personnel		#/bed	
		Health personnel	Nurses	Physicians	Pers. other than nurses and physicians	GP/ spec.	Nurses/ physicians	Nurses	Physicians as a whole	Personnel	Nurses
United States	14.10	31.40	7.00	2.30	22.10	0.19	3.07	22.70	7.40	3.61	1.57
Canada	10.20	24.38	8.10	2.20	14.08	1.14	3.80	38.80	9.00	2.80	0.82
Switzerland	9.90	50.19	13.80	3.00	33.39	0.56	4.68	26.70	5.90	2.04	1.04
France	9.80	28.83	5.50	2.80	20.53	1.02	2.01	19.10	9.50	1.16	0.41
Austria	9.30	–	7.80	2.30	–	0.91	3.31	–	–	0.85	0.66
Finland	8.80	35.53	11.30	2.60	21.63	0.75	4.22	31.80	7.50	2.10	0.70
Netherlands	8.70	23.48	–	2.50	–	0.72	–	–	11.30	2.24	0.87
Germany	8.60	23.96	5.20	3.20	15.56	0.72	1.70	20.90	12.20	1.31	0.54
Australia	8.50	30.82	8.50	2.20	20.12	1.91	3.78	26.90	7.10	1.90	1.35
Italy	8.50	17.97	4.10	1.70	12.17	–	2.47	22.60	9.20	1.43	0.60
Belgium	8.30	21.02	–	3.60	–	1.02	1.98	32.80	17.10	1.46	0.82
Norway	8.20	43.69	13.70	3.20	26.79	5.19	4.24	32.20	5.50	2.78	0.87
New Zealand	7.70	16.81	7.30	2.00	7.51	1.25	3.74	45.50	11.20	2.00	1.20
Sweden	7.50	43.16	9.90	3.00	30.26	0.26	3.31	22.90	6.90	–	1.04
Japan	7.30	12.75	6.40	1.70	4.65	–	3.76	47.00	12.80	0.80	0.42
United Kingdom	7.10	20.61	4.30	1.50	14.81	–	3.12	19.40	7.10	3.27	1.63
Denmark	6.70	22.93	6.70	2.80	13.43	4.16	2.40	29.10	12.10	3.10	0.99
Mean	8.78	27.97	7.97	2.51	18.36	1.41	3.22	29.23	9.49	2.05	0.91
Standard deviation	1.64	10.26	2.94	0.58	7.92	1.41	0.87	8.59	3.01	0.84	0.35

Table 6 (cont.)

	% GDP	#/1,000 pop.				Ratio		% health personnel		#/bed	
		Health personnel	Nurses	Physicians	Pers. other than nurses	GP/ spec.	Nurses/ physicians	Nurses	Physicians as a whole	Personnel	Nurses
		Relative index (country/mean)									
United States	8.60	1.12	0.88	0.92	1.20	0.14	0.95	0.78	0.78	1.76	1.72
Canada	8.50	0.87	1.02	0.88	0.77	0.81	1.18	1.33	0.95	1.36	0.90
Switzerland	9.30	1.79	1.73	1.20	1.82	0.40	1.45	0.91	0.62	0.99	1.14
France	8.30	1.03	0.69	1.12	1.12	0.72	0.62	0.65	1.00	0.57	0.45
Austria	10.20	–	0.98	0.92	–	0.64	1.03	–	–	0.41	0.72
Finland	6.70	1.27	1.42	1.04	1.18	0.53	1.31	1.09	0.79	1.02	0.77
Netherlands	8.80	0.84	–	1.00	–	0.51	–	–	1.19	1.09	0.95
Germany	9.80	0.86	0.65	1.28	0.85	0.51	0.53	0.72	1.29	0.64	0.59
Australia	8.50	1.10	1.07	0.88	1.10	1.35	1.17	0.92	0.75	0.93	1.48
Italy	7.30	0.64	0.51	0.68	0.66		0.77	0.77	0.97	0.70	0.66
Belgium	8.20	0.75	–	1.44	–	0.72	0.61	1.12	1.80	0.71	0.90
Norway	7.70	1.56	1.72	1.28	1.46	3.67	1.31	1.10	0.58	1.35	0.95
New Zealand	8.70	0.60	0.92	0.80	0.41	0.88	1.16	1.56	1.18	0.97	1.31
Sweden	7.10	1.54	1.24	1.20	1.65	0.18	1.03	0.78	0.73	–	1.14
Japan	7.50	0.46	0.80	0.68	0.25	–	1.17	1.61	1.35	0.39	0.46
United Kingdom	9.90	0.74	0.54	0.60	0.81	–	0.97	0.66	0.75	1.59	1.78
Denmark	14.10	0.82	0.84	1.12	0.73	2.94	0.75	1.00	1.28	1.51	1.08
Mean		1.00	1.00	1.00	1.00	1.00	1.00	1.00	1.00	1.00	1.00
Standard deviation		0.37	0.37	0.23	0.43	0.99	0.27	0.29	0.32	0.41	0.39

Table 7 shows that the gross income of physicians in Canada is 35 percent higher than that of their colleagues in the other countries as a whole ($96,513 PPP compared to $71,433 PPP).[3] Although the income of Canadian physicians is almost half that of their colleagues in the United States, it still ranks fourth. The spread between nurses' salaries is less but Canada ranks second, after the United States, with an income that is 15 percent higher than the average ($29,802 compared to $25,856). Unfortunately, there is no data on the income of health workers as a whole in Canada. It can be assumed, however, that this figure too would be higher than the average, but probably to a lesser degree.

Table 7 can also be used to evaluate the relative income level in the health sector compared to the economy as a whole and workers in each country. We can see, for example, that the GDP per capita in Canada is only slightly higher than the average GDP for the 15 countries included in the sample, while the average income of Canadian workers in the economy as a whole is 13 percent higher than the average. Canada ranks sixth. The income levels of all workers are higher in Canada, but the ratio of the income of physicians and nurses to the average salary for the country is much higher than that of the countries as a whole: in the case of physicians, 3.6 times higher compared to 2.8, and in the case of nurses, 1.11 times higher compared to 0.95. Only four countries have a higher ratio than Canada for physicians and only one is higher in the case of nurses.

A relative index of these ratios can be used to measure the spread in the variation in the ratios of each country compared to the average. Consequently, the Canadian ratio between physicians and workers as a whole is 28 percent higher than the average (3.2/2.8) and that of nurses is 17 percent higher (1.11/0.95). In other words, if Canada wanted the gap between the income of its physicians and workers as a whole to be the same as that of the average of the countries studied, then it would have to reduce the income of its physicians by 28 percent. But to achieve the level of the United States, physicians' salaries would have to be increased by 54 percent (82–28).

---

3. The fact that in countries such as Canada and the United States, the payment of physicians in private practice also includes the operating expenses for their offices does not impact significantly on the results. In Quebec, incomes from private practice represent 39 percent of all physicians' incomes and, according to the Fédération des médecins omnipraticiens, operating costs would account for 30 percent to 35 percent of incomes or 13.7 percent of total incomes. It should be pointed out that the Ontario Medical Association estimates private practice operating expenses at 38 percent. If this percentage is removed from the figures for Canada, the United States and a few other countries, the average also declines, therefore the spread between Canada and the average for other countries remains practically unchanged.

The cost of labour in general, and especially in the health field, therefore appears to be one of the reasons why health expenditures account for a large percentage of the GDP. A rough estimate of this cost can be obtained by considering that expenditures for physicians represent 15 percent of health expenditures and consequently, 1.5 percent of the GDP (15 percent × 10.2 percent). If the ratio between the income of Canadian physicians and workers was to be lowered to the average for the OECD countries as a whole, the income for Canadian physicians would have to be reduced by 28 percent, which represents 0.4 percent of the GDP (28 percent × 1.5 percent). The impact on the GDP of the cost of nurses and the other categories of workers can be estimated by taking the case of Quebec where public health expenditures account for 7.2 percent of the GDP (6.9 percent in Canada). Expenditures on personnel account for 78 percent of total public health expenditures, of which 28 percent is spent on nurses.[4] The labour cost of nurses therefore represents 1.6 percent of the GDP (7.2 × .78 × .28); the labour cost of the other categories of workers represents 4.0 percent (7.2 × .78 × .72). Therefore, reducing the income of nurses by 17 percent would reduce the percentage of the GDP allocated to health expenditures by less than 0.3 percent (1.6 × .17); for the other categories of personnel, the reduction would be 0.7 percent (4 × .17) if we apply the same rate to them as to the nurses.

To summarize, these estimates show that, in relation to the average of the other developed countries, the spread of income between health sector workers in Canada could account for less than 10 percent of health expenditures (or 1 percent of the GDP), while the number and mix of personnel would have little impact. Since health expenditures in Canada are 1.4 percent higher than the average for other countries in terms of their percentage of the GDP (10.2 percent compared to 8.8 percent), part of this gap would appear to be attributable to causes other than the level of remuneration or mix and number of personnel, as mentioned in the previous section.

---

4. Personal conversation with André Matte, Ministère de la Santé et des Services sociaux, Quebec.

Table 7

Income levels ($PPP) of physicians, nurses, and health workers compared with the average income of workers in the country as a whole. Last year available. Data adjusted for 1991

	% exp./ GDP	GDP/p.c. 1993 ($PPP)	Workers (country as a whole)	Average income ($PPP)			Ratio on average salary		
				Physicians	Nurses	Health workers	Physicians	Nurses	Health workers
United States	14.10	23,358	33,019	168,539	33,349	31,038	5.10	1.01	0.94
Canada	10.20	19,271	26,849	96,513	29,802	–	3.59	1.11	–
Switzerland	9.90	23,033	32,500	128,224	–	–	3.95	–	–
France	9.80	18,764	27,576	56,351	–	–	2.04	–	–
Austria	9.30	–	–	–	–	–	–	–	–
Finland	8.80	15,530	23,600	40,096	19,116	19,824	1.70	0.81	0.84
Netherlands	8.70	17,602	27,816	–	–	23,365	–	–	0.84
Germany	8.60	21,163	26,060	101,661	–	16,157	3.90	–	0.62
Australia	8.50	17,555	22,155	59,244	25,035	–	2.67	1.13	–
Italy	8.50	17,865	27,340	–	–	33,081	–	–	1.21
Belgium	8.30	–	–	–	–	–	–	–	–
Norway	8.20	19,467	20,325	31,541	19,309	19,715	1.55	0.95	0.97
New Zealand	7.70	15,409	16,301	67,457	–	–	4.14	–	–
Sweden	7.50	16,828	21,541	36,941	16,371	14,432	1.71	0.76	0.67
Japan	7.30	20,550	24,171	46,350	19,337	–	1.92	0.80	–
United Kingdom	7.10	17,152	22,964	52,794	20,668	24,801	2.30	0.90	1.08
Denmark	6.70	19,340	21,890	42,924	23,860	25,174	1.96	1.09	1.15
Mean	8.78	18,859	24,940	71,433	22,983	23,065	2.81	0.95	0.92
Standard deviation	1.64	2,322	4,314	39,362	5,268	5,920	1.13	0.13	0.19

Table 7 (cont.)

	% exp./GDP	GDP/p.c. 1993 ($PPP)	Workers (country as a whole)	Average income ($PPP) Relative index (country/mean)			Ratio on average salary		
				Physicians	Nurses	Health workers	Physicians	Nurses	Health workers
United States	1.61	1.24	1.32	2.36	1.45	1.35	1.82	1.06	1.02
Canada	1.16	1.02	1.08	1.35	1.30	–	1.28	1.17	–
Switzerland	1.13	1.22	1.30	1.80	–	–	1.40	–	–
France	1.12	1.00	1.11	0.79	–	–	0.73	–	–
Austria	1.06	–	–	–	–	–	–	–	–
Finland	1.00	0.82	0.95	0.56	0.83	0.86	0.60	0.85	0.91
Netherlands	0.99	0.93	1.12	–	–	1.01	–	–	0.91
Germany	0.98	1.12	1.04	1.42	–	0.70	1.39	–	0.67
Australia	0.97	0.93	0.89	0.83	1.09	–	0.95	1.19	–
Italy	0.97	0.95	1.10	–	–	1.43	–	–	1.31
Belgium	0.95	–	–	–	–	–	–	–	–
Norway	0.93	1.03	0.81	0.44	0.84	0.85	0.55	1.00	1.05
New Zealand	0.88	0.82	0.65	0.94	–	–	1.47	–	–
Sweden	0.85	0.89	0.86	0.52	0.71	0.63	0.61	0.80	0.72
Japan	0.83	1.09	0.97	0.65	0.84	–	0.68	0.84	–
United Kingdom	0.81	0.91	0.92	0.74	0.90	1.08	0.82	0.95	1.17
Denmark	0.76	1.03	0.88	0.60	1.04	1.09	0.70	1.15	1.24
Mean	1.00	1.00	1.00	1.00	1.00	1.00	1.00	1.00	1.00
Standard deviation	0.19	0.12	0.17	0.55	0.23	0.26	0.40	0.14	0.21

CONFIGURATIONS OF COUNTRIES SUCCESSFUL AND UNSUCCESSFUL IN CONTROLLING EXPENDITURES

We need to ask ourselves two questions to better understand the impact of human resources on health expenditures: (1) do number and mix of personnel and income levels explain the differences between the successful and unsuccessful countries?; (2) how can physicians, and the mechanisms by which they are regulated, help account for the differences in expenditure levels not explained by income levels?

In this section, we will try to identify what distinguishes the most successful countries from the least successful ones. We will also try to define these countries in terms of certain organizational mechanisms which affect one of the key intervenors in all health systems: the physician.

Comparisons between the Two Groups of Countries

Table 8 presents a synthesis of the results found in tables 1 to 7 of the preceding section for the four countries in which health expenditures as a percentage of the GDP are the highest, and the four in which they are the lowest.

The first thing we find is that, for all of the indicators used and in spite of the reservations expressed concerning the quality of the data, the two groups of countries have relatively homogenous results: the successful countries generally have scores higher than or equal to the average, while the less successful countries have scores that are lower. The biggest differences between the two groups occur in the areas of the number of health workers (except for physicians), the percentage of public funding, the length of stay, the percentage of the population hospitalized and the number of contacts per patient in ambulatory care services. The income level of workers in the economy as a whole and the relative income level of health workers, especially that of physicians, is much lower in those countries with lower health expenditures, with the exception of Denmark.

However, there are significant differences between the countries in the same group. In the United States, there is a relatively low number of beds and they are underutilized (low occupancy rate) and funded and managed primarily by the private sector; the number of personnel is high. The ambulatory care sector is extensive and the medical profession is highly specialized with a high income level. Canada has a greater number of beds, a higher occupancy rate and longer length of stay, and a lower staff per bed ratio— but one which is composed mainly of nurses whose level of income is relatively higher. The ambulatory care sector is less developed in Canada than in the United States. Sweden and Denmark, two countries with low health expenditures, have very different labour strategies. In Sweden, there are a greater number of workers in the health sector but the remuneration level is low, while the opposite is true in Denmark.

Table 8
Relative position (country/mean) of selected countries in which health expenditures/GDP are the highest or the lowest; selected indicators

	% exp./GDP	% health expenditures			#/1,000 pop.				Ratio		% on health personnel		Income — Ratio on workers/country			
		Hospitals	Ambulatory	Long term	Health personnel	Nurses	Physicians	Personnel other than nurses and physicians	GP/spec.	Nurses/ physicians	# nurses	# physicians	Workers/ country (SPPP)	Physicians/ country	Nurses/ country	Health workers/ country
Highest expenditures																
United States	14.10	=	++	-	=	=	=	+	-	=	-	-	++	++	=	=
Canada	10.20	+	--	=	=	=	-	-	=	+	++	=	+	+	++	
Switzerland	9.90	+	=	-	++	++	+	++	-	++	=	--	++	++		
France	9.80	=	=	--	=	-	-	=	=	--	--	=	+	-		
Lowest expenditures																
Sweden	7.50	+		++	++	+	+	++	-	=	-	-	-	--	--	--
Japan	7.30	--	=	--	--	--	--	--		+	++	++	=	-	--	--
United Kingdom	7.10	+	=	+	-	-	--	-	-*	=	--	-	-	-	-	+
Denmark	6.70	++	--	++	-	-	+	-	++	--	=	+	-	-	++	++

Table 8 (cont.)

	Hospital									Ambulatory	
	% priv. beds	% priv. hosp.	# beds/ 1,000 pop.	Length of stay	Occupancy rate	% hosp. pop. and physicians	# hosp. days/ pop.	Personnel/ bed	Nurses/ bed	# services/ physician	# acts/ pers.
Highest expenditures											
United States	++	++	- -	=	- -	- -	- -	++	++	+	=
Canada	- -	-	-	+	=	-	=	+	=	-	=
Switzerland	=	=	++	++	=	-	++	=	=	=	++
France	=	-	=	-	=	++	=	- -	- -		=
Lowest expenditures											
Sweden	- -		- -	-	=	=	- -	=	=	++	- +
Japan	++		-					- -	-	+	++
United Kingdom	- -	-	- -	- -		+	- -	++	++		-
Denmark		-	+	-	++	+	=	++	=		- +

Source: Tables 1 to 7

* Based on Contandriopoulos et al. 1989.

Note: + or – means the result for that country is between one half and one standard deviation from the mean for all countries.

++ or – – means it is over one standard deviation.

Organizational Strategies Relating to Physicians

The dynamics therefore appear to be different in these two groups of countries. One of the key distinguishing features is the type of control exercised over the medical profession, through the status of physicians in the system (contractor or employee), and the incentives associated with methods of payments.

Table 9 shows that there is a very obvious gap between the two groups but that there is also strong homogeneity within each group in terms of the methods of control and method of payment of physicians. In countries with high health expenditures, there is little control over the number of physicians (at least there was up to the early 1990s), except through incentives to limit the number of admissions to medical faculties; physicians can set up practice wherever they choose or wherever the market allows, and they are paid on a fee-for-service basis as an independent contractor. In countries with low health expenditures, the number of new physicians who enter the system depends on the number of students trained, but primarily (as for all other workers) on the number of vacant positions to be filled; moreover, in all of these countries except Japan, physicians are employees or paid on a per capita basis (with a per-service supplement) in the ambulatory care sector.

It would appear that the degree of autonomy given to physicians is linked to the level of total expenditures in the health sector, both in terms of ability of physicians to generate their own incomes and to prescribe tests or treatments, and also in terms of the power their status gives them to influence the inflationary forces of the health care system. Table 10 uses the data from table 2 to calculate an index of health expenditures for each sector compared to the average of all the countries. It shows that the four least successful countries (those with a high level of expenditure) differ from the four most successful countries not only because, overall, their level of expenditure (in $PPP per inhabitant) is higher in the labour-intensive sectors (hospitals and ambulatory care), but also because expenditures are higher in the other sectors (medication, medical aids and appliances).

Table 9

Characteristics of the most and the least successful countries in terms of control of entry in system and method of payment of physicians (in early '90s)

	% exp./ GDP	Method of control		Method of payment	
		# of physicians	Place, type of practice	GP	Specialists
Highest expenditures					
United States	14.10	Market	Market	Fee for service + per capita	Fee for service
Canada	10.20	# of admissions to faculties	Market (limited)	Fee for service	Fee for service
Switzerland	9.90	# of admissions to faculties	Market	Fee for service	Fee for service
France	9.80	# of admissions to faculties	Market	Fee for service	Salary + fee for service
Lowest expenditures					
Sweden	7.50	# of vacant positions	# of vacant positions	Salary	Salary
Japan	7.30	# of vacant positions	?	Fee for service	Salary
United Kingdom	7.10	# of vacant positions	# of vacant positions	Per capita + fee for service	Salary
Denmark	6.70	# of vacant positions	# of vacant positions	Per capita + fee for service	Salary + fee for service

Source: Contandriopoulos et al. 1989

Table 10

**Current health expenditures per capita ($PPP),
selected OECD countries, by type of expenditure, 1988**

	% exp./ GDP	Total	Hosp.ª	Ambulatory physicians	Drugsᵇ	Long-term care	Dental services	Medical aids and appliances	Other services
United States	14.1	2,007	868	419	170	193	119	82	156
Canada	10.2	1,495	725	159	183	184	86	59	99
Switzerland	9.9	1,385	679	232	145	117	121	49	42
France	9.8	1,158	531	186	201	57	75	48	60
Austria	9.3	999	460	175	93	125	93	29	24
Netherlands	8.7	1,062	461	108	98	197	54	52	92
Germany	8.6	1,201	408	194	198	93	156	87	65
Italyᶜ	8.5	997	425	242	180	73	–	45	32
Belgium	8.3	918	324	194	148	78	32	47	95
Sweden	7.5	1,330	623	137	90	213	77	52	138
Japan	7.3	989	326	156	173	108	55	46	125
United Kingdom	7.1	856	406	117	116	111	36	19	51
Denmark	6.7	1,091	552	80	83	212	51	36	77
Mean	**8.92**	**1,191**	**522**	**185**	**144**	**135**	**73**	**50**	**81**

Table 10 (cont.)

	Total	Hosp.[a]	Ambulatory physicians	Drugs[b]	Long-term care	Dental services	Medical aids and appliances	Other services
			Relative index (country/mean)					
United States	1.68	1.66	2.27	1.10	1.40	1.62	1.64	1.92
Canada	1.25	1.39	0.86	1.20	1.30	1.17	1.18	1.22
Switzerland	1.16	1.30	1.26	1.00	0.80	1.65	0.98	0.52
France	0.97	1.02	1.01	1.30	0.40	1.02	0.96	0.74
Austria	0.84	0.88	0.95	0.60	0.92	1.27	0.58	0.30
Netherlands	0.89	0.88	0.59	0.68	1.45	0.74	1.04	1.13
Germany	1.01	0.78	1.05	1.37	0.69	2.12	1.74	0.80
Italy[c]	0.84	0.81	1.31	1.25	0.54	–	0.90	0.39
Belgium	0.77	0.62	1.05	1.02	0.58	0.44	0.94	1.17
Sweden	1.12	1.19	0.74	0.62	1.57	1.05	1.04	1.70
Japan	0.83	0.62	0.85	1.20	0.80	0.75	0.92	1.54
United Kingdom	0.72	0.78	0.63	0.80	0.82	0.49	0.38	0.63
Denmark	0.92	1.06	0.43	0.57	1.57	0.69	0.72	0.95
Mean	1.00	1.00	1.00	0.98	1.00	1.00	1.00	1.00

Source: Beratungsgesellschaft für angewandte Systemforschung (BASYS) Ltd.; Rublee and Schneider 1991.

[a] Includes physician services provided in hospitals.

[b] Excludes drugs prescribed in hospitals.

[c] Ambulatory physician services included dental services.

CONCLUSION

In spite of the limits imposed by the comparability of the data, certain observations can be made from our analysis.

Compared to the average of the other developed countries, Canada has a relatively large hospital system, which belongs almost exclusively to the public sector, with a measurable share of private funding, a relatively low number of acute care beds but slightly longer lengths of stay, and an ambulatory care sector that is not well developed.

Canada does not stand out from the other countries in terms of the number and mix of its personnel, except that it has a proportionately slightly higher number of nurses. However, the level of income of its health workers is higher in relation to the average salary for Canada in the other sectors of the economy. This characteristic is particularly important given that this average salary is also much higher than the average of the countries as a whole. The higher income level of health personnel in Canada compared to the average of the other developed countries could account for less than 10 percent of total health expenditures (or 1 percent of the GDP). Since health expenditures in Canada are 1.4 percent higher in terms of a percentage of the GDP (10.2 percent compared to 8.8 percent), part of this gap is apparently attributable to factors other than the level of remuneration.

Overall, there is a significant difference in the configurations of the four most successful countries (in terms of cost control) and the four least successful countries. The first group does better in terms of the quantity of health personnel (except for physicians), the percentage of public funding, the length of stay, the percentage of the population hospitalized, and the magnitude of the ambulatory care sector. The income level of workers in the economy as a whole and the relative income level of health personnel, and especially physicians, is much lower in countries with lower health expenditures.

There are however some differences between countries in the same group. Consequently, there is no one recipe for controlling costs. Sweden and Denmark, for example, the two countries with the lowest health expenditures, have adopted totally different labour strategies: Sweden has many workers with a low income level, while Denmark has the inverse.

In general, the two groups of countries appear to have different dynamics. The distinguishing features are the type of control exercised over the medical profession, the status of physicians in the system (contractor or employee), and the incentives associated with the methods of payment. In countries with high expenditure levels, there is little control over the number of physicians; they can choose the site of their practice and what type it will be, and they are paid on a fee-for-service basis as an independent contractor. In countries with low expenditures, the growth in the number of physicians and their distribution depends primarily on vacant positions; moreover, in all of these countries except Japan, physicians are employees or are paid on a per capita basis (with a per-service supplement) for ambulatory care services.

Therefore, there appears to be a link between the level of autonomy given to physicians in a health system and the level of total expenditures in the health sector.

Marc-André Fournier *is a doctoral student in public health at the University of Montreal. He has also studied economics and demography. He has worked as a research assistant with GRIS (Interdisciplinary Research Group on Health) at the University of Montreal for many years. His main research interests are medical manpower planning, health care system regulation, and service utilization.*

BIBLIOGRAPHY

ARWEILER, D. 1998. International comparisons of health expenditures. International Comparison Series Paper. Papers commissioned by the National Forum on Health. Ottawa (ON). Published in this volume.

BROUSSELLE, A. 1998. Controlling health expenditures: What matters. International Comparison Series Paper. Papers commissioned by the National Forum on Health. Ottawa (ON). Published in this volume.

CONTANDRIOPOULOS, A.-P., M.-A. FOURNIER, M. CASTONGUAY, and A.-S. PREKER. 1989. *Comparaisons des effectifs médicaux au Québec avec ceux de certains pays développés.* Report R89–05, GRIS, University of Montreal.

CONTANDRIOPOULOS, D. 1998. How Canada's health care system compares with that of other countries: An overview. International Comparison Series Paper. Papers commissioned by the National Forum on Health. Ottawa (ON). Published in this volume.

HEALTH CANADA. 1995. *Health Personnel in Canada.* Ottawa (ON).

_____. 1996. *National Health Expenditures in Canada: 1975–1994.* Ottawa (ON).

OECD. 1995. *Health Data.* Paris: OECD.

RUBLEE, D. A., and M. SCHNEIDER. 1991. International health spending: Comparisons with the OECD. *Health Affairs,* fall: 188–198.

Health Care Expenditures and the Aging Population in Canada

ELLEN LEIBOVICH, ARCH., M.SC.
HOWARD BERGMAN, M.D.
FRANÇOIS BÉLAND, PH.D.

Research Group on Integrated Care for the Frail Elderly,
Division of Geriatric Medicine, McGill University
Department of Health Administration, University of Montreal

PUZZLING ISSUE NO. 2

Differences in the relative age of populations across OECD countries do not explain variations in health expenditures. Countries with populations older than ours do not spend any more, and in many cases, spend less than Canada. Do other countries spend health care dollars differently or does their social/economic environment reduce pressure on the health system? What long-term strategies should Canada be considering to deal with an aging population?

TABLE OF CONTENTS

Introduction 288

The Aging Population and the Cost of Health Care in Canada 288

    Intensity of Treatment 291

    Technology 291

    Social Changes 291

    Drug Therapy 291

    System Inefficiencies 296

System of Care for the Elderly in Sweden and
the United Kingdom 296

Care of the Elderly in Canada 299

Strategy for the Development of a System of Care for the Frail
Elderly in Canada 300

Conclusion 302

Bibliography 304

FIGURE

Figure 1   Cost index by percentage of population over 80
            (1963–1993) 289

LIST OF TABLES

Table 1   Sources of increased per capita utilization by specific
          age group 1969–1978 292

Table 2   Sources of increased per capita utilization by specific
          age group 1979–1980, 1985–1986 294

INTRODUCTION

The National Forum on Health has identified a number of "puzzling issues" which surfaced from six technical papers (NFOH-TP) prepared for its working group. Our mandate is to respond to one of these issues. The rising costs associated with Canada's health care system are often directly associated with the growing percentage of elderly within the population. However, some OECD countries with a higher proportion of elderly are spending less on health care. What methods do these countries use to care for their aging population? Can we derive some inspiration from their systems and apply it to a long-term care strategy for Canada?

THE AGING POPULATION AND THE COST OF HEALTH CARE IN CANADA

The technical documents prepared for the National Forum on Health draw no correlation between the age of a population and its health care expenditures. The percentage of Canadians over the age of 65, at 11 percent, is lower than that of countries such as Sweden (17.7 percent), Norway (16.3 percent), and the United Kingdom (15.1 percent).[1] The health status of the Canadian population is considered to be one of the best in the world, with a life expectancy of 77.6 years, fifth in the world behind Japan (79.1 years), Iceland (78.1 years), Sweden (77.9 years), and Switzerland (77.6 years).[1] However, Canada spends the equivalent of 9.8 percent of its gross domestic product (GDP) on health care services, the third highest rate in the world behind the United States and Switzerland. By comparison Sweden spends 8.2 percent of GDP and the United Kingdom 6.5 percent on health. As such, while the quality of care dispensed may be good, the cost control performance of Canada's system is best described as mediocre (NFOH-TP1). These differences are not due to differences in per capita GDP. The NFOH technical papers reveal that Canada has the third highest cost index (.97), indicating one of the highest levels of spending amongst the 24 OECD countries (NFOH-TP1). The United States has the highest cost index (3.13) and Switzerland has the second highest cost index (1.12). However, when assessing the quantity of care consumed, Canada's rank is average. This suggests that the price of care in Canada is higher than the other OECD countries (NFOH-TP2). Canada has approximately 2.3 physicians per 1,000 inhabitants, Sweden has approximately 2.8 and the United Kingdom approximately 1.45. Canada ranks seventeenth lowest out of the 24 OECD countries on physician availability. The NFOH papers also reveal that for expenditures on income security, Canada spends 11.9 percent of GDP which is well below the average. Sweden

---

1. The data given is the calculated average between the years 1989–1993 (NFOH-TP1).

ranks the highest and the United Kingdom close to the average (NFOH-TP6).

The graph in figure 1 (Brousselle 1996) illustrates that Canadian spending on health care is double that expected given its proportion of the population aged 80+ (note where the horizontal line located at the highest point on the Canadian curve meets the line of regression). The graph illustrates, as well, that for all of the countries except two (one of which is Canada—see the curves included in the rectangle of the graph in figure 1) costs increase linearly with respect to the proportion of elderly persons greater than 80 years old (see line of regression).

Why is the relationship between costs and the proportion of elderly over 80 in Canada and in one other country so off the mark? A number of possibilities can be considered:

- The health of the population in Canada is lower than that of other countries. Data on life expectancies and infant mortality do not support this hypothesis.
- The system is the source of the problem and is affected by either producer or consumer behaviour. The latter possibility is true only if it is the demand for care that drives the system, which is not the case. Our working assumption is that the problems stem from the production side.

Figure 1

Cost index by percentage of population over 80 (1963–1993)

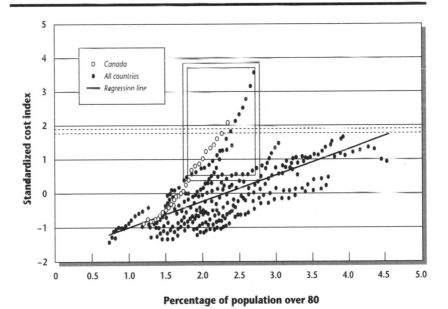

Percentage of population over 80

Source: Brousselle 1996.
Note: The rectangle and the horizontal line have been added to Brousselle's graph.

In comparative terms, there are ample resources being spent on health care in Canada (figure 1). The real problem is the increasing intensity and manner in which services are given to the elderly and in the incentives built into the system of care that pushes the Canadian rate of expenditures on health care to such levels. In Canada, many individuals attribute the escalating cost of health care to the increase in the proportion and absolute numbers of elderly over 65 and particularly over 75 years of age. The more the population of a country ages, the more likely it is that the country will have higher health care expenses (figure 1). The more the average age increases, the greater the impact on health care expenses (Brousselle 1996). However, it is not only the increasing number of elderly which is problematic, rather it is also and even principally the intensity with which the system delivers treatment to them (Barer et al. 1995). It has been demonstrated that the demographic shift towards an aging population is responsible for only a relatively small portion of growing health care costs. According to Barer, this demographic shift will result in an annual 1 percent rise in per capita use of the health care system when spread over the entire population base (Barer et al. 1987). Such a shift may be supported by sustained economic growth. The increased number of elderly, as well as their increasing average age, account for one-third of their increased share of hospital use (Barer et al. 1995). Changes in per capita utilization rates amongst the elderly account for the remaining two-thirds increase, and this does not take into consideration increases related to use of long-term and chronic care facilities (Barer et al. 1995). Barer's findings have been confirmed by a recent study in Quebec (Demers 1996).

Analyzing data for the province of British Columbia, Hertzman et al. (1990) show that the increasing utilization rates for the ≥ 65 age group is clearly associated with treatment of relatively few (±10) medical conditions (on average, utilization rates actually dropped for all other discharge diagnoses when combined). All medical conditions showing increased utilization by the elderly also involve a corresponding dramatic increase in the average length of stay in hospital extended care and rehabilitation beds. Significant increases in utilization rates were associated with conditions of dementia, personality, thought, and mood disorders and are significantly higher than the remaining medical conditions identified by Hertzman (i.e., arthritis, osteomyelitis, etc.; Hertzman et al. 1990; tables 1 and 2). Studies do not indicate that these increased utilization rates are the result of a parallel increase in the prevalence of these conditions within the elderly population (Hertzman et al. 1990). This suggests that the elderly are receiving extensive care for conditions for which they were generally not hospitalized 25 years ago. This suggests important changes have occurred both within the health care system and the community's value system. Given the interrelational nature of utilization rates, morbidity and treatment practices, it is difficult to draw direct cause and effect conclusions regarding these changes. However, the following factors clearly influence the tendency towards increased utilization among the elderly:

Intensity of Treatment

This trend is demonstrated by increased per capita patient separation rates[2] and number of patient days for the elderly, both contrary to trends in the younger adult population (Barer et al. 1995). Similarly, the rate of increase for the average medical fee per service per capita is greatest for the elderly (Barer et al. 1987).

Technology

The elderly occupy an increasing share of acute care beds, principally illustrated by a rapidly rising per capita surgery rate. Also their per capita separation rate for acute care beds is increasing. Both of these statistics are contrary to the trend for the rest of the population (Barer et al. 1995). The elderly's per capita patient day use of acute care beds is down due to reduced lengths of stay; however, the rate of reduction is lower than that of the general population. This statistic is likely influenced by the high percentage of extended (≥ 60 days) average length of stay for patients in the ≥ 80 age category (Evans et al. 1989).

Social Changes

The above-mentioned increase in cases pertaining to dementia and behavioral disorders amongst the elderly without a corresponding increase in morbidity suggests that priorities within the health care system and society have changed. For a segment of the elderly population, hospital extended care beds have become a permanent home (Barer et al. 1995). The hospital has inherited problems of a sociocultural nature which are more directly related to community issues such as social isolation, housing, women in the work force, welfare, etc. (Hertzman et al. 1990).

Drug Therapy

The elderly account for approximately 30 percent of medication use even though they make up only 11 to 12 percent of the population. This could be partially related to their greater relative needs. However, studies show that there is a significant trend towards inappropriate prescription of medication for the elderly which leads to greater costs for medication as well as the treatment of complications that result from this inappropriate use (Tamblyn et al. 1994).

---

2. Separations are defined as "the total of live discharges plus in-hospital deaths during a year" (Evans et al. 1989).

Table 1

Sources of increased per capita utilization by specific age group 1969–1978

3-digit chapter heading, ICD 8*	Age 65+ Number of days		% increase per 100 population	% increase per 100 population 1969–1978		
	1969	1978		65–74	75–84	85+
Females						
Senility and ill-defined diseases	1,019	31,155	2,048.68	923.87	4,547.56	1,415.18
Psychoses	7,213	76,276	643.17	205.39	990.75	915.56
Neuroses; personality disorders	7,077	55,406	450.21	67.62	527.40	1,413.30
Osteomyelitis	11,362	79,986	394.74	12.24	514.38	1,280.81
Other diseases of central nervous system	8,873	55,999	343.54	595.47	215.81	408.20
Cerebrovascular disease	74,583	348,160	228.06	141.85	281.09	252.68
Arthritis and rheumatism	27,055	100,435	160.89	103.56	170.03	222.21
Diseases of other endocrine glands	19,030	38,914	43.71	1.42	34.23	445.43
Ischemic heart disease	82,355	162,735	38.87	−37.27	34.03	139.69
Diseases of arteries and capillaries	20,866	37,564	26.52	8.38	−10.10	126.87
Total days, selected categories	259,433	986,630	167.27	67.30	178.81	292.73
Total days, other categories	322,017	439,211	−4.15	−19.82	3.08	21.90
Overall totals	581,450	1,425,841	72.34	12.96	87.46	162.36

Table 1 (cont.)

3-digit chapter heading, ICD 8*	Age 65+			% increase per 100 population 1969–1978		
	Number of days		% increase per 100 population	65–74	75–84	85+
	1969	1978				
Males						
Senility and ill-defined diseases	692	15,963	1,669.46	28.63	4,220.08	1,948.18
Psychoses	8,165	43,228	306.11	134.73	385.83	1,775.00
Osteomyelitis	8,404	22,247	103.06	2.72	133.81	384.56
Other disease of respiratory system	5,386	13,382	90.58	32.38	163.28	348.34
Arthritis and rheumatism	17,878	40,801	75.06	14.06	88.51	541.33
Cerebrovascular disease	95,603	205,638	63.28	35.84	73.28	174.99
Other diseases of central nervous system	27,216	53,670	51.27	15.88	131.79	77.84
Ischemic heart disease	101,184	112,991	−14.34	−21.49	−23.89	42.59
Total days, selected categories	265,528	507,920	46.73	13.79	70.89	152.30
Total days, other categories	498,158	508,928	−21.64	−28.39	−16.13	9.31
Overall total	763,886	1,016,848	2.11	−14.51	11.87	61.70

Source: Hertzman et al. 1990.

* International classification of diseases (version 8). The 3-digit chapter headings refer to categories of diseases.

Table 2

Sources of increased per capita utilization by specific age group 1979–1980, 1985–1986

3-digit chapter heading, ICD 9*	Age 65+ Number of days		% increase per 100 population	% increase per 100 population 1979–1980, 1985–1986		
	1979–1980	1985–1986		65–74	75–84	85+
Females						
Health services in other circumstances	2,069	106,176	3,910.02	1,601.52	3,416.98	7,729.45
Ill-defined and unknown causes of morbidity	13,813	67,406	281.32	2,373.35	408.32	240.13
Other forms of heart disease	25,478	93,010	185.26	104.75	140.55	293.20
Psychoses	8,490	29,630	172.71	76.70	322.93	892.68
Malignant neoplasm	35,128	22,147	153.53	189.22	274.31	−1.85
Neuroses, personality disorders	6,826	113,692	152.90	18.41	129.35	354.63
Pneumonia and influenza	15,905	46,853	130.19	23.97	127.16	252.28
Other diseases of central nervous system	16,547	47,664	125.09	15.96	153.35	6,310.01
Symptoms	9,406	26,158	117.31	67.77	151.66	182.35
Hereditary diseases of central nervous system	65,538	142,932	70.42	−10.27	96.52	193.64
Late effects of injuries	23,114	39,367	33.09	−85.64	−1.97	130.96
Organic psychotic conditions	153,652	247,469	25.85	−37.79	−1.13	72.65
Total days, selected categories	375,966	982,504	104.20	25.56	89.27	186.16
Total days, other categories	1,355,169	1,240,800	−28.45	−21.51	−27.59	−32.32
Overall totals	1,731,135	2,223,304	0.36	−11.45	−1.93	15.08

Table 2 (cont.)

3-digit chapter heading, ICD 9*	Age 65+ Number of days 1979–1980	Age 65+ Number of days 1985–1986	% increase per 100 population	% increase per 100 population 1979–1980, 1985–1986 65–74	% increase per 100 population 1979–1980, 1985–1986 75–84	% increase per 100 population 1979–1980, 1985–1986 85+
Males						
Health services in other circumstances	1,119	55,478	3,959.13	1,971.94	4,145.80	11,118.59
Other diseases of central nervous system	9,374	62,361	444.67	213.25	3,786.81	135.53
Health services for specific procedures	1,864	9,707	326.36	219.45	231.83	2,576.76
Ill-defined and unknown causes of morbidity	6,448	26,422	235.49	482.44	572.06	218.65
Malignant neoplasm	4,157	13,950	174.75	147.02	268.06	116.47
Symptoms	7,130	21,270	144.24	118.85	151.22	225.71
Other forms of heart disease	20,200	58,109	135.52	117.22	95.83	282.57
Pneumonia and influenza	20,032	46,326	89.34	41.55	140.28	96.21
Hereditary diseases of central nervous system	35,359	79,769	84.70	13.63	84.54	279.96
Neuroses and personality disorders	16,458	36,604	82.09	−11.45	95.65	516.36
Total days, selected categories	122,141	409,996	174.83	94.72	215.49	301.49
Total days, other categories	994,915	856,250	−29.82	−31.17	−20.36	−35.99
Overall totals	1,117,056	1,266,246	−7.52	−16.23	5.11	−3.59

Source: Hertzman et al. 1990.
* International classification of diseases (version 9). The 3-digit chapter headings refer to categories of diseases.

System Inefficiencies

The use of acute and extended care beds by persons awaiting transfer to alternative facilities is significant among the elderly (Hertzman et al. 1990). Inadequately allocated resources have a domino effect on the entire system.

In conclusion, it does not appear that the aging of the population or changing characteristics of the aging population such as increased morbidity are the main causes of escalating health care costs in Canada. However, it is quite clear that increased pressure on the health care system and on costs from an aging population will continue unless we address the factors that influence the tendency towards increased utilization by the elderly. A central issue is the question of appropriate care for the frail elderly. The fact that other OECD countries such as Sweden and the United Kingdom have a higher percentage of elderly but lower costs of health care suggests that we should look at their health care systems.

SYSTEM OF CARE FOR THE ELDERLY IN SWEDEN AND THE UNITED KINGDOM

We have chosen to examine the system of care in Sweden and the United Kingdom. Sweden and the United Kingdom are two OECD countries which have a higher proportion of elderly and whose percentage of GNP spent on health care is lower than that of Canada. Both Sweden and the United Kingdom are two countries with a long tradition of developing social security policies as well as an organized system of health care where emphasis is placed on primary care, community services for the elderly, and integration of care.[3]

The Swedish government and society strongly support expenditures for programs for the elderly (Thorslund and Parker 1994). The system provides both social services and medical care. Included in the social services sector are home help services, transportation, access to day centres and institutional care. The medical side includes services such as: medical care provided by physicians who visit patients in their home, prescription drugs and medical care provided in the hospital (Thorslund and Parker 1994). Government policies attempt to maintain the elderly in the community by giving large pensions, housing allowances, and strongly subsidized home help services. The use of these services is not influenced by socioeconomic status. In Sweden, alternative housing in the form of apartment dwellings is also available (Sundstrom and Thorslund 1994).

---

3. Because of the difficulty in obtaining and comparing figures on costs of spending levels of care, on rates of hospitalization and institutionalization, it is difficult to explain why relative spending is lower in other countries.

An important problem in Sweden which contributed to rising costs was an escalating rate of institutionalization. The Adel reform was a major reform of long-term care services. Implemented in January 1992, it shifted clinical and financial responsibility for long-term care services from the counties to the municipalities which are closer to the patients and thus more able to discern their needs. These long-term care services include health care services for the elderly within institutions (not including physician care) as well as social and home care services. The municipalities now have responsibility for nursing homes and institutional housing and all other care facilities for the elderly. The municipalities are financially responsible for all long-term care patients including those in acute care hospitals. This financial responsibility, along with an increase in housing for the elderly, is the main reason for the decrease in the number of "bed-blockers" in hospitals. The decentralization of responsibilities to the municipalities has led to an improved coordination and integration with social and home care services which have always been financed and provided at the municipal level. The Adel reform also changed the manner in which the municipalities were financed. A budget based on the number of elderly persons served replaced financing according to the volume of services produced. This change in policy gave the municipalities the incentive to develop alternatives to traditional methods of treating the elderly (Thorslund and Parker 1994).

Similar to Sweden, concerns regarding the care for the elderly have been raised in the United Kingdom. The British health care system has always been known for its emphasis on primary care, community care, and extensive geriatric services.

Increased demands from an aging population and limited funds to develop home care have led to a new policy for community care. A local single-source financing agency was established for social care (in the United Kingdom, social services and medical services are under the responsibility of two different local authorities). Since 1989, the focus has been to better integrate services and caregivers through case management. Studies show that fragmentation of services can be reduced through case management which increases coordination between services. There is a tendency toward "downward substitution by moving away from institutional to enhanced home care and developing improved coordination at the client level" (Challis 1993). The 1989 policy on community care established an organization financially responsible for the social care of the elderly. This agency is expected to improve the integration and coordination of social and personal care services to the elderly through the development of case management models (Challis 1993).

Other reforms in the United Kingdom brought about the creation of independent NHS trusts, public organizations that are responsible for the provision of hospital and community health services. These organizations are independent but financially accountable to the NHS Management

Executive. Previously, hospital services were provided directly by the managed district health authority (DHA) who was directly accountable to the department of health (Smee 1995). By creating these independent trusts, a competitive element was introduced into the British system. The main element behind this reform is the separation of provider (NHS trusts) and purchaser (district health authorities) of services. Providers are responsible for the provision of services and district health authorities, appointed by the government to run local health care services, have been modified to take on a purchasing role (Saltman 1991, 1994, 1995). Hospital and community health services are now run by the NHS trusts. Rather than be given a fixed budget, the NHS trusts and hospitals are placed in the position of competing for contracts and resources from district health authorities and GP Fundholders (Ham and Brommels 1994). Therefore the creation of trusts introduced market incentives into the health care system by separating purchaser from provider as well as encouraging managerial innovation now free from political interference (Smee 1995).

Another important reform is the creation of GP Fundholders. Group practices of private physicians have been formed which are composed of groups of GPs that serve 7,000 or more patients and that choose to manage a budget with which to buy services for their patients (Ham and Brommels 1994). These GP Fundholders act as purchasers and providers of services. They are responsible financially for providing patients with a range of primary as well as specialty outpatient and elective inpatient services. As well, they negotiate with NHS trusts for the best possible contracts that take into account both price and quality. Therefore, in contrast to the NHS trusts, the second allocative mechanism combines the purchaser and provider role into one entity (Saltman 1995).

Pilot projects are underway in which Total GP Fundholding practices are given budgets for all primary and secondary care including acute hospital care. These incentives encouraged the Total GP Fundholders to develop primary care services and to emphasize alternative solutions and new programs for the elderly (Bosanquet and Zajdler 1993).

According to Ham (Ham 1996a) the reforms mentioned earlier were intended to create open competition within the health care system. In reality, however, these reforms resulted in yardstick competition or contestability measures (Saltman and von Otter 1995; Ham 1996a) which is sufficient to increase organizational performance and effectiveness. Ham suggests that the possibility of movement of patients and resources from one establishment to another, rather than the actual movement of patients and resources, is what is needed to improve performance and decrease inefficiency in health care systems (Ham 1996a).

CARE OF THE ELDERLY IN CANADA

Canadian Medicare is essentially a system of insurance for payment of physicians and acute hospital services. It was originally based on a cost-sharing agreement between the federal government and the provinces which did not cover services such as long-term and community care. As a result, provincial governments were less inclined to develop programs and alternative ways of treating the elderly. The tendency was to expand the acute care system because federal financing could be easily obtained. This explains, in part, the increased intensity of acute hospital services to the elderly. Because of this, no overall Canadian health care policies or objectives were developed for the long-term care sector and each province was left to manage on its own. With the 1977 Established Programs Financing Act, the federal government extended its coverage to include other services such as home care and long-term care (Shapiro 1994).

However, the increasing number of services available to the elderly has resulted in important problems. The delivery of the complex combination of services necessary to care for the frail elderly is presently under the responsibility of many different agencies and jurisdictions. For example, in Quebec primary medical care is generally under the responsibility of the family physician in private practice but may also be under that of the physician working in a CLSC (Clarfield and Bergman 1991). Nursing and home care services are the responsibility of the CLSC but community and private organizations are heavily involved. Day centres and day hospitals are generally the responsibility of long-term care institutions, rarely the same one for both. Alternative housing is private. Geriatric services and specialty medical services are hospital based.

Since each institution is a distinct administrative entity with its own global budget, jurisdiction and criteria for patient selection, services are not coordinated based on patient needs. The efforts to maintain the elderly person in the community are fragmented and no single institution or organization can be held accountable. Each component of the system tends to work in parallel and functions within its own budget. These components have separate and distinct responsibilities that can either overlap or leave important needs unmet. There is no one institution which has both the clinical and the financial responsibility to reduce inappropriate hospitalizations and to maintain the dependent elderly in the community (*Rapport de la commission d'enquête sur les services de santé et les services sociaux* 1988; Trahan and Bélanger 1993). The reduction of inappropriate acute and long-term care admissions is a matter of professional conscience because negative incentives encourage institutions to send the more serious cases to other institutions even though this may entail unnecessary, more costly, and potentially harmful services (i.e., institutionalization in a nursing home or hospitalization). The most striking effect of this situation is the number of elderly patients in acute care hospitals waiting to be placed in a long-term care institution. This group of elderly occupies between 10 to 25 percent of acute care beds in Quebec (Régie régionale de la santé et des services sociaux 1995). With some variation, the fragmentation of care is similar in other Canadian provinces.

STRATEGY FOR THE DEVELOPMENT OF A SYSTEM OF CARE FOR THE FRAIL ELDERLY IN CANADA

The need to reduce costs often leads to the discussion of obvious but simplistic solutions such as the rationing of services, the pros and cons of privatization, or fiscal control via salary freezes and user fees. It is not within the objectives of this paper to discuss such possible changes given their implicit negative effect on the quality of services. Any proposed solution must reduce cost without sacrificing quality or compromising the fundamental principles upon which the Canadian health care system is based.

Canada's response, in the 1970s, to the aging population was to increase the number of long-term care institutional beds as well as to introduce some community services for the elderly. In the 1980s, with the development of an increasing number of services, and due to the increasing cost and use of acute care hospital beds for elderly patients awaiting discharge or placement, the coordination of services became an important objective.

There have been a number of important developments in Canada. In many Canadian jurisdictions this has taken the form of single entry point systems with case management for continuing care services in the community and for admission to a long-term care institution. The single entry point system developed in the 1990s represents a significant development in British Columbia, Manitoba, and New Brunswick. Alberta and Quebec are in the process of enacting these reforms (Régie régionale de la santé et des services sociaux 1995; Hollander and Pallan 1995; Béland and Shapiro 1993; Béland and Lemay 1995). The objectives of these systems are to ensure the evaluation and selection of patients, the allocation and coordination of community services, as well as improved communication and coordination when patients are admitted or discharged from acute care (Hollander 1994; Hollander and Pallan 1995).

Key elements of the single entry point system which is referred to as the "best practices system" in British Columbia include: the single entry point, coordinated assessment and placement, coordinated case management, a single administration, consistent care level classification (Hollander and Pallan 1995).

This single entry point system represents an important development and has resulted in reduced fragmentation and an improved use of resources. However, there are still significant limitations to the Canadian system. Institutions remain autonomous with their own jurisdiction and budget. Acute hospital and continuing care, medical and social care as well as community and institutional long-term care remain separate and as such cannot sufficiently respond to the complex health and social needs of the elderly.

It is clear that significant room for improvement lays in the organization and coordination of both health and social services. For the frail elderly population, integration of medical and social care, acute and long-term care is essential in order to reduce the expensive and inappropriate use of hospital and nursing home services and to improve quality of care (Kane et al. 1992; Kane 1995). It is also clear that such a system must be combined with the introduction of financial incentives based upon performance. Our analysis points to the need for an integrated system of care for the frail elderly within the Canadian health care system.

There has been increasing interest in the past several years in integrated systems of care, particularly for the frail elderly, with an emphasis on case management and clinical responsibility throughout the spectrum of care. A number of projects, with varying degrees of integration, have demonstrated this interest although many of them are still in the demonstration phase. These are: the On Lok/PACE projects (Branch et al. 1995; Kane et al. 1992) and the Social/Health Maintenance Organizations (S/HMO) (Finch et al. 1992) in the United States, GP Fundholders in Britain (Ham 1996a, b; Ham and Brommels 1994), the Darlington (Challis et al. 1991a, b) and EPICS projects (Davies et al. 1994) in Britain, as well as the Adel reform in Sweden (Johannson 1995).

The On Lok/PACE projects utilize the most complete system of integrated care. *On Lok* is Chinese for "happy, peaceful abode" and is a project implemented in San Francisco's Chinese community. It has been replicated in the United States with funding from the Health Care Financing Administration as the Program of All-Inclusive Care for the Elderly. With a capitated budget for nursing home–eligible patients, the interdisciplinary team is responsible for the evaluation of the patient, the allocation of resources and the delivery of care to the patient in all settings, including hospital and nursing home. Although a preliminary study (Yordi and Waldman 1985) suggested reduction in costs, hospitalization, length of stay, and institutionalization as well as some increase in functional autonomy, the On Lok/PACE projects have not yet been rigorously and completely evaluated (Branch et al. 1995; Kane et al. 1992). However, Yordi and Waldman's study demonstrated a reduction in the number of hospitalizations as well as the length of stay. A reduction in hospitalizations from 10.5 days in 1980 to 8.5 days in 1982, to 6.5 days in 1988 was seen. In 1981, 9 percent of the On Lok patients resided in a nursing home and by 1987 this was reduced to 5.4 percent (Zawadski and Eng 1988). This change in service utilization showed a consequential reduction in the cost of services (Zawadski and Eng 1988). Planning is underway for the second-phase S/HMO projects with more complete integration of acute and long-term care (Finch et al. 1992). As well, through the utilization of waivers, many states are developing integrated systems of care for elderly eligible for Medicare and Medicaid (Kane and Starr 1996). In Britain, the Darlington project (Challis 1991a, b) utilized a geriatric team, case management with a devolved budget, and multipurpose community workers to discharge long-stay elderly patients from the hospital back to the community. The evaluation demonstrated that the project decreased length of stay, increased patient and family satisfaction, and was cost effective.

In Canada, there have been a number of developments in integrated systems of care for the frail elderly. The Choice project in Edmonton established by the Capital Health Authority is a replicate of the On Lok/PACE model and began in January 1996. It is being monitored but there are no evaluations as of yet. The evaluation has been partially built into the pilot project design.

Our research group has developed a conceptual model of integrated care for the frail elderly based on the following essential characteristics (Bergman, Béland, Lebel, et al. 1996; Bergman, Béland, Leibovich, et al. 1996):

– community primary care–based system offering a full range of primary and secondary health and social services including acute hospital care as well as long-term community and institutional care;
– responsibility for the care of a defined population;
– case management with clinical responsibility for the entire range of services provided;
– prepayment based on capitation with financial responsibility for the entire range of services provided.
– publicly managed respecting the fundamental principles of the Canadian health care system.

CONCLUSION

The five principles outlined above signify important changes to the way health and social services for the elderly are organized, delivered, and financed by the existing system. It is expected that these changes will lead to improved quality of life for the frail elderly as well as increased patient satisfaction, more appropriate use of resources, increased accountability of providers of care and cost-effectiveness.

The challenge is to implement a model of integrated care for the frail elderly in Canada within its publicly funded health care system based on global budgets. Such an integrated system of care for the frail elderly raises several important issues: quality of care; patient choice; the relationship among providers of care; capitation and the target population (Bergman and Béland 1996).

Before proposing a major change to the present system, these issues need to be addressed. It would, therefore, be appropriate to organize demonstration projects on different sites both in order to develop the experience of integrated care in the Canadian context and to evaluate the model as an effective and cost-efficient system of care.

Ellen Leibovich *is an architect and holds a master's degree in health administration from the University of Montreal. She is working for the Research Group on Integrated Care for the Frail Elderly, a joint initiative of the McGill University Division of Geriatric Medicine and the University of Montreal Department of Health Administration.*

BIBLIOGRAPHY

ARWEILER, D. 1998. International comparisons of health expenditures. International Comparisons Series Paper. Papers commissioned by the National Forum on Health. Ottawa (ON). Published in this volume.

BARER, M. L., R. G. EVANS, and C. HERTZMAN. 1995. Avalanche or glacier? Health care and the demographic rhetoric. *Canadian Journal on Aging* 14(2): 193–224.

BARER, M. L., R. G. EVANS, C. HERTZMAN, and J. LOMAS. 1987. Aging and health care utilization: New evidence on old fallacies. *Social Science and Medicine* 24(10): 851–862.

BÉLAND, F., and A. LEMAY. 1995. Quelques dilemmes, quelques valeurs pour une politique de services de longue durée. *Canadian Journal on Aging* 14(2): 263–293.

BÉLAND, F., and E. SHAPIRO. 1993. Dix provinces appellent de leurs vœux la même politique de services de longue durée. *Journal of Canadian Studies*, 28(1): 166–191.

BERGMAN H., and F. BÉLAND. 1996. Vers une intégration des soins de santé. *Le Devoir*, section Idées, May 24.

BERGMAN, H., F. BÉLAND, E. LEIBOVICH, A. P. CONTANDRIOPOULOS, P. LEBEL, Y. BRUNELLE, T. KAUFMAN, P. TOUSIGNANT, R. RODRIGUEZ, R., and G. SCOTT. 1996. Care for the frail elderly in Canada: Fragmentation or integration. Manuscript in preparation. Research Group on Integrated Care for the Frail Elderly, Division of Geriatric Medicine, McGill University and Department of Health Administration, University of Montreal.

BERGMAN, H., F. BÉLAND, P. LEBEL, A.P. CONTANDRIOPOULOS, Y. BRUNNELLE, T. KAUFMAN, P. TOUSIGNANT, E. LEIBOVICH, R. RODRIGUEZ, R., and G. SCOTT. 1996. *A System of Integrated Care for the Frail Elderly*. Research Group on Integrated Care for the Frail Elderly, Division of Geriatric Medicine, McGill University and Department of Health Administration, University of Montreal. (Available in French.)

BOSANQUET, N. and A. ZAJDLER. 1993. Health care policies in the U.K. *Reviews in Clinical Gerontology* 3: 399–405.

BRANCH, L. G., R. F. COULAM, and Y. A. ZIMMERMAN. 1995. The PACE evaluation: Initial findings. *The Gerontologist* 35(3): 349–359.

BROUSSELLE, A. September 1996. 14 Fact Sheets. Working paper prepared for the National Forum on Health.

BROUSSELLE, A. 1998. Controlling health expenditures: What matters. International Comparison Series Paper. Papers commissioned by the National Forum on Health. Ottawa (ON). Published in this volume.

CHALLIS, D. 1993. The effectiveness of community care. *Reviews in Clinical Gerontology* 3: 97–104.

CHALLIS, D., R. DARTON, L. JOHNSON, M. STONE, and K. TRASKE. 1991a. An evaluation of an alternative to long-stay hospital care for frail elderly patients: I. The model of care. *Age and Ageing* 20: 236–244.

_____. 1991b. An evaluation of an alternative to long-stay hospital care for frail elderly patients: II. Costs and effectiveness. *Age and Ageing* 20: 245–254.

CLARFIELD A. M., and H. BERGMAN. 1991. Medical home care services for the housebound elderly: A program description. *CMAJ* 144: 41–45.

CONTANDRIOPOULOS, D. 1998. How Canada's health care system compares with that of other countries: An overview. International Comparison Series Paper. Papers commissioned by the National Forum on Health. Ottawa (ON)). Published in this volume.

DAVIES, B., D. HOBMAN, R. HOLLINGBERY, and A. NETTEN. 1994. *Building on EPICS Principles. New Models Combining the Provisions and Financing of Care and Their Costing*. London: Helen Hamlyn Foundation.

DEMERS, M. 1996. Factors explaining the increase in cost for physician care in Quebec's elderly population. *Canadian Medical Association Journal* 155 (11): 1555–1560.

EVANS, R. G., M. L. BARER, C. HERTZMAN, G. M. ANDERSON, I. R. PULCINS, and J. LOMAS. 1989. The long good-bye: The great transformation of the British Columbia Hospital System. *Health Services Research* 24(4): 435–459.

FINCH, M., R.A. KANE, R. KANE, J. CHRISTIANSON, and B. DOWD. 1992. *Design of the 2nd Generation S/HMO Demonstration: An Analysis of Multiple Incentives.* Minneapolis (MN): Institute for Health Services Research.

HAM, C. 1996a. Contestability: A middle path for health care. *British Medical Journal* 312: 70–71.

_____. 1996b. Managed markets in health care: The U.K. experiment. *Health Policy* 35: 279–292.

HAM, C., and M. BROMMELS. 1994. Health care reform in the Netherlands, Sweden, and the United Kingdom. *Health Affairs* 13(5): 106–119.

HERTZMAN C., I. R. PULCINS, M. R. BARER, R. G. EVANS, G. M. ANDERSON, and J. LOMAS. 1990. Flat on your back or back to your flat? Sources of increased hospital services utilization among the elderly in British Columbia. *Social Science and Medicine* 30(7): 819–828.

HOLLANDER, M. J. 1994. *The Costs and Cost-Effectiveness of Continuing Care Services in Canada.* Ottawa (ON): Queen's–University of Ottawa Economic Projects.

HOLLANDER, M. J., and P. PALLAN. 1995. The British Columbia continuing care system: Service delivery and resource planning. *Aging: Clinical and Experimental Research* 7(2): 94–109.

JOHANSSON, L. November 15–19, 1995. *Swedish Elder Care in Transition—Results from an Ongoing Evaluation of Legal Reforms.* Paper presented at the 48th GSA meeting in Los Angeles.

KANE, R. L. 1995. Health care reform and the care of older adults. *Journal of the American Geriatrics Society* 43: 702–706.

KANE, R. A., and L. STARR. February 1996. *Managed Care, Medicaid and the Elderly—The Minnesota Experience* (report 4 in a series of state case studies). The National Resource Centre, University of Minnesota, Institute for Health Policy Research. Sponsored by the Administration on Aging.

KANE, R. L., L. H. ILLSTON, and N. A. MILLER. 1992. Qualitative analysis of the Program of All-Inclusive Care for the Elderly (PACE). *The Gerontologist* 32(6): 771–780.

Rapport de la commission d'enquête sur les services de santé et les services sociaux. 1988. Les publications du Québec.

RÉGIE RÉGIONALE DE LA SANTÉ ET DES SERVICES SOCIAUX, MONTRÉAL-CENTRE. 1995. *Recommendations – The Organization of Health and Social Services on the Island of Montreal. Achieving a New Balance.*

SALTMAN, R. B. 1991. Emerging trends in the Swedish health system. *International Journal of Health Services* 21(4): 615–623.

_____. 1994. Patient choice and patient empowerment in Northern European health systems: A conceptual framework. *International Journal of Health Services* 24(2): 201–229.

_____. 1995. The role of competitive incentives in recent reforms of Northern European health systems. In *Health Care Reform through Internal Markets—Experience and Proposal,* eds. JÉROME-FORGET et al. Canada: Institute for Research on Public Policy. pp. 75–94.

SALTMAN, R. B., and C. VAN OTTER. 1995. Balancing social and economic responsibility. In *Implementing Planned Markets in Health Care—Balancing Social and Economic Responsibility,* eds. R. B. SALTMAN and C. VAN OTTER. Buckingham: Open University Press, pp. 239-251.

SHAPIRO, E. 1994. Community and long-term health care in Canada. In *Limits to Care—Reforming Canada's Health System in an Age of Restraint,* eds. A. BLOMQUIST, and D. M. BROWN. Toronto (ON): McGraw-Hill Ryerson Limited. pp. 327–362.

_____. 1995. Case management in long-term care—Exploring its status, trends, and issues. *Journal of Case Management* 4(2): 43–47.

SMEE, C. H. 1995. Self-governing trusts and GP fundholders: The British experience. In *Implementing Planned Markets in Health Care—Balancing Social and Economic Responsibility,* eds. R. B. SALTMAN, and C. VON OTTER. Buckingham: Open University Press. pp. 177–208.

SUNDSTROM, G., and M. THORSLUND. 1994. Caring for the frail elderly in Sweden. In *The Graying of the World. Who Will Care for the Frail Elderly?*, ed. L. K. OLSON. New York (NY): The Haworth Press. pp. 59–81.

TAMBLYN, R. M., P. J. MCLEOD,M. ABRAHAMOWICZ, J. MONETTE, D. C. GAYTON, L. BERKSON, W. D. DAUPHINEE, R. M. GRAD, A. R. HUANG, L. M. ISSAAC, et al. 1994. Questionable prescribing for elderly patients in Quebec. *Canadian Medical Association Journal* 150(11): 1801–1809.

THE CENTRE FOR INTERNATIONAL STATISTICS AT THE CANADIAN COUNCIL ON SOCIAL DEVELOPMENT. 1998. Health spending and health status: An international comparison. International Comparison Series Paper. Papers commissioned by the National Forum on Health. Ottawa (ON). Published in this volume.

THORSLUND, M., and M. G. PARKER. 1994. Care of the elderly in the changing Swedish welfare state. In *Community Care: New Agendas and Challenges from the U.K. and Overseas*, eds. D. CHALLIS, B. DAVIES, and K. TRASKE. Great Britain: British Society of Gerontology. pp. 249–263.

TRAHAN, L., and L. BÉLANGER, L. 1993. *Une évaluation de la prestation de services dans les CLSC et les centres hospitaliers pour des services de qualité aux personnes âgées en perte d'autonomie* (Collection Études et Analyses, no 19). MSSS. Direction générale de la planification et de l'évaluation.

YORDI, C. L., and J. WALDMAN. 1985. A consolidated model of long-term care: Service utilization and cost impacts. *The Gerontological Society of America* 25(4): 389–397.

ZAWADSKI, R. T., and C. ENG. 1988. Case management in capitated long-term care. *Health Care Financing Review*, annual supplement: 75–81.

Puzzling Issues in Health Care Financing

RAISA DEBER, PH.D.

Professor of Health Policy
University of Toronto

BILL SWAN

Queen's Health Policy
Kingston

PUZZLING ISSUE NO. 3

1. Canada is among the lowest third of OECD countries in terms of its share of public funding for health care. Public funding is also more skewed towards hospital and physician services in Canada than in most European countries. Would/could a more even distribution of public funding across the health service continuum (hospitals, physicians, drugs, community-based care, etc.) improve overall cost control without compromising access?
2. (Supplementary question) Why have some countries such as England been able to maintain a fairly constant private sector without the predicted "downward spiral" to an American-type system?

TABLE OF CONTENTS

Question One: Introduction and Summary 310

Overview of Data 310

Hypotheses 311

    Choosing the Comparator Matters 311

    Measurement of Health Expenditures Is Hardly
    an Exact Science 318

Discussion 329

Question Two (Supplementary Question):
The Case of the United Kingdom 331

Conclusions 335

Bibliography 338

APPENDIX

Working with Cross-National Data... 341

LIST OF TABLES

Table 1   Expenditure on health care in OECD countries as a %
of GDP, 1960–1995 312

Table 2   International health care spending, % publicly funded,
1960–1995 314

Table 3   Metrics matter: Value and rank of total health spending
(1993) in OECD countries under different measurement
approaches 316

Table 4   The public-private mix in Canadian health expenditures,
by subcategory of expenditure, 1992 320

Table 5   The public-private mix in Canadian health expenditures,
by subcategory of expenditures, 1975–1994 322

Table 6   Percentage of public expenditure in OECD countries,
selected categories, 1991–1995 327

QUESTION ONE: INTRODUCTION AND SUMMARY

> *Canada is among the lowest third of OECD countries in terms of its share of public funding for health care. Public funding is also more skewed towards hospital and physician services in Canada than in most European countries. Would/could a more even distribution of public funding across the health service continuum (hospitals, physicians, drugs, community-based care, etc.) improve overall cost control without compromising access?*

Following the review of six papers commissioned for the "Striking a Balance" working group of the National Forum on Health, a number of "puzzling issues" were identified. As will become evident, the brief answer to puzzling question one is "no." The puzzle arises in part from difficulties in defining costs in a manner that allows for meaningful comparisons across health care systems, and in part from the paucity of data clarifying funding by sector. In particular, the evidence suggests that the best cost control is precisely within the areas with the highest proportion of public financing; to the extent a "more even" distribution implies taking money away from the hospital and physician sectors and diverting it to other sectors, evidence suggests that this would worsen both access and cost control. However, to the extent that "more even" implies maintenance of the current support for needed services within the hospital and physician sectors but also broadening the scope of services so qualifying, there may indeed be scope for improvement.

OVERVIEW OF DATA

Much of the concern about cost control (or the lack thereof) in Canadian health care has arisen from an examination of OECD data (OECD 1996). Table 1 depicts the widely cited OECD comparison of health expenditures as a percentage of gross domestic product (GDP) in industrialized countries; examination shows that by 1992, Canada's spending had risen to 10.3 percent, second only to the United States. Although this ranking can be partially attributed to the role of two back-to-back recessions in the 1980s (Evans 1993), and although cost-cutting efforts coupled with economic recovery had reduced this ratio to 9.5 percent by 1995, Canada still appeared to be one of the most expensive public health care systems in the world. Less widely noticed is the fact that over the past 25 years Canada has seen a long-term—although slow—decline in the percentage of the system which is publicly funded, and has consistently ranked below the OECD average on this measure (table 2). In 1975, the system was 75.9 percent publicly funded; by 1994 that had declined to 71.8 percent.

However, when making international comparisons of health data, it is important to be aware that there are often significant data incompatibilities across countries. Indeed, the papers commissioned by the Forum and reviewed here in draft form (Contandriopoulos 1998; Arweiler 1998; Brousselle 1998; CIS 1998; Scott 1998; Kennedy 1998), as well as a number of consultations made for this review, stress that international comparisons of expenditures must be treated with caution. Moreover, although a detailed review of data was beyond the scope of this paper, consultation with both developers and users of Canada's health expenditures data has shed light on a number of questions regarding both the creation of the health expenditures data set in Canada and inconsistencies between that data and the data available from the OECD. In addressing this "puzzling issue," it is accordingly prudent to discuss a number of the assumptions which underlie the data.

HYPOTHESES

Choosing the Comparator Matters

As noted above, policy analysts have gotten into the habit of looking at health expenditures as a proportion of GDP. Consequently, the revelation that Canada had risen to the rank of number two internationally (10.2 percent in 1993), second only to the United States (14.3 percent), and considerably worse than such countries as Japan (6.6 percent) and the United Kingdom (6.9 percent), evoked cries of alarm and pessimism.

The paper by Arweiler (1998) gives a clear explanation of alternative and arguably more reliable methods of measuring health expenditure and consequently ranking countries internationally, illustrated with comparative data from 24 OECD countries for 1993. We have used these observations and the OECD data set to note how Canada's ranking changes depending upon how one chooses to measure health spending (table 3).

According to Arweiler, the simplest way of comparing expenditures across countries is "nominal" health expenditures per capita, in which all series are converted using the current exchange rate (the price of the national monetary unit in foreign currency) into a common metric (usually U.S. dollars). Nominal expenditures therefore reflect some combination of the strength of the currency, the differences in quantities of goods and services provided, and price differences—although it is hard to disentangle the contribution of each element. Based on this method, Canada ranked ninth ($1,943 per capita), with the United States first ($3,299 per capita), followed by such countries as Switzerland ($3,294 per capita), Japan ($2,463 per capita), and Germany ($2,308 per capita). By this measure, Canadian spending would not appear to be out of line, and Japan's performance is not nearly as impressive.

A more subtle measure, purchasing power parity (PPP) per capita, is computed by comparing the prices of identical products in various countries and dividing by population. This eliminates price disparities between countries. With this comparator, Canadian performance is less impressive, ranking fourth

Table 1

Expenditure on health care in OECD countries as a % of GDP, 1960-1995

	1960	1965	1970	1975	1980	1985	1990	1991	1992	1993	1994	1995
Australia	4.9	5.1	5.7	7.5	7.3	7.7	8.3	8.6	8.7	8.6	8.5	8.4
Austria	4.4	4.7	5.4	7.3	7.9	8.1	8.4	8.5	8.9	9.4	9.7	9.6
Belgium	3.4	3.9	4.1	5.9	6.6	7.4	7.6	8.0	8.1	8.3	8.2	8.0
Canada	5.5	6.0	7.1	7.3	7.3	8.5	9.2	9.9	10.3	10.2	9.8	9.5
Czech Republic	–	–	–	–	–	–	5.3	5.4	5.4	7.7	7.6	–
Denmark	3.6	4.8	6.1	6.5	6.8	6.3	6.5	6.5	6.7	6.8	6.6	6.5
Finland	3.9	4.9	5.7	6.4	6.5	7.3	8.0	9.1	9.3	8.8	8.3	8.2
France	4.2	5.2	5.8	7.0	7.6	8.5	8.9	9.1	9.4	9.8	9.7	9.9
Germany	4.8	5.1	5.9	8.1	8.4	8.7	8.3	9.0	9.3	9.3	9.5	9.6
Greece	2.4	2.6	3.4	3.4	3.6	4.1	4.3	4.3	4.5	4.6	5.2	–
Hungary	–	–	–	–	–	–	6.6	6.6	6.8	6.9	7.0	–
Iceland	3.3	3.9	5.0	5.8	6.2	7.3	7.9	8.1	8.2	8.3	8.1	8.1
Ireland	3.8	4.2	5.3	7.6	8.7	7.8	6.7	7.0	7.3	7.4	7.9	–
Italy	3.6	4.3	5.1	6.2	6.9	7.0	8.1	8.4	8.5	8.6	8.3	7.7
Japan	–	–	4.4	5.5	6.4	6.7	6.0	6.1	6.4	6.6	6.9	7.2
Luxembourg	–	–	3.7	5.1	6.2	6.1	6.2	6.2	6.3	6.2	5.8	–
Mexico	–	–	–	–	–	–	–	–	4.9	5.0	5.3	–
Netherlands	3.8	4.3	5.9	7.5	7.9	7.9	8.4	8.6	8.8	9.0	8.8	8.8
New Zealand	4.3	–	5.2	6.7	7.2	6.4	7.4	7.8	7.8	7.3	7.5	–

Table 1 (cont.)

	1960	1965	1970	1975	1980	1985	1990	1991	1992	1993	1994	1995
Norway	3.0	3.6	4.6	6.1	6.1	5.9	6.9	7.2	7.4	7.3	7.3	–
Portugal	–	–	2.8	5.6	5.8	6.3	6.6	7.1	7.2	7.4	7.6	–
Spain	1.5	2.6	3.7	4.9	5.7	5.7	6.9	7.1	7.2	7.3	7.3	7.6
Sweden	4.7	5.5	7.1	7.9	9.4	8.9	8.6	8.4	7.6	7.6	7.7	7.7
Switzerland	3.3	3.8	5.2	7.0	7.3	8.1	8.4	9.0	9.4	9.5	9.6	–
Turkey	–	–	2.4	2.7	3.3	2.2	2.9	3.4	2.9	2.6	4.2	–
United Kingdom	3.9	4.1	4.5	5.5	5.6	5.9	6.0	6.5	7.0	6.9	6.9	6.9
United States	5.2	5.8	7.2	3.2	9.1	10.7	12.7	13.5	14	14.3	14.3	14.5
Mean	3.9	4.4	5.1	5.3	6.8	7.1	7.4	7.7	7.7	7.8	7.9	8.6
Mean w/o U.S.	3.7	4.3	4.9	6.2	6.7	6.9	7.1	7.4	7.4	7.6	7.6	8.2

Source: OECD Health Data 1996.

Table 2

International health care spending, % publicly funded, 1960–1995

	1960	1965	1970	1975	1980	1985	1990	1991	1992	1993	1994	1995
Australia	47.6	54.0	56.7	72.8	62.9	71.7	68.1	67.8	67.8	67.3	68.5	–
Austria	69.4	70.3	63.0	69.6	68.8	66.7	66.1	65.5	65.8	65.1	63.4	–
Belgium	61.6	75.3	87.0	79.6	83.4	81.8	88.9	88.1	88.9	88.9	87.9	87.8
Canada	42.7	52.1	70.2	75.9	75.1	75.1	74.6	74.6	74.1	73.1	71.8	–
Czech Republic	–	–	–	–	–	–	–	–	–	–	–	–
Denmark	88.7	85.9	86.3	91.9	85.2	84.4	82.3	83.3	83.0	82.9	83.0	–
Finland	54.1	66.0	73.8	78.6	79.0	78.6	80.9	81.1	79.6	77.1	75.2	–
France	57.8	68.1	74.7	77.2	78.8	76.9	74.5	74.7	74.6	74.2	78.4	78.4
Germany	66.1	70.8	69.6	77.2	75.0	73.6	71.8	73.1	74.2	73.0	73.5	73.5
Greece	64.2	71.1	53.4	60.2	82.2	81.0	84.2	75.7	76.1	75.8	–	–
Hungary	–	–	–	–	–	–	–	–	–	–	–	–
Iceland	76.7	81.1	81.7	87.2	88.2	87.0	86.8	87	85.1	83.7	84.0	84.1
Ireland	76.0	76.2	81.7	79.0	82.2	77.4	74.7	77.2	77.8	77.8	76.0	–
Italy	83.1	87.8	86.9	84.5	80.4	77.1	78.1	78.3	76.3	72.9	70.6	70.0
Japan	60.4	61.4	69.8	72.0	71.3	70.7	77.1	77.2	76.9	78.4	79.1	–
Luxembourg	–	–	–	91.8	92.8	89.2	98.5	97.3	98.8	100.0	–	–
Mexico	–	–	–	–	–	–	–	–	58.0	58.0	58.0	–
Netherlands	33.3	68.7	84.3	73.4	74.7	75.1	72.4	73.8	77.4	78.2	77.6	77.5
New Zealand	80.6	–	80.3	83.9	83.6	86.3	82.2	79	76.6	75.9	76.9	–

Table 2 (cont.)

	1960	1965	1970	1975	1980	1985	1990	1991	1992	1993	1994	1995
Norway	77.8	80.9	91.6	96.2	98.4	96.5	94.5	94.2	94.8	93.3	94.5	–
Portugal	–	–	59.0	58.9	64.3	54.6	54.6	55.5	56.0	55.7	55.8	56.0
Spain	58.7	50.8	65.4	77.4	79.9	81.1	78.7	78.9	78.8	78.6	78.6	78.2
Sweden	72.6	79.5	86.0	90.2	92.5	90.2	89.7	88.3	85.2	83.5	83.4	–
Switzerland	61.3	60.8	63.9	68.9	67.5	66.1	68.4	68.6	70.1	71.8	71.8	–
Turkey	–	–	37.3	49.0	27.3	50.2	35.6	65.7	46.1	52.3	58.1	–
United Kingdom	85.2	85.8	87.0	91.1	89.4	85.8	84.1	83.7	84.5	84.8	84.1	–
United States	24.8	25.0	37.8	42.1	42.4	40.7	40.8	42.1	42.8	43.4	44.3	48.4
Mean	63.9	68.6	71.6	76.2	76.1	75.7	75.3	76.3	74.8	74.6	73.7	72.7
Mean w/o U.S.	66.9	71.8	73.9	77.9	78.2	77.5	77.2	78.2	76.5	76.3	75.3	75.7

Source: OECD Health Data 1996.

per capita ($1,971), following the United States ($3,299 per capita), Switzerland ($2,283 per capita), and Luxembourg ($1,993 per capita). Again, factors such as quantity of care consumed, prices paid to doctors, and global costs of care, cannot be disentangled. A variant measure, PPP (health) looks at the cost of an equivalent basket of health goods and services across countries. On this measure, Canada ranked tenth ($3,020), with France highest ($4,128), followed by Japan ($3,858). Clearly the choice of comparator changes the international rankings of health expenditures substantially. In addition, absolute differences are often not large, meaning that relatively small shifts can have a fairly major effect upon international rank.

Table 3

Metrics matter: Value and rank of total health spending (1993) in OECD countries under different measurement approaches

	% of GDP		Nominal ($) per capita		PPP per capita		PPP health per capita	
	Value	Rank	Value	Rank	Value	Rank	Value	Rank
United States	14.3	1	3,299	1	3,299	1	3,299	5
Canada	10.2	2	1,943	9	1,971	4	3,020	10
France	9.8	3	2,129	6	1,835	5	4,128	1
Switzerland	9.5	4	3,294	2	2,283	2	3,801	3
Austria	9.4	5	2,117	7	1,777	7	3,157	6
Germany	9.3	6	2,308	4	1,815	6	3,076	8
Netherlands	9.0	7	1,760	11	1,631	8	2,842	12
Finland	8.8	8	1,449	16	1,363	15	2,355	15
Italy	8.6	9	1,485	15	1,523	12	3,008	11
Australia	8.6	9	1,392	17	1,493	14	2,733	13
Iceland	8.3	11	1,902	10	1,564	11	3,100	7
Belgium	8.3	11	1,727	13	1,601	9	3,061	9
Sweden	7.6	13	1,598	14	1,266	17	2,157	17
Ireland	7.4	14	884	21	922	21	1,473	21
Portugal	7.4	14	630	22	866	22	1,368	22
Norway	7.3	16	1,962	8	1,592	10	2,702	14
New Zealand	7.3	16	961	19	1,179	19	2,092	19
Spain	7.3	16	890	20	972	20	1,925	20
United Kingdom	6.9	19	1,161	18	1,213	18	2,328	16
Denmark	6.8	20	1,756	12	1,296	16	2,097	18
Japan	6.6	21	2,463	3	1,495	13	3,858	2
Luxembourg	6.2	22	2,284	5	1,993	3	3,777	4
Greece	4.6	23	402	23	500	23	1,059	23
Turkey	2.6	24	79	24	146	24	333	24

The continued insistence on the use of the ratio of expenditures for health care services to GDP as the "gold standard" for measuring costs appears to play a part in the perception that there has been a cost explosion in Canada's health care system. As a guide to policy action, however, this ratio is misleading for several reasons.

First, as Evans (1993) has pointed out, a GDP ratio has both a numerator and a denominator. One of the clearest relationships is between national wealth and health spending, a finding reiterated by most of the six papers reviewed. For example, Arweiler's regressions (1998) noted that per capita GDP explained over 90 percent of the variance in care expenditures across OECD countries, and that Canadian consumption (in quantity of care) fell within the confidence interval (i.e., it was what would be predicted on the basis of national wealth). Contandriopoulos' regressions (1998) yielded similar findings. In a well-performing economy, even relatively high spending can form a small percentage of GDP. For example, Japan's per capita spending appears considerable, although their very healthy economy made it appear that their costs were under control; Alberta showed similar results during the oil boom. Conversely, a poor economy can make relatively stable costs a growing proportion of national wealth. Much of Canada's seemingly poor performance arose from a recession, which meant a diminished ability to sustain the levels of spending derived from previous economic performance, rather than from health spending itself being "out of control." Arweiler noted that the combination of economic improvements and increased provincial willingness to use their regulatory power has caused health expenditures in Canada to have grown more slowly than GDP since 1991 (4.19 percent vs. 4.42 percent) (Arweiler 1998).

Next, the ratio of spending to GDP is an aggregate, which hides significant variations. Attempts to control health care costs have often been compared to "pushing on a balloon." Squeezing one sector (e.g., hospitals) may just cause costs to balloon in other sectors (e.g., ambulatory care) as patterns of care shift to accommodate the availability of resources. Unfortunately, existing data is not strong enough to make these sorts of computations (certainly the papers reviewed do not even try to do so). To fully address this "puzzling issue," data on spending growth by sector is necessary. For such data to be meaningful, cost shifting (eg., from hospitals to home care, pharmaceuticals, etc.) would have to be minimal, and definitions of what belonged in each sector would have to be stable over time. (For example, is day surgery classified as hospital or ambulatory care? What of mental health services?)

Next, if one wishes to focus upon population health, it must be recognized that a very small proportion of health spending can be expected to show up in the sorts of health outcomes commonly used for analysis. How many interventions would be expected to directly affect life expectancy or alter infant mortality? Existing measures capture morbidity only imperfectly, and therefore may considerably understate health benefits. For example, the paper by the Centre for International Statistics at CCSD (1998) found no strong link between spending and health status (at least as measured by life expectancy and infant mortality). This is not surprising, given how few medical interventions are intended to directly affect these outcomes. However, the same paper also found no correlation between these health outcomes and such factors as income security, education, or labour market programs, even though these are clearly related to the determinants of health. One likely explanation is that the existing ways of measuring health outcomes miss most of the picture, and policy made on this basis may similarly miss significant improvements (or harms) to the health of a population.

Next, many spending decisions relate to policy goals totally unrelated to health outcomes, even if they were more measurable. A decision to pay health workers at a higher rate, or introduce pay equity, or sustain a facility in a rural community, is justified on grounds other than those of health. To that end, the Contandriopoulos paper (1998) notes its suspicion that prices are a key factor in Canadian performance.

Finally, political science has recognized a series of "governing instruments" whereby government can influence private activity (Doern and Phidd 1992). These include "exhortation," "expenditure," "regulation," and "public ownership." The political science literature would stress that government can achieve cost control in many ways, and that regulatory authority over sectors may be a more powerful lever than merely spending the money. (Public expenditure itself does not control costs; it merely eases the task of enforcing regulatory controls once government has chosen to exert its monopsony buying power.)

Measurement of Health Expenditures Is Hardly an Exact Science

While choosing a proper comparator is certainly important, the intricacies of producing health expenditures data at a national level and the problems with translating these for international study may cause more potential for misinterpretation. As a result, it is very difficult to be confident about cross-national comparisons. Arweiler (1998) notes that the data is not necessarily comparable, as it is difficult to allow for the sociocultural, economic, and medical characteristics of each country, and that this not reflected in calculation of price indices. "In effect, since the definitions of care expenditures vary from country to country, as do the variables, the same relationships are not being measured in all of the countries."

As a result, differing definitions of care may lead to potential misinterpretations in a number of areas. For example, study of the health expenditures data produced by Health Canada (Health Canada 1996) suggests that the differing interpretation used by the OECD may underestimate the size of the public share of funding for international comparison by up to 2 percent. When the expenditures data is disaggregated more problems become apparent. In the drug sector, for example, the OECD database estimates 25 percent of pharmaceuticals come from public funds (Kennedy 1998), whereas Health Canada puts the figure closer to 33 percent.

Perhaps more interestingly, the OECD interpretation of data may also lead to underestimation of the public share of the drug sector. In Canadian health expenditure data, drug expenditures in hospitals, drugs provided directly by physicians, and immunization expenditures are not counted as part of the overall drug expenditure. While this does not change the public component of total health care, it can lead to misinterpretation of the data on both a sectoral and subsectoral level. For example, the percentage of drug expenditure in hospitals has been estimated at five percent. If this was included as public drug expenditures (rather than hospital expenditure) the percentage of public drug expenditure would be closer to 40 percent, rather than 33 percent as suggested by initial scrutiny of Health Canada's expenditure data.

There are a number of other potential problems which may undermine the stability of health expenditures data in Canada. The source of the data becomes an issue particularly when data is disaggregated to private expenditures (Phillips, personal communication). Data from hospitals, physicians, and workers' compensation has been largely accepted as high-quality data as its source is well regulated. Similarly, data from private insurance companies has been useful for augmenting the private insurance expenditures data (although the quality of the data can vary depending on company and insurance plan). Unfortunately, data is not nearly as robust for private out-of-pocket expenses. These data rely primarily on surveys and other tabulations to estimate the amount spent out-of-pocket in a number of areas, such as alternative providers, prescribed drugs, home care, and ambulances. As can be seen in table 4, a number of the "other" expenditure categories do not include breakdowns for private spending, and intuitively seem underestimated.

As the working group requested, we have constructed tables giving the breakdown in such spending by sector for Canada (table 5) and for the OECD countries (table 6). Caution must be exerted in their interpretation (see appendix).

Table 4

The public-private mix in Canadian health expenditures, by subcategory of expenditure, 1992

Subcategory	Public sector (million $)	Private sector (million $)	Public %	Private %	Total (million $)
Hospitals	24,369.1	2,408.9	91.0	9.0	26,778.0
Other institutions	4,944.2	1,889.9	72.3	27.7	6,834.1
Physicians/psychologists	10,368.7	95.2	99.1	0.9	10,463.9
Other professionals	965.7	4,947.2	16.3	83.7	5,912.9
of which:					
Dentists/denturists	326.8	4,269.8	7.1	92.9	4,596.6
Other professionals	638.9	677.4	48.5	51.5	1,316.3
of which:					
Chiropractors	198.2	–			
Optometrists/orthopists	205.6	–			
Podiatrists	18.7	–			
Osteopaths/naturopaths	2.4	–			
Private duty nurses	4.5	–			
Physiotherapists	209.4	–			
Drugs	2,862.6	5,589.0	33.9	66.1	8,451.6
of which:					
Drugs—prescribed	2,862.6	3,187.5	47.3	52.7	6,050.1
Drugs—nonprescribed	0	1,122.7	0	100.0	1,122.7
Health personnel supplies	0	1,278.8	0	100.0	1,278.8

Table 4 (cont.)

Subcategory	Public sector (million $)	Private sector (million $)	Public %	Private %	Total (million $)
Capital	**1,721.4**	**557.1**	**75.5**	**24.5**	**2,278.5**
Other expenditures	**6,646.2**	**2,666.8**	**71.4**	**28.6**	**9,313.0**
of which:					
Home care	915.6	–			
Ambulance	783.2	–			
Eyeglasses	18.1	1,295.3	1.4	98.6	1,313.4
Hearing aids	11.9	–			
Health appliances	294	–			
Unspecified services	216.9	–			
Prepayment administration	416.3	808.2	34.0	66.0	1,224.5
Public health	3,280.5	–			
Health research	463.8	264.2	63.7	36.3	728.0
Miscellaneous health care	245.8	–			
Other private health care	–	299.2			
All categories	**51,877.9**	**18,154.1**	**74.1**	**25.9**	**70,032.0**

Source: Health Canada. 1996. *National Health Expenditures in Canada 1975–1994.* Table 13A.

Table 5

**The public-private mix in Canadian health expenditures,
by subcategory of expenditures, 1975–1994**

Year	Total (million $)	Public (million $)	Public (%)	Private (million $)	Private (%)
		Hospitals			
1975	5,512.0	5,196.2	94.3	315.7	5.7
1976	6,406.0	6,029.0	94.1	377.0	5.9
1977	6,838.7	6,421.5	93.9	417.2	6.1
1978	7,441.2	6,924.2	93.1	517.0	6.9
1979	8,172.7	7,549.6	92.4	623.0	7.6
1980	9,395.2	8,650.0	92.1	745.2	7.9
1981	11,131.0	10,231.2	91.9	899.8	8.1
1982	13,234.7	12,147.4	91.8	1,087.3	8.2
1983	14,557.6	13,317.5	91.5	1,240.1	8.5
1984	15,449.4	14,043.6	90.9	1,405.8	9.1
1985	16,383.6	14,863.7	90.7	1,519.9	9.3
1986	17,737.1	16,099.9	90.8	1,637.2	9.2
1987	19,111.3	17,340.6	90.7	1,770.7	9.3
1988	20,471.1	18,652.2	91.1	1,818.9	8.9
1989	22,361.0	20,454.0	91.5	1,907.0	8.5
1990	23,870.5	21,811.8	91.4	2,058.6	8.6
1991	25,725.1	23,499.0	91.3	2,226.1	8.7
1992	26,778.0	24,369.1	91.0	2,408.9	9.0
1993	27,138.8	24,543.2	90.4	2,595.6	9.6
1994	26,999.1	24,206.0	89.7	2,793.1	10.3
		Other institutions			
1975	1,124.3	795.9	70.8	328.4	29.2
1976	1,367.8	998.2	73.0	369.6	27.0
1977	1,575.9	1,174.1	74.5	401.8	25.5
1978	1,850.4	1,366.0	73.8	484.4	26.2
1979	2,169.7	1,579.2	72.8	590.5	27.2
1980	2,536.6	1,818.0	71.7	718.6	28.3
1981	2,882.4	2,138.9	74.2	743.6	25.8
1982	3,336.2	2,482.5	74.4	853.7	25.6
1983	3,694.9	2,747.5	74.4	947.5	25.6
1984	3,886.2	2,893.5	74.5	992.6	25.5
1985	4,076.9	3,037.1	74.5	1,039.8	25.5
1986	4,066.6	2,961.1	72.8	1,105.5	27.2

Table 5 (cont.)

Year	Total (million $)	Public (million $)	Public (%)	Private (million $)	Private (%)
Other institutions (cont.)					
1987	4,308.1	3,110.2	72.2	1,197.9	27.8
1988	4,715.5	3,445.5	73.1	1,270.0	26.9
1989	5,117.5	3,805.2	74.4	1312.3	25.6
1990	5,720.3	4,139.1	72.4	1,581.2	27.6
1991	6,315.9	4,547.7	72.0	1,768.2	28.0
1992	6,834.1	4,944.3	72.3	1,889.9	27.7
1993	7,007.9	4,991.7	71.2	2,016.2	28.8
1994	7,090.3	4,952.0	69.8	2,138.3	30.2
Physicians/psychologists					
1975	1,839.9	1,813.2	98.5	26.7	1.5
1976	2,071.0	2,041.5	98.6	29.5	1.4
1977	2,284.4	2,252.1	98.6	32.3	1.4
1978	2,566.7	2,528.4	98.5	38.3	1.5
1979	2,857.0	2,804.5	98.2	52.5	1.8
1980	3,287.5	3,236.0	98.4	51.5	1.6
1981	3,824.8	3,775.1	98.7	49.7	1.3
1982	4,420.8	4,353.2	98.5	67.6	1.5
1983	5,052.6	4,973.3	98.4	79.3	1.6
1984	5,525.8	5,444.6	98.5	81.2	1.5
1985	6,046.7	5,963.2	98.6	83.5	1.4
1986	6,675.3	6,598.4	98.8	76.8	1.2
1987	7,342.4	7,265.8	99.0	76.5	1.0
1988	7,948.0	7,868.1	99.0	79.9	1.0
1989	8516.5	8,432.1	99.0	84.4	1.0
1990	9,258.3	9,169.8	99.0	88.6	1.0
1991	10,219.6	10,127.7	99.1	91.9	0.9
1992	10,463.9	10,368.7	99.1	95.2	0.9
1993	10,362.6	10,264.0	99.0	98.6	1.0
1994	10,322.6	10,222.2	99.0	100.4	1.0
Other professionals					
1975	901.7	135.2	15.0	766.5	85.0
1976	1,052.7	160.4	15.2	892.3	84.8
1977	1,240.2	184.8	14.9	1,055.4	85.1
1978	1,426.9	226.4	15.9	1,200.5	84.1
1979	1,649.1	284.3	17.2	1,364.8	82.8

Table 5 (cont.)

Year	Total (million $)	Public (million $)	Public (%)	Private (million $)	Private (%)
Other professionals (cont.)					
1980	1,906.6	360.7	18.9	1,545.9	81.1
1981	2,183.3	475.5	21.8	1,707.7	78.2
1982	2,514.0	494.4	19.7	2,019.5	80.3
1983	2,737.0	519.9	19.0	2,217.1	81.0
1984	2,959.3	554.4	18.7	2,404.8	81.3
1985	3,312.0	594.9	18.0	2,717.0	82.0
1986	3,631.2	657.9	18.1	2,973.3	81.9
1987	3,956.4	684.7	17.3	3,271.7	82.7
1988	4,310.2	712.4	16.5	3,597.8	83.5
1989	4,752.9	792.6	16.7	3,960.3	83.3
1990	5,179.5	865.5	16.7	4,314.0	83.3
1991	5,636.8	960.6	17.0	4,676.2	83.0
1992	5,912.9	965.7	16.3	4,947.2	83.7
1993	6,056.1	901.8	14.9	5154.2	85.1
1994	6,192.9	846.9	13.7	5,346.0	86.3
Drugs					
1975	1,073.5	157.5	14.7	916.0	85.3
1976	1,194.8	214.3	17.9	980.6	82.1
1977	1,305.8	263.6	20.2	1,042.1	79.8
1978	1,438.4	324.5	22.6	1,114.0	77.4
1979	1,651.5	383.3	23.2	1,268.2	76.8
1980	1,877.5	461.9	24.6	1,415.6	75.4
1981	2,324.7	563.7	24.2	1,761.0	75.8
1982	2,631.6	680.4	25.9	1,951.2	74.1
1983	2,945.6	814.0	27.6	2,131.6	72.4
1984	3,305.6	939.5	28.4	2,366.0	71.6
1985	3,788.7	1,109.8	29.3	2,678.9	70.7
1986	4,401.0	1,307.8	29.7	3,093.3	70.3
1987	4,896.0	1,477.9	30.2	3,418.0	69.8
1988	5,502.0	1,689.0	30.7	3,813.0	69.3
1989	6,213.9	1,951.5	31.4	4,262.5	68.6
1990	6,903.1	2,255.7	32.7	4,647.4	67.3
1991	7,670.6	2,578.6	33.6	5,092.0	66.4
1992	8,451.6	2,862.6	33.9	5,589.0	66.1
1993	8,841.7	2,908.5	32.9	5,933.2	67.1
1994	9,179.3	2,929.0	31.9	6,250.3	68.1

Table 5 (cont.)

Year	Total (million $)	Public (million $)	Public (%)	Private (million $)	Private (%)
Capital					
1975	536.9	377.2	70.3	159.6	29.7
1976	545.3	368.2	67.5	177.1	32.5
1977	564.7	386.4	68.4	178.3	31.6
1978	672.5	455.1	67.7	217.4	32.3
1979	786.9	609.6	77.5	177.3	22.5
1980	1,054.4	698.9	66.3	355.4	33.7
1981	1,206.7	827.4	68.6	379.3	31.4
1982	1,467.1	978.0	66.7	489.1	33.3
1983	1,510.0	1,138.6	75.4	371.4	24.6
1984	1,560.9	1,196.6	76.7	364.3	23.3
1985	1,839.0	1,424.6	77.5	414.4	22.5
1986	2,026.2	1,576.3	77.8	449.9	22.2
1987	2,058.4	1,577.7	76.6	480.7	23.4
1988	2,022.7	1,436.9	71.0	585.8	29.0
1989	2,197.9	1,622.0	73.8	575.9	26.2
1990	2,231.9	1,717.3	76.9	514.6	23.1
1991	2,092.0	1,610.7	77.0	481.3	23.0
1992	2,278.5	1,721.4	75.5	557.1	24.5
1993	2,290.7	1,755.6	76.6	535.1	23.4
1994	2,074.3	1,549.7	74.7	524.6	25.3
Other					.
1975	1,266.6	886.5	70.0	380.1	30.0
1976	1,461.4	1,059.5	72.5	401.9	27.5
1977	1,687.9	1,213.8	71.9	474.1	28.1
1978	1,772.7	1,281.6	72.3	491.1	27.7
1979	2,001.6	1,464.7	73.2	536.9	26.8
1980	2,340.7	1,726.3	73.8	614.4	26.2
1981	2,888.7	2,103.3	72.8	785.4	27.2
1982	3,305.7	2,464.7	74.6	840.9	25.4
1983	3,667.3	2,698.7	73.6	968.6	26.4
1984	4,123.4	2,961.3	71.8	1,162.1	28.2
1985	4,591.3	3,304.8	72.0	1,286.6	28.0
1986	5,017.0	3,610.4	72.0	1,406.6	28.0
1987	5,351.2	3,865.9	72.2	1,485.2	27.8
1988	6,081.5	4,311.7	70.9	1,769.8	29.1
1989	7,074.9	4,899.2	69.2	2,175.7	30.8

Table 5 (cont.)

Year	Total (million $)	Public (million $)	Public (%)	Private (million $)	Private (%)
Other (cont.)					
1990	7,878.0	5,558.0	70.6	2,320.0	29.4
1991	8,630.3	6,117.5	70.9	2,512.8	29.1
1992	9,312.9	6,646.1	71.4	2,666.8	28.6
1993	10,077.7	7,087.2	70.3	2,990.5	29.7
1994	10,604.2	7,355.6	69.4	3,248.6	30.6
Total					
1975	12,254.8	9361.7	76.4	2,893.1	23.6
1976	14,099.0	10,871.1	77.1	3,227.9	22.9
1977	15,497.6	11,896.4	76.8	3,601.2	23.2
1978	17,168.8	13,106.1	76.3	4,062.6	23.7
1979	19,288.5	14,675.2	76.1	4,613.3	23.9
1980	22,398.4	16,951.7	75.7	5,446.6	24.3
1981	26,441.5	20,115.0	76.1	6,326.5	23.9
1982	30,910.1	23,600.6	76.4	7,309.5	23.6
1983	34,165.1	26,209.5	76.7	7,955.6	23.3
1984	36,810.4	28,033.6	76.2	8,776.8	23.8
1985	40,038.2	30,298.1	75.7	9,740.1	24.3
1986	43,554.4	32,811.8	75.3	10,742.7	24.7
1987	47,023.6	35,322.9	75.1	11,700.8	24.9
1988	51,050.9	38,115.8	74.7	12,935.1	25.3
1989	56,234.7	41,956.6	74.6	14,278.1	25.4
1990	61,041.6	45,517.3	74.6	15,524.4	25.4
1991	66,290.3	49,441.8	74.6	16,848.4	25.4
1992	70,032.1	51,878.0	74.1	18,154.1	25.9
1993	71,775.3	52,451.9	73.1	19,323.5	26.9
1994	72,462.6	52,061.4	71.8	20,401.2	28.2

Source: Health Canada. 1996. *National Health Expenditures in Canada 1975–1994.* Tables 10A, 11A, and 2A.

Table 6
Percentage of public expenditure in OECD countries, selected categories, 1991–1995

	Prescriptions					Acute care hospitals					Physicians				
	1991	1992	1993	1994	1995	1991	1992	1993	1994	1995	1991	1992	1993	1994	1995
Australia	42.5	46.6	46.7	–	–	76.3	75.7	75.7	–	–	80.7	81.6	82.8	–	–
Austria	60.7	62.6	63.1	64.3	–	–	–	–	–	–	–	–	–	–	–
Belgium	48.9	48.3	43.7	45.3	–	–	–	–	–	–	–	–	–	–	–
Canada	33.6	33.9	32.9	31.9	–	91.3	91	90.4	89.7	–	99.1	99.1	99.0	99.0	–
Czech Republic	–	–	–	–	–	–	–	–	–	–	–	–	–	–	–
Denmark	48.7	52.8	50.4	51.1	–	100.0	100.0	100.0	–	–	–	–	–	–	–
Finland	47.8	45.4	44.3	45.6	–	93.9	92.7	97.7	89.8	–	–	–	–	–	–
France	61.6	61.9	61.6	61.0	–	90.1	90.8	90.4	89.9	–	62.9	61.8	60.1	59.4	–
Germany	69.7	70.0	66.1	–	–	–	–	–	–	–	88.5	88.3	88.0	87.9	–
Greece	24.9	24.1	–	–	–	–	–	–	–	–	–	–	–	–	–
Hungary	–	–	–	–	–	–	–	–	–	–	–	–	–	–	–
Iceland	68.5	67.5	63.0	66.1	66.0	100.0	100.0	100.0	100.0	100.0	78.0	71.9	73.6	73.6	73.4
Ireland	58.2	61.1	62.5	–	–	–	–	–	–	–	–	65.6	–	–	–
Italy	63.1	56.9	48.9	41.0	38.4	–	–	–	–	–	68.5	67.1	60.9	57.5	55.0
Japan	–	–	–	–	–	–	–	–	–	–	85.6	85.5	85.8	–	–
Luxembourg	84.6	–	–	–	–	–	–	–	–	–	–	68.5	86.8	–	–
Mexico	–	–	–	–	–	–	–	–	–	–	–	–	–	–	–

Table 6 (cont.)

	Prescriptions					Acute care hospitals					Physicians				
	1991	1992	1993	1994	1995	1991	1992	1993	1994	1995	1991	1992	1993	1994	1995
Netherlands	66.7	94.3	94.4	91.2	–	69.3	72.4	74.1	73.0	–	52.9	51.2	51.4	53.1	–
New Zealand	67.7	70.9	66.2	–	–	98.0	98.0	87.6	–	–	80.1	80.1	–	–	–
Norway	39.2	–	–	–	–	–	–	–	–	–	–	–	–	–	–
Portugal	63.0	61.4	61.8	62.5	–	–	–	–	–	–	–	–	–	–	–
Spain	73.3	76.1	–	–	–	80.8	–	–	–	–	–	–	–	–	–
Sweden	71.7	70.6	68.9	70.8	–	–	–	–	–	–	–	–	–	–	–
Switzerland	56.5	60.1	–	–	–	–	–	–	–	–	79.5	79.0	–	–	–
Turkey	–	–	–	–	–	–	–	–	–	–	–	–	–	–	–
United Kingdom	64.8	63.6	63.4	64.3	–	85.7	86.1	85.8	–	–	–	–	–	–	–
United States	11.6	11.5	12.2	12.7	–	–	–	–	–	–	31.0	30.2	30.9	32.1	–

Source: OECD Health Data 1996.

DISCUSSION

At present, there is policy pressure to shift activities outside of the more heavily controlled sectors to those sectors where the ability to control costs appears to be less effective. One cannot rule out the hypothesis, on the basis of this data, that the price problem may be localized in those sectors with less regulatory control. With these caveats in mind, subject to data limitations, the papers reviewed appear to suggest that cost control has been best precisely in the sectors where there is significant public funding (e.g., hospitals), and most problematic where the private role is greatest (e.g. pharmaceuticals).

However, this conclusion may not apply equally to different sectors. It may also cloud the impact of the price of medical care. Consider, for example, the three conclusions in the Contandriopoulos paper from their examination of the relative performance of Canada and 24 other OECD countries:

- The state of health of the population in Canada is among the best in the world.
- There are fewer medical resources—number of beds and physicians— than the average for the OECD countries. The report noted that Canada ranked sixteenth of 24 in beds per inhabitant and seventeenth in number of physicians per inhabitant, which they argue "is not an indication of insufficient resources but rather a sign of efficient management."
- Canada is one of the three OECD countries which spends the most on health.

(Adapted from Contandriopoulos 1998.)

This paper inferred that the problem is "the price of these resources." Similarly, the Arweiler paper notes, "Since Canada has high real health expenditures and average quantities of care consumed close to the average for OECD countries, it can be concluded that Canada's relative prices of care appear to be higher than the average for OECD countries" (Arweiler 1998).

One trouble with this inference, however, is that it assumes homogeneity across sectors. The aggregate data may instead hide considerable variation in costs and outcomes. For example, it is possible that the costs of resources in the publicly financed and regulated sectors may be under control, but that prices may be high in the "private" components. Although no good data exists in the material given to test this hypothesis, some inferences can be made from the reviewed papers which examined two specific sectors— hospitals, and pharmaceuticals.

The paper by Scott (1998) concentrates upon an international comparison of the hospital sector. However, the key variable examined is relative share of health expenditures rather than hospital spending per se. This introduces a definitional issue (e.g., to which sector are particular activities allocated in particular nations) which could severely complicate such analysis. For example, the use of bed ratios may not capture variations in the use of ambulatory care or day surgery as substitutes for inpatient care. In addition, the focus of this paper is on methods of paying (reimbursing) hospitals; since most countries use global budgets, there was not a lot of variance. The paper concluded that the share of total health expenditures going to short-term hospitals is decreasing over time, but is still the dominant component of spending, and noted that Canada has fewer beds per thousand, but more personnel resources per occupied bed (Canada went from 2.56 staff per bed in 1980 to 3.31 in 1990, vs. the OECD average of 1.8 in 1980 to 2.4 in 1992). In particular, Canada had about double the number of nursing staff, which may reflect, in part, the growth in outpatient care. Canada had reduced the share of total expenditures going to hospitals (all types of institutions) from 54 percent in 1975 to 48 percent in 1991. The paper concluded that "Canada appears to spend on average 5 percent less than the other OECD countries."

In contrast, Kennedy examined the pharmaceutical sector (Kennedy 1998). She first noted the caveat that it is hard to make generalizations, since programs differ across provinces. In addition, "Certain portions of the Canadian market are subject to some price control pressures, resulting for example from the negotiation of provincial formulary prices and the tender purchasing practices of many hospitals and hospital groups." However, two key observations were made. First, "Canada has clearly been the poorest performer in terms of cost control over the decade studied." Using PPP, Canada was at the median in terms of spending, but showed the steepest overall increase in proportionate expenditure on pharmaceuticals (as a percentage of total health care expenditures from all sources, 1980–1993). Second, "at 25 percent, Canada's public funding proportion is well below that of most of the comparator countries" (note that these figures are inconsistent with table 5). The paper clearly suggests that there is a connection between increased spending and a smaller public share of funding. It is also suggested that the best efficiency in controlling pharmaceutical costs would be with global budgets, which implies a shift away from fee for service; enforcing global budgets is clearly difficult with a wide variety of payers. If the public proportion of spending is not going to increase, then, there will have to be some regulatory mechanisms for controlling both quantity (utilization) and price. This paper also notes that there may be access, equity, and health consequences in the current system. For example, will underutilization of necessary medications have long-term effects on the health of the individuals affected?

QUESTION TWO (SUPPLEMENTARY QUESTION):
THE CASE OF THE UNITED KINGDOM

Why have some countries such as England been able to maintain a fairly constant private sector without the predicted "downward spiral" to an American-type system?

Before attempting to address this issue, it is important to clarify what is meant by the "private" sector in the United Kingdom. Until recently, the National Health Service (NHS) was publicly financed, and publicly delivered. Consultants (specialists) working within hospitals were state employees. General practitioners received capitation payments from government to care for a roster of patients. Much of what is referred to as "privatization" has occurred within delivery—that is, transforming care providers from state employees into employees of private "trusts" who nonetheless operate with public money. As noted by Deber et al. (1998), there is no reason to predict any downward spiral from such activities.

Possible difficulties can be predicted from two sets of practices:
- Private financing. A market for privately financed care will exist only if the publicly financed care were somehow inadequate. There thus might be incentives to allow the public sector to deteriorate. Access and equity problems might also arise, and costs would be predicted to increase.
- Multiple purchasers (even with public money) if there were not safeguards against "cream skimming" of low-risk populations.

It is important to recognize that the private sector has not sought to duplicate the NHS. It occupies a niche market for the relatively simple, usually elective, procedures, leaving everything else to the NHS. To date, there is little desire to alter the basis of financing the system (the U.K. system had 83.7 percent public financing, as compared to 74.6 for Canada in 1991). As Klein has noted (1995, 141), the Thatcher government "had sent a civil servant round Europe to examine different systems of funding health care; the resulting analysis confirmed the conclusion that 'in many ways our centrally financed system was the most effective in controlling costs.' In addition, the government recognized the strong public support for the NHS. The main element of private medicine in the NHS therefore arose at the margins.

The recent "privatization" within the NHS, as Klein (1995) notes, is "more complex than political stereotypes or rhetoric would suggest" (155). It includes an element of user charges for public services, which do not amount to a large proportion of costs (note table 2, showing that the United Kingdom had a higher degree of public financing than most countries). It also includes contracting out or other ways of allowing the private sector to deliver services paid for from the public purse (including private hospitals, should they be allowed to compete for business with hospital trusts).

The key issue, then, is the existence of private insurance to pay for care which otherwise might have been available within the NHS. This has grown, from a small base, along with the British middle class. Klein notes that in 1980, only 6.4 percent of the population were covered by private insurance schemes, but that by the end of the decade this had increased to 11.5 percent (27 percent among professionals, and 23 percent among employers and managers; 155–156). Current estimates are that it now covers about 12 percent of the population (Law, personal communication).

In earlier writings about the NHS, the private issue was often considered within the rubric of "pay beds," often located within NHS hospitals, to which consultants (specialists) could admit their private fee-paying patients. These were not new, but had been in place since the inception of the NHS as a result of Bevan's 1946 compromise with the medical profession (Klein 1995, 106–107). In 1974, there were 4,500 pay beds handling about 120,000 patients a year; this represented just over 1 percent of the NHS beds and 2 percent of the nonpsychiatric cases handled in the NHS (107). For the most part, they were a part-time activity by specialists who spent the rest of their time in the NHS; private general practice was basically nonexistent. This private minitier was a concession to the class nature of British society. The NHS did not offer choice of physician; what the private payment purchased was not a choice of treatment, but "only the right to be treated by a consultant of their own choice in a room of their own" (107). In other words, the public system was seen as inadequate for most middle-class individuals with respect to the amount of choice offered regarding elective procedures, but perfectly adequate for most other things.

In the mid-1970s, the pay bed issue became politicized, with concern expressed that queue jumping could result if consultants admitted their private patients ahead of other people on the waiting list. Again, this is a recognition of the inadequacy of the public system, if queues had become unmanageable.

However, even this limited tolerance for a private tier evoked problems. By definition, doctors with whole-time contracts would not be allowed to have a private practice. There were also distributional issues. Klein notes that less than 50 percent of specialists had part-time contracts by the mid-1970s, but that these tended to be concentrated in particular specialties (e.g., less than 15 percent of general surgeons had whole-time contracts vs. 94 percent of those in geriatric medicine). Doctors also tended to move into those parts of the country—such as London—where opportunities for private practice were greatest, but which did not have a shortage of physicians. For a limited number of doctors, this private tier allowed sizeable income gains. Klein notes the case of one consultant who could double his NHS income by carrying out 24 private operations a year (110).

Klein argues that, for several reasons, the growth of private insurance did not represent exit from the NHS. First, the demand for private health care remained, predominantly, for the treatment of those conditions requiring elective surgery where there were long queues in the NHS. The private sector, in short, continued to offer treatment to improve the quality of life for people of working age rather than dealing with life-threatening conditions in the population as a whole. In the mid-1980s, an estimated 16.7 percent of all nonabortion elective surgery in England and Wales was carried out in the private sector, with the proportion rising to over 28 percent in the case of hip replacement. Second, the evidence suggests that the growth of the private sector reflected not just frustrated access but also a demand for consumer control over the nonmedical aspects of treatment—personal privacy, the timing of an operation, and the right to insist on being treated by a consultant. Third, an increase in such demands (and in the financial ability to satisfy them) might have been expected to follow from the social and economic changes in the population, and may simply have reflected the spreading capacity to do what the wealthiest had always done during the entire history of the NHS, which was to exit into the private sector when it suited them. There had always been a two-tier health care system in the United Kingdom; the difference in the 1980s lay in the fact that the private tier, rather like holidays abroad, became more widely accessible. Fourth, the fears that the increasing use of the exit option would erode support for the principle of a universal, tax-financed health care system were contradicted by the experience of the 1980s. Even those with private insurance coverage continued to use the NHS for much of the time; more than half of their inpatient stays, and four-fifths of their outpatient attendances, were as NHS rather than as private patients. In short, "consumers did not exit into the private sector; they commuted between it and the NHS" (156–157).

The private sector has a market only if the publicly provided services are somehow inadequate. In the United Kingdom, the private tier still takes a very limited role, concentrating upon those services with long waiting lists, and for desires to have more choice of physician (aspects which the current Canadian system already meets). The primary care system is strong—and public—and may play a role in maintaining commitment to the ideals of the NHS. The purchaser-provider split has led to more information about processes and outcomes, and the greater visibility of inadequacies has led to pressure to correct these within the public system. The government response in the United Kingdom was instructive; they increased public resources into the NHS to alleviate the worst of these problems, including strong performance expectations for decreasing waiting time. Klein notes that in the three years from 1985–1986 to 1988–1989, the NHS budget rose by a total of 1.8 percent, whereas in the three years from 1989–1990 to 1991–1992, the increase was 10.4 percent (218). Private hospitals have not done particularly well, and there were some well-publicized bankruptcies (e.g., the private hospital in the north).

The United Kingdom does, however, appear to be showing some of the predicted downsides of a private tier. First, there are access issues, particularly with respect to quality of care. Klein concluded that "the NHS remained a multitiered service, accurately mirroring the multitiered nature of the society in which it operated" (225). Law observes that issues have arisen about what GP Fundholders have access to, in comparison to those patients not covered by Fundholders. "There is concern that an emphasis on developing local priorities and contracts for health services, in general, will lead to greater inequity" in the absence of "any national/central plan to safeguard services for the most vulnerable" (Law, personal communication). She notes that "there are conferences sprouting up this autumn on equity in the NHS—an indicator that concern is mounting."

Second, costs appear to have increased. Spending on the NHS increased from 6 percent of national income in 1989 to 7.1 percent by 1992 (Klein 1995, 240). Klein noted that consultant salaries in the NHS tended to lag behind earnings in many comparable occupations, and be supplemented from private fees. In 1980, the insurers paid out just over £57 million in fees to doctors, which rose to almost £245 million by 1988 (157). In that period, the income tax limits for tax relief on group health insurance were lowered, significant given that about half of private health insurance is provided by employers. Schemes therefore expanded to include white-collar and even some manual workers (often through union schemes). These workers made heavier calls on their insurance, the insurance companies made losses, and subsequently took a more cautious approach to expansion (Ranade, personal communication).

Third, there may be some erosion of services within the NHS, although data is not good. For example, about half of abortions are performed privately, which may dissipate public interest in improving such services in the public sector. Another problematic area is long-term care, which has largely disappeared from the NHS. However, the expansion in private long-term care arose from what Klein terms "an inadvertent policy slip which made funding through social security available on demand. It was this which financed the expansion of the private sector. And much of the private sector provision continues to be funded by local authorities (to whom responsibility has been switched from social security)" (Klein, personal communication).

To date, these concerns are embryonic. Law comments that "the biggest reason the United Kingdom has not spiralled is the overwhelming public, political and professional commitment to a national health service," an ideology under strain from financial constraints and imposed efficiency targets. She also notes that it is very difficult to obtain data on activity or prices from private sector providers, and that the situation is not being well monitored. However, there are considerable geographic differences in the extent of the private market; Glouberman argues that it reflects a "target income" hypothesis, being important primarily where physicians need the extra earnings to maintain a middle-class lifestyle (personal communication). He collected data showing that 53 percent of specialists' incomes in London comes from the private sector.

Fourth, far from improving access, privately financed care appears to worsen it. Glouberman has found that the size of waiting lists is correlated with the extent of private care. He refers to private medicine as a "carbuncle" on the public system, being staffed by physicians from the NHS working privately who draw their customers through the public system. They might indicate that "I can see you in 3 months in the public system, or tomorrow in Harley Street."

In summary, privately financed health care still takes a limited role within the United Kingdom; however, they do appear to be getting some of the spiral problems (including much higher administrative costs, and concerns about access). To that end, the Labour Party has already promised to put more resources into the NHS and to curb the internal market should they be elected.

CONCLUSIONS

Consideration of the question of would or could a more even distribution of public funding across the health service continuum improve overall cost control without compromising access depends upon a number of assumptions.

Publicly funded services are intended to be those most "medically necessary"; services for which price elasticity is likely to be lowest (since people will sacrifice much to obtain services which they believe to be required for the health and survival of themselves and their families). Greater private financing is likely to evoke access problems for those to whom the costs are a significant barrier. Those expected to incur high costs (e.g., those with preexisting conditions) may be unable to purchase insurance at all. If public subsidy remains to ensure that no one can be priced out of such markets, then price can no longer act to balance supply and demand, and costs are likely to escalate. As pointed out in a paper for the National Forum on Health by Deber et al. (1998), single-source public financing for those services deemed "medically necessary" would thus seem appropriate for reasons of equity, security, and efficiency.

While we believe that this rationale is still correct, we have also noted that the basis for the current distribution of funding is no longer fully appropriate. The Canada Health Act builds upon previous legislation (the 1957 Hospital Insurance and Diagnostic Services Act, and the 1966 Medical Care Act) in privileging interventions done by doctors and in hospitals. At the time, it was believed that most serious illness would be treated in that way; technological change has meant that more and more needed care can be delivered in other sites by other providers, but that such care need not be deemed an insured service. Better use of evidence-based medicine and better attention to patient wishes may indeed find considerable room for economy in what care is delivered by doctors and hospitals, thus freeing resources— if desired—to incorporate medically necessary services delivered in the community which are not covered, but probably should be.

An improbable solution is adding funding for health services in general; no one argues that the current proportion of GDP needs to be raised. A plausible, but politically difficult, approach is to shift some costs from private to public sector—e.g., by augmenting pharmaceutical coverage for serious conditions. As suggested by the international research, this would likely improve cost control in the added sectors, due to reduced reliance on multiple funding sources, while maintaining accessibility, as the need for cost sharing would be minimal. This does not, however, address many of the other efficiency concerns which have predicated health reform in the last decade.

If a "more even distribution" led to cutting the public proportion of spending on current services, all available data suggests that the simple answer to the first question is NO. Indeed, diminishing public funding to the hospital and physician portion of the health service continuum is likely to produce the worst of both worlds—worse access and worse cost control. Reduced public funding in these sectors would introduce the need for multiple payers, thereby creating an environment with little capacity for cost control and decreased accessibility due to the likely introduction of user fees and similar devices. We also believe that improving public funding for other portions of the continuum should not be at the expense of necessary care for the acutely ill.

On the other hand, as pointed out above, the same evidence suggests that increasing the proportion of public funding in the other sectors may introduce better control over prices and utilization in those sectors (either directly or indirectly through global budgets) and may be essential to attain cost control. Ultimately, gaining cost control of those sectors currently "out of control" may reduce the overall health expenditure in Canada. For example, prescription drugs—which appear to have the worst record of cost control—are largely privately financed. It would appear that those medications which are not very discretionary (i.e., we would not like recipients to avoid taking them because they cannot afford them) could benefit from the cost control inherent in a publicly administered (although not necessarily publicly financed) system. These benefits could be achievable in a number of ways, from monopsony control over financing to various regulatory mechanisms.

The most promising approach would appear to be "freeing up" current public funds by "breaking down the silos"—that is, by extending the envelope of services intended to be covered by a global budget to encompass such services currently outside of the public sphere deemed to be "medically neces-sary," with full recognition of the difficulty of drawing such demarcations. Moreover, some of these services may provide overall cost saving in the long run. If this is the case, an argument can be made that they should be publicly funded. For example, is it more cost effective to provide primarily private prescription therapy to an asthmatic or to rely on the public, hospital-based system. By focusing on the therapy rather than the sector, it may be possible to redefine public coverage to include that which is effective and appropriate by covering the care regardless of the sector. A number of models and gate-keepers are possible (for example, including key pharmaceuticals in primary care budgets), but their consideration is beyond the scope of this paper.

This also begs the question of what to do about interventions deemed to be useless or harmful. In the name of liberty, one could argue for retaining the ability of individuals to purchase these in the private market, assuming that there is truth in advertising. We confess our own belief that if something is ineffective, inappropriate, and unwanted, it is not worth purchasing by anyone. However, there are clearly a number of marginal interventions which offer small benefits which society does not feel need be universal; for such cases, we find little difficulty in allowing these to remain consumer items distributed according to the same market forces as much of the rest of the economy. Again, the measurement issues arise—to what extent are these things included as health expenditures, and to what extent should health policy concern itself with them? There are many ways to achieve wellness, and not all require public expenditure. Private financing for such activities—which are likely to be disproportionately located at certain parts of the continuum of care—may thus be perfectly appropriate.

At present, therefore, we advise careful attention to the public-private mix, retaining and strengthening our current reliance upon public financing for that care deemed medically essential, for reasons of both cost control and access.

Raisa Deber *is a professor of health policy in the Department of Health Administration at the University of Toronto. She holds a Ph.D. in political science from the Massachusetts Institute of Technology. She has written, taught, and consulted on many aspects of Canadian health policy. Her current research focuses on the public-private mix, implications of purchase models for specialized services, shared decision making, and patient empowerment.*

Acknowledgements

We appreciate the help of the following individuals who were willing to give us timely information, but should not be held responsible for our interpretation (or misinterpretation) of their wisdom. Prof. Rudolf Klein (Bath), Susan Law (Oxford), Prof. Wendy Ranade (Newcastle), Prof. Sholom Glouberman (King's Fund and U. of Toronto), Andre Grenon (Health Canada), Gary Holmes (Health Canada), and Karen Phillips (Health Canada).

BIBLIOGRAPHY

ARWEILER, D. 1998. International comparisons of health expenditures. International Comparisons Series Paper. Papers commissioned by the National Forum on Health. Ottawa (ON). Published in this volume.

BROUSSELLE, A. 1998. Controlling health expenditures: What matters. International Comparison Series Paper. Papers commissioned by the National Forum on Health. Ottawa (ON). Published in this volume.

CONTANDRIOPOULOS, D. 1998. How Canada's health care system compares with that of other countries: An overview. International Comparison Series Paper. Papers commissioned by the National Forum on Health. Ottawa (ON). Published in this volume.

DEBER, R.B., L. NARINE, P. BARANEK et al. 1998. *The Public-Private Mix in Health Care*. Papers commissioned by the National Forum on Health. Ottawa (ON). Published in this volume.

DOERN, G. B., and R. W. PHIDD. 1992. *Canadian Public Policy: Ideas, Structure, Process*. 2nd ed. Toronto (ON): Nelson Canada.

EVANS R. G. 1993. Health care reform: "The issue from hell". *Policy Options* 14(6): 35–41.

HEALTH CANADA. January 1996. *National Health Expenditures in Canada 1975–1994, Full Report*. Health Canada, Policy and Consultation Branch.

KENNEDY, W. 1998. Managing pharmaceutical expenditures: How Canada compares. International Comparison Series Paper. Papers commissioned by the National Forum on Health. Ottawa (ON). Published in this volume.

KLEIN, R. 1995. *The New Politics of the National Health Service*. 3rd ed. New York (NY): Longman.

OECD. 1996. *OECD Health Data 96* (on CD Rom). Paris: OECD Health Policy Unit.

SCOTT, G. 1998. International comparison of the hospital sector. International Comparison Series Paper. Papers commissioned by the National Forum on Health. Ottawa (ON). Published in this volume.

THE CENTRE FOR INTERNATIONAL STATISTICS AT THE CANADIAN COUNCIL ON SOCIAL DEVELOPMENT. 1998. Health spending and health status: An international comparison. International Comparison Series Paper. Papers commissioned by the National Forum on Health. Ottawa (ON). Published in this volume.

APPENDIX

Working with Cross-National Data

Attempting to work with cross-national data is notoriously tricky, and a few caveats must be noted about the papers reviewed, with the understanding that the review has been very cursory, and the authors may have been well aware of these issues.

It is not always clear that purportedly similar data series measure the same thing. This becomes more problematic the more disaggregated they get. For example, close scrutiny of the tables derived from both OECD and Health Canada data (tables 1 to 6) reveals strange anomalies, such as Luxembourg's 100.2 percent public share of spending in 1993 in table 2 (which we arbitrarily changed to 100 percent).

Any consideration of time series must also ask whether things change over time. To be a valid comparison, it is necessary to understand the fine print and know whether items have shifted categories. Again, these data series tend to revise series retrospectively, meaning that attempts to compile data from multiple sources can be hazardous. Indeed, the most recent OECD data (OECD 1996) differs somewhat from that reported by Arweiler (1998) and employed by us in this paper to retain consistency with earlier work.

Although linear regression is an established technique for attempting to predict one variable (e.g., total spending on health care) through knowledge of other variables, the technique makes a large number of assumptions, including that observations are not correlated with each other (e.g., knowing about John should not tell us much about Mary). This assumption is particularly problematic when referring to time series, since knowing the value of spending in year t usually tells us quite a bit about the value in year t+1. Accordingly, a number of corrections are usually necessary. In some papers, the authors appear to have mixed time series and cross-sectional data within their regression equations. For example the version we reviewed of the paper by Brousselle (1998) appears to have run regressions on 13 countries between 1960 and 1993, reporting 434 degrees of freedom for the resulting regressions. Dealing with cross-sectional time series data can be error prone; although some statistical packages (such as SAS-PC) include specific procedures for handling this sort of data, others do not, and it is unclear the extent to which the paper incorporated the necessary corrections. At the very least, the approach taken has inflated the degrees of freedom. If corrections were not made, then the strong autocorrelation characteristic of most time series (and certainly of time series of expenditure data) would have skewed the results. Caution is accordingly urged in interpreting these findings. However, the other papers appear to use their data correctly, and are appropriately cautious in the conclusions they draw. For example, the Scott paper on hospitals ran regressions on total spending, and found a strong autoregressive component, in which policy changes within the hospital sector tended to get swamped by the national wealth effect (Scott 1998). From a technical standpoint, alternative estimations might have been interesting (e.g., would there have been any significant findings if they had tried difference equations?)

Because of data consistency issues, the sector breakdowns we (rather reluctantly) included at the request of the Task Force as tables 5 and 6 are, in our view, quite problematic, and we would urge caution in any attempts to talk about the public-private mix strictly on the basis of secondary analysis of this data.

Commentary on Health Care Expenditures, Social Spending and Health Status

TERRENCE SULLIVAN, PH.D.

President
Institute for Work & Health

PUZZLING ISSUE NO. 4

Health expenditures and social spending are not correlated with health status, and social indicators such as income distribution and education are only weakly correlated with health status. Stronger associations can be found with a small sample of countries (e.g. Canada, United States, Japan), but not in larger samples. Apart from conveying the complexity of these phenomena across countries with vast social, economic and cultural differences, what does this tell us about the appropriate allocation of public spending and social/fiscal policies to achieve better health outcomes?

TABLE OF CONTENTS

Introduction 346

Overview of the Data 346

Hypotheses 347

Conclusions 352

Bibliography 354

APPENDICES

Appendix 1   Model of State- and Firm-Level Effects on Labour
               Market, Income, and Health Pathways 359

               Figure 1   Firm and state influences, income
                          distribution and health relationships,
                          macro-/microdynamics 360

Appendix 2

               Table 1   Level and trend in child poverty and
                          income inequality rates, 1967–1992 361

               Figure 2   Real income distribution comparisons 363

INTRODUCTION

I have summarized key points from the previous papers in this volume on Canada's international position in the health field in the following way: (1) although not the leader among OECD comparator nations with respect to the conventional health outcome indicators, Canada ranks consistently among the top ten depending on the year and measure used; (2) our country ranks in the top four (depending on the year and measure used), with respect to spending on its delivery system; (3) Canada is solidly average with respect to OECD neighbours in the portion of public expenditure vs. private spending on health care; (4) Canada spends more on its health care resources owing to higher health care prices as a function of its southern neighbour and relatively poor control of physician costs associated with reliance on fee-for-service medicine; (5) Canada has exercised a reasonable degree of control of its hospital expenditures in the last decade, faced with significant fiscal pressure; (6) Canada has seen a significant growth in ambulatory care; (7) a growing expenditure pressure in the area of pharmaceuticals where Canada has been climbing rapidly to one of the top spenders per capita; (8) of particular relevance to this commentary, the analyses of social spending (nonhealth care) shows limited and equivocal relationships between social spending and health outcomes. This last point will draw most of the attention for the purposes of this commentary, but some preliminary comments first.

OVERVIEW OF THE DATA

The previous papers all make extensive use of the 1995 OECD *Health Data*. Although an excellent source of international comparisons, there are serious problems inherent in the comparison of data reported from different OECD countries as originally detailed by Jean Pierre Poullier and his colleagues at the OECD. The data are not always comparable and a more detailed understanding of the respective delivery systems is required to render sensible international comparisons. In several cases, OECD data are truncated for presentation purposes, and sometimes outliers are removed to illustrate certain relationships. Nevertheless, at least much of the data comes from the same source, the OECD.

Contandriopoulos (1998) makes interesting and creative use of derived performance measures, in particular, a composite index of costs of the system's performance based on health outcomes and cost. This indicator provides for a kind of administrative efficiency approach to different delivery systems, and suggests that Canada's system, while producing reasonably good health outcomes may not be performing as well as other less developed economies within the OECD by way of dollar spent for health outcome received. Of course some might argue for the very limited effects of health care systems on overall health outcomes (McKeown 1979) but some effect is certainly there (Bunker et al. 1994). In the case of Brousselle's paper (1998), another simple scoring method was used to calculate a cost control ranking for physician compensation methods. In both cases, the use of indices is imaginative and interesting, if difficult to interpret.

In all cases, the health-related indicators were restricted to mortality and morbidity data from the OECD. This source does not yet contain any comparable data on health "fullness" or positive health indices such as might be found in the Ontario Health Survey and/or elsewhere.

In the Centre for International Statistics (CIS) paper (1998), other sources of data were introduced including the UN Human Development Report, the OECD Education Expenditure files (1991–1992) and the OECD Employment Outlook (1994) for labour market expenditure, the Luxembourg Income Study database (no year given), and no clearly specified source for the income security data. A serious constraint in the CIS paper is that it makes very little reference to the significant literature on the links between social spending, income inequalities, and health (Gough and Thomas 1994; Vagero 1995; Wennemo 1993; Whitehead 1995). Table 2 in the CIS paper lists a number of rank order correlations for selected expenditure areas, itemizing four health outcomes against 11 related social spending measures. Chance alone might dictate that two of these 44 would be spurious, so it may not be surprising that not all of the correlations are immediately interpretable. Four correlations are significant at the .05 level. Total and public health care spending are linked to life expectancy for women. Interestingly, total labour market expenditure is correlated with infant mortality (but labour market compensation falls just short of significance at $p < .1$). Family poverty (no specified indicator) is significantly correlated with infant mortality, although only 9 countries have available data for this unspecified variable. Income security and infant mortality are highly correlated ($r = -.73$, $p < .001$) if the three outliers (Japan, Luxembourg, and Australia) are removed from the correlation. A weak association is shown between life expectancy at birth and income share of the bottom 40 percent. This last indicator touches on the study of health outcomes and income distribution in the population.

HYPOTHESES

The distribution of income may in fact be a more direct link to health outcomes than social spending, such as education, labour market spending, or income security, since it pools the distributive effects of earned income with state-determined income buffers (various social transfers, investment income, and tax effects), and it is a reasonable proxy for the kind of social environment in which people actually live and work.

With respect to the absence of strong relationships between health status and indicators of income disparities, two observations are warranted. The relationships between health and income distribution remain controversial, although in my view nonetheless compelling (Judge 1995; Wilkinson 1994, 1996). The relationship between absolute living standard and mortality, on the other hand, is by now fairly indisputable (Townsend et al. 1992; Wilkinson 1992; Eames et al. 1993; Evans et al. 1994). Controversy surrounds the relationship between health and income dispersion, not only because of the usual ideological problems, but also because of challenging methodology. Measurement issues are challenging in two respects: (1) serious and variable reporting problems tracking the real incomes of the top earners and sometimes the bottom income groups, (2) specifying the appropriate measure of income dispersion (Kaplan et al. 1996; Smeeding and Gottschalk 1996; Kawachi and Kennedy 1997). Nevertheless, these relationships hold much promise for those interested in understanding the nonhealth care pathways by which health is determined (I have included in appendix 1 an abbreviated conceptual diagram borrowing ideas from Kaplan, which sketches out how firm- and state-level policies may drive income and income dispersion effects on health).

In a recent U.K. study, Ben-Shlomo et al. (1996) set out to examine the relationships between social deprivation, income, and income variation in the 8,464 wards of England. They looked at mortality and computed the Townsend deprivation index from the 1981 census (Eames et al. 1993). They sorted the wards into larger aggregations at the level of 369 local authorities. Each authority was divided into quartiles of deprivation and variation. Mortality was regressed on quartile of variation within each quartile of deprivation. Mortality was positively associated with average deprivation and also positively associated with variation in deprivation: the average fully adjusted trend was 7 per 100,000 per quartile of variation (4 to 9, p <. 001).

Recently, Kaplan et al. (1996) showed a very powerful link between the proportion of income earned by the bottom 50 percent of the population within all U.S. states for a variety of health and social indicators, while the share of total income received by the least well-off 10 percent was predictive of lower mortality declines over the decade from 1980–1990. Interestingly, a parallel study in the United States using two other dispersion measures, the Robin Hood index and the Gini coefficient (Kennedy et al. 1996), found a similar set of correlations between income dispersion and health and concluded that the Gini coefficient provides a greater measure of sensitivity to extreme deprivation, depending on how it is specified. Kennedy et al. also concluded that inequality in the distribution of income suggested a significant cross-state variance in a number of mortality causes, independent of poverty and smoking; that the size of the gap between the top and the bottom was related to mortality, and that policies dealing with the growing inequities in income dispersion may have considerable impact on the health of the population. This view has been echoed by others in the European jurisdictions (Wennemo 1993; Whitehead 1995).

In *New Atlantis*, Francis Bacon (1630) identified the prospect of a state in which all scientific research was incorporated into decisions about the health and well-being of all its citizens. Notwithstanding our wholesale enthusiasm for evidence-based decision making in the health field, there is naïveté in believing that data-driven rational processes are the important factors in state-level decision making regarding health. We recently argued that a more advanced understanding of institutional arrangements is necessary to understand the pathways by which health policy has been influenced by social actors in the health care delivery system, and in order to bring intentional processes to influence health outcomes through non-health-related expenditures (Lavis and Sullivan, forthcoming).

In the new world of market globalization, OECD countries face a choice between a high-wage, high-productivity economy—with consequent high unemployment, income security, and fiscal pressures—and low-wage competition with higher employment rates, the price of which seems to be a large group of working poor (Kapstein 1996; Dahrendorf 1995). The high-wage solution has been the European solution, and the low-wage option has characterized the American solution, with expected consequences for levels of unemployment. Pursuing the three goals of fiscal discipline, wage equality, and employment growth form a political "trilemma" where only two of these goals seem achievable at the same time (Iversen and Wren 1996).

Already among the most unequal of OECD countries with respect to the distribution of wealth (see data by Smeeding 1996 in appendix 2), Canada faces increasing dispersion in individual market incomes (Betcherman 1996) as a function of globalization and segregation of employment categories (Sullivan et al. 1998). Although we are arguably more communitarian and statist than our southern neighbours (Lipset 1990), Canada has always been something of a residualist welfare state committed more to reducing regional disparities than income disparities (Esping-Anderson 1990). The redistributive challenge to sustain our health status and social cohesion is enormous when confidence in our governments has waned for a variety of reasons. Moreover, Canada does have a more serious debt problem than many of our OECD counterparts, although we are on our way to putting our fiscal house in order federally, and in most of the provinces. Although when taking into account the additive effects of market incomes, the cash equivalents of social transfers, and investment income, total household income distribution has remained very stable in the decade ending in 1993 (Wolfson 1996). This is owing in large measure to the historically progressive nature of Canadian social transfers. With the massive reductions in income security and social transfers taking place federally and provincially, greater household income dispersion appears inevitable.

The bottom tenth of U.S. workers are paid 38 percent of median earnings, whereas their European counterparts earn 67 percent of median earnings (Hutton 1995). These differences derive in part from historically different institutional solutions to similar challenges. In the United States, the financial system is highly market based, and the importance of workforce flexibility is also high. In the United States, unions are weak and employment regulation is weak. Social spending, corporate, and personal income taxes are low. In Western Europe, the political, economic, and social institutions hang together to form an interdependent net. Cooperation exists between business and labour. The financial system, less market based, is more committed to supporting its enterprises, and the welfare structure is more inclusive allowing for greater power sharing at both the firm and state level of decision making. At the heart of the European model of the state is the notion that the capacity to generate wealth is intimately linked to social cohesion. It is what Hutton (1995) calls the "social market."

Dahrendorf (1995) has argued that health care has become a useful institutional lens with which to assess the institutional capacity and civic nature of modern economies. Fukuyama (1995) has written compellingly on the manner in which culture and social trust interact to generate prosperity. He argues that high-trust societies (such as Japan and Germany) manage to find the institutional cooperation necessary to spawn and support large multinational corporations, remain competitive, and link capital with industrial adjustment. Similarly, in Putnam's analysis of Italy's civic tradition, civic engagement and the capacity to compromise and work together appear to produce prosperity and regional governments that work in a kind of virtuous cycle (Putnam 1993; Putnam, Leonardi, and Nanetti 1993). While prosperity is something which Fukuyama ties closely to culture across nations and time, Putnam's work highlights the important interdependence between civic engagement, effective government, and prosperity. Putnam's message may be important for a nation which prides itself on Peace, Order and Good Government.

Prosperity has been forcefully and effectively argued by the CIAR to be at the root of improvements in human health in the dramatic case of Japan (Evans et al. 1994) and the basis of some historical jumps in the health of populations (Frank and Mustard 1994). Likewise, a relative decline in prosperity and social instability appear to be at the root of the compelling and important decline in the health of middle-age men in Central and Eastern Europe (Hertzman 1995).

However, the relative distribution of prosperity, whether it is through market income dispersion or lifetime earnings (Wolfson et al. 1993), appears to have an important bearing on population health status, even when median incomes are controlled for (Kaplan et al. 1996). Labour market and social transfer changes in Canada which drive income dispersion are, in turn, likely to generate health consequences for our populations. Kawachi et al. (1997), recently concluded a path analysis which built on earlier income disparity work. Their analysis shows a relationship between social trust, group membership, and income inequality. Social trust and group membership are also associated with total and some cause-specific mortality. They conclude that income inequity leads to increased mortality via a dis-investment in social capital.

Although little Canadian data exist, the recent work in the United Kingdom and the United States in this previously murky area is producing interesting and fruitful results which illuminate the health differences between populations associated with income distribution (Ben-Shlomo et al. 1996; Davey-Smith 1996; Kaplan et al. 1996; Kennedy et al. 1996; Watt 1996; Wilkinson 1992, 1994, 1995).

The (CIS) puzzling finding—that income disparities and social spending are only weakly correlated with health status—cannot be held to be true if we look beyond the limited Canadian data and beyond the advanced economies of the OECD. Income and health have been shown to be linked to major health advances across the development spectrum, and in the developing world education has played a major role in health advances (World Bank 1993). As pointed out in Contandriopoulos (1998), once social and health spending "level off" at a fairly rich threshold level of spending in advanced economies, noticeable improvements in health status may be harder to achieve. This is in part because of the relatively narrow range of variation in public spending, as well as the inherent "flat of the curve" limits to both medical, technological efficiencies, and social arrangements on human biological realities such as aging.

Prosperous market economies and limited inequality may be the two keys to good health, but they constitute a policy tightrope (Stoddart 1995), given differences between the political culture and institutional arrangements of our national and provincial governments. In a small state like Canada, institutional solutions to our economic and social problems cannot be addressed adequately by a fleet-footed market sector or solely through the voluntary associations of the nonmarket community sector (civic society). We cannot export the costs of market globalization through selective protectionism (as does the United States) nor can we preempt the costs of change through internal restructuring of our economy (as has Japan). Small states like Canada must devise a variety of economic and social policies to minimize the political and social costs of economic change (Katzenstein 1985). In essence, we must live with change by compensating for it, implying once more an important role for government.

Which policy pathways are likely to generate the greatest health return through greater income equality is a question which moves us into the world of conjecture. Almost any move to shift income distribution through tax and social transfers involves resource and transaction costs, and there will be different short- or long-horizon solutions which may be argued. There are, nonetheless, a number of possible policy paths worthy of some consideration and further research. Income and social enrichment in the early years of life appear to have important economic returns (Romer 1994) and may have long-term health consequences (Power et al. 1996) throughout the lifespan. We have argued elsewhere that social transfers which buffer the most vulnerable are essential to prevent deprivation in a time of major market adjustment, as are active labour market programs which support a flexible and adjustable labour force (Sullivan et al. 1998).

CONCLUSIONS

Far from the modernist utopia of Francis Bacon's *New Atlantis*, the key preconditions for producing health in Canada in an era of globalization may be met if:

- government, firms, and civic society set the conditions for economic growth and prosperity; in a small state like Canada, home to few trans-national corporations and little firm-level commitment to the home market, the role of government will continue to be important in helping us adjust to global markets;
- national prosperity is distributed with fairness through a mixture of income security, social transfers, flexible labour market policies, pro-gressive tax measures, and investment opportunities;
- health care spending does not exceed a portion of national resources which cannot be justified by internal and international cost-effectiveness indicators.

The Canadian health care management objectives required to 'strike a balance' arising from the papers might be summarized in the following fashion:

- To sustain and manage health care expenditures near the OECD average, since there is no immediately apparent benefit from U.S.-level health care expenditures.

Based on the papers in this volume, this will require, among other actions:

- a coordinated, national approach to controlling pharmaceutical costs;
- moving away from excessive reliance on fee-for-service payments for physician service (through primary care reform or integrated delivery systems);
- resisting the enlargement of private financing in the delivery system, while preserving a role for private delivery and innovation.
- To sustain and improve the health of Canadians by promoting a mixture of tax, income security, labour market, social transfer, and investment levers to halt or reduce the dispersion of income and wealth, in order that social cohesion and the social pathways to health be strengthened.

Terrence Sullivan, *Ph.D., is president of the Institute for Work & Health. The Institute is a nonprofit corporation formally affiliated with the University of Toronto, McMaster University, and the University of Waterloo. The Institute conducts innovative population-based health studies investigating the determinants of modern workplace health and the effective treatment and management of musculoskeletal injury. He maintains appointments at the Department of Health Administration at University of Toronto and at the Department of Sociology at York University.*

BIBLIOGRAPHY

BACON, F. 1630. *New Atlantis*. London.

BEN-SHLOMO, Y., R. WHITE, and M. MARMOT. 1996. Does the variation in socioeconomic characteristics of an area affect mortality? *British Medical Journal* 312: 1013.

BETCHERMAN, G. 1996. Globalization, labour markets and public policy. In *States Against Markets*, eds. P. BOYER, and D. DRACHE. New York (NY): Routledge.

BROUSSELLE, A. 1998. Controlling health expenditures: What matters. International Comparison Series Paper. Papers commissioned by the National Forum on Health. Ottawa (ON). Published in this volume.

BUNKER, J., H. FRAZIER, and F. MOSTELLER. 1994. Improving health: Measuring effects of medical care. *The Millbank Quarterly* 72(2): 225–258.

CONTANDRIOPOULOS, D. 1998. How Canada's health care system compares with that of other countries: An overview. International Comparison Series Paper. Papers commissioned by the National Forum on Health. Ottawa (ON). Published in this volume.

DAHRENDORF, R. 1995. A precarious balance: Economic opportunity, civil society, and political liberty. *The Responsive Community* (summer).

DAVEY-SMITH, G. 1996. Income inequality and mortality: Why are they related? *British Medical Journal* 312: 987–988.

EAMES, M., Y. BEN-SHLOMO, and M. G. MARMOT. 1993. Social deprivation and premature mortality: Regional comparison across England. *British Medical Journal* 307: 1097–1101.

ESPING-ANDERSON, G. 1990. *The Three Worlds of Welfare Capitalism*. Princeton (NJ): Princeton University Press.

EVANS, R. G., M. L. BARER, and T. R.MARMOR. 1994. *Why Are Some People Healthy and Others Not? The Determinants of Health in Populations*. New York (NY): Aldine de Gruyter.

FRANK, J. W., and J. F. MUSTARD. 1994. The determinants of health from a historical perspective. *Daedalus* 123(4): 1–19.

FUKUYAMA, F. 1995. *Trust: The Social Virtues and the Creation of Prosperity*. London: Hamish Hamilton.

GOUGH, I., and T. THOMAS. 1994. Why do levels of human welfare vary among nations? *International Journal of Health Services* 24: 715–748.

HERTZMAN, C. 1995. *Environment and Health in Central and Eastern Europe*. Washington (DC): The World Bank.

HUTTON, W. 1995. *The State We're In*. London: Jonathan Cape.

IVERSON, T., and A. WREN. 1996. *Equality, Employment and Fiscal Discipline: The Trilemma of the Service Economy*. Paper presented at the American Political Science Association Meeting, San Francisco (August).

JUDGE, K. 1995. Income distribution and life expectancy: A critical appraisal. *British Medical Journal* 311: 1282–1285.

KAPLAN, G. A., E. PAMUK, J. W. LYNCH, R. D. COHEN, and J. L. BALFOUR. 1996. Inequality in income and mortality in the United States: Analysis of mortality and potential pathways. *British Medical Journal* 312: 999–1003.

KAPSTEIN, E. 1996. Workers and the world economy. *Foreign Affairs* (May–June): 16–37.

KATZENSTEIN, P. J. 1985. *Small States in World Markets*. Ithaca (NY): Cornell University Press.

KAWACHI, I., and B. KENNEDY. 1997. In press. The relationship of income inequality to mortality— Does the choice of indicator matter? *Social Science and Medicine*.

KAWACHI, I., B. KENNEDY, K. LOCHNER, and D. PROTHROW-SMITH. 1997. In press. Social capital, income equality, and mortality. *American Journal of Public Health*.

KENNEDY, B. P., I. KAWACHI, and D. PROTHROW-SMITH. 1996. Income distribution and mortality: Cross-sectional ecological study of the Robin Hood Index in the United States. *British Medical Journal* 312: 1004–1007.

LAVIS, J., and T. SULLIVAN. Forthcoming. Health improvements and the state: Past policies, current constraints and the possibility of political change. In *Health Promotion: Linking Theory and Practice*, eds. GREEN, ROOTMAN, and POLAND. Sage.

LIPSET, T. 1990. *Continental Divide: The Values and Institutions of the United States and Canada*. New York (NY): Routledge.

MCKEOWN, T. 1979. *The Role of Medicine*. Oxford: Basil Blackwell.

POWER, C. M., BARTLEY, G. DAVEY-SMITH, G., and D. BLANE. 1996. Transmission of social and biological risk across the life course. In *Health and Social Organization*, eds. D. BLANE, E. BRUNNER, and R. WILKINSON. London: Routledge.

PUTNAM, R. 1993. The prosperous community: Social ccapital and public life. *The American Prospect* 13: 13–42.

PUTNAM, R., R. LEONARDI, and R. Y. NANETTI. 1993. *Making Democracy Work: Civic Traditions in Modern Italy*. Princeton (NJ): Princeton University Press.

ROMER, P. 1994. Economic growth and investment in children. *Daedalus* (Health and Wealth Issue) 123(4): 141–154.

SMEEDING, T., and P. GOTTSCHALK. 1996. *The International Evidence on Income Distribution in Modern Economies: Where Do We Stand?* Paper presented at the Population Association of America, May, 26 p.

STODDART, G. 1995. *The Challenge of Producing Health in Modern Economies*. International Workshop on Health Economics, French national Institute of Statistics and Economic Studies, July.

SULLIVAN, T., O. UNEKE, J. LAVIS, D. HYATT, and J. O'GRADY. 1998. Labour adjustment policy and health: Considerations for a changing world. Paper commissioned by the National Forum on Health, Ottawa (ON). Published in volume 3.

THE CENTRE FOR INTERNATIONAL STATISTICS AT THE CANADIAN COUNCIL ON SOCIAL DEVELOPMENT. 1998. Health spending and health status: An international comparison. International Comparison Series Paper. Papers commissioned by the National Forum on Health. Ottawa (ON). Published in this volume.

TOWNSEND, P., M. WHITEHEAD, and N. DAVIDSON. Eds. 1992. *Inequalities in Health: The Black Report and the Health Divide*. London: Penguin Books.

VAGERO, D. 1995. Health inequalities as policy issues—reflections on ethics, policy and public health. *Sociology of Health and Illness* 17: 1–19.

WATT, G. C. M. 1996. All together now: Why social deprivation matters to everyone. *British Medical Journal* 312: 1026–1029.

WENNEMO, I. 1993. Infant mortality, public policy and inequality. A comparison of 18 industrialized countries 1950–1985. *Sociology of Health and Illness* 15: 429–444.

WHITEHEAD, M. 1995. Tackling inequalities: A review of policy initiatives. In *Tackling Inequalities In Health*, eds. M. BENZEVAL, K. JUDGE, and M. WHITEHEAD. London: The King's Fund. pp. 22–72.

WILKINSON, R. G. 1992. Income distribution and life expectancy. *British Medical Journal* 304: 165–168.

_____. 1994. The epidemiological transition: From material scarcity to social disadvantage? *Daedalus* 123(4): 61–77.

_____. 1995. Commentary: A reply to Ken Judge: Mistaken criticisms ignore overwhelming evidence. *British Medical Journal* 311: 1285–1287.

_____. 1996. *Unhealthy Societies: The Afflictions of Inequality*. London: Routledge.

WOLFSON, M. 1996. *Three Views of Income Equity*. Robarts Centre Conference on Globalization, State Choices and Citizen Participation in Health Care Reform. York University.

WOLFSON, M., G. ROWE, J. F. GENTLEMAN, and M. TOMIAK. 1993. Career earnings and death: A longitudinal analysis of older Canadian men. *Journal Of Gerontology: Social Sciences* 48: 167–179.

WORLD BANK. 1993. *World Development Report 1993: Investing in Health*. Oxford: Oxford University Press.

APPENDICES

APPENDIX 1

Model of State- and Firm-Level Effects on Labour Market, Income, and Health Pathways

The proposed model represents a simplified functional and conceptual diagram delineating some of the important interactive forces between labour market factors and income inequality, and their effects on health and human function. It is essentially an elaboration of a model developed by Professor George Kaplan at the University of Michigan. In this model the macroeffects of globalization, trade, and technology are experienced through both firm-level behaviour and government actions in the area of social, tax, and labour market policy.

Firms in Canada and elsewhere have moved toward an approach of retaining a small core of trained workers and relying more on a contingent "labour force." In addition, there has been a significant rise in so-called nonstandard employment. Added to this we have seen a segregation between higher-end knowledge workers on the one hand, and lower-end service workers on the other hand. Taken together these firm-level behaviours have resulted in segregation of the labour market. This greater segregation of the labour market is reflected in some income segregation as well, resulting in greater income insecurity for many, a high level of structural unemployment, and increasing inequality.

At the level of governments, the retrenchment of the welfare state is underway. Social transfers are being constrained by virtually all Western jurisdictions, and the forces of competitive globalization have resulted in the establishment of a "tax wall" and tax cuts to ensure favourable foreign direct investment decisions in local and national markets. The consequences of all of this is that income distribution is affected by the redistributive functions of the tax system, the redistributive and buffering functions of a social safety net and income security system, and the scope and scale of labour adjustments and training programs. Thus, the actions of governments have had, and will continue to have, important effects on the distribution of income, and on dealing with those at the margins of the labour market.

These macroeffects of both firm-level behaviour, and government tax, social, and labour market policy, are expressed through the microenvironment of the occupational experience and decisions on where to live and work. Position in the occupational hierarchy appears to be strongly correlated with individual resilience in response to a range of diseases and conditions. These are then buffered, or modulated, by the health care system resulting in the consequential expression of disease distribution in the population.

This brief functional and conceptual model is intended to highlight the pathways by which labour market factors influence firm-level and government-level decision making, income, the distribution of income, and consequently, health and human function. Although highly speculative, this model may have useful explanatory power for connecting the competitive pressures of globalization with local labour markets and health status.

360

Figure 1

Firm and state influences, income distribution and health relationships, macro-/microdynamics

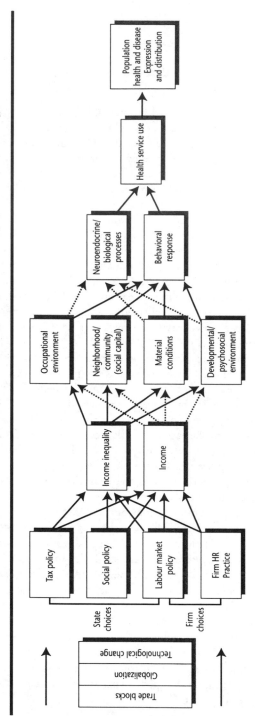

Source: Author's adaptation.

APPENDIX 2

Table 1

Level and trend in child poverty[1] and income inequality rates 1967–1992

Nation	Year of survey	Period 1 < 1971	Period 2 1971–1975	Period 3 1976–1981	Period 4 1982–1985	Period 5 1986–1988	Period 6 1989+	Change[2] in child poverty	Change in inequality
United States and Anglo									
United States	69, 74, 79, 86, 91/94	13.1	17.3	18.5		22.9	21.5/22.7	++++	+++
Australia	82, 86, 90			14.0	13.1	14.0		0	++
Canada	71, 75, 81, 87, 91	15.2	14.6	13.9		13.6	13.5	− −	0
Western Europe									
Belgium	85, 88, 92				3.4	3.1	3.8	+	+
Finland	87, 91					2.9	2.5	− −	0
Denmark	87, 92					5.3	3.3	− −	++
France	79, 84			6.3	6.5			0	0
Germany (West)	73, 78, 83/84, 89[3]		4.0	3.2	4.8/6.4		6.8	+	0
Italy	86, 91					10.8	9.6	− −	− −
The Netherlands	83, 87/91[4]				2.5	2.6	/6.2	+	+
Norway	79, 86, 91			3.8		3.8	4.6	++	+
Spain	80, 90			12.3		12.4		0	0
Sweden	67, 75, 81, 87, 92	3.5	1.9	3.9		3.0	2.7	− −	+++
United Kingdom	69, 74, 79, 86	5.3	7.0	8.5		9.9		+++	++++
Other									
Israel	79, 86			8.2		11.1	10.6	+	0
Taiwan				9.7		9.8	10.4	+	0

Table 1 (cont.)

Sources: Luxembourg Income Study; T. Smeeding, CIAR Presentation, Montreal, April 26, 1996.

1. Poverty is defined as the percentage of children living in households with adjusted disposable income less than 50 percent of median-adjusted disposable income for all persons. Income includes all transfers and tax benefits.

2. Degree of change in child poverty and overall inequality from earliest to latest year is coded as follows:

Designation	Interpretation	Range of change in estimates
– –	small decline	– 5 percent or more
0	zero	– 4 to + 4 percent
+	small increase	5 to 10 percent
++	moderate increase	10 to 15 percent
+++	large increase	16 to 29 percent
++++	extremely large increase	30 percent or more

Source of change in overall inequality is Smeeding and Gottschalk. 1996. "The International Evidence on Income Distribution in Modern Economics: Where Do We Stand" in M. Kaser and Y. Mundlak, eds., *Contemporary Economic Development Reviewed*, Vol 2, *Labour, Food and Poverty* (Oxford University Press), table 2.

3. The slash (/) for Germany indicates that the German Survey for 1973–1983 is different from that of 1984 and 1989, hence one cannot derive overall trend estimates from 1973 through 1989 from these figures.

4. The slash (/) for the Netherlands indicates that the survey for 1983 and 1987 differs from the 1991 survey, hence one cannot derive trend estimates for 1983–1991 from these figures.

Figure 2

Real income distribution comparisons (all figures in 1991 U.S. dollars)

A: The real dollar gap between high- and low-income individuals (United States median = 100)

Country	Low disposable income[1]	Length of bars represents the gap between high- and low-income individuals	High disposable income[2]	Ratio of high to low incomes
Finland, 1991	45		122	2.74
Belgium, 1992	49		135	2.76
Sweden, 1992	49		136	2.77
Norway, 1991	46		128	2.79
Denmark, 1992	48		136	2.84
The Netherlands, 1991	45		134	2.94
Italy, 1991	42		132	3.14
Canada, 1991	45		174	3.86
Australia, 1989	38		161	4.26
United States, 1991	37		207	5.67
Average[5]	45		146	3.12

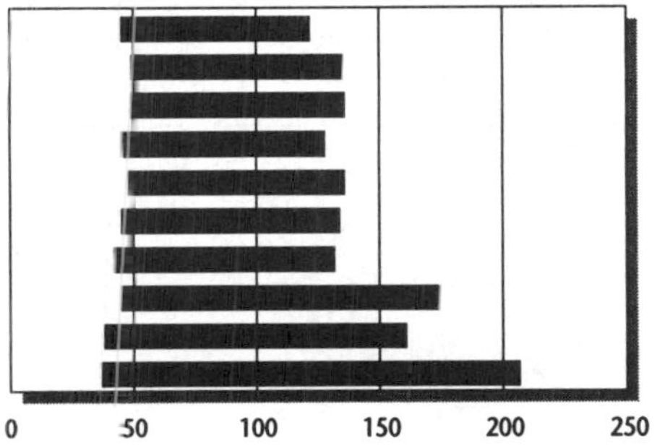

Chart axis: 0, 50, 100, 150, 200, 250

Figure 2 (cont.)

B: Ratio of real income to United States real income (United States = 100 at each point)

Country	Low disposable income (P10)	Incomes at the median[3] (P50)	High disposable income[2] (P90)	Income of the rich[4] (P95)
Finland, 1991	122	77	59	57
Belgium, 1992	133	83	65	62
Sweden, 1992	134	85	65	63
Norway, 1991	125	81	62	59
Denmark, 1992	131	88	66	62
The Netherlands, 1991	124	78	64	64
Italy, 1991	115	75	64	63
Canada, 1991	123	95	84	82
Australia, 1989	103	83	78	77
United States, 1991	100	100	100	100
	123	83	67	65

Source: Author's tabulation of data in the Luxembourg Income Study.

1. Relative income for individuals who are below 90 percent of the individuals in the country and more affluent than 10 percent of the individuals in the country. Numbers give real income (1991 U.S. dollars) as a percent of the United States median.

2. Relative income for individuals who are more affluent than 90 percent of the individuals in the country and below 10 percent of the individuals in the country. Numbers give real income (1991 U.S. dollars) as a percent of the United States median.

3. Numbers give real income (1991 U.S. dollars) of the median individuals in each country as a percent of the United States median.

4. Numbers give real income (1991 U.S. dollars) at the 95th percentile (individuals who are more affluent than 95 percent of the population as a percent of the United States 95th percentile).

5. Simple average, excluding United States.

International Comparisons

National Goals and the Federal Role in Health Care

ALLAN M. MASLOVE, PH.D.

School of Public Administration
Faculty of Public Affairs and Management
Carleton University, Ottawa

SUMMARY

The series of restraints on fiscal transfers to the provinces imposed by the federal government over the last decade have raised questions about the federal role in the field of health.

This paper provides a context and framework for consideration of federal policy levers in the field of health. It describes roles and limits of existing federal levers, and presents potential alternatives. Of particular interest are fiscal instruments—existing, proposed, and potential—given their importance and the scrutiny to which they are subjected.

It is the thesis of this paper that a role exists for the federal government to support national health care standards and to provide policy leadership in the field of health. It can also provide a more efficient substitute for interprovincial coordination with respect to specific components of the health system.

The key policy insrument to maintain national standards is federal financial participation. However, the structure of the Canada Health and Social Transfer (CHST), as revealed to date, does not address most of the central issues surrounding federal financial participation in health care.

A conceptual framework is developed for considering national goals and the federal role in health, followed by a description of the general types of policy instruments or levers that might be used in pursuit of these goals. We then describe the structure of the current federal health policy levers and examine a range of nonfinancial instruments. Finally, we consider several models for federal financial participation beyond the existing fiscal arrangements and the CHST.

TABLE OF CONTENTS

Introduction 371

National and Provincial Goals in Health Care 372

    Efficiency 374

    Equity 377

    Constraints 379

    National Objectives and the Canada Health Act 379

Federal Levers in Health Care 380

    Summary 383

National Goals and Federal Instruments: Options for Upholding
National Health Care Principles 384

    Federal Legal Authority 387

    Potential Nonfinancial Routes for Federal Intervention 388

    Other Levers 390

Models of Financial Partnership 391

    Option 1 – Maintaining a Cash Transfer 393

    Option 2 – Conditional Revenue Sharing 395

    Option 3 – Direct Funding 396

    Option 4 – Tax Credit/Reimbursement Arrangements 397

Conclusion 398

Bibliography 400

APPENDICES

Appendix 1   Review of Federal-Provincial Financial Arrangements
                with Respect to Health Care 405

Appendix 2   Experiences of Other Federal Systems 417

LIST OF TABLES

Table 1   CHA principles and national goal 380

Table 2   Federal health policy instruments by "partner"
            and purpose 385

Table 3   Chronology of major federal financial initiatives with
            respect to health care, 1948–1996 413

Table 4   Federal cash transfers to the provinces relating to health
            care (millions of dollars) 415

INTRODUCTION

The series of restraints on fiscal transfers to the provinces imposed by the federal government over the last decade, and the recent announcement of the Canada Health and Social Transfer, have raised questions about the federal role in the field of health. Among these are questions about maintaining the federal presence, and the policy instruments available to the federal government to do so. A particular focus has been to ask whether there is some minimum level for cash below which federal leverage disappears and what other instruments or arrangements the federal government might rely upon in order to uphold national health care principles as its cash contributions to the provinces decline.

To shed light on these and other related questions, this paper provides a context and framework for consideration of federal policy levers in the field of health, examines roles and limits of existing federal levers within this framework, and considers potential alternatives. Of particular interest are fiscal instruments—existing, proposed, and potential—given their importance and the scrutiny to which they have recently been subjected.

It is the thesis of this paper that a role exists for the federal government to support national health care standards and to provide policy leadership in the field of health. It also can provide a more efficient substitute for interprovincial coordination with respect to specific components of the health system. The key policy instrument to maintain national standards is federal financial participation (in some form). In addition, the demonstration of federal commitment through these contributions may well be a prerequisite for the government to play an effective role with respect to the other aspects of health. The structure of the Canada Health and Social Transfer (CHST), as revealed to date, does not address most of the central issues surrounding federal financial participation in health care.

There are four main sections following this introduction. In the first section, a conceptual framework is developed for considering national goals and the federal role in health care. The general types of policy instruments or levers that might be utilized in pursuit of these goals are then described. The section "Federal Levers in Health Care" organizes the current federal health policy levers in terms of this framework. In the section "National Goals and Federal Instruments," a range of nonfinancial instruments (some generic, other specific) potentially available to the federal government to uphold national goals are identified and discussed. Because financial levers are arguably the key element of virtually all federal activity in the health field, the section "Models of Financial Partnership" provides a general discussion of several models for federal financial participation. This discussion is to prompt consideration of fiscal alternatives beyond the existing arrangements and the CHST.

Two appendices provide background information. The first presents a brief survey of federal financial participation with respect to health care beginning in 1948. The second provides a flavour for levers exercised by central and regional (state) governments in other industrialized federal countries and for the emerging arrangements in the European Community.

To enable the paper to focus more directly on the core issues, several assumptions and limitations are accepted from the outset. First, the continued existence of a publicly funded health care system under the primary jurisdiction of the provinces, and its basic structure are not called into question. Second, the focus is on the health care system itself as distinct from broader federal programs which impact on health status (e.g., environmental protection). These two conditions permit the paper to concentrate directly on federal instruments relevant to the health care system rather than becoming involved in related, but less immediately relevant questions. Finally, the federal role in direct health care delivery with respect to specific groups such as Aboriginal peoples, military personnel, and federal prisoners is not discussed in the paper. *The focus is on the general health care system where federal and provincial roles and their interactions are at issue.* It is recognized, however, that the direct health care delivery activities of the federal government may open opportunities for demonstration effects relevant to the general health care system, and that federal activities in areas outside the health care system per se can have important impacts on the health status of Canadians.

NATIONAL AND PROVINCIAL GOALS IN HEALTH CARE

The fact that health care is primarily under provincial jurisdiction does not mean that national goals do not exist in this field, or that they are always completely coincident with provincial goals. Neither does the existence of distinct national goals necessarily call forth a federal role in the area of health. In this section a framework of policy goals is developed, the areas of convergence and divergence between national and provincial goals are identified, the role for federal action is defined, and the officially stated federal policy goals are situated within this framework.

In this paper the existence of publicly funded health care is taken as given. The arguments for public health care systems are well established, and it is not necessary to develop them here.[1] There are two points we can take from these arguments that provide helpful entry points to a discussion of federal and provincial roles in health care. These relate to the familiar concerns of equity and economic efficiency. While people with few resources

---

1. The arguments for publicly provided health care are addressed in other work of the National Forum on Health.

are disadvantaged in other markets as well, health care merits special concern as a basic form of social security. Health care heads the (short) list of items (along with basic education and perhaps housing) that all advanced societies have judged to merit special concern with respect to equity (specific equity).[2] Economic efficiency is promoted by public funding of health care largely because of serious inefficiencies inherent in private insurance markets for medical services and because of health care linkages with other markets, particularly labour markets.

Given these rationales for public provision of health care insurance, are the efficiency and equity goals national or regional (provincial) in scope?[3] Two possibilities are relevant for this discussion. First, there is a set of objectives or goals for public action that are shared by the national and provincial communities. Second, there is a set of national goals that diverge from provincial goals. As will become evident, this divergence most often occurs in the sense that national goals are broader than (subsume) provincial goals or because provinces, facing different demands and constraints, interpret or order national health care goals differently, rather than being in direct conflict with them. While provinces are unlikely to be overtly opposed to national objectives, this divergence implies that a provincial government, *on its own*, would not choose to spend resources to achieve the particular goal or objective.[4]

It is relatively uncontested (and is already assumed) that a provincial government would have the primary responsibility to pursue provincial or regional goals. When provincial and national goals diverge, is the federal government necessarily the appropriate authority to assume primary responsibility to articulate and pursue the national objectives? National concerns need not necessarily be federal concerns. It is possible, at least in theory, that the provinces acting in concert can address national concerns, even though it would not be in the interest of any one province acting alone to do so. By the same token, there may also be a rationale for federal action in areas where provincial and national goals coincide. To address each of these possibilities it is necessary to identify these efficiency and equity goals more precisely along with their provincial and national dimensions.

---

2. Even the United States, which has no universal publicly funded health care system, offers special public programs in health to the poor, disabled, and elderly.

3. In the conceptual discussion in this section, this issue is addressed in functional terms rather than in terms of the constitutional division of authority.

4. This may be true even while recognizing that the goal may be desirable from the perspective of all the provinces collectively. This is the classic dilemma of externalities or spillovers between jurisdictions (provinces).

Efficiency

Over the years the importance accorded to efficiency in health care has increased and the particular focus it has taken has shifted. The traditional issues can be categorized as either microefficiency concerns—to achieve the efficient allocation of resources *within* the health care system—and macroefficiency concerns—the interaction of the health care system with the larger economy.

Microefficiency involves using the least-cost combination of resources to perform a given activity, selecting the appropriate activity to achieve a result, and achieving quality improvements (e.g., through technological advances) at minimum cost. Microefficiency concerns include the direct provision of medical services (e.g., physicians' services, hospital care) but also broader activities such as filling information gaps (e.g., providing information on the safety and efficacy of pharmaceuticals, information on the health effects of tobacco use, surveillance of disease threats) and public health measures (e.g., immunization programs).

While aspects of microefficiency were not a high-priority concern in the earlier years of Medicare, in recent years they have increasingly become a preoccupation of governments and health care delivery agencies as budget restraints have become more severe. Achieving microefficiency would appear to be an objective shared by both levels of government. A provincial government, that pays the full cost of these services, would presumably have a strong interest in realizing these efficiencies without any prodding or inducement from the federal government.

Is there then any role for the federal government to play with respect to these objectives? To answer this, imagine first what might occur if there was no federal government, or at least if the federal government remained completely out of the field of health. In some areas, such as the organization of the health care delivery system, a province would likely choose to act on its own to address efficiency issues. In other areas, the provinces, in their pursuit of microefficiency, would likely find it mutually advantageous to cooperate. Examples might include the establishment of an interprovincial pharmaceutical evaluation and regulatory agency to provide information to practitioners and consumers on the safety and efficacy of various drugs[5] and information-sharing arrangements (say) with respect to communicable diseases. There would clearly be economy of scale gains from which all provinces could benefit if these functions were performed once collectively rather than for each province to provide the services independently. Similarly, there would be mutual advantages to establishing institutions for the sharing of information to facilitate one province learning from the experiences of others.

---

5. For example, in Switzerland, pharmaceutical authorization and regulation are the responsibility of an intercanton (interstate) agency. See appendix 2.

Federal participation in these areas can be viewed as providing a substitute for these interprovincial arrangements that would foster additional efficiencies (beyond those available from interprovincial cooperation)—even if the activities themselves were identical. An important aspect of the federal contribution in situations such as these is the reduction in the costs that the provinces would otherwise incur in identifying problems or needs, negotiating arrangements with other provinces, and administering these arrangements over time. These costs, all of which are distinct from and additional to the direct costs of providing the actual services themselves, are collectively described as transactions costs. Experience with interprovincial relations in other policy domains—such as securing freer interprovincial trade—suggests that these transactions costs potentially may be quite substantial.[6] The federal contribution—directly providing catalyst/brokerage and regulatory services, or establishing "arm's-length" organizations to do so—eliminates (or reduces) these provincial transactions costs, replacing them with lower federal costs. Transactions costs would be lower by virtue of federal leadership substituting for provincial coordination. The provinces would benefit from this federal activity and, as a consequence, they would be expected to be supportive of these federal initiatives.

The other aspect of efficiency, macroefficiency, has also been the object of increasing and shifting attention. In the past, the primary focus was on labour market issues. If health care systems offered substantially different benefits from province to province, the Canadian economic market could be adversely affected. Health care system differences can inhibit the mobility of labour by creating deterrents to move between provinces when, for labour market reasons, such moves would otherwise be desirable and efficient. (Similarly, health system differences may induce interprovincial moves when there is no labour market reason for them.) There is, therefore, a clear benefit to the Canadian economy as a whole if provincial health care systems offer sufficiently similar services not to affect labour mobility.[7] Avoidance of such barriers to mobility is (implicitly) addressed in section 36(1) of the 1982 Constitution Act, which notes the commitment of governments to "furthering economic development ...."

Despite this general national benefit, it may not be in the interest of a single province to ensure that labour mobility is maintained across provinces.[8]

---

6. Trebilcock and Schwanen 1995.
7. This does not mean identical services; there could still be a large measure of provincial variation. This condition should be read as being more in the nature of minimum service standards.
8. This is not to deny that mobility may be in the interest of *a* province at *some* time.

For example, a province offering a "superior" health care system to its citizens may, on its own, act to "protect" that system by excluding migrants, thereby restricting portability. Therefore, interprovincial portability is desirable to prevent artificial barriers to mobility. Interprovincial portability is, however, only one facet of mobility. Another is the establishment of minimum levels of service (minimum standards and comprehensiveness) in order not to create artificial barriers/inducements to move.

In the absence of federal action it is not impossible to envisage a scenario in which all provinces would jointly agree to maintain such conditions. However, it is also the case that such agreements would be very difficult to arrive at and to maintain over time. Unlike the prospects for provincial cooperation in the case of microefficiency where every province could benefit, in this case it would often not be in the interest of an individual province to bind itself to an agreement, and may very well be in its interest to act in a contrary fashion. Therefore, to address this national concern adequately would require federal action.

More recently, macroefficiency attention has shifted to a concern with the share of national production (income) accounted for by medical services, and with health care and health care expenditures as they affect the international competitive position of Canadian industries. The discussion centers on achieving some "acceptable" level of health care spending relative to GDP, and the impacts of health care financing on industrial costs of production. An interplay of several considerations is involved.

First, a healthy workforce enhances productivity. In addition to the medical care system, its achievement is related to government activities in areas such as health promotion and healthy lifestyles. Second, health care spending levels that are "too high" (according to some standard, usually unspecified) lead to higher levels of taxation, which may inhibit productivity through a depressing impact on investment and labour force participation. But restricting public health care spending is not sufficient, and indeed may be counterproductive, if it results in more private sector spending on health. Third, therefore, there is an interest in restraining medical costs outside the publicly financed system since these costs tend to increase costs of production as they become part of employer-paid insurance plans. Maintaining a single-payer system for Medicare is an important factor in achieving these efficiency objectives.

These, more recently prominent macroefficiency issues, create further possible roles for federal action. Renewed emphasis on prevention and lifestyle choices, which involve governments mainly as information providers, suggest a federal role because of economy of scale and coordination cost considerations. Perhaps more to the point, maintaining the integrity of the public Medicare system, as one factor in restraining private sector insurance costs and maintaining the integrity of a single-payer system, is addressed in the Canada Health Act, an act of the Parliament of Canada.

Equity

The pursuit of equity in health care was arguably the dominant driving force behind the original development of the public health care system and it remains a central objective today. As with efficiency, however, the focus of equity has shifted somewhat over time. In the early years of Medicare, equity of access was the primary concern. While that remains a central objective of Medicare, it is also noteworthy that, more recently, achieving a more equitable distribution of health status has become a prominent consideration as well. This later concern is correlated with the heightened emphasis on lifestyle issues and emphasizes the links with policy domains other than health care.

Equity has two dimensions, horizontal and vertical equity. In the present context horizontal equity refers to reasonably equal access to medical services to individuals irrespective of factors such as location and age. Vertical equity refers to reasonably equal access irrespective of income or wealth.[9] While horizontal and vertical equity are both national and provincial goals, they may nonetheless result in different policy choices as differing priorities and constraints are reflected in decisions.

Further, the (implicit) redistribution involved in publicly funded health care may be accomplished more effectively at the national than the regional level. Moreover, the involvement of the federal government may be justified in terms of a national commitment to equity in health care as an expression of national community. The pursuit of a national equity goal based on these rationales implies the existence of at least some national standards *and* the presence of federal financial resources in support of the health care system.

While not without controversy, national redistribution, which involves both interpersonal and interregional redistribution, is well established in Canada. Direct income redistribution programs such as Old Age Security/ Guaranteed Income Supplement and Unemployment Insurance redistribute explicitly among people and implicitly among regions. Federal programs such as the Fiscal Equalization Program, the Canada Assistance Program

---

9. The general interpretation of vertical equity is usually read as a prescription for income redistribution from high- to low-income individuals and families, for example, through the tax transfer system. Equal access to health care for high- and low-income individuals fits this general interpretation in the sense that the service is a greater relative benefit to low- than to high-income people, *even if their actual use of services is the same.*

and the Established Programs Financing arrangements redistribute explicitly among regions and implicitly among individuals.[10]

This commitment to national redistribution has been asserted repeatedly over the years. As recently stated:

> Canadians as Canadians have obligations to each other that go beyond an inter-regional laundering of money. For us, the Canadian community is meaningful if it directly engages important social issues that touch Canadians deeply. For us, Canada is made more meaningful if there are important spheres of shared experience, critical programs such as health care and social welfare the parameters of which we set in common.[11]

National equity goals are similarly recognized in the 1982 Constitution Act (section 36). Whether these equity goals are interpreted as relating to access or outcomes (health status), a potential divergence between national and provincial conceptions of the goal arises, and a potential for (at least indirect) regional redistribution arises.

An illustration of a possible divergence between provincial and national interpretations of equity involves the issue of user fees in health care (including extra-billing by physicians and user fees in hospitals). If we accept the argument and evidence that reliance on user fees does not significantly affect the quantity of resources devoted to health care, the decision to permit or encourage such fees, or to prohibit them is essentially based on distributional considerations.[12] Raising part of the revenues required to finance medical care services through user fees shifts a portion of the costs from general taxpayers to direct users of the system. Given the different populations, income distributions, revenue mixes, and potentially different philosophical interpretations of what constitutes vertical and horizontal equity and the importance that should be accorded to these goals, it is not difficult to imagine the federal government

---

10. The current EPF arrangements redistribute across provinces in the sense that each province receives an equal per capita grant from the federal government, if one includes the tax point transfer undertaken in 1977. If one only considers the cash transfer, poorer provinces receive somewhat more in per capita terms than do the richer provinces. For example, in 1995–1996, the four Atlantic Provinces receive about $372 per capita in cash under EPF, Ontario receives $328, and Alberta receives $345. (Quebec receives less cash per capita than other provinces because it received an additional tax point transfer as part of a special abatement.) A review of federal-provincial financial arrangements as they apply to health care over the last fifty years is provided in appendix 1.
11. Keith Banting and Robin Boadway, "Presentation to the Standing Committee on Finance, House of Commons", May 9, 1995.
12. See, for example, the series of papers by Evans et al. prepared for the Ontario Premier's Council on Health, Well-Being and Social Justice (1994).

arriving at an interpretation of national equity that differed from one province's interpretation of provincial equity.

Constraints

Generally speaking, the identification of distinct national goals in health care will almost certainly imply some divergence between (some of) the national goals and (some of) the provincial goals. If the federal government is to be the agent representing the national goals, one must acknowledge the potential for a certain degree of tension between the federal and provincial orders of government,[13] because of differences in preferences (interpretation of goals), differences in constituencies, or differences in resources (different budget constraints). At the same time the maintenance of harmonious federal-provincial relations is a concern that may constrain federal interventions in the field of health. In part, the extent to which it is possible to achieve national health care goals, while cognizant of this constraint, will depend upon the methods or policy instruments used by the federal government.

Other constraints also shape the methods of federal intervention. It is generally accepted that under the Constitution, the organization and delivery of health care is a matter of local concern and thus comes under the jurisdiction of the provinces (section 92). Further, the federal government cannot regulate the provinces in their areas of jurisdiction and therefore must rely on indirect methods of intervention (such as financial inducements) in order to modify provincial policies. While financial levers (the federal "spending power") are available to the federal government constitutionally, the use of these levers is, nevertheless, constrained by federal budgetary concerns. In addition, the federal government assumes obligations resulting from its international commitments relating to health and its participation in international organizations.

National Objectives and the Canada Health Act

To summarize, federal and provincial interests are likely to coincide with respect to the goal of microefficiency, but they are likely to diverge to varying degrees with respect to the other public goals, namely macroefficiency, and vertical and horizontal equity. The differences between the national and provincial goals often are a function of the differing priorities and constraints,

---

13. This is not to say that there is only one set of provincial goals. Thus, there may be friction between the federal government and some provinces and, at the same time, an overall consensus over health policy between the federal government and other provinces.

rather than outright conflict between inconsistent views of what is desirable. Rationales for federal action may exist when national and regional objectives coincide as well as when they diverge, but the rationales differ as does the potential for tension between the federal and provincial orders of government. The choice of federal instruments is likely to be a function of these differences and of constraints faced by the federal government.

Finally, this section concludes with a brief note on the correspondence between the broad goal areas as they have been discussed here, and the objectives of federal policy as they are stated in the Canada Health Act. The five principles enunciated in the act can, in fact, readily be understood in terms of their efficiency and equity properties. These relationships are presented briefly in table 1. As is apparent, with the partial exception of the last condition, the national objectives that have been enunciated in the CHA are primarily in the areas where it has been argued that national and provincial goals likely diverge. This is as one might expect, because it is where the goals diverge that statements of federal intent with respect to influencing provincial actions are most required. In other areas of health, where federal action may be seen as supportive of or a substitute for interprovincial coordination, such statements are less necessary.

Table 1

CHA principles and national goals

CHA principles	Conceptual national goals
• Portability	Horizontal equity; macroefficiency
• Accessibility	Vertical equity; horizontal equity (e.g., no exclusion based on preexisting conditions)
• Comprehensiveness	Macroefficiency; vertical equity; horizontal equity
• Universality	Vertical equity; horizontal equity
• Public administration	Microefficiency; macroefficiency

FEDERAL LEVERS IN HEALTH CARE

The purpose of this section is to classify the policy instruments or levers currently utilized by the federal government in the field of health in terms of the framework developed in the previous section. This classification[14] will link the federal instruments to the national goals in health care, and will facilitate the analytical discussion of these and other potential federal

---

14. This classification is based on a detailed enumeration provided in an internal working paper prepared by the National Forum on Health, July 1995.

instruments in the next section. This classification is not intended to be a detailed enumeration of all relevant federal programs. Rather, the exercise is intended to canvas the types of instruments (several specific programs may be variants of the same type) and to link them to the national goals which they advance.

Table 2 provides a summary of this classification. The table is arranged to link three variables: the type of federal instrument, the first "point(s) of impact" or federal "partner" affected by the instrument, and the national goal(s) which the instrument is intended to advance.[15] Though, as stated above, the discussion is in terms of instrument types rather than individual specific federal programs, the federal department or agency responsible for each instrument type is also indicated.

Four instrument types are identified. Spending (grants and contributions) includes direct cash payments to other governments or their agencies, organizations, and individuals. Spending (direct) comprises programs on which the federal government spends resources to provide services directly. Taxation instruments are those that utilize provisions in the income and other tax laws to provide benefits to institutions, firms, and individuals. Controls over the domain of permissible activities, products, and services are included in the regulation instrument grouping. Regulatory controls (levers) may range from requirements to provide product information and licensing to the use of criminal code sanctions to ensure product safety. Finally, information services are meant to encompass a variety of federal activities to demonstrate alternatives, provide guidelines, promote discussion, and provide information to other actors in the health care field. It also includes actions that fill the role of broker in coordinating interested parties in the establishment of goals and agreements to guide future activities.

In some cases an individual program (lever) can be included under more than one instrument type. For example, an information/advertising campaign to promote healthy lifestyles could be included under the spending (direct) category and under the information services category. Similarly, instruments may be substitutes for one another. Thus, research and development can be promoted through a program of direct grants and through tax measures that permit special treatment of research expenses. The current exercise does not focus on these aspects because its main purpose is to draw the links between federal levers and national goals.

Grants to the provinces (item 1) are by far the largest of all the spending instruments. In 1995–96 total Established Programs Financing (EPF) cash

---

15. Where a goal is identified as simply efficiency it is meant to include both micro- and macroefficiency. Similarly, the single designation equity is meant to include both vertical and horizontal equity.

payments to the provinces will amount to just over $9 billion.[16] These grants contribute to national equity objectives and to macroefficiency objectives in that they redistribute resources across provinces and provide the mechanism by which the federal government can uphold the principles in the Canada Health Act. (See appendix 1 for more detailed information on the EPF grants.)

Health promotion (items 2, 7, and 19) activities include information, education, and public relations activities that the federal government undertakes directly or helps to finance through grants to provinces, health care providers, and other organizations and individuals. These activities advance microefficiency goals through the generation and dissemination of information that might not otherwise be readily available to health care professionals and consumers. They also promote vertical and horizontal equity to the extent they are focused on specific groups who, for whatever reasons, are at a relative disadvantage in accessing information necessary to making informed decisions about their health and health care. In part, the mandate of the recently established Canadian Institute for Health Information fits into these categories.

Similar descriptions apply, at least in part, to the programs for children (item 3) and seniors (item 4) undertaken by Health Canada. To the extent they promote the dissemination of information concerning special needs individuals in these groups, they contribute to microefficiency and equity. To the extent they support research on related health issues, they contribute to microefficiency.

Research grants funded by Health Canada (item 5) and by the Medical Research Council (item 6), or tax incentives for research and development (item 14) contribute to microefficiency. Because of the externality benefits often associated with research outputs (i.e., benefits that the individual or institution undertaking the research cannot capture), public subsidies are required to stimulate an optimal level of research activity. Because the benefits are not restricted to any one province, federal subsidies may promote additional efficiency gains compared to a variety of incentives offered individually by provinces or collectively through interprovincial coordination.

Surveillance and disease control activities (item 8) are a prime example of the economy of scale benefits available from some forms of federal participation. Presumably even in the absence of federal action, provinces would find it mutually advantageous to cooperate and exchange information

---

16. About $7 billion of this amount is designated in the federal budget as support for provincial health care systems (table 4). If one accepts the federal position that the 1977 tax point transfer to the provinces is part of the current EPF transfer, the revenue yield plus the actual federal cash transfer amount to $22 billion.

on changing health and disease patterns; such coordination would clearly be more efficient (exploit economies of scale) compared to activities that each province might undertake independently. The additional advantage of federal participation is that the "overhead costs" (transactions costs) of arriving at and administering provincial agreements would be reduced.

Similar arguments can be made with respect to programs of food research, standards and inspection (items 9 and 17), pharmaceutical regulations (item 16), and the assessment of medical devices (items 10 and 18).

Through the income tax system the federal government offers a number of provisions[17] to assist individuals with large medical expenses (item 11) or disabilities (item 12), primarily for reasons of equity (primarily horizontal). The charitable donations credit offers tax incentives for individuals (and firms) to contribute to hospitals and health service organizations (item 13). This incentive is a substitute for (increased) direct government funding of these institutions that would otherwise likely occur, and in that context if it results in an allocation of funds that is closer to individual preferences than would be achieved through government budgeting, efficiency is enhanced. Finally, in the taxation category, GST legislation allows for a rebate of 83 percent of GST paid by hospitals, 57.14 percent paid by municipal long-term care facilities, and 50 percent paid by nonprofit long-term care facilities (item 15).

Finally, as an example of political leadership, under the mandate of the National Forum on Health (item 21), the federal government promotes public consultations and discussions on health care alternatives, and methods to promote increased efficiency.

Summary

Table 2 suggests a number of regularities in the use of federal instruments that are worthy of note. Most of the instruments or levers address the goal of microefficiency, and relate to specific areas in which one can assume there is no significant divergence between provincial and national perspectives. Many of these federal programs are relatively narrow in terms of their focus or targets. Further, all of the nonfinancial federal levers (regulation and information services) address these concerns. In addition, a number of federal financial levers (mainly spending, to a lesser extent

---

17. As previously noted, the federal government maintains the position that the 1977 personal and corporate income tax room vacated in favour of the provinces is part of its contribution to health care (and postsecondary education). Virtually all independent observers of federal-provincial fiscal relations regard this tax room as being firmly in the provincial domain and unavailable to the federal government for any policy purpose. That is the view taken throughout this paper as well.

taxation) have this focus, though the amounts of money involved are relatively small.

Where national and provincial goals diverge—macroefficiency and (some aspects of) equity—the federal government relies almost entirely on grants to the provinces to advance the national perspective. Recalling the earlier comments on the constraints relating to the use of federal levers, there are both political and constitutional reasons for this. Politically, potential tensions arising from the divergence in goals can be avoided or minimized if the federal government modifies provincial policies through positive inducements or incentives rather than through negative controls such as regulation. Colloquially stated, "carrots" work better than "sticks." Constitutionally, the federal government does not possess the authority to regulate provincial behaviour in areas of provincial jurisdiction, and therefore can only rely on nonregulatory inducements to achieve national policy objectives. This constraint is underlined by the absence of any entries in table 2 in the provincial column for the taxation and regulation instruments.

NATIONAL GOALS AND FEDERAL INSTRUMENTS: OPTIONS FOR UPHOLDING NATIONAL HEALTH CARE PRINCIPLES

Two general comments on the federal role in health should be made at this point. First, it is important to note that the characterization of the federal role developed thus far leaves a great deal of room for interprovincial variation in health care policies and programs. Many provincial actions in these areas, which generally do not involve significant interprovincial aspects, might be expected to vary considerably as each government makes decisions in accordance with the needs and concerns of its own population. Thus, coordinated national action and the maintenance of national standards are fully compatible with a large measure of interprovincial variation.

Second, several analysts have reached the conclusion that the case for federal involvement to sustain national standards is not all that compelling. Widespread public support for the established Medicare principles, and common interests of health care professionals across provinces will constrain any moves by provincial governments to deviate from or dilute these principles. Thus, while national goals do exist, federal intervention is not necessarily warranted.[18] While this is not the thesis of this paper, it is a credible position that will appear in the following discussion of potential federal policy instruments.

---

18. Explicitly or implicitly this is the position adopted by Hobson and St. Hilaire 1993; and Norrie 1994, among others.

385

Table 2

Federal health policy instruments by "partner" and purpose

Instrument type/partner	Provinces (and agencies)	Professionals/ institutions	Private sector/ consumers
Spending (grants and contributions)			
Health Canada			
1. Grants (EPF)	Equity; macroefficiency		
2. Health promotion	Microefficiency	Microefficiency	Microefficiency; equity
3. Children's initiatives		Microefficiency	Microefficiency; equity
4. Seniors' initiatives		Microefficiency	Microefficiency; equity
5. NHRDP		Microefficiency	
Medical Research Council			
6. Research grants		Microefficiency	
Spending (direct)			
Health Canada			
7. Health promotion	Microefficiency	Microefficiency	Microefficiency; equity
8. Surveillance/disease control	Microefficiency	Microefficiency	
9. Food			Microefficiency; equity
10. Medical devices		Microefficiency	Microefficiency; equity

Table 2 (cont.)

Instrument type/partner	Provinces (and agencies)	Professionals/institutions	Private sector/consumers
Taxation			
Finance Canada			
11. Medical expense credit			Equity
12. Disability tax credit			Equity
13. Charitable donations credit		Equity; microefficiency	
14. Research tax incentives		Microefficiency	Microefficiency
15. GST rebates		Equity	
Regulation			
Health Canada			
16. Drugs		Microefficiency	Microefficiency
17. Food		Microefficiency	Microefficiency
18. Medical devices		Microefficiency	Microefficiency
Information services			
Health Canada			
19. Health promotion	Microefficiency	Microefficiency	
20. Health services	Microefficiency	Microefficiency	
NFH			
21. Action areas re: health	Efficiency; equity	Efficiency; equity	

This section begins by drawing together the sources of federal "authority" in the field of health, and how this authority is closely linked to federal financial participation which has been, in many ways, the linchpin to overall federal participation in health. It then explores whether and how federal leverage over national health care goals might be maintained through mechanisms other than financial participation. The conclusion is that these nonfinancial instruments are not viable, and that continuing financial participation is necessary. The section "Models of Financial Partnership" then turns to a discussion of alternative models for financial participation.

Federal Legal Authority

While the section "National and Provincial Goals in Health Care" developed functional rationales for federal involvement in health care, it still remains to discuss the source of legal, political, and moral authority that allows the federal government to play its role.

From a constitutional or legal perspective, the two major bases for federal activity in the health field are its spending power and its criminal law power. The spending power permits a federal presence in policy areas where it does not have power to regulate directly. It has been well established and broadly interpreted over the years, leading to a federal presence in a variety of areas and involving federal contributions to provinces, institutions, and individuals. The federal power consists of placing conditions on eligibility for receipt of its financial contributions as distinct from regulating the activity directly. To date, the government's ability to support the principles in the Canada Health Act has rested entirely on its spending power and the conditions it places on its cash grants to the provinces.

To maintain public health and safety, the federal government has the authority to use its criminal law power. Thus, for example, federal health-related activities occur through criminal sanctions against unauthorized use of narcotics (Narcotics Control Act), misleading labeling and unsafe handling practices (Food and Drugs Act), and control of hazardous products.[19]

Other legal bases for federal intervention with respect to health have been supported by the "peace, order and good government" clause in the Constitution, and federal powers to regulate trade and commerce between provinces. Federal authority extends to entering into agreements on international health care matters and to health concerns of people entering Canada. Finally, the federal government has explicit responsibilities for

---

19. Recently, the Supreme Court held that the federal government did have authority under the criminal law power to control the sale of tobacco products. (*RJR-MacDonald v. Canada*, S.C.C., September 21, 1991.) This affirmation of this federal power was noted by Peter Hogg in comments on an earlier draft of this paper.

providing health care to Aboriginal peoples, military personnel and veterans, and public servants.

Potential Nonfinancial Routes for Federal Intervention

Three nonfinancial alternative routes or classes of options for federal maintenance of national health care goals are assessed.

The first might be characterized as the regulatory route. It might involve a combination of steps. A starting point would be to amend the Canada Health Act to specify more precisely the definitions of national goals; for example, there is some pressure on the government to produce a list of "covered" ("medically required") health care services that would give sharper definition to the comprehensiveness principle.[20] Enforcement would be pursued through the federal government's criminal law authority or via the national concern doctrine of the "peace, order, and good government" (pogg) clause. This (or a similar) route is unlikely for several reasons. It seems well established in law that direct federal regulation of provincial programs in their areas of jurisdiction is not possible. Politically, such aggressive action by the federal government is certain to prompt strong negative reactions from the provinces and to seriously disrupt federal-provincial relations more generally. Further, legal and political barriers aside, federal actions of this type, by themselves, would not advance the equity goal, the achievement of which requires federal financial participation.

A second possible route is a constitutional or legal route. One possibility is to add to the Charter of Rights and Freedoms a right to health care.[21] Another would be to add to the Constitution a Social Contract as was proposed in the Charlottetown Accord. In that proposal a number of non-justiciable objectives relating to the Canadian economic and social union were enumerated, including one that reiterated the principles of the CHA.

While constitutional provisions such as these would presumably influence the decisions of the provincial governments, it is important to point out that they would not provide the federal government with any new form of leverage over provincial health systems. Such provisions would be interpreted by the provinces (and perhaps the courts, in the case of Charter amendments), albeit subject to an important new constraint. Still, in the final analysis, proposals such as these return to the argument that federal intervention is not required to maintain national objectives in health care. While provincial discretion

---

20. The question addressed here is whether this move, in combination with other nonfinancial initiatives, would be sufficient to maintain federal leverage in health care. A separate argument can be made for beefing up the act as part of an initiative that maintains the federal fiscal presence. Maslove 1995.

21. For example, see the discussion in Canadian Bar Association 1994.

would be presumably narrowed (to an extent depending upon whether the new constitutional clause was justiciable), ultimately provincial interpretations of the national objectives would prevail.[22]

The third potential nonfinancial route for federal involvement in support of national objectives might be termed grand politics or (capital M) Moral Suasion. Besides its legal authority, the federal government possesses considerable political and moral authority by virtue of strong public support for the national health care system. The Medicare system and, by extension, the Canada Health Act consistently receives overwhelming approval and support in public opinion samplings.[23] Moreover, the historical role played by the federal government in the establishment of Medicare (appendix 1) and the federal financial presence with respect to health care (though very often misunderstood) create the perception that federal involvement is important to its preservation. This accords the federal government strong moral authority to act.

One could envisage the federal government becoming more involved in providing information and perhaps even mobilizing political pressure in attempting to ensure provincial compliance with national health care objectives. But the effectiveness of these interventions, *by themselves*, may well be limited. If provincial public sentiments are basically supportive of the federal position, then these sentiments, rather than this federal intervention itself, may be the determining factors in provincial policy. In other words, this route, even more so than the set of constitutional options, may ultimately reduce to an argument that provinces, given the political pressures they face, are likely to adhere to national objectives without federal involvement.

Arriving at essentially the same conclusion from a somewhat different line of reasoning, one might point out that Moral Suasion by itself is likely to have only limited impacts. Its effectiveness requires that it be backed up by the "persuader's" ability/power to resort to more direct instruments (e.g., regulation, spending). In the case of the federal government, its political and moral authority in health is to a large extent predicated on its financial participation. While the regulatory and criminal powers that the federal government can exercise in health-related areas are important to maintaining and protecting the health status of Canadians, the most visible component of the broad health system is medical care, and here federal money is seen as the main lever of government policy. Without this financial presence one might reasonably question whether Moral Suasion would be successful.

---

22. A similar result might be expected if each of the provinces incorporated the CHA principles into their own health legislation. Essentially all arrangements of this sort would be more or less significant according to the extent that they constrained or limited the range of discretion within which the provinces interpreted national goals.

23. Tuohy 1994.

One might be tempted to argue further, that in addition to being necessary to advance national goals with respect to Medicare per se, federal financial partnership with the provinces is a prerequisite for the federal government being able to play a leadership/moral suasion role in other areas relating to health care. This argument suggests that, in other areas, where federal and provincial health goals may coincide, the political and moral (but not legal) authority behind federal participation is a strong federal financial presence. Moreover, if the relationship between federal financial contributions and federal moral authority is direct, more money may permit the federal government to attach fewer and looser conditions to achieve national goals, because its financial contribution will strengthen its moral suasion levers. The two broad categories of goals and associated instruments may therefore be interrelated. If so, financial levers take on an even greater significance than is often attributed to them.

The foregoing discussion leads back to federal financial participation as the linchpin of federal involvement in health. While nonfinancial mechanisms can be contemplated, it would appear that they would either be unworkable (e.g., direct regulation of provincial programs) or indirect, tacit arguments that meaningful federal intervention is not necessary for the maintenance of national goals in health. If one accepts that federal involvement is required, fiscal instruments must continue to exist. Indeed, virtually every analysis that argues that a federal role exists also argues that money is the only effective lever.[24] It is also noteworthy that even in other federal countries, which accord greater regulatory powers in health to the central government than does Canada, financial participation is generally the most or one of the most important instruments of the national government (appendix 2).

Other Levers

For goals shared with the provinces, federal levers are in many ways substitutes for provincial levers and therefore might be expected to correspond, more or less, to actions the provincial governments would undertake for the same purposes. In essence therefore, the federal government could be expected to use the full range of policy instruments for these purposes as it acts in concert with the provinces (explicitly or implicitly) to modify the behaviour of other agents. These include fiscal levers (direct spending and taxation measures), regulation, and the range of activities summed by the term information services.

---

24. See, for example, Battle and Torjman 1995b; Mendelson 1995; Osberg 1995; HEAL 1995; and other submissions to the House Standing Committee on Finance.

Potential may exist for the federal government to become even more active in these areas. In recent years the establishment of new institutions such as the Canadian Institute for Health Information (CIHI) has been a recognition of the need for improved information and monitoring and stronger promotion of preventative health care procedures.[25] Moving further in this direction, federal activity could be supportive of the provinces in areas such as developing health status goals, producing comparative health status reports, conducting research on medical practice organization (HMOs, etc.), economic analysis (benefit-cost) of medical intervention alternatives, assessment of new technologies, etc. These activities could be performed by the CIHI under a liberal interpretation of its mandate. CIHI could serve a role in the field of health care comparable to the public education, research, and policy evaluation role in economic policy formerly played by the Economic Council of Canada.[26]

MODELS OF FINANCIAL PARTNERSHIP

Given the central role of the federal fiscal lever(s) in health care, this section considers alternative models by which federal financial participation can be effected, including the government's proposed Canada Health and Social Transfer. As background to this discussion, appendix 1 provides a brief history of federal financial participation in health care over the last half century.

The current principal federal financial contribution to the provinces relating to health care is the Established Programs Financing (EPF) transfer. (For details of EPF, see appendix 1.) The EPF transfer serves three purposes:

- it contributes to the total fiscal resources available to the provinces. Without federal contributions, provinces would presumably levy higher taxes (and the federal government presumably lower taxes, or run a lower deficit) in order to finance the same level of services. As suggested earlier, there are both general efficiency and equity reasons why it may be preferable to have the federal rather than the provincial governments raise these revenues;[27]
- it equalizes (though not completely) the fiscal capacities of the provinces;

---

25. Though established as an independent nonprofit organization, the federal government was the main catalyst behind the emergence of CIHI.
26. The idea for a Health Council of Canada was advanced in 1985 in the "Health and Sports Program Study Team Report" of the Task Force on Program Review (Nielson Task Force). CIHI could effectively become such an institution.
27. Tax incidence studies generally conclude that the federal tax system is more progressive than the provincial systems.

- it provides the federal government with leverage over the health care system. Specifically, the EPF cash transfer constitutes the mechanism for the enforcement of the Canada Health Act.

The first two of these purposes are not directly related to health care or any other particular policy domain. Enhancing provincial financial resources enables the provincial governments to increase their spending levels and/or to reduce their own rates of taxation. Based on the overall composition of provincial expenditures, one might expect that typically one-quarter to one-third of any spending increase would be allocated to health care, but there is no direct link to any national health care goals.

Similar comments apply to the equalization aspect of the EPF grant. If one takes the "total entitlement" (cash transfer plus the revenue from the 1977 tax point transfer) as the relevant measure, all provinces receive equal per capita amounts. If one regards only the cash as being the relevant measure, the lower-income provinces actually receive more in per capita terms (as noted in the section "National and Provincial Goals in Health Care").

It is the third aspect of the EPF cash transfer that directly relates to provincial health care provision. It is the conditionality in the EPF transfer as authorized by the Canada Health Act that provides for limited federal leverage over this policy field. The conditionality is not in the form of matching funding for eligible provincial expenditures, but rather in the prospect of discretionary financial penalties (cash transfer reductions) for the failure to observe the CHA principles. As such, as appendix 1 demonstrates, this represents the minimum degree of conditionality since the federal government began its financial participation in health care half a century ago.

The primary fiscal problems facing the EPF transfer are its lack of stability (the decline in real value over time) and predictability (subject to unanticipated and unilateral federal changes).[28] Because of these factors, at some point (in the absence of further change in the structure of the grant) the amount of cash remaining in the EPF transfer would no longer be sufficient to provide the ability to uphold the CHA principles.

It is difficult to specify a precise minimum level for the EPF transfer, below which the federal government loses its leverage. This threshold will vary from province to province depending on the agendas of the provincial governments (as suggested earlier, some may choose to subscribe to the CHA principles even without federal sanctions), and the constraints they face. It is possible, however, to note benchmarks that may be relevant to this question. The most obvious one is the point when the total cash transfer would fall to zero. Another potential break point is where the cash transfer reaches zero for a particular province. Most estimates indicate this would

---

28. The inherent ambiguities in the program constitute another serious problem. Maslove 1995.

begin to occur in about a decade, depending on the particular province.[29] At that point, where the federal government loses its fiscal leverage over one province, it may find it politically impossible to exert leverage over any of the other provinces as well.

A third reference point would be the time at which the grant to a province is comparable to what that province could realize if it instituted reasonable user fees (fees for hospital patients and extra-billing for physician services) for medical care services. (One could imagine the user fee revenues flowing directly to the province or to physicians and hospitals with a corresponding reduction in direct payments from the provincial treasury.) This comparison is relevant because the CHA permits reductions in the cash transfer equal to the amount generated by fees; the point at which the latter begins to exceed the former is therefore a potential threshold point.

Finally, but with even less precision, one might refer to an amount of cash sufficient to demonstrate a federal political commitment to health care and to maintain public appreciation of and support for a continuing federal role. This last potential threshold amount relates to the earlier point that financial contributions, in addition to providing an "enforcement" lever vis-à-vis the CHA, also create a cachet for the federal government to play a broader role in the Canadian health care system. This moral authority, which extends to the issues addressed in the CHA as well as other aspects of health, is dependent upon public support for federal participation and that, in turn, may well be related to federal financial contributions.[30]

To maintain its presence as a financial partner in health care, and the accompanying direct and indirect leverage, the federal government has several options. Four are raised and discussed here in order to provide a sense of the range of financial alternatives available. Public discussion of alternatives should not be artificially restricted to a comparison of EPF and the proposed CHST.

Option 1 – Maintaining a Cash Transfer

This is the alternative that would continue the traditional form of support over the last half century and that is represented by the proposed Canada Health and Social Transfer (CHST). The federal government would continue to provide cash transfers to the provinces. The CHST, or a similar program,

---

29. The Caledon Institute estimates that if the EPF formula was applied to the new CHST, cash transfers would run out beginning in the year 2010. Quebec would arrive at the zero cash position first because it received an additional special tax abatement (and thus less cash) under previous arrangements. See appendix 1.

30. While the institutional contexts are quite different, it is interesting to note (appendix 2) that with the exception of Switzerland, in other federal countries, the federal government's share of the public health care costs exceeds 50 percent.

would continue to address the three purposes outlined above: it would contribute to the fiscal capacities of the provinces collectively; it would incorporate a measure of equalization, by contributing more, in per capita terms, to the poorer provinces; and it would provide the federal government with an enforcement lever by making the transfer contingent upon provinces continuing to observe the five conditions specified in the CHA.

As implied above, the key requirements that must be incorporated into the CHST are first, stabilizing the amount of cash in the transfer, and second, securing its value over time. The details available about the CHST at this time provide only vague suggestions about the former and nothing about the latter. While the February budget itself was silent on the issue, recent statements by government members indicate that the amount of cash available in the transfer will be stabilized and not permitted to shrink to zero. Whether this stabilized amount will be sufficient in terms of any of the potential thresholds suggested above is an open question. The question of the "optimal" or "correct" level for the transfer is beyond the scope of this paper (and it may well be a question for which there is no definitive answer), but it is clear that a continued federal partnership in health care demands that this issue be settled.

Further, no indication has been forthcoming as to how the real value of the transfer will be maintained over time. Essentially this is an issue of the formula established to determine provincial entitlements and the security of the formula. A secure formula that incorporates adequate growth provisions is required to facilitate budgetary management and planning by provincial governments. The EPF formula has been effectively disregarded through its frequent manipulation by the government to achieve its overall fiscal objectives. The result has been fiscal disruptions for the provinces which are reflected in health care, and calling into question the federal presence in the field.

Recent commentaries on the CHST have addressed the core issue of stabilizing and ensuring the continuation of the federal cash transfer. For example, Courchene has called for stabilizing or "flat-lining" the CHST cash transfer at its 1997–1998 level (approximately $12.5 billion) and making a commitment to its continuation. Letting the cash dwindle, he argues, would be tantamount to Ottawa abandoning its social policy commitments and would "risk turning the CHST into an unmitigated disaster."[31]

Mendelson argues for an infusion of additional federal money in the CHST after 1997–1998 to bring the entitlement of all provinces up to the per capita level of the highest (Quebec) gradually over the next two decades.[32] The Health Action Lobby (HEAL), in submissions to the Commons

---

31. Courchene 1995a, p. 62.
32. Mendelson 1995.

Standing Committee on Finance argued that a minimum cash transfer must be established and firm five-year commitments made to the provinces. The HEAL coalition also advocates treating health separately from the other programs included in the CHST: a separate health transfer would enhance parliamentary accountability with respect to how federal funds are spent. (We return to this last point below.)

Option 2 – Conditional Revenue Sharing

An alternative to renovating the existing model of fiscal transfers might be to establish the cash transfer to the provinces by designating the revenue generated by a specified set of tax points as being for the support of provincial health care systems.[33] This is not the same as making more tax room available to the provinces; the federal government would continue to levy and collect these taxes but would undertake that the resulting revenue would be distributed as cash transfers to the provinces on an equal per capita basis, subject to the CHA conditions. The "revenue pool" from which these cash transfers would be made, could be drawn from Personal Income Taxes, from the GST, or from some combination of both.[34]

An arrangement such as this would continue to meet the three purposes initially met by EPF. The provinces would continue to receive funds from the federal government to enhance their fiscal capacities. The transfer would be equalizing. And finally, the federal government would maintain leverage with respect to the CHA principles. Further, the problems of stability and predictability would be addressed. The transfer would be stabilized in that the amount would be determined by the revenue generated by the designated taxes. It would be predictable to the same extent as would be the growth of the designated revenue pool. At the same time, because the transfer is determined by revenue generated by designated taxes, its relative claim on the federal budget would also tend to be stabilized.

A conditional revenue-sharing arrangement would differ in a subtle but significant way from previous grant programs. Because the transfer to the provinces is determined by designated tax revenues rather than being a conventional spending item in the federal government's expenditure budget, it would be somewhat more insulated from normal budgetary pressures. Provincial revenues from the revenue sharing would thus enjoy a corresponding greater degree of security than has been experienced under EPF,

---

33. It is worth reiterating that this is *not* related to the tax room vacated in favour of the provinces at the outset of EPF.
34. A similar proposal was suggested recently by Paul A. Hobson and France St. Hilaire, 1993. However, unlike the suggestion here, the Hobson-St. Hilaire proposal for income "tax abatement" was not conditional on meeting the terms of the Canada Health Act.

and the federal presence in health care would be similarly more secure. This distinction between conditional revenue sharing and traditional grant programs (such as EPF and the CHST) is, however, one of degree; it should not be overstated. A federal government that was intent on changing the terms or structure of the revenue-sharing arrangement could still do so.

One could designate this revenue-sharing plan as a CHT or CHST, and if desired even attach such a label to the federal taxes used to generate the revenue pool. As already noted, HEAL has advocated a separate health transfer. From the perspective of federal fiscal leverage, there is probably little to commend one choice over the other. As long as the potential monetary penalty is sufficient, it would not seem to make much difference if one or two social assistance conditions were added to the five CHA conditions. From the perspective of accountability (the HEAL proposal) and federal political visibility, there would likely be some benefit to clearly identifying a separate transfer for health. Certainly the magnitude of the federal commitment to health care would be clearer. One should recognize, however, that these federal grants would not flow to health care directly. The money paid to the provinces would flow to the provincial Consolidated Revenue Funds (as EPF now does), some portion of which is allocated to health care in the budget-making process.

Option 3 – Direct Funding

Rather than provide revenue to the provinces, another alternative would be to provide funding directly to health care agencies that meet criteria established by the federal government. Thus, for example, the government could make grants to regional health authorities that operate in line with federal objectives. Potentially, the grants could be directed even more finely to actual delivery agencies such as health maintenance organizations, or similar institutions conforming to a delivery model which the government wished to foster. Obviously, one might expect that if federal cash was directed to these institutions rather then to provincial governments, provincial funding to these agencies would correspondingly decline. In other words, there would not be a net increase in resources available, but a partial substitution of one funding government for another.

Presumably, the attractiveness of this option to the federal government would be a more direct role in the health care system and correspondingly greater opportunity to influence and guide its evolution. Legally, the federal spending power enables it to provide such direct funding to provincially established and regulated institutions.[35] Politically, however, they clearly

---

35. Until 1958 the federal government provided operating grants directly to universities, though no conditions were attached.

would be highly contentious. Earlier, the maintenance of generally harmo–nious federal-provincial relations was identified as a constraint on federal action in the field of health care. Clearly, a direct funding option along the lines sketched here would run headlong into this broader concern.

Option 4 – Tax Credit[36]/Reimbursement Arrangements

A still more radical alternative would be for the federal government to create a direct link or partnership between itself and individual Canadians rather than with provincial governments. The federal government would no longer provide cash grants (or revenue sharing) to provinces and instead would provide refundable tax credits or direct reimbursements to individuals claiming medical expenses. As noted earlier (in the section "Federal Levers in Health Care"), the government already offers a medical expense tax credit for relatively large otherwise unreimbursed medical expenses; this arrangement would involve making that credit refundable, and beginning reimbursement with the first dollar of expense (or perhaps after some low threshold). Alternatively, a direct federal reimbursement scheme would operate analogously to private insurance reimbursement.[37]

The radical aspect of this alternative relates to the system of health care finance that it implies. Rather than discourage user fees, a tax credit/reimbursement scheme would be a virtual invitation to the provinces to intro–duce user fees in health care as a means of cutting their spending, to recoup the lost transfers from the federal government. Patients would thus make direct payments for services received in the knowledge that they would be reimbursed for these costs by the federal government.

The principal advantages of this arrangement are two. It would, more than most other conceivable models, maximize public awareness of the federal government's role in and contribution to health care. If it is indeed this perception that is the cachet for the effective operation of other federal levers, the heightened public awareness would strengthen the ability to exercise these other levers as well. For example, federal leadership and moral suasion/authority in health would be enhanced. The second advantage is that public awareness of the costs of health care would be increased.

On the other hand, there are several administrative difficulties and other disadvantages that would be encountered. Administratively, there would be a need to determine eligible health care providers, a list of services/

---

36. Discussions of taxation-based instruments are sometimes linked to the federal financial contribution embodied in the 1977 income tax point transfer to the provinces. This linkage is unhelpful for reasons already made clear.

37. Operationally, a scheme such as the one sketched here would be very similar to the "voucher" systems sometimes proposed for health care and education.

procedures eligible for tax credit or reimbursement,[38] and reimbursement rates. To avoid cash flow difficulties, individuals would have to receive payments regularly. In a direct reimbursement system this would be presumably straightforward; in a refundable tax credit system it becomes more difficult.[39] In either case there would be a need for monitoring and audit activities. In addition, there would be compliance costs imposed on individuals filing claims, possibly resulting in the emergence of commercial services to perform this activity. Finally, in this model the efficiency benefits of a single-payer system would be lost.

CONCLUSION

In general in the area of health, the federal government has access to a broad range of policy instruments or levers. This array is necessary because not only are there several goals or policy objectives, but also a variety of constitutional, political, and financial constraints. In some instances, the national and provincial goals coincide and the federal role is one of being a facilitator or catalyst of national action, a leader or initiator of provincial cooperation, or a more efficient substitute for provincial coordination. In other instances, the federal role is to promote national goals as embodied in the CHA that provinces would not, on their own, always pursue. Here, the federal financial levers—primarily grants to provinces—are really the only viable options available to the federal government. In addition, it may well be the case that federal financial participation underlies the federal government's ability to play the leadership/catalyst role in the other areas of health care.

Given the central role of federal participation, there is ample reason to consider how this role can best be filled. Public discussion tends to be confined to comparing the relative merits of the status quo—EPF, with some repairs—and the recently proposed CHST. But other options exist. In particular, the idea of conditional revenue sharing merits consideration. Such a program would contribute to and equalize the fiscal capacities of the provinces, maintain it over time, and provide the inducement to the provinces to maintain the CHA principles. It would thus meet the fiscal needs of the provinces, while simultaneously enhancing and securing the federal presence in support of national health care objectives.

---

38. This list may well differ by demographic groups. For example, pharmaceutical costs of elderly and/or low-income individuals may be covered, but not of other groups.

39. As Peter Hogg pointed out on an earlier draft of this paper, the current refundable credits are based on the taxfiler's income in the previous year. This arrangement would likely be unsuitable for medical expenses reimbursements.

Allan M. Maslove *is a professor in the School of Public Administration at Carleton University in Ottawa. An economist specializing in public finance, Dr. Maslove is the author or editor of more than fifteen books and has written numerous articles in the areas of public policy, public finance, and federal-provincial relations. Most recently, Dr. Maslove has continued his work in the area of federal-provincial fiscal arrangements with a particular focus on the financing of the Canadian health care system. Dr. Maslove is currently Dean of Faculty of Public Affairs and Management at Carleton University.*

Acknowledgements

I wish to thank the National Forum on Health and in particular members of the working group on "Striking a Balance" for helpful discussions and comments on earlier drafts. Marie Fortier, John Marriott, and Marcel Saulnier of the Forum secretariat provided much-appreciated assistance and feedback along the way.

Helpful discussions with officials from Health Canada, the Ministry of Health in Ontario, Michael Decter, and several colleagues in the Carleton School of Public Administration are also acknowledged. Professor Peter Hogg reviewed an earlier draft and provided valuable guidance in general and with respect to constitutional and legal issues in particular.

Finally, I thank Kevin Moore who provided excellent research assistance in support of this paper.

BIBLIOGRAPHY

BATTLE, K., and S. TORJMAN. 1995a. *How Finance Re-Formed Social Policy.* Caledon Institute for Social Policy.

_____. 1995b. *Can We Have National Standards?* Caledon Institute for Social Policy.

CALEDON INSTITUTE FOR SOCIAL POLICY. 1995. *Constitutional Reform By Stealth.*

CANADIAN BAR ASSOCIATION. 1994. *What's Law Got to Do with It? Health Care Reform in Canada.* CBA Task Force on Health Care.

COURCHENE, T. J. 1995a. *Celebrating Flexibility: An Interpretive Essay on the Evolution of Canadian Federalism.* C.D. Howe Institute, Benefactors Lecture.

_____. 1995b. *Redistributing Money and Power: A Guide to the Canada Health and Social Transfer.* C.D. Howe Institute, Observation 39.

DEBER, R. B. 1991. *Regulatory and Administrative Options for Canada's Health Care System* (HEAL).

EVANS, R., G., M. L. BARER, and G. L. STODDART. 1994a. *Charging Peter to Pay Paul: Accounting for the Financial Effects of User Charges.* Premier's Council on Health Well-Being and Social Justice, Ontario.

_____. 1994b. *User Charges, Snares and Delusions: Another Look at the Literature.* Premier's Council on Health Well-Being and Social Justice, Ontario.

EVANS, R. G., M. L. BARER, G. L. STODDART, and V. BHATIA. 1994a. *It's Not the Money, It's the Principle: Why User Charges for Some Services and Not Others?* Premier's Council on Health Well-Being and Social Justice, Ontario.

_____. 1994b. *The Remarkable Tenacity of User Charges.* Premier's Council on Health Well-Being and Social Justice, Ontario.

_____. 1994c. *User Charges in Health Care: A Bibliography.* Premier's Council on Health Well-Being and Social Justice, Ontario.

_____. 1994d. *Who Are the Zombie Masters, and What Do They Want?* Premier's Council on Health Well-Being and Social Justice, Ontario.

HOBSON, Paul A. R., and F. ST. HILAIRE. 1993. *Reforming Federal-Provincial Fiscal Arrangements: Toward Sustainable Federalism* (IRPP).

MASLOVE, A. M. 1992. Reconstructing fiscal federalism. In *How Ottawa Spends 1992–93: The Politics of Competitiveness,* ed. F. ABELE. Carleton University Press.

_____. 1995. Time to fold or up the ante: The federal role in health care. John F. Graham Memorial Lecture, Dalhousie University, March.

MASLOVE, A. M.and B. RUBASHEWSKY. 1986. Cooperation and confrontation: The challenges of fiscal federalism. In *How Ottawa Spends 1986–87: Tracking the Tories,* ed. M. J. PRINCE. Methuen.

MENDELSON, M. 1995. *Looking for Mr. Good-Transfer: A Guide to the CHST Negotiations.* Caledon Institute of Social Policy, October.

NATIONAL COUNCIL OF WELFARE. 1995. *The 1995 Budget and Block Funding.*

NORRIE, K. 1994. Social policy and equalization: New ways to meet an old objective. In *The Future of Fiscal Federalism,* eds.K. G. BANTING, D. M. BROWN, and T. J. COURCHENE. Queen's University: School of Policy Studies.

OSBERG, L. 1995. The equity, efficiency and symbolism of national standards in an era of provincialism. 8th Annual Health Policy Conference, McMaster University.

PERRY, J. H. 1989. *A Fiscal History of Canada—The Postwar Years.* Canadian Tax Foundation.

SCOTT, G. 1995. Inventory of federal levers in the field of health. National Forum on Health, internal working document, July.

TASK FORCE ON PROGRAM REVIEW (Neilson Task Force). 1985. *Improved Program Delivery: Health and Sports.*

TAYLOR, M. G. 1978. *Health Insurance and Canadian Public Policy*, McGill-Queen's University Press.
THOMPSON, A. 1991. *Financing Health Care* (HEAL).
TREBILCOCK, M. and D. SCHWANEN (Eds.). 1995. *Getting There: An Assessment of the Agreement on Internal Trade*. C. D. Howe Institute.
TUOHY, C. 1994. Health Policy and Fiscal Federalism. In *The Future of Fiscal Federalis*, eds. K. G. BANTING, D. M. BROWN, and T. J. COURCHENE. Queen's University: School of Policy Studies.

Submissions to the House of Commons Standing Committee on Finance. 1995.

- Assn. of Universities and Colleges of Canada
- Keith Banting and Robin Boadway
- Canadian Association of University Teachers
- Canadian Health Coalition
- Canadian Hospital Association
- Canadian Teachers' Federation and Canadian School Boards Assn.
- Citizens for Public Justice, "Will Ottawa Preserve National Equity?"
- Health Action Lobby (HEAL) (and letter to Minister of Finance, February 1, 1995)
- National Council of Welfare
- Nova Scotia Provincial Health Council

Comparative international experience

FIELD, M. Ed. 1989. *Success and Crisis in National Health Systems*. New York (NY): Routledge.
OECD. 1994. *The Reform of Health Care Systems: A Review of Seventeen OECD Countries*. Paris: OECD.
OECD. 1992. *The Reform of Health Care: A Comparative Analysis of Seven OECD Countries*. Paris: OECD.
OECD. 1992. *U.S. Health Care at the Crossroads*. Paris: OECD.
PHELPS, C. 1992. *Health Economics*. New York (NY): Harper Collins Publishers Inc.
ROEMER, M. 1991. *National Health Systems of the World*. New York (NY): Oxford University Press.

European Community

FLYNN, P. Towards a European Health Policy. Speech given at the London School of Economics and Political Science, London, January 27, 1995.
COMMISSION OF THE EUROPEAN COMMUNITIES. *Social Europe*. (Office for Official Publications of the European Communities, Luxembourg, no. 2, 1993)
COMMISSION OF THE EUROPEAN COMMUNITIES. *Official Journal of the European Communities* (Office for Official Publications of the European Communities, Luxembourg, no. C 191, July 1992)
ECONOMIC AND SOCIAL COMMITTEE OF THE EUROPEAN COMMUNITIES. "Opinion on the Communication from the Commission and Proposal for a European Parliament and Council Decision on health promotion, information, education and training within the framework for action in the field of public health" (Brussels, January 25©26, 1995). (COM(94) 202 final).

APPENDICES

APPENDIX 1

Review of Federal-Provincial Financial Arrangements with Respect to Health Care

Financial partnerships have been the linchpin of federal participation in health care in the half century since World War II. In the (not altogether approving) words of one analyst of and participant in many of the federal-provincial arrangements during this period: "It is through the use of the superior money power of senior levels of government that politicians have implemented their own concepts of the ideal society and impressed on the citizens the unquestionable merits of a particular brand of politics."[40] In no area of concern was the emergence of the postwar welfare state more marked than in the area of health care. This appendix reviews and analyzes the major financial initiatives because of their importance as federal instruments over this period. They tend to fall into three distinct phases, though drawing sharp divisions between them is obviously not possible. Table 3 provides a summary of these initiatives.

Phase One

The first significant use of the power of the federal treasury in the health field came in 1948 with a program of grants to the provinces to subsidize hospital construction[41] and cancer control programs, and grants for a range of other specified health service activities. Other activities, including child and maternal health care, were added in 1953. The program emerged as part of a larger initiative to address pressing social needs that built up during the 1930s and the war years. Sentiments in favour of federal action were strong as a result of the nationalism that developed during the war, and coincided with the emerging Keynesian consensus on economic policy which generally implied a larger role for the federal government. That these "demands" provided support for federal efforts to hang on to the income tax revenues the federal government acquired from the provinces to finance the war was likely more than coincidental. This program of grants, most of which supported hospital construction, was in place until 1972.

During this first phase, federal grants to the provinces tended to be for specific purposes, in some cases quite detailed (at least relative to conditions in later periods). The grants were often of fixed amounts (e.g., per unit of activity) and payment was contingent on provincial reporting to the federal government.

---

40. Perry 1989, p. 441.

41. Initially, hospital construction grants were set at $1,000 per active treatment bed and $1,500 per chronic care bed. These amounts were increased in 1958.

Phase Two

The first major federal step towards a publicly funded comprehensive health care system came with the Hospital Insurance and Diagnostic Services Act in 1958. It followed four provinces which had already commenced some form of public hospital insurance. The federal program offered to reimburse participating provinces roughly one-half the costs of specified hospital services provided under provincially administered plans. More precisely, the federal reimbursement was calculated as 25 percent of average national per capita costs plus 25 percent of per capita costs in the particular province, all multiplied by the population of that province. No limits were established with respect to the total size of the grant and no conditions were specified as to how the province could finance its share of the costs. In January 1961, Quebec became the last province to join the plan. As table 4 shows, the federal contributions relative to total provincial spending grew rapidly in the years following 1958.

The structure of the federal grant meant that a province spending less than the national average per capita on insured services would be compensated more highly (relative to its total spending on the service) than a province spending more than the national average. While this could be seen as inequitable towards the provinces that faced unavoidably higher cost structures, it did not seem to be an object of provincial complaint. Rather, the generally accepted view was that by making part of the grant dependent upon national average expenditure levels, the incentive for provinces to contain expenditure levels and costs that were controllable would be strengthened. At any rate, that reasoning shaped the next major innovation, Medicare, even more strongly.

In 1968, the Medical Care Act came into effect (after being passed by Parliament in late 1966) to provide to Canadians medical care insurance comparable to the hospital insurance already in place. The federal contribution to each province was 50 percent of the average national per capita cost multiplied by the province's population. Provincial expenditure levels were not taken into account directly and no ceiling was imposed on the amount of the grant. Initially provinces were required to meet four conditions to be eligible for reimbursement: the provincial plans had to provide universal coverage, be comprehensive in the range of services covered, be administered by the province or an agency of the province, and be portable between provinces.

All this was accomplished over the opposition of several provinces. Ontario was particularly opposed; Premier Robarts response was that "Medicare is a glowing example of a Machiavellian scheme that is in my humble opinion one of the greatest political frauds that has been perpetrated on the people of this country."[42] Nonetheless, the combination of the substantial amounts of money being offered by Ottawa and the evident popularity of Medicare among voters proved irresistible to the provincial governments. While only two provinces were included in Medicare at its inauguration on July 1, 1968, by January 1971 all ten provinces had signed on. Federal Medicare payments amounted to about one-half of the payments Ottawa was making under the hospital insurance program.

---

42. Quoted in Perry 1989, p. 645.

Two additional federal programs were launched in the early years of Medicare. Through the Health Resources Fund the federal government provided 50 percent of the costs of construction for health care training and research facilities. The Extended Health Care program was introduced in 1977 to provide for federal grants (initially $20 per capita) in support of services not included under Medicare such as some types of nursing home care.

The introduction of Medicare marked the high point of the second phase of federal participation. The dominant model which characterized this phase was that of cost-sharing arrangements through which the federal government used its spending power to lead the establishment of a comprehensive, universal health care system and to participate fully as a financial partner with the provinces. The main players to this point were officials in the federal Department of National Health and Welfare (NHW) and their counterparts in the corresponding provincial ministries. The creation of the public health care system was thus to a large extent guided by officials with common professional backgrounds and interests in the field.

The first decade of Medicare was characterized by rapidly growing medical and hospital costs. Because of the open-ended nature of both the hospital and Medicare grants, Ottawa quickly became concerned over the demands being placed on the federal revenue system. As is shown in table 4, in the decade following the introduction of Medicare, federal cash commitments grew to about one-third of total provincial health care expenditures. It was not many years into the system before Ottawa began to talk about incorporating ceilings into the grant programs to accommodate "normal" growth but not the extraordinary increases. Reflecting these growing concerns, this period also marked the gradual shift in the centre of federal activity away from NHW to the Department of Finance.

In the budget of 1975 the federal Minister of Finance announced that the growth in the federal contribution for Medicare would be limited to the rate of population growth plus 13 percent and 10.5 percent respectively for 1976 and 1977 (amounting overall to about 14.5 percent and 12 percent). A rate of 8.5 percent was announced for subsequent years, but this latter limit never became effective because of subsequent changes. From the perspective of the 1990s these growth ceilings seem laughable in their generosity. However, the move was significant because it marked the first time that the federal government unilaterally restrained an existing health care financing arrangement with the provinces. It turned out to be a forerunner of much more consequential restraints to come.

Phase Three[43]

Even with the ceiling on the growth of the transfer announced in 1975, the federal government was becoming increasingly concerned that a growing portion of its annual expenditures was tied up in health care grants over which it had no effective control. High rates of inflation contributed to this expenditure growth pressure.

---

43. The discussion of EPF in this section draws heavily upon Maslove and Rubashewsky 1986; and Maslove 1992.

At the same time, federal revenues were becoming less buoyant, particularly as the impact of the indexing of the Personal Income Tax in 1974 became more evident.

On the other side, provincial dissatisfaction with the existing arrangements (principally the HIDS and Medicare Acts) mainly focused on the degree of federal intrusion into provincial affairs. In part this was a continuation of the original provincial opposition to Medicare; in part it reflected increased assertiveness on the part of provincial governments of their constitutional powers. The nature of the argument that was enunciated more explicitly was that the shared cost arrangements distorted provincial priorities, both between health care in general and other provincial areas of responsibility, and within the health care field between services that were subsidized by the federal program and those that were not.

Thus, mutual dissatisfaction with the status quo, though for quite different reasons, led to the federal-provincial negotiations that resulted in the Established Programs Financing (EPF) arrangements of 1977[44] which replaced the separate federal grant programs for hospital insurance, Medicare and postsecondary education. The federal EPF transfer to the provinces was composed of two parts. First, the federal government withdrew from a portion of the Personal and Corporate Income Tax, creating room for the provinces to raise their income tax rates. The tax transfer amounted to 13.5 Personal and one Corporate Income Tax points, equalized according to the general equalization formula.[45] The second portion, the cash transfer, was an equal per capita payment to each province set initially at approximately 50 percent of the federal contribution to the three "established" programs in 1975–76. The federal cash payment for extended health care was added to the EPF cash transfer. The cash grant was to grow in future years in accordance with provincial population and GNP (three-year moving average). Initially, the tax and cash portions of the transfer accounted for roughly equal amounts of revenue for the provinces.

The important changes incorporated in EPF were seen differently by the provinces and Ottawa, just as their dissatisfactions with the previous arrangements differed. From the federal perspective, the major innovation was that its cash grant would no longer be determined by provincial spending on health and education. Federal transfers, which were now tied to GNP growth, would henceforth increase roughly in step with federal revenues which were also closely related to economic growth. Moreover, the provinces would now have a stronger incentive to control costs in these programs because they were no longer spending "50-cent dollars."[46]

---

44. Formally passed by Parliament as the Federal-Provincial Fiscal Arrangements and Established Programs Financing Act.

45. This amount included points previously transferred to the provinces with respect to postsecondary education and a revenue guarantee portion to protect the revenues of the provincial governments necessitated by the income tax reform of 1971.

46. This often repeated phrase overstated the actual situation in that the replaced grants were more closely tied to national average expenditures than they were to the expenditures within any one province. However, a large province could noticeably affect the national average through its own expenditure levels.

From the provincial perspective, the meddling and conditions imposed by Ottawa were greatly diminished. Further, they were free to allocate the EPF funds according to their own priorities; the division of the EPF transfer into health and education components was purely an artifact of federal accounting.

Thus, the phase three model is characterized by block funding in place of matching grants, significantly fewer and looser conditions, and virtually no reporting requirements on the part of the provinces. As will become evident below, while significant structural changes have occurred and are in the offing at the time of this writing, these basic characteristics remain in place.

Satisfaction with the new arrangement, at least on Ottawa's part, was short-lived. The tax room Ottawa had vacated in favour of the provinces did not generate as much revenue for them as predicted at the outset and, as a result, under transitional arrangements Ottawa found itself providing larger cash transfers than anticipated. (Federal cash as a percent of provincial health expenditures grew in the years following 1977; table 4.) Further, the federal government was dissatisfied with the relatively little visibility and credit it was receiving for the relatively large financial commitment to the program.[47] For Ottawa, this was the downside of the block-funding arrangement that broke the link between provincial spending on health care (and postsecondary education) and the size of the federal grant.

The principal argument that the federal government advanced publicly was slightly different, however. This was the argument that the provinces had not lived up to the spirit of the EPF agreement, because they did not maintain their spending shares in the notionally associated programs, particularly postsecondary education. In fact, the provinces were taking advantage of the increased flexibility EPF offered to adjust their spending priorities.

In 1982, when the EPF arrangement was renewed, the federal government sought to limit further its financial exposure through an alteration in the formula. This change, which to many observers first appeared as a technical adjustment without great significance, has proved to be—in combination with subsequent events—of great consequence. Rather than separate determinations of the tax point transfer and the cash transfer (the latter being an equal per capita amount for all provinces) amounts, the revised EPF was based on a single equal per capita entitlement. The cash transfer was determined as a residual amount by subtracting the revenue generated by the designated tax points from the total entitlement. Each province thus receives a different (per capita) amount in cash, depending on the amount of revenue it receives from the tax points.[48]

The import of this change soon became apparent, as the federal government entered into a period of severe restraint from which the EPF transfer did not escape.

---

47. While "visibility" is difficult to measure, it was clear that federal officials felt that the government's perceived presence in the health care field suffered as a result of the move to block funding.

48. As noted in the section "National and Provincial Goals in Health Care," this, in fact, means that the poorer provinces, because they generate less revenue per capita from the tax points, actually receive more per capita in cash.

In 1983–84 and 1984–85 as part of the "six and five" anti-inflation program, the growth escalator for the portion of the total entitlement the government notionally designated as being for postsecondary education, was limited to 6 percent and 5 percent respectively. In the May 1985 budget, the escalator for the full EPF entitlement was reduced from the GDP growth rate to GDP minus two percentage points beginning in 1986–87. In the April 1989 budget, the escalator was reduced by another percentage point beginning in 1990–91. In the budget of February 1990, the escalator was frozen for two years (1990–91 and 1991–92) and limited to GDP minus three thereafter. Ultimately this freeze was extended through to 1995–96.[49]

This succession of restraints and freezes applied to the total entitlement of each province. Therefore, when the (generally) growing revenues from the designated tax points were subtracted, the residual cash payment to the provinces declined each year. Table 4 shows the rather dramatic decline in the relative size of cash transfers since the mid-1980s as a consequence of the successive (and cumulative) restraint measures. By 1995, most independent estimates suggested that shortly after the turn of the century the cash transfer would begin to disappear entirely, the precise year varying somewhat by province.

During this same period, in 1984, the Canada Health Act was passed (replacing the Hospital Insurance and Diagnostic Services Act and the Medical Care Act) which enunciated the (now) well-known five principles or criteria that provincial health systems must meet in order to receive the full EPF cash transfer. These are:

- accessibility – reasonable access to health care without financial or other barriers;
- comprehensiveness – all medically necessary hospital and medical services are covered;
- universality – all legal residents of a province (after 3 months residency) must be covered;
- portability – residents are entitled to coverage when temporarily absent from their province or when moving between provinces;
- public administration – health plans must be administered by an agency of the province on a nonprofit basis.

To preserve accessibility, the CHA gave to the federal government the authority to reduce the cash transfer to a province on a dollar-for-dollar basis any amount that the province allowed physicians to bill their patients or that hospitals charged in the form of user fees for medical services. Unspecified authority also exists for the federal government to withhold cash for violations of the other CHA principles as well. The inconsistency between the CHA and the declining EPF cash is readily apparent and by now, well known. As the cash transfer dwindles, the power that Ottawa has to

---

49. The restraints and freezes were applied to the per capita entitlements. Therefore, the total entitlement continued to grow at the same rate as population growth, generally about 1 to 1.5 percent annually.

enforce the terms of the Canada Health Act dwindles with it.[50] At some point even before the cash transfer reaches zero, the amount involved will not be sufficient to deter a province that wishes to allow user fees or to take some other action counter to the CHA[51].

Finally, in the budget of February 1995, the government announced the end of the EPF arrangement and the creation of the Canada Health and Social Transfer (CHST) effective in 1996–97.[52] The CHST will combine the cash transfers made under EPF and under the Canada Assistance Plan (CAP) into one block fund cash transfer. For 1996–97 and 1997–98 the total amounts available to the provinces under the CHST were announced in the budget. Beyond that, a formula is to be determined through negotiations with the provinces. While statements made in the budget and elsewhere suggest that the government intends to maintain an EPF-type formula (that is, the cash transfer would be determined residually as the difference between a total entitlement and a revenue amount generated by—by now completely artificially—designated tax points), other recent statements by the Minister of Health and the Parliamentary Secretary to the Minister of Finance have indicated the government's intention to maintain the cash transfer.

The CHST has become the subject of considerable hostility and criticism from groups with concerns in the fields of health care, education, and social assistance. Many of these groups have made submissions to the Commons Standing Committee of Finance during the course of public hearings on the bill to enact the budget measures[53]. They are unanimous in their opposition, though for different reasons.

In the present context, the question to be addressed is how the CHST alters the federal position vis-à-vis health care. It appears to do very little. Assuming a continuation of an EPF-type formula as suggested above with an escalator for total entitlement that grows more slowly than GDP, the problem of the disappearing cash transfer and the loss of enforceability that accompanies it, remains. At most, the new arrangement would alter the amount of cash currently in the "pool" and

---

50. Enforcement in this context refers to the leverage Ottawa has by virtue of its spending power. The federal government has no direct constitutional authority to regulate provincial health care systems.

51. Recognizing this dilemma, in December 1991 Parliament passed legislation authorizing the federal government to withhold other money owed to a province when the so-called health component of the EPF cash transfer runs out or is no longer adequate. This measure has yet to become relevant, but if and when Ottawa resorts to this legislation there is little doubt that its legality will be challenged by the provinces. Even if upheld in the courts, this measure would prove so damaging to federal-provincial relations in a broad range of fields that it is difficult to conceive it being viable.

52. In the budget speech this new program was identified as the Canada Social Transfer. The word "health" was added in government documents emerging several weeks later.

53. See bibliography.

may, by a few years, affect when the transfer falls to zero.[54] If, on the other hand, a minimum cash transfer is to be maintained, the key issues will be the level of this minimum and how its value is maintained over time. At this point, the most one can safely say is that the CHST serves notice to the provinces that major changes in financial arrangements are in the offing.

---

54. The Caledon Institute estimates that a GDP-3 formula would lead to the disappearance of the cash transfer by 2011–12. Battle and Torjman 1995a.

Table 3

Chronology of major federal financial initiatives with respect to health care, 1948–1996

Year*	Initiative	Comment
1948	Grants for hospital construction and some general services	• First significant postwar program to provide funding to provinces for health
1958	Hospital Insurance and Diagnostic Services Act	• (25% of national per capita cost + 25% of per capita costs in the specific province) x provincial population • Specified expenditures • No ceiling and no conditions on provincial financing arrangements
1968	Medical Care Act (Medicare)	• 50% of national per capita cost x provincial population • 4 conditions: universality, comprehensiveness, provincial public administration, portability • Last province in January 1971
1976	Ceilings placed on growth of Medicare grant (announced in federal budget 1975)	• Ceiling limit = population growth + 13% in 1976 and 10.5% in 1977 (14.5% and 12% respectively)
1977	Extended Health Care	• Replaced several other programs • Cash payment of $20 per capita escalated by GNP growth
1977	Established Programs Financing (EPF)	• Vacated tax points in favour of provinces (equalized) plus cash payment = about 50% of 1975–76 per capita expenditure on hospitals, Medicare, and postsecondary education escalated by GNP growth (3-year moving average)

Table 3 (cont.)

Year*	Initiative	Comment
1982	EPF restructured	• Total entitlement determined for each province; cash grant calculated as total entitlement minus revenues from designated tax points
1984	Canada Health Act	• Conditions for receipt of full cash transfer
1983–1995	Series of restraints imposed on EPF total entitlement	• Significantly reduced cash transfer
1996	Canada Health and Social Transfer (CHST)	• Amalgamated EPF and Canada Assistance Plan into one cash transfer • Fixed cash transfer for 1996–97 and 1997–98 • Formula for future years to be determined

* Year of initiation

Table 4

Federal cash transfers to the provinces relating to health care
(millions of dollars)

Fiscal year-end	General cash[1]	As % of provincial health expenditure	As % of provincial total expenditure	"Health cash" (EPF + EHCS)[2]	As % of provincial total expenditure	As % of provincial total expenditure	Health costs under CAP	As % of provincial health expenditure	As % of provincial total expenditure
1958	28	7.8	1.2				–		
1959	64	14.7	2.5				–		
1960	158	23.9	5.2				–		
1961	207	26.8	6.0				–		
1962	295	31.1	7.7				–		
1963	337	31.8	7.7				–		
1964	384	33.4	8.1				–		
1965	434	33.0	8.0				–		
1966	390	25.7	5.9				–		
1967	454	24.9	5.7				–		
1968	530	24.4	5.6				–		
1969	671	26.6	6.3				–		
1970	915	28.6	7.3				62	1.9	0.5
1971	1,249	31.4	8.3				85	2.1	0.6
1972	1,524	33.0	8.7				103	2.2	0.6
1973	1,639	31.6	8.5				110	2.1	0.6
1974	1,834	31.7	8.3				129	2.2	0.6
1975	2,195	31.2	7.9				166	2.4	0.6
1976	2,680	31.2	7.9				264	3.1	0.8

Table 4 (cont.)

Fiscal year-end	General cash[1]	As % of provincial health expenditure	As % of provincial total expenditure	"Health cash" (EPF + EHCS)[2]	As % of provincial total expenditure	As % of provincial total expenditure	Health costs under CAP	As % of provincial health expenditure	As % of provincial total expenditure
1977	3,083.0	31.8	8.0				329	3.4	0.9
1978	3,570.6	33.9	8.3	2,573.0	24.4	6.0	139	1.3	0.3
1979	4,124.8	35.7	8.6	2,366.9	20.5	5.0	146	1.3	0.3
1980	4,695.8	36.5	8.6	3 371.0	26.2	6.2	182	1.4	0.3
1981	5,123.6	33.9	8.3	3,686.8	24.4	6.0	159	1.1	0.3
1982	5,725.5	31.8	7.9	4,121.2	22.9	5.7	140	0.8	0.2
1983	6,448.8	30.8	7.6	4,644.0	22.2	5.5	183	0.9	0.2
1984	7,489.6	32.7	8.2	5,463.5	23.9	6.0	207	0.9	0.2
1985	7,941.8	32.6	8.2	5,981.7	24.6	6.2	229	0.9	0.2
1986	8,433.7	32.0	7.9	6,283.0	23.8	5.9	265	1.0	0.2
1987	8,722.4	30.2	7.8	6,483.7	22.4	5.8	266	0.9	0.2
1988	8,698.4	28.3	7.4	6,499.8	21.1	5.5	299	1.0	0.3
1989	8,879.6	26.6	7.0	6,657.0	19.9	5.2	354	1.1	0.3
1990	9,119.9	24.9	6.6	6,861.0	18.7	5.0	395	1.1	0.3
1991	9,075.4	22.9	6.1	6,841.8	17.3	4.6	398	1.0	0.3
1992	9,530.9	22.1	5.8	7,163.3	16.6	4.4	477	1.1	0.3
1993	9,919.5	22.2	5.9	7,462.2	16.7	4.4	582	1.3	0.3
1994	9,831.5	21.4	5.7	7,459.9	16.2	4.3	552	1.2	0.3
1995	9,637.5	21.1	5.6	7,277.1	15.9	4.2	–		
1996	9,076.0			6,956.7			–		

1. Cash transfers after 1977 include all EPF cash.
2. Includes only EPF cash designated for health care.

APPENDIX 2

Experiences of Other Federal Systems

This appendix presents a brief overview of the allocation of powers and responsibilities with respect to health care in several other federal countries and of the emerging structure in the European Community. Its purpose is to provide some indication of the relative degree of (de)centralization of the Canadian health care system.

Four federal countries with comparable levels of economic development are included in this overview—Australia, the United States, Germany, and Switzerland. In addition, because in some aspects the European Community represents an emerging federal structure, the role of the EC in health care policies is also briefly reviewed.

There has been substantial reform in each of the four countries in the last decade, generally intended to restrain health care costs, or at the very least, those falling on the public sector. Reform initiatives range from increases in user fees, to reductions in benefits provided by public health care systems, to price controls on pharmaceuticals, to changes in methods by which hospitals are funded and physicians and other health care providers are remunerated.

With one exception, these reforms do not seem to have changed the balance of responsibilities between federal and state governments, although in some instances this balance may have been indirectly affected. The exception was in Germany where in 1986 all investment in hospitals was made the responsibility of state governments, an obligation that was previously shared by the two levels. In Switzerland the federal government has reduced its commitments to health care financing, but this has been replaced by increased private health care insurance rather than increased state participation.

Australia

While Canada and Australia are similar in many ways—small open economies, federal systems, and British parliamentary traditions—Australia is a considerably more centralized federation than is Canada. One illustration of this difference, relevant for current purposes, is that the central (Commonwealth) government collects a substantially larger share of total tax revenues than does the Canadian federal government, and provides correspondingly more to the states through a system of general- and specific-purpose grants. Some of the latter have conditions attached which are quite controlling compared to conditional federal grants to the provinces in Canada.

In the field of health care, the Commonwealth government plays the dominant role in financing, and has assumed a strong leadership role in planning and policy as well. The Australian Medicare system is similar to Canada's to the extent that it relies on public compulsory insurance to cover the costs of privately provided services. Australian Medicare (under federal government regulation) covers all ambulatory medical care and prescription drugs plus private hospital care costs. Most hospital treatment, however, is provided by public institutions at no charge to patients; public hospitals are the responsibility of state governments.

Ambulatory medical care is provided on a fee-for-service basis by practitioners who may bill either the central government or patients directly. Government payments to physicians or to reimburse patients are made in accordance with a regulated fee schedule. (Physicians are free to bill over scheduled amounts if they choose.) The Commonwealth government also subsidizes pharmaceuticals (at 100 percent for pensioners and welfare recipients) according to a schedule which regulates prices and eligible drugs. Private hospital fees are also regulated by the Commonwealth as are private insurance funds. Grants are provided to state governments on a conditional basis in support of public hospitals and other state health care services.

State governments have primary responsibility for the provision of public hospital services, community health services, nursing homes, and home support services for the elderly. In addition, states license private hospital beds and thus control their number, location, and, through their input to the Commonwealth, influence the rates they charge. States receive specific-purpose grants from the Commonwealth on a block-funding basis in support of their health care activities. They also rely on general-purpose transfers from the Commonwealth and own-source tax revenues.

United States

While most American health care is provided through private sector arrangements, two important programs do involve government. Medicare is managed and financed solely by the federal government to provide health insurance for the aged and disabled (about 13 percent of the population). It is primarily a program to cover acute care costs, with patients paying a deductible and a portion of the covered amounts (coinsurance). Federal payroll taxes and general revenues and premiums cover the public sector costs. Fees paid to physicians and hospitals under Medicare are regulated.

Medicaid is a health insurance program for certain low-income groups (about 10 percent of the population) which is operated by the state governments but funded and regulated jointly by the two levels. Federal shares of total costs vary from 50 to 80 percent of total expenditures, depending on the average personal income level in the states. The federal government regulates the program by setting guidelines covering the scope of services, payment rates, and eligible population groups. States have some scope to design and operate their own Medicaid programs within the guidelines established by the federal government.

In the United States, the federal government, through the Food and Drug Administration, is responsible for the regulation of prescription drugs, including what drugs can be offered for sale, the uses to which they can be put, and the information that must accompany each package. The Office of the Surgeon General provides national leadership on health issues and the Centre for Disease Control provides specialized laboratory facilities. State governments regulate some aspects of private health insurance, and license hospitals, doctors, and other medical professionals.

Germany

In Germany, compulsory health insurance is provided through approximately 1,100 "sickness funds" usually controlled by employee and employer representatives. The funds negotiate on a regional level with physicians' associations and with individual hospitals to provide services to their members at agreed rates. These negotiations are guided by a committee, the members of which include federal and state governments. Compulsory premiums paid by employees and employers finance the sickness funds.

The central government is responsible for the overall regulation of the sickness funds, including regulating the minimum basket of services which the funds must offer their members. The federal government also regulates the premiums and pays the contributions on behalf of the unemployed, pensioners, and the disabled. Given its regulatory and financial powers, the federal government is able to rely quite extensively on moral suasion to direct the operation of the sickness funds and the rates negotiated between the funds and the health care providers. Regulation of drugs is also a federal government responsibility.

The state governments are responsible for local regulation of the sickness funds and the regional physician associations, for managing state-owned hospitals, and for regulation of other hospitals. Capital investments undertaken by hospitals are financed by grants from the state governments almost exclusively (since 1986). Public health services are provided mainly by local governments with financial support from the federal and state levels.

Switzerland

Switzerland relies on a system of private health insurance provided under federal regulation. The national government supervises the health plans and provides subsidies to them where required as a result of regulations (e.g., accepting all applicants, providing specified minimum benefits). Insurance fees are regulated by the central government which also subsidizes premiums for low-income persons. Patients are required to pay some user fees as part of the federal regulations.

The states (cantons) are responsible for public health measures within the state and, as well, coordinate with other states. Some cantons have made health insurance compulsory. Cantons are responsible for subsidies to and regulation of hospitals and other institutions. They also monitor prices set between providers and insurance funds and regulate these charges, at least within ranges (i.e., minimum and maximum charges allowed).

An interesting feature of the Swiss system is that the regulation of medical training and pharmaceuticals (authorization and risk assessment) is delegated to intercanton bodies, which perform these functions on behalf of all cantons.

European Community

While not a federal country, the EC is interesting because of the emerging powers and responsibilities of the Community relative to its member states. Responsibility for health care policy clearly rests primarily with the member countries. However, the Community is becoming increasingly involved in a number of health care programs.

The Treaty on European Union (Maastricht Treaty), which came into effect in 1993, delineated the scope of EC involvement in health care and the types of policy instruments on which it could rely (Article 129). In particular:

1. The Community shall contribute towards ensuring a high level of human health protection by encouraging cooperation between Member States and, if necessary, lending support to their action.

    Community action shall be directed towards the prevention of diseases, in particular the major health scourges, including drug dependence, by promoting research into their causes and their transmission, as well as health information and education.

    Health protection requirements shall form a constituent part of the Community's other policies.

2. Member States shall, in liaison with the Commission, coordinate among themselves their policies and programs in the areas referred to in paragraph 1. The Commission may, in close contact with the Member States, take any useful initiative to promote such coordination.

3. The Community and the Member States shall foster cooperation with third countries and the competent international organizations in the sphere of public health.

4. In order to contribute to the achievement of the objectives referred to in this Article, the Council

    –   … shall adopt incentive measures, excluding any harmonization of the laws and regulations of the Member States

    –   acting by qualified majority on a proposal from the commission, shall adopt recommendations.

Thus, the EC's role is largely limited to public health issues, health promotion, and preventative policies rather than treatment of disease, and its available policy instruments are largely promoting cooperation, supporting actions of member states, and providing information and data and offering leadership. It can help states to achieve synergies and economies of scale where possible, especially in research.

Priority areas for Community action that have been identified to date include: cancer; drug dependency; health promotion, education, and training; health data and indicators and surveillance of diseases; AIDS and other communicable diseases; accidents and injuries; and pollution-related diseases.

Conclusion

In the four federal countries examined, spending and regulation are the dominant policy instruments in health care policy, and both the federal and state levels of governments utilize these levers extensively. Spending is particularly important at the federal level in Australia and the United States; in these countries the federal government spends at least two dollars for every health care dollar spent by the states. In Germany it appears that the federal government outspends the states (but by a smaller margin), and in Switzerland the cantons appear to spend more than the federal government. In all cases, the federal governments play a leading financial role to promote equity in health care (e.g., spending on behalf of low-income people, the unemployed, seniors).

While both levels of government extensively use regulatory levers in the area of health care, it is difficult to draw conclusions about the relative use of regulation. No standard unit of measure exists by which such comparisons can be drawn.

Taxation seems to be a significant policy instrument only in the United States. This is as one might expect, given the heavy reliance on private health care arrangements. Tax expenditures for health care purposes are primarily federal initiatives. It was difficult to get a sense of the use of moral suasion/political leadership by the federal government in these countries, in part because such levers are often "less formal." It does appear, however, that the federal government in Germany does use moral suasion (backed up by a readiness to regulate) to influence the sickness funds and health care provider associations.

In general, Australia, Germany, and the United States (at least in terms of its public programs) are clearly more centralized in their health care systems than is Canada. The central governments have leading financial and regulatory roles and levers and are involved in the design and the delivery of their health care programs. While it is more decentralized, in Switzerland, the federal government does control the operation of health insurance. Canada is the most decentralized country of the group in terms of the power of the provinces to determine the organization of the health care system, and to regulate its operation.

Only the European Community, which is still an international superstructure rather than a federal state, displays less central control over health care levers than Canada.

The Public-Private Mix in Health Care

RAISA DEBER, PH.D.
LUTCHMIE NARINE, PH.D.
PAT BARANEK, M.SC., Ph.D. candidate
NATASHA SHARPE, Ph.D.
KATYA MASNYK DUVALKO, M.SC., Ph.D. candidate
RANDI ZLOTNIK-SHAUL, LL.B., Ph.D. candidate
PETER COYTE, PH.D.
GEORGE PINK, PH.D.
A. PAUL WILLIAMS, PH.D.

Department of Health Administration
University of Toronto

SUMMARY

What is the appropriate mix between public and private roles and responsibilities for health care? We begin by defining our terms. Public can refer to the national (federal), provincial (or state), regional or local levels. Private may refer to corporate for-profit entities, small businesses, individuals and their families, or charitable not-for-profit entities, which in turn may rely on a mixture of volunteers and paid labour and act as mediating structures to carry out public objectives. Much current policy activity thus relates to movement within rather than between public and private. It is also important to define which dimensions of health services are being referred to. In this paper, we concentrate on three:
— financing—how services are paid for
— delivery—how services are provided to recipients of care
— allocation—how resources flow from those who finance care to those who deliver it.

A series of possible models, drawn from the international literature, are noted. The current Canadian system is composed of public financing for "medically necessary" care, coupled with private (usually not-for-profit) delivery. In evaluating these models, we note that the international literature strongly suggests that single-source (public) financing is optimal for financing required services—that is, services that public policy suggests should not be denied to individuals who cannot afford to pay for them. The arguments for public financing rest not only on equity grounds, but on considerations of economic efficiency. If care recipients cannot be priced out of the market, then one cannot rely on market mechanisms to achieve cost control. Multiple financers are less likely to achieve monopsony bargaining power in bargaining with providers and are likely to have more difficulties in achieving cost control (which is one reason why providers are likely to favour pluralistic funding arrangements). To the extent that private insurance is allowed, costs are likely to be shifted to employers, with negative effects on economic competitiveness. Multiple financers also have strong incentives to shift costs by avoiding clients who are likely to require services, which in turn implies both higher costs for government (if it is the payer of last resort), and equity concerns. For all of these reasons, models with single-source (public) financing for medically required care—the approach used for services insured under the Canada Health Act—are strongly preferred.

In contrast, the literature suggests that public delivery of care is less likely to be client responsive. However, for-profit private delivery appears acceptable only when outcome standards can be clearly specified and monitored, a condition often difficult to meet in providing complex services. Where outcome criteria are not clear cut and monitorable, not-for-profit delivery appears optimal. Again, this is the general Canadian pattern, albeit with exceptions for particular services in particular jurisdictions.

The literature is less clear about an optimal approach to allocation. Allocation mechanisms for publicly financed care can be arrayed on a continuum from planned models (in which patients follow money, i.e., patients can go for care only to those organizations that have received funding to offer a particular service) through to market models (in which money follows patients, i.e., money flows to those organizations that can attract clients). Planned allocation models have the virtue of easing cost control (since the total amount to be spent can be specified). Market allocation models are more likely to be client responsive (since organizations are paid only if they can attract clients). Considerable international experimentation is under way with mixed models (e.g., managed competition, public competition, etc.), which seek to combine the virtues of both, although these models have not yet been well evaluated. Room remains for experimentation with allocation and reimbursement measures that tailor incentives to desired outcomes; such efforts are likely to accelerate.

Following a description of the legislative and regulatory framework for hospital and medical care insurance in Canada and the presentation of selected data on the extent of the public-private mix in Canada, we briefly describe a series of case studies of some experiences with different models. These cases include hospitals, private clinics, physician services, the deinsurance of medical procedures, automobile insurance and rehabilitative services in Ontario, travel health insurance, pharmaceuticals, and private insurance in Australia. The presumption that cost control is more likely under public spending is confirmed, both by the overall spending figures and by the specific case examples. Multiple sources of funding do appear to give rise to the postulated problems of cost control, as well as presenting difficulties for equity.

We then suggest values by which any policy framework can be evaluated (i.e., equity, efficiency, security, and liberty). Next, we review a number of potential frameworks for making decisions about what should and should not be insured: the Canada Health Act approach (current system), the Oregon model, the proposed Netherlands four-sieve model and two approaches proposed for Canada: the four-screen model and the Canadian Medical Association Core and Comprehensiveness Project. Most attention is paid to the four-screen model, which consists of the following four screens:

1. *Effectiveness: Does it work?*
2. *Appropriateness: Is it needed?*
3. *Informed choice: Is it wanted?*
4. *Public provision: Should the public pay?*

The four-screen model has the advantage of encouraging flexibility and appropriateness, but the difficulty of not giving rise to hard and fast rules about coverage. A modification, the global four-screen model, whereby this more nuanced approach could be compatible with both the Canada Health Act and global (regional) funding, is then suggested. The report concludes with four recommendations:

1. *Public financing for medically required services*
2. *Public competition allocation*
3. *Mixed (largely private not-for-profit) delivery*
4. *Client-sensitive determination of medical necessity (no lists).*

TABLE OF CONTENTS

Objectives 431

Understanding the Basis for the Current Public-Private Mix
of Services 431

  Appropriate Role of the Public Sector versus the Private Sector 431
    Public and Private 432
    How Does Health Care Differ from Other Markets? 436
    Financing 440
    Delivery 449
    Allocation 452
    Interrelationship among Financing, Delivery, and Allocation 456

Legislative and Regulatory Framework 457

  Historical Roots: The Constitution and the Growth of
  Shared-Cost Programs 457

  Current Legislative and Regulatory Framework 460
    The Canada Health Act 460
    Canadian Charter of Rights and Freedoms 464
    Provincial and International Legislation and Regulations 467

The Case of Canada: Selected Data on the Extent of
the Public-Private Mix 469

  Financing 469
    Total Health Spending 470
    Total Public Spending for Health 472
    Total Provincial Spending for Health 474
    Total Private Spending for Health 478
    Health Spending by Particular Sectors 479

  Delivery 482

  Allocation 482

Case Studies of Some Experiences with Different Models 485

  Hospitals 485

Private Clinics 488

Physician Services 492

Deinsurance of Medical Procedures 494

Automobile Insurance and Rehabilitative Services in Ontario 495

Travel Health Insurance 498

Paying for Pharmaceuticals 499

Private Insurance in Australia 501

Evaluating the Models: Equity, Efficiency, Security, and Liberty 503

Conceptual Issues and Historical Debate 503

Balancing Social and Political Values with Technical and
Administrative Values 504

Evaluation Criteria 505

Financing 507

Delivery 510

Allocation 511

Frameworks for Making Decisions about What Should and
What Should Not Be Insured 512

Canada Health Act Model 513

    Adequacy of CHA Definitions of Comprehensiveness 513

    Views of the Private Role 515

    Services That Governments Believe They Should Not Be
    Paying For 516

    Services That Would Ideally Be Insured 517

    Processes for Insuring and Deinsuring 518

    Examination of Canada Health Act Model 519

Oregon Model 520

Netherlands Model 521

Four-Screen Model (Deber-Ross) 522

    Cost Minimization 524

    Social Values 524

    Advance Knowledge 525

The Model in Practice 525

CMA Core and Comprehensiveness Project 527

Examination of Four-Screen Model and CMA Approaches 528

Summary of Models 529

Policy Implications and Recommendations 531

Recommendations 531

Recommendation 1 – Public Financing for Medically
Required Services 531

Recommendation 2 – Mixed (Largely Private Not-for-Profit)
Delivery 533

Recommendation 3 –Public Competition Allocation 533

Recommendation 4 – Client-Sensitive Determination
of Medical Necessity (No Lists) 534

Endnotes 537

LIST OF FIGURES

Figure 1   Models of relationship between service and payment 437

Figure 2   Distribution (%) of national health expenditures
by sector of finance, Canada, 1984 and 1994 470

Figure 3   Distribution (%) of national health expenditures
by category, Canada, 1984 and 1994 472

Figure 4   Per capita total health expenditure by province, 1994 478

Figure 5   Health expenditures as a percentage of provincial GNP,
1994 479

Figure 6   Health spending as a percentage of GDP vs. private
spending 480

LIST OF TABLES

Table 1   Categories of public and private 433

Table 2   Classification of health care systems 439

Table 3   Allocation models for publicly financed services 453

Table 4   Total health expenditures by sector of finance,
Canada, 1975–1994 471

Table 5   Total health expenditures by category of expenditure,
            Canada, 1975–1994 473

Table 6   Federal health transfers by type of transfer, Canada,
            1975–1994 475

Table 7   Provincial government health expenditures by category,
            Canada, 1975–1994 476

Table 8   Workers' compensation health expenditures by category,
            Canada, 1975–1994 481

Table 9   Health expenditures by subcategory of expenditure,
            Canada, 1992 483

Table 10   Interprovincial comparison of number of cataract
            surgeries provided by all specialties per 1,000 covered
            population, 1983–1991 493

Table 11   Estimates of auto insurers payments for rehabilitation
            policies, 1991–1994 497

Table 12   Supplementary health benefit payments by type
            of benefit ($), 1984–1993 501

Table 13   The four-screen model...523

Table 14   Summary of model characteristics...530

OBJECTIVES

In September 1995, the National Forum on Health released a discussion paper, *The Public and Private Financing of Canada's Health System*,[1*] which sought to clarify the terms of the impending debate about how best to fund health care services. To augment the discussion, the working group on "Striking a Balance" commissioned us to write a follow-up background paper. The main objective was "to develop a framework to help determine the extent to which various types of services should be publicly or privately funded, and to outline options for mechanisms which could bring more coherency and consistency to health care financing in the Canadian context."

We were asked to examine the basis for the current public-private mix of services—with particular attention to the historical roots of the present configuration of services and to the legislative and regulatory framework within which decisions about private and public funding are now made—and to identify the advantages and disadvantages of the current framework. Building on our findings, we were then to develop a decision-making framework that encompasses notions of medical necessity, appropriateness of care, effectiveness and access to services, and that could be used to determine whether services qualify for full, partial or no public funding. Finally, we were asked to discuss the policy implications of the framework and to make recommendations.

Accordingly, we begin this paper with a conceptual framework, in which we examine notions of public and private. Next, we describe the situation in Canada, including several case studies. We then discuss several decision-making frameworks. Following a discussion of evaluation criteria, we conclude with recommendations.

The question of the appropriate roles of the public and private sectors is a complex one, which is evoking considerable discussion. To date, this discussion has been characterized by more heat than light. We hope that this background paper assists in the debate.

UNDERSTANDING THE BASIS FOR THE CURRENT PUBLIC-PRIVATE MIX OF SERVICES

Appropriate Role of the Public Sector versus the Private Sector

What is the proper role for government in health and social policy? The purpose of this paper cannot be to give the answer. We instead seek to clarify the question, distinguishing the factual and ideological components, noting possible models and their implications, and providing a few case studies.

---

* Notes are found at the end of the document.

The public-private mix is at the root of current ideological debate.[2] Arguments from the right see a minimal role for governments and a maximal role for the market; these theorists tend to place the highest values on individual choice and liberty, and to presume that government involvement breeds inefficiency. Arguments from the left claim that collective values and the public interest cannot be left to market mechanisms; these people place a high value on social equity and redistribution to those seen as being in need. We do not mediate among these clashing ideologies, but do deal with their implications in the section "Evaluating the Models", which discusses evaluation criteria that can be used to select policies.

A necessary first step is clarification of what is meant by the terms "public" and "private." The public-private distinction is a complicated one; there are many levels of the public and private sectors, and movement can occur within as well as between them.

A further complication is that health policy differs in several crucial ways from many other areas of public policy. Health care also has several dimensions—the issues involved in determining how to pay for care are not the same as those involved in deciding how to deliver it. In addition, health care systems are made up of many sectors, and the way in which they are organized can vary considerably; it is not meaningful to speak of Canada's health care system without specifying which aspects are being addressed.

Accordingly, we begin by building a conceptual framework with two key elements: (1) definitions of "public" and "private", and (2) features characteristic of health systems, including the three key dimensions of financing, delivery, and allocation.

Public and private

Paul Starr, a leading U.S. health policy analyst, has written on the meanings of privatization, cautioning that the terms "public" and "private" do not have consistent meanings and concluding that it is risky to generalize about the merits of privatization as public policy beyond a particular institutional or national context. He notes that the terms "public" and "private" are usually paired to describe a number of related oppositions in our thought, where "public" is to "private" as "open" is to "closed," as "the whole" is to "the part," or as governmental or official activities are to activities beyond the state's boundaries (i.e., in the market or in the family).[3]

Just as there are many gradations between open and closed, there appears to be a continuum between public and private (table 1). As Richard Saltman has noted, "public" may refer to a wide variety of structural arrangements (from branches of government to semiautonomous agencies). These may operate at the national, provincial, regional or local level, may be managed by elected or appointed administrators, and may be accountable for day-to-day decisions or only for long-term outcomes.[4] The term "private" is even less precise, including not only for-profit concerns, but also a wide variety of not-for-profit voluntary organizations. Accordingly, classification can be somewhat arbitrary. For example, workers' compensation premiums are not formally part of the public sector and are not usually classified as taxes, but such contributions are often mandatory and statutory. Canadian hospitals may be run by private boards, but be heavily regulated and receive most of their operating funds from public sources. Even the distinction between not-for-profit and for-profit is blurred, sometimes being separated only by whether an excess of revenues to expenditures should be called "profit" or "surplus." As U.S. practice has made clear, not-for-profit organizations such as hospitals can engage in many antisocial practices commonly associated with the for-profit sector, such as patient dumping or "cream skimming." One has to look not only at the ownership structure, but also at the broad framework of incentives that determine how these institutions behave.

Table 1

Categories of public and private

Category	Levels
Public	Nation
	Province or state
	Region
	Local
Private	Corporate (for-profit)
	Small business/entrepreneurial
	Charity/nonprofit (paid employees or volunteers)
	Family or personal

Although the charitable or nonprofit sector is nominally private, it often works closely with government and may even provide services free of charge. To the degree that government delegates functions to this sector, often accompanied by financing or regulation of its activities, these institutions may be referred to as mediating structures. Examples are Germany's Sickness Funds, which, although nominally private, represent a quasi-public funding mechanism, and Ontario's hospitals, which can be viewed as quasi-public, quasi-private delivery mechanisms.

There has been an extensive, if not always illuminating, debate over the relative merits of public versus private roles. Among the justifications offered for a public (government) role in providing goods and services are public goods, externalities, market failure, the provision of order, and social justice.

Public (collective) goods – The term "public good" is used to refer to items that cannot be managed by market mechanisms because it is impossible to exclude people who have not paid from consuming them. For example, once pollution controls have been implemented, everyone can breathe the resulting clean air. All residents of a territory, not only those who choose to pay for a military defence, are equally protected from foreign invasion. Inevitably, some people become what economists call free riders, refusing to pay, since they cannot be denied the resulting benefits.[5] In a world of rational decision makers, the consequence is that too few of such public goods are provided (where "too few" is defined in economic terms as the quantity that such rational decision makers would be willing to pay for if free riding did not exist). Accordingly, even those people most ideologically opposed to government involvement tend to accept that the state has a legitimate economic role in ensuring an optimal provision and financing of public goods. Although pure public goods are rare, a number of public health activities (e.g., prevention of epidemic disease) clearly fall within this rubric.[6]

Externalities – Another category of goods can lead to negative or positive external consequences (e.g., polluting a river has consequences for those downstream; educating a professional can provide benefits and costs to other members of the society). Most political philosophies recognize a role for government intervention (often to police or regulate) to ensure that the costs and benefits of externalities are fairly borne.

Market failure – In economic terms, it is recognized that all markets need a market manager to ensure fairness.[7] In some cases, governments can assist markets by enforcing rules and standards. In others, governments may be able to improve efficiency by interfering in failed markets (e.g., by regulating private monopolies, or even by themselves becoming providers). Although there is considerable debate about the extent and causes of market failure in health care and the extent (if any) of government involvement that can be justified on these grounds, the phenomenon of risk selection (when insurers avoid insuring people at high risk of needing health care services) is often thought to justify government intervention.

Provision of order – The state's monopoly of force and its sovereign authority ensure that social and economic order are maintained. One justification for the welfare state has been that, by "buying off" workers with social programs, one can prevent social instability.

Social justice – The outcomes of markets may be unjust or unfair. Social justice is an argument used primarily for redistributive purposes. For example, one may argue that all citizens of a nation are entitled to a certain level of benefits by right, and that the state has a role in ensuring that these benefits are received. Clearly, the extent to which social justice is a legitimate concern of the state is a highly ideological issue. Among the reasons for rejecting a public role are inefficiency, overuse, and lack of innovation.

Inefficiency – Orthodox economists often note that competition weeds out the inefficient, whereas protected markets tend to propagate inefficiency.

Overuse – If price is the signalling device linking supply and demand, pure economic theory suggests that there will be an infinite demand for "free" goods, leading to overuse and waste.

Lack of innovation – Organizations not facing competition—whether these be in the public or the private sector—can grow complacent and stagnant.

For all these reasons, privatization has emerged as a serious counter-movement to the growth of government. Starr distinguishes among four types of privatization:[8]

- the cessation of public programs and the disengagement of government from specific kinds of responsibilities (implicit privatization) (This form of privatization may also happen indirectly, through restricting the volume, availability, or quality of public services such that consumers shift toward privately produced and purchased substitutions. Starr calls this process "privatization by attrition.")
- the transfer of public assets (e.g., airports, hydro) to private ownership
- the replacement of direct government services with public financing of private service delivery (through contracting out or vouchers)
- the deregulation of entry by private firms into activities that were previously treated as a public monopoly.

Bendick makes a similar distinction between "government load shedding" and the "empowerment of mediating institutions."[9] "Load shedding" refers to arrangements wherein both the means of financing and the means of delivery are divorced from government—for example, budget reductions, the introduction of user fees, and the increased use of volunteers. Canadian health policy analysts have noted the growth of this approach, which they refer to as passive privatization; government policy in recent years has resulted in an increasing share of total health care expenditures coming from the private sector (particularly employers) and a greater reliance on private insurance.[10] In contrast, the empowerment of mediating institutions involves arrangements wherein government delegates the production and delivery of services while retaining some or all responsibility for financing—for example, the use of vouchers, contracting out of services, and public-private partnerships. Osborne and Gaebler have described a number of such efforts in New Zealand, Australia, Britain, and the United States.[11]

The justifications for privatization reflect several different views of what is meant by "private." For example, justifications based on laissez-faire capitalism assume that free markets and the profit motive can yield innovation, greater efficiency, improved management and responsiveness to individual choice. Another vision, however, is grounded in a return of power to individuals and communities through a greater reliance on families, churches, and nonprofit institutions. Yet another view merely sees private as "not public," and privatization as a political strategy for diverting demands away from the state and reducing the size and scope of government.

Although many advocates of privatization speak in terms of increasing competition, it is important to recognize that these terms are not synonymous.[12] Competition is a particular methodology for allocating scarce resources, employing a variety of operating mechanisms (including consumer choice, open bidding, and negotiated contracts), in which the performance of multiple players is compared, resulting in winners and losers. Clearly, monopolies can exist with private ownership. Conversely, competition can exist within a system of public ownership and administration. Indeed, the popular movement of reinventing government grants the validity of a public interest, but seeks to take advantage of the presumed efficiencies of the private sector for service delivery by encouraging competition for provision of publicly funded services.[13]

How Does Health Care Differ from Other Markets?

All markets assume a supply of goods, a demand for them, and some mechanism to bring together seller and buyer. Three parties are thus potentially involved in the process by which an individual receives services: the provider (who sells the available supply), the recipient (who demands the product or service), and the payer. A pure market assumes that price acts as the signalling device to bring supply and demand into balance, increasing if there is too much demand, and decreasing if there is an excessive supply.

Figure 1 depicts two potential relationships between receiving services and paying for them. The top diagram depicts the simplest market transaction, in which the recipient is also the payer. A two-way relationship results, in which the provider gives services in exchange for payment.

The bottom diagram in figure 1 depicts a possible response to fluctuating costs—for example, if there is a small likelihood of a large cost. Under such circumstances, it is rational to pool risks—that is, for each individual in a group to pay an affordable premium to ensure coverage in the unlucky event of catastrophe. Insurance principles thus can lead to the growth of third-party payers. Under this model, potential care recipients pay the third-party agent, who in turn reimburses providers. Price no longer directly links supply and demand, because the purpose of insurance is to insulate the insured person from the costs of catastrophe.

Health care services present major dilemmas for believers in markets. Consider the issue of how resources should be allocated for health care services. A pure market model assumes that resources should go to the people willing to pay the highest price, following the well-known law of supply and demand. Yet despite the superficial attractiveness of market metaphors, there is ample evidence that much of health care does not fit this model. The features that differentiate supply and demand in the health services

Figure 1

Models of relationship between service and payment

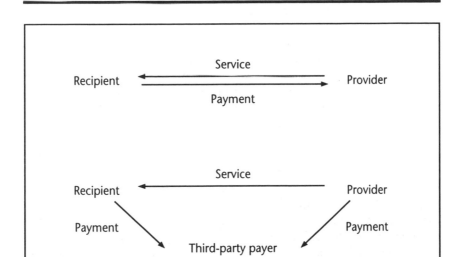

sector from supply and demand in other sectors have been well docu-mented.[14]

One set of violations of pure markets can potentially be addressed through better provision of information to consumers. Information issues include the uncertainty of risks for both consumers and insurers, information asymmetry between consumers and providers and between insurers and providers, and imperfect information, most health care consumers not having the economic resources, the time, or the interest to apply rational self-interest, particularly under circumstances where they require urgent or emergency care. As a result, providers rather than consumers have tended to determine what services are recommended. One set of reforms thus seeks to preserve the market by producing a perfectly informed consumer. Our research on medical decision making suggests that the pure form of this goal is both unwise and unattainable, because it does not distinguish between two ele-ments of choice, which we refer to as problem solving and decision making. Problem solving—the search for the correct answer—requires a high degree of technical knowledge. Preferences are irrelevant. It does not matter if someone would prefer that his leg not be broken, or would like a surgical procedure to guarantee a cure—the results are what they are. Research by Deber and colleagues has shown that few people wish to perform medical problem-solving tasks, particularly when the consequences of error can be severe.[15] Decision making, in contrast, requires individuals to weigh advantages and disadvantages and decide on a course of action; only the person living with chest pain can decide whether the symptoms are tolerable, or whether it is preferable to risk cardiac surgery. Given appropriate information, many patients do wish a role in decision making, usually shared with the physician.

A physician-patient partnership, which we believe is both feasible and highly desirable, therefore differs fundamentally from the relationship between buyer and seller. It is built on the assumption that professionals will solve the problem and then support patients and their families in making the decision. Accordingly, the partnership is built on trust that the information is accurate and that the provider is acting in the best interest of the patient.[16]

Important as these informational aspects are, the fundamental difference between the market for health services and that for other commodities is the role of need. The statement that people should receive the care that they need has two implications. First, it postulates that the price signal cannot operate, since it has been agreed that no one can be priced out of the market and denied necessary care. Second, it suggests that it is not ethical to market unnecessary care. This constraint is in striking contrast to other markets; there is no problem if customers purchase an unnecessary pair of shoes. Because medical services can do harm, provision of unnecessary care is considered to be a violation of professional ethics. This role of need further distorts markets, because many services are not "price elastic," and because there can be negative consequences for underconsumption of services that are price elastic. For example, price is not usually a consideration if an individual collapses with a stroke; thus, hospital admissions tend to be "price inelastic." Nor are people likely to shop around for the cheapest neuro-surgeon. However, individuals may well be deterred from visiting a family doctor if a user fee is imposed. Therefore, in the long run, the user fee strategy can be counterproductive: for example, a person could forgo the opportunity to detect and treat high blood pressure, and thus incur the far higher costs of a stroke. Neither can goods be fully substituted—for example, one cannot compensate for a shortage of hip replacements by pointing to an excess of pediatricians. For all of these reasons, reliance on the seemingly logical predictions of neoclassical economics tends to lead to distorted and erroneous predictions in the health policy arena, particularly when considering matters of life and death.[17]

However, not all health care deals with life and death, and hence classical economic models may prove more valid in some areas than in others. As Adams and colleagues[18] indicate, Canada's health system can be divided into at least 16 different sectors: acute hospital care; chronic hospital care; ambulatory or outpatient care (including physician's services); laboratories and radiology; capital costs; ancillary benefits (dental, vision, physiotherapy, chiropractic, and podiatry); ambulance and transportation; nursing homes or homes for the aged; home care; rehabilitation care; drugs; assistive devices; mental health; public health and health promotion; education and training of health professionals; and planning, research, and management. These sectors vary considerably in how they are treated by provincial insurance plans (we note the legal constraints on Canada's health care system in the section "Legislative and Regulatory Framework"), and in whether they deal with surviving or thriving.[19] Appropriate policy responses are likely to vary depending on what sorts of health services are being discussed.

At the most general level, health care systems can be divided into three dimensions. Although there are many ways of characterizing health systems,[20] we have found it helpful to focus on *financing* health systems, the *delivery* of health services, and the *allocation* of resources to providers.

Three broad categories of health care systems arise from the cross-classification of public and private against delivery and financing (table 2).

Table 2

Classification of health care systems

Delivery	Financing	
	Public	**Private**
Public	National health service	–
Private	Public insurance	Private insurance

The national health services (such as the old National Health Service in Britain or those in Scandinavia) are examples of public financing and public delivery. Private insurance systems, such as what the United States likes to believe operates in that country, use private financing and private delivery (although, in fact, U.S. health care financing is heavily government subsidized through the tax code, as well as through direct government-funded plans). Public insurance systems, such as those in Canada and much of Europe (e.g., France, Germany, the Netherlands), employ the combination of public (or quasi-public) financing with private delivery. We know of no complete system using private financing with public delivery, although many national health services do allow limited private purchase of publicly delivered services.

It must be recognized that it is an oversimplification to classify a country's health system as either public or private. Virtually every country employs some combination of financing and delivery models, relying on various public-private combinations in various sectors of the health system or for various groups of the nation's population. Cost shifting also varies by country, group, and service (e.g., use of copayments and deductibles and supplementary insurance). Similarly, the public and private sectors are involved to a lesser or greater extent in service delivery, depending on the health sector within which services are provided (e.g. dental, vision, rehabilitation, long-term care), on the population group for which services are geared (e.g., state employees, veterans, the elderly) or on the perceived urgency of the services (acute versus chronic care, elective versus urgent surgery). Even Sweden's system and the pre-1989 British NHS, long considered prototypically public delivery systems, included elements of private sector involvement in service delivery. The descriptions below thus paint with a fairly broad brush, drawing on the analysis performed in a study for the Ontario Task Force on the Financing and Delivery of Health Care.[21]

Financing

The first dimension of health systems is the question of how services should be financed. This issue is receiving particular attention in the current era of slow economic growth and resulting pressure on resources.

A wide array of participants can be involved in financing health services, and mixed models abound. For example, copayments or deductibles represent a sharing of costs between individuals and insurers. Tax deductibility represents a sharing of costs with all other taxpayers. On average, 80 percent of health care expenses in OECD countries (but less than 72 percent in Canada) come from the public sector. As the following models clarify, the distribution between public and private sector is usually based on some combination of the segment of the population (who is insured) and the particular services being provided (what is insured). Since it is easier to shift costs than to control them, many measures purporting to be cost saving prove instead to be cost shifting—that is, they move costs from government to the private sector or among governments, but do not decrease (and often increase) the total amount spent for health care services.

Saltman makes a number of distinctions: between public and private financing sources, between voluntary premiums and mandatory social insurance and taxation schemes, between single source and multiple payers (competing or complementary), and between policies that provide primary coverage and supplementary insurance policies that duplicate or extend a basic package of services.[22] A similar categorization based on financing dichotomies is presented by Appleby.[23] The Canadian Medical Association offers the following as possible sources of financing: public sources such as consolidated revenue funds, earmarked taxes, intergovernmental transfers, employer-based taxes, vouchers and direct federal expenditures, and private sources such as private insurance, point-of-service charges, philanthropic donations, lotteries, and premiums.[24] They propose two conclusions based on their review of financing options: that the form of funding should follow its spending function, and that the one who spends should tax. They argue that as health programs are decentralized or regionalized, focus will turn to clear lines of responsibility, authority, and accountability for tax and spending decisions.

Although most industrialized countries finance their health care through more than one model depending on health sector, population group and type of care, Saltman's four major financing-related dichotomies (public/private, voluntary/compulsory, single payer/multiple payers, and comprehensive/supplementary) have aligned into several dominant health system types.[25] Two represent public financing—the clearly public, tax-based, single-source financing found in Australia, Canada, New Zealand, Sweden, and the United Kingdom; and the quasi-public, highly regulated, social insurance, multiple-source financing found in France, the Netherlands, and Germany. The remaining categories are classified as private financing—the compulsory, competing multiple-payer model proposed (but not implemented) to complement basic public insurance in the Netherlands' Dekker reforms, and the voluntary, competing private plans characteristic of the United States.

The multiple levels of public and private sectors described in table 1 can then be combined with these financing approaches to create a wide array of health financing options. For example, compulsory public financing of health services through taxation can occur at the level of the national government (e.g., England's NHS), at the local level (e.g., Sweden's county councils), or at multiple levels (e.g., federal-provincial or federal-state cost sharing as in Canada, Australia, and the U.S. Medicaid program).

Tax-based financing is, in theory, related only to ability to pay. However, many systems choose to meet at least a portion of their costs through insurance premiums. Insurance is a logical response to situations in which risks must be spread over time and over a large number of people by pooling resources. However, if the only reason for health insurance were protection against risk, there would be little rationale for comprehensive coverage. Insurers would offer only catastrophic coverage, on the logical grounds that no one purchases insurance against routine costs; there is no market for "food insurance." There would also be no role for government beyond provision of sufficient income to the poor to allow them the option of purchasing insurance. A pure insurance model must also be concerned with abuse and the issue of "moral hazard"; that is, individuals who know that they are likely to need services are more likely to purchase insurance against those costs and to engage in risky behaviour. The availability of flood insurance may encourage people to build on flood plains, while people at low risk of flooding are unlikely to purchase such insurance.

The applicability of such concepts to health care is debatable. In our view, people are not likely to abuse their health solely because they will not have to pay for the resulting care; poor health has too many other non-monetary costs. However, it may well be the case that people who perceive their risk of illness to be low (e.g., people who are young and in good health) may decide to run the risk of going without insurance, although this calculation appears most likely if incomes are either very high or very low. Insurers, on the other hand, have a clear incentive to be selective in making decisions about which individuals they will cover. As insurers become more skilled at risk selection, a problem arises—often referred to by such food analogies as cream skimming, cherry picking, or picking the raisins—in which insurers can identify and refuse to insure people at high risk of requiring costly services. Because voluntary plans cannot and will not guarantee that everyone can purchase coverage, governments often assume a role in ensuring that everyone will be able to join a plan, sometimes even acting as an insurer of last resort.

One approach is to charge everyone the same premium, a process known as community rating. Community rating represents a subsidy of those likely to incur high charges by those likely to remain healthy. If a competitive market is allowed, insurers have an incentive to cream skim those at lower risk by charging them lower premiums. Plans with community rating will then tend to retain the higher-risk population, increasing the costs to that plan and causing a spiral referred to as adverse selection—that is, as costs increase, low-risk individuals leave the plan seeking cheaper coverage, which further increases premiums for the people remaining. For these reasons, the competitive market approach to financing fails the people most in need; those in poorest health may become uninsurable. Most systems therefore retain a role for government in regulating how premiums will be set and who must be covered.

Accordingly, as noted, the charitable and private not-for-profit sectors, although nominally private, may work so closely with government that they become what theorists refer to as mediating structures, performing duties delegated to them by the public sector, often financed by the public sector and strictly regulated by public legislation.[26] De facto, insurance companies in such systems remain private, but the line between the public and private sectors is blurred by the facts that they are performing a public function and that individuals have no choice but to contribute.

The literature and international experience both strongly suggest that public or quasi-public single-source financing of health services is optimal, not only on equity grounds, but to achieve cost containment.[27] First, administrative costs are far lower in single-payer systems than in health systems with multiple, competing insurers.[28] Second, there is little incentive to try to shift the cost of care for high-risk, elderly, or other high-cost patients onto other payers. Thus, the inevitable inequities of unequal insurance coverage resulting from multiple insurers are avoided.[29] Third, with one tax-based public insurance system, the costs of financing health care are more evenly distributed throughout the economy—no one particular sector carries the bulk of the financial burden. In countries that rely on employers to pay premiums for their workers, the disincentive of the heavy cost burden for each person added to a payroll is thought to increase unemployment, while people with good medical benefits may be reluctant to change jobs and risk interruption or loss of coverage. Fourth, with one public insurance system, the single payer retains monopsony (single purchaser) bargaining power over service providers, which it can use (should it choose to do so) to achieve greater control over total health care expenditures.[30] This last feature clearly has disadvantages for providers, who will find it more difficult to evade cost controls. To ensure that overly stringent cost control does not erode quality and access, it is important to ensure that accountability and monitoring mechanisms exist; how best to achieve these mechanisms is beyond the scope of this paper.

In light of these advantages of a single source of financing, most reasons advanced in favour of allowing competing insurers or financers appear to be based on ideology rather than evidence. The primary justification is usually based on the assumptions that markets promote efficiency and that competition is more responsive to innovation and patient choice. There is good justification for these arguments when speaking of delivery, but none when speaking of financing. As noted, multiple-source financing is associated with considerable overhead costs: plans must compete (and absorb the costs of advertising); providers must absorb the costs of dealing with multiple payers; regulators must absorb the costs of ensuring that plans remain solvent and dealing with adverse selection; individuals have the costs of reviewing and selecting plans and filing claims, and may face potential exposure to considerable financial risks. Mixed funding sources make it harder to deal with risk selection and more difficult to achieve monopsony bargaining power over providers. (Accordingly, such arrangements may be attractive to providers, precisely because they make it easier to avoid stringent cost controls.) For these reasons, governments usually attempt to regulate the multiple sickness funds in countries such as Germany or the Netherlands, while the plans themselves have formed consortia to bargain collectively with providers. In addition, although people clearly find it important to be able to select their own care provider, it is less clear that they place a high value on being able to select their own insurer.

There are a variety of ways of financing health services in any given country. Although most of the countries of Western Europe have provided for universal health care coverage for all of their citizens (in fact, the United States is the only country in the industrialized world that does not provide for universal health care coverage), many have different methods of financing care for different groups of people.

Some countries, such as Canada, divide coverage on a geographical basis (e.g., by province). In other countries, the method of financing health services varies according to the income level of the individual covered, usually covering core medical and hospital services for most of the population through general taxes or sickness fund premiums, but allowing those individuals with higher incomes to opt out of the public system, either partially (e.g., in England when jumping queues) or entirely (e.g., in Germany the most wealthy can choose to purchase private insurance). The United States instead relies on private financing of services for the mainstream of the population (although with considerable cross-subsidization from tax exemptions) and then provides public coverage as a safety net for those individuals whose incomes are low enough to qualify for government aid, with those too poor to pay for their own insurance but not poor enough to qualify for public coverage falling between the cracks.

A second way of differentiating who is covered in various insurance plans is through the notion of social entitlements. Most often these variations occur with groups of individuals seen to have a particular call on government resources. Public servants often have special health insurance plans financed by their employer (government). Such special insurance may also exist for individuals with difficult but valuable occupations that might make them uninsurable, such as firefighters or miners.[31] Other groups who commonly have some claim to public financing (or at least public subsidy) may include war veterans, the disabled, the blind, and the elderly.[32]

A third way of differentiating health services financing centres on occupational category. This distinction is most frequently found in countries with sickness funds (e.g., France, Germany). In these countries, the choice of sickness fund (and the concomitant premium rate) depends on occupation; people employed in industries having primarily young and healthy workers may pay considerably less than people in industries having an aging labour force. Such employment-based plans may present difficulty in dealing with such groups as farmers, other agricultural workers, the unemployed, and the self-employed; government may choose to play a role in serving those groups.

It is important to recognize that actuarial principles require a large enough pool of individuals in any insurance plan to even out the inevitable peaks and valleys. "Small is beautiful" may work well with delivery (in terms of ensuring closeness to clients, although often not with respect to maintaining a critical mass of expertise), but financing requires larger pools. Small insurance plans are inherently unstable, and indeed the U.S. market is characterized by a wave of mergers. Most Canadian provinces are relatively small as insurance plans; as long as geography remains a primary basis for determining coverage (i.e., as long as health care remains a provincial responsibility), any moves away from single payers are thus likely to evoke actuarial and efficiency problems as well as the equity issues more commonly raised.

A distinction commonly made is between insurance policies that provide primary coverage and supplementary insurance policies that duplicate or extend a basic package of services.[33] The dominant model in industrialized countries other than the United States is to provide universal coverage for basic, "medically necessary" services; however, the content of these basic services packages varies considerably. For example, the Canadian package of medically necessary services evolved in such a way that it includes only services provided in hospitals or by physicians in its basic coverage.[34] Other countries such as Sweden, Germany, and the Netherlands include a much broader range of services, including pharmaceuticals, in their basic packages.[35] (We analyze approaches taken to determining what should be included in the section "Frameworks for Making Decisions.") Accordingly, we can distinguish a number of possible financing models.

I. Public sector as sole financer of comprehensive mix; private sector not permitted

The maximum role for the public sector in health services financing exists where financing is the responsibility of the public sector alone, with the private sector prohibited from financing the same services. A good example of this model is found in Canada for insured medical and hospital services under the Canada Health Act; among the national conditions that must be complied with is the requirement that patients not be charged directly for insured health services. Consequently, provinces generally prohibit the private sector from insuring services that are financed through provincial health insurance plans. (The rationale for such provisions is noted in the section "Evaluating the Models.")

II. Public sector as financer of basic core services, with mandatory or voluntary private coverage of other services

A. Mandatory private coverage of services not covered in the public plan

In Canada, certain medical services are now covered outside provincial plans. In Ontario, for example, much rehabilitative care for patients injured in automobile accidents is no longer paid for through Ontario Health Insurance Plan billings, but rather through car insurance premiums. Each individual who wants to drive is required to purchase car insurance from the private insurance industry and pay for this insurance through actuarially based premiums. A different level of services is therefore available to people injured in automobile accidents and deemed to be covered by this private insurance than to people with comparable injuries acquired in other ways. Similarly, workers' compensation plans can offer an additional tier of services; participation is mandatory for covered workplaces. (We look at automobile insurance in the section "Case Studies.")

B. Voluntary private coverage of services not covered in the public plan (extended coverage and top-up insurance), with or without tax breaks

In this model, the public sector finances a basic tier, of varying comprehensiveness. Private health insurance is voluntary and can be purchased (usually financed through premiums) by individuals who desire supplementary coverage for services not covered under the public plan. This model, commonly employed for such services as long-term care, pharmaceuticals and dental services, is palatable for people most concerned with universal coverage in that every citizen in a country receives what is seen to be necessary medical care at an affordable price (levels of copayments and deductibles for the basic plan vary from country to country). At the same time, public costs are controlled to some extent because not every service is included in the funding envelope. Rather, the financial burden for luxury or elective care is passed on to the consumer.

There are two complications. First, definitions of "luxury" clearly vary; for example, many countries are publicly debating how long-term care should be financed. Second, in many cases, employers are induced to offer such additional coverage as an employment benefit. There is an ongoing debate about whether such benefits are ultimately paid for by employers or passed along to their employees through reduced wage levels. However, to the extent that such benefits are tax deductible, a large proportion of such benefits is also borne by taxpayers, including many who never receive similar benefits. To the extent that such benefits are not tax deductible, fewer employers will offer them. The importance of tax preferences in encouraging employers to provide such plans is illustrated by the recent experience of Quebec. Its 1993 budget taxed employees on the employer's contribution to health insurance plans; a similar measure was widely discussed in the consultations preceding the 1994 federal budget. A paper by the Canadian Life and Health Insurance Industry maintains that such taxation "would impair the viability of private health insurance."[36] According to William Tholl (personal communication, 1995), the proportion of employers offering supplementary health insurance has decreased dramatically, which may in turn present equity problems in obtaining access to such services.

The clearest examples of this type of financing model are Blue Cross and other supplementary insurance plans available in most Canadian provinces for people who prefer to have extra coverage for such noninsured services as private hospital accommodation, home care, ambulance services, dental care, or prescription drugs. (The precise nature of the plans varies according to what the province provides under its own insurance plans.) Similarly, the United Kingdom allows individuals to purchase private insurance for prescription drugs and eyeglass frames more elaborate than the basic model provided by the NHS. (Data on private coverage in Canada are included in the section "The Case of Canada.")

The proposed Dekker reform plan in the Netherlands also sought to create a supplementary private insurance model. The majority of the population would be covered by a compulsory insurance plan covering basic services, and people who wanted to and had the financial resources would be able to purchase supplementary insurance as a top-up.

It is important to note that the existence of a market for private insurance under this model depends on public coverage not being comprehensive, such that potentially beneficial care is not available as a basic service. Such markets cannot be restricted to purely elective procedures (e.g., cosmetic surgery), because moral hazard would certainly come into play—only people planning to use such services would purchase insurance, meaning that it would not be economical for insurers to offer such coverage. This model would therefore create incentives for delisting benefits, both because public plans would wish to seize the opportunity to shift costs and because providers would welcome the opportunity to escape from expenditure caps by providing uninsured services. To the extent that private insurance premiums were tax deductible, such models would also create equity concerns (because people who did not have access to supplementary insurance would be forced to subsidize people who did). In addition, a vibrant supplementary tier would give rise to the disadvantages already noted as being characteristic of multiple funding sources: risk shifting, lack of cost control, and burden on employers.

Travel health insurance in Canada and private insurance in Australia are examined in the section "Case Studies."

III. Public sector as one of many financers of basic core services alongside private sector financers (complementary and competing)

A. Voluntary private coverage of services that are covered by the public plan, but with a requirement that all continue to support the public plan through compulsory contributions or through taxes

Under this model of health services financing, an alternative to the mainstream public sector exists, but not as an option covering all medical care. Individuals who have the resources can choose to seek care through the private sector, where they will be individually responsible for paying for their medical care. However, these individuals are not allowed to opt out of the public system. They continue to pay for the mainstream public system through their taxes or compulsory sickness fund contributions. Tax breaks for this type of coverage vary.

A recent example of this model existed in Alberta, where private clinics were becoming available to wealthier individuals who do not wish to wait in a queue for similar services provided by the public system. Elective surgery in England for people who want to jump the queue is another example. These models present an interesting dilemma. In theory, the public plan should ensure that all medically necessary procedures are available in a timely fashion. To the extent that delivery problems are the result of poorly organized systems of care, the solution would appear to be to fix delivery (e.g., through setting up registries, improving management practices, increasing the efficiency of service delivery, or reallocating money from lower-priority activities) rather than to manipulate financing. To the extent that the problem is underfinancing of the system as a whole, it would appear more cost effective to provide the additional resources through public financing. The popularity of the private clinic as a financing alternative (rather than as a delivery option) appears in many ways to reflect a confusion in defining the issues. If private clinics can really provide high-quality, needed care more efficiently than existing delivery mechanisms (which in the Canadian context are usually also private), there appears to be no reason why they cannot do so within the existing public system, either as a substitute for less valuable current providers or—should there be insufficient resources for those particular services—through resource reallocation. (The private clinic example is discussed in the section "Case Studies.")

B. Voluntary private coverage of services that are covered by the public plan

In this model, individuals can choose to opt out entirely and no longer make contributions to the public system. Assuming that high quality is retained (i.e., that the public system has not opted for privatization by attrition), the bulk of the population is likely to remain in the publicly funded system.

In Germany, the approximately 10 percent of the working population in the top income bracket is allowed to opt out of the sickness fund system and purchase health insurance from private insurance companies instead of having payroll taxes deducted each month. This option is available only to families in the highest paying and most stable job categories. If unregulated, this option would appear to present risk selection issues (particularly if people who opted out tended to be healthier) and ultimately could erode public support for maintaining a healthy public sector.

C. Mandatory or voluntary private coverage of services, with public financing for people meeting certain conditions

1. Public employees – In certain health systems, such as in the Netherlands, financing of health services through mandatory insurance contributions is the norm. However, public employees in certain income categories are exempt from the requirements to purchase private health insurance coverage or to contribute to sickness funds. Instead, because they work for the state, they are covered through a publicly financed health insurance system as part of their wage-and-benefit package. In the United States, federal, state, and local governments may also contribute to the financing of insurance for their employees.

2. Income related – In other models, public financing may be provided to certain individuals based on their income level. In the Netherlands, individuals with an income over a certain level are not permitted to have their care financed through the mainstream system. Instead they must purchase special insurance coverage from private, for-profit insurance companies. In the U.S. Medicaid program, public financing of health services is means tested and covers only the poor. A similar approach has been proposed in the past by the Canadian Medical Association; the majority of the population would be covered through purchases of private health insurance, while the public sector would be limited to the safety net role of financing care for the poor or disabled. The following exchange between Mr. John Tanti of Mutual Benefit insurance company and an Ontario legislative committee in 1955, culminating in a comment from then premier Leslie Frost, is cautionary:[37]

Mr. Tanti:　　Just a minute, Mr. MacDonald. If the cost of health services is to be distributed evenly, let those who are un-insurable, let the government provide benefits for the un-insurable; in other words, we will insure the insurable.

Mr. Whicher: The "cream of the crop"?

Mr. Tanti: That is true. We will insure them and let the government provide for the uninsurable.

Mr. Frost: That sounds like a bad deal for the government.

What was recognized by the Progressive Conservative Premier of Ontario seems equally true today.

3. Group related – Still other models with generally private sector financing of health services have group-related exemptions for financing. Public financing of health services for those groups occurs as a social entitlement. For example, in the United States the public sector pays for care for veterans through the Veterans Administration, for the elderly and disabled through Medicare, and for public employees through various public plans. The quasi-private sickness funds in the Netherlands and Germany finance health services for most of the population, with the state financing care for individuals who are no longer in the workforce (e.g., the unemployed, the disabled, retired people).

IV. Public sector has minimal role

At the very least, the public sector usually covers public health services— such as environmental health protection (e.g., clean water, clean air, safe food), immunizations, prenatal and perinatal care, school health, and the detection and control of infectious diseases and epidemics. Although none of the OECD countries has such a minimal role for the public sector, countries such as Singapore have chosen to follow this route and rely on Medisaver accounts by which most individuals can, in theory, save for their own care. This model is supported by some U.S. Republicans. It tends to be most attractive for people who are young, affluent, and in good health. This model abandons insurance principles in favour of a retirement model, in which individuals save what would be actuarially predicted to cover their needs; some provisions for catastrophic expenses are usually attached to such models.

Delivery

Frequently, the literature talks about "owning and operating" health services[38] as synonymous with delivery. The international literature indicates that countries usually adopt a combination of service delivery models. Public delivery approaches emphasize plans that provide universal coverage, uniform services, uniform quality, and uniform prices. They have such advantages as fewer overlapping facilities, reduced administration costs, and greater equity of access (including maintenance of services to populations, such as small towns, even if such services are not economically efficient). Their purported disadvantages are tendencies to be bureaucratic, unresponsive to individual choice, and slow to change and innovate.

As a result, recent years have witnessed increased debating about the privatization of the public delivery of health services. Much of the literature claims that the private sector is more efficient in producing services than is the public sector and attributes the difference to profit motives, competition, and incentives. However, many of these works can be criticized on the grounds that similar goals and services are not being compared in the two sectors. Judge compared private sector provision of residential care for the frail elderly to public provision in England and Wales. His tentative conclusion was that private provision is good value for money.[39] Knapp compared the relative efficiency of public, voluntary, and private producers in the provision of residential child care in the United Kingdom.[40] In Britain, child care is publicly financed but may be publicly or privately delivered (i.e., contracted out from the public sector). After controlling for technologies of care and characteristics of clients, he tentatively concluded that the private and voluntary sectors were more cost effective than the public sector. However, the study looked only at short-term outcomes and did not consider the long-term effects of care on children and their families. The cheaper costs in the private and voluntary sectors arose from a number of sources, including tax concessions (i.e., cost shifting to the public purse), low wages, long hours, and charitable giving. To the extent that wage rates reflect policy choices unrelated to service provision (e.g., to encourage pay equity or boost employment in smaller communities), cost comparisons to sectors not bound by those considerations can be misleading.

An important caveat arises from the work of Bendick, who reviewed the efficacy of the privatization of publicly delivered services within a framework of public financing.[41] Bendick concluded that privatization to for-profit organizations tended to be efficient for services for which goals are measurable, easily monitored, and easily evaluated (e.g., garbage collection). However, nonprofit deliverers had a better record in providing services in the interest of clients beyond what is precisely specified in contracts. Accordingly, where problems are complex, as in health and social welfare programs, and where the processes to be employed are not well understood, he recommended that programs be privatized to the nonprofit sector rather than to the for-profit sector, a strategy he refers to as the empowerment of mediating institutions.

Saltman indicates that the advantages of public providers are the assurance of equal access to all citizens (geographically and economically), the greater accountability to public officials, and the tendency to provide better preventive care and coordination of services across subsectors.[42] The disadvantages are as outlined earlier—public providers tend to be bureaucratic, inflexible, inefficient in the utilization of resources and time, lacking innovation, and unresponsive to individual need. Private providers, on the other hand, are seen as flexible, innovative, efficient and responsive to patients, but also as unwilling to treat difficult or undesirable patients, tending to practice in large urban areas, difficult to control in terms of costs, and inequitable because services are provided based on ability to pay rather than on need. The following delivery models can thus be described.

I. Public sector as sole entity responsible for delivery of a comprehensive mix of services

This model is the well-known national health service, in which the state owns and operates most service delivery institutions and providers are considered employees of the state. It existed at the national level in the former Soviet Union, and in the NHS of Britain before the 1989 reforms. The Scandinavian countries are also dominated by this model of health services delivery, except that in Sweden and Finland ownership is at the subnational level.

II. Public sector responsible for delivery of comprehensive array of services, with voluntary private sector delivery of specialized or elective services

In this model, the public and private sectors do not compete, but are supplementary.

In France, Australia, New Zealand and the United Kingdom, private hospitals exist alongside public hospitals. The two sectors, however, do not compete. Public hospitals are large and well equipped and provide a comprehensive array of medical services. Private hospitals are limited in number and in scope of activity; indeed, they may exist as private wards within public hospitals. Rather than providing comprehensive care, private hospitals provide elective surgery or specialized services such as obstetric or long-term care. Serious illnesses are left to the public sector, which also has most responsibility for training health human resources.

III. Public sector as one of many providers of health services alongside and competing with private sector

A. Public sector delivery as income related

In the United States, most people who have insurance or sufficient resources receive services delivered by the private sector; the public sector provides subsidized care to the very poor through community care clinics or state hospitals as a social safety net function.

B. Public sector delivery for special groups

In certain models of service delivery, the public sector's involvement in service delivery is limited to special groups. Examples of such care are the remaining provincial psychiatric hospitals in Canada (whose employees are civil servants) and Veterans Administration hospitals in the United States.

C. Competing public and private delivery

In this model of service delivery, public hospitals and private hospitals coexist and compete for contracts or individual business. One example is the competition between public homes for the aged (municipally owned) and private nursing homes to provide long-term care in Ontario. This competition model is also typical of the vast majority of health services delivery in the United States. It also now exists in the United Kingdom, New Zealand (which is following a reform quite similar to the United Kingdom's), and the Netherlands. In this model, public and private hospitals compete to win contracts from purchasing agents (e.g., regional authorities or GP fundholders in the United Kingdom; sickness funds and insurance companies in the Netherlands and the United States). The private hospitals can be either for-profit (as are many in the United States) or not-for-profit (as in England or the Netherlands) and can exist in varying proportions in comparison with public hospitals. For example, in the United States and the Netherlands, most hospitals are private, while in the United Kingdom most hospitals are still public.

IV. Predominantly private delivery, but heavily regulated by the public sector

As with the financing dimension, there exists a model of service delivery wherein delivery is the responsibility of de facto private institutions run by autonomous boards of directors. However, the degree of government regulation and control of these institutions is so high that they are actually quasi-public mediating structures. This model is characteristic of Canadian hospitals. The extent of government regulation is even stronger in Western Europe; in countries such as the Netherlands, state involvement in private hospital functioning is extensive. The trend toward regional models in most Canadian provinces is further decreasing the autonomy of providers, but they remain legally autonomous (e.g., their employees are not classified as government workers).

V. Public sector having only minimal role in health services delivery

A truly minimal role would eschew regulation; purchasers of services would be expected to follow the rules of *caveat emptor*, and providers would be curbed only by legal prohibitions against false advertising or demonstrable harm. Owing to fairly ubiquitous concerns about quality of care, there are no examples of a true laissez-faire market for medical services in advanced industrial societies, and this model is accordingly limited to nontraditional sectors of their health care systems. These sectors may include such providers of alternative medicine as acupuncturists, chiropodists or natural healers, or those delivering counselling services.

Allocation

Once decisions have been made about the financing and delivery of health services, health policy turns to the link between the two: allocation. Allocation is not so much a public-private issue as an issue of degree of government control and the sorts of incentives built into reimbursement policies. Saltman and von Otter describe allocation mechanisms as lying along a continuum ranging from fully planned systems to pure, neoclassical market systems.[43] We have adapted their models (table 3).

Table 3

Allocation models for publicly financed services

Clients follow money				Money follows clients
Centrally planned	Regionally planned	Managed competition	Public competition	Market

The two most traditional means of allocating finances within health care systems are located at the extremes of the allocation continuum. *Centrally planned allocation* is associated with a command-and-control model in which the patient follows the money: planners decide where particular services will be provided and supply a global budget; patients must go wherever the services happen to be. Examples include the health system of the former Soviet Union, the National Health Service in Britain before the 1989 reforms, and specialized hospital services in Canada. *Market allocation,* not to be confused with market-based financing, is a mechanism for allocating available resources (which may well be from public sources) to providers based on the ability of providers to attract clients (patients): the money follows the patients. Examples include physician services in Canada, as well as in the nonmanaged care portions of the U.S. system, where physician income depends on how many patients can be attracted. The clear advantage of the planned allocation models is cost control. The clear advantage of the market allocation mechanisms is increased sensitivity to patient choice and therefore presumably to client needs and wishes.

The models found in the middle of the continuum represent various attempts to create a compromise between planning and markets that would ideally obtain the benefits of each without the corresponding flaws. Most of these models are relatively new and untested.

The regional reforms being adopted in many Canadian provinces are examples of what Saltman terms adaptive planning; they represent a shift toward the planned end of the allocation continuum. In contrast, the reforms being implemented in the United Kingdom, New Zealand, and Sweden represent the intentional creation of a new market consciously designed to achieve state policy objectives through the limited and selective use of market instruments.

Some of the most active debates currently under way over allocation concerns these middle-ground models within publicly financed systems.[44] There are a variety of ways to structure a planned market for health services, but the primary ways are for providers to compete on the basis of price or quality. Price competition has the advantage of encouraging innovations and efficiencies, which would presumably lower prices; preferred by economists, it is usually based on negotiated contracts between purchasers and providers. This type of market, however, can lead to risk selection of patients, has higher administrative and transaction costs, and reduces patient choice of provider in that the patient must follow prior allocations of money. With planned markets based on quality, fees tend to be negotiated and to approximate real costs; there may be few incentives to achieve economic efficiency, but there are also fewer problems in ensuring universality of access, and lower administrative and transaction costs. However, quality is far more difficult to measure than are costs.

The two basic types of planned markets fall on either side of the public-private divide.[45] In public competition models, all providers are publicly funded and politically accountable. Providers have an incentive to attract and satisfy patients, because budgets are determined on the basis of the number of patients and through bonuses based on increased productivity and efficiency. The central agents of change in this model are patients, whose choices of physician and treatment site have budgetary consequences for providers. Through modifying incentives, the specifics of this public market can, in theory, be consciously configured by elected officials to ensure that allocation of health care resources reinforces rather than undermines broader social objectives.

In contrast, managed competition models (which Saltman also refers to as mixed market models) create a mixed public-private market in which existing and new privately capitalized providers can bid for contracts against present publicly capitalized facilities. The central agent for change in this model is the administrative agent managing the health plan, who is responsible for overseeing service contracts to providers. Managers are expected to balance questions of quality and cost in the search for less expensive forms of care. The extent of patient choice is reduced to the selection of an administrative agent, who then makes choices on the patient's behalf. If dissatisfied, the patient's main option is to switch to another plan. The NHS reforms are an example of managed competition.

Allocation issues are at the heart of the debate about separating the functions of purchasing and delivery (the purchaser-provider split). It is important to recognize that the concept of a split between purchaser and provider can apply only under one of these two conditions:

- The third-party payers have disappeared, leaving the patient as the sole purchaser of services. This condition implies relinquishing the insurance model and forgoing protection against catastrophic risks, and as such seems both undesirable and unlikely.
- The patient has relinquished his role in making decisions about where to receive services and delegated this decision making to a purchasing agent. However, choice has always been seen as important in Canada.

Similarly, the Netherlands has been unwilling to implement reforms that would deny patients their choice of provider; to date, all their insurance plans contract with all providers rather than seeking to achieve U.S.-style savings through designating preferred providers. It should also be noted that any fusion between financing and delivery, as is characteristic of many managed care models, can in theory give rise to the same sort of risk selection issues found in pluralistic financing models. Such models accordingly have major requirements for determining how to adjust the payment attached to each patient according to risk, and for ensuring that high-risk patients are not abandoned. Although such calculations may ultimately be possible, current techniques appear inadequate to the task and post hoc adjustments are usually needed.

Despite the importance of choice as a value in the Canadian health system, there have been recent tendencies to restrict it. For example, the Capital Health Authority in Edmonton cut funding for physiotherapy services by 30 percent and shifted to a preferred provider network. Only 17 of the 56 private clinics in the region received contracts. At the same time, a new system of assessing needs was implemented, which will disqualify people with "low needs" from publicly financed treatment. Presumably, those clients and clinics will form an alternative private market (S. Lowry, personal communication, 1995). Any move in this direction for medical treatment currently insured under the terms of the Canada Health Act, however, would represent a significant departure (and a highly unpopular one) for the Canadian system.

I. Command and control planning (patient follows money)

This model involves centrally determined health system budgets, which in theory should be based on health needs. It was typical of the former Soviet Union and of the British NHS before the 1989 reform. To some extent, a command-and-control system still exists for French hospital capacity, which is based on a nationally derived needs map. Similar approaches can also be undertaken at a regional or local level; for example, in Sweden, allocations were made by county councils. Canada has funded hospital services on this model; decisions were made about where services should be located and budgets given to operate them. Individuals seeking care would follow the money to gain access to services. The regional models being implemented in most Canadian provinces extend this planned approach to encompass a wider variety of services than hospital care within a single budgetary envelope.

II. Internal markets, managed competition, and public competition

Although Sweden is experimenting with public competition models,[46] the most commonly cited examples of internal markets are the current British NHS reform and the similar measures in New Zealand. The precise arrangements are still undergoing some change, but the purchaser of services (usually a district health authority or a GP fundholder) makes contracts with providers (including self-governing hospital trusts). The purchaser contracts for the types and volumes of services required and the fees to be paid. General practitioners are paid on a capitation basis, which rewards them for successfully competing for patients but creates disincentives to acceptance of high-needs individuals. Purchasers act on behalf of patients, but the only elements of patient choice are the ability to select a physician or to complain if not satisfied. Evaluation of these reforms is limited as yet.[47] Managed competition was also at the core of the abortive Clinton reform in the United States.

One goal of these models is to create incentive structures that will restructure delivery arrangements in local communities and increase efficiency. One risk can be seen in the United States, in which the private insurers are indeed competing in the marketplace, but with few guarantees that savings will not be made by cutting benefits and shedding high-needs beneficiaries rather than by improving efficiency and appropriateness of care, and few controls over who will capture the resulting savings. As noted in the above dialogue between Mr. Frost and Mr. Tanti, not only may costs not be controlled, but government may end up with responsibility for those shed, while private insurers reap windfall profits.

III. Market allocation (money follows patient)

To a large extent, market allocation is still the most common form of allocation in health systems worldwide. Most physicians are still paid on a fee-for-service basis in an open-ended budgetary system (e.g., Australia, Canada, France, and nonmanaged care settings in the United States). Money follows patients in a fairly uncontrolled way, although total budgets can be capped. However, allocation among providers still depends on relative drawing power, and the formulae may result in considerable conflict, because physicians churning higher volumes gain a comparative economic advantage over colleagues with different practice styles. As noted in the section "Case Studies." many Canadian reforms are directed at altering this allocation pattern.

Interrelationship among Financing, Delivery, and Allocation

Although there is little direct evidence, it appears likely that the three dimensions of financing, delivery, and allocation and the public and private sector distinctions cannot be randomly combined; certain models of allocation may go better with certain models of financing and delivery. For example, command-and-control allocation systems would appear to function best in health systems having a high level of involvement of the public sector in both financing and delivery, because of practical considerations (fewer players to be coordinated), ideological acceptance of a government role, and the strong political benefits in being accountable for where public money is spent. Conversely, systems having many sources of funding may balk at command-and-control types of allocation, both because enforcing control may be difficult and because social values may oppose state intrusion in private business. For this reason, health systems having high levels of private sector involvement tend to locate on the market side of the allocation continuum, although individual managed care plans might use planned mechanisms for their own internal allocations. Most systems occupy a middle ground, accepting extensive private sector involvement in delivery with an active role for government in financing and regulating (e.g., France, Germany, the Netherlands, and Canada).

LEGISLATIVE AND REGULATORY FRAMEWORK

Medicare—the term commonly used for universal hospital and medical care insurance—is among Canada's most popular programs. It has arisen as a partnership between the federal and provincial governments, a partnership now under strain from the impact of economic and constitutional factors. An excellent account of the growth of Canadian medicare can be found in Taylor.[48]

Historical Roots: The Constitution and the Growth of Shared-Cost Programs

Section 92 of the Constitution Act, 1867, assigns certain exclusive powers to the provincial legislatures; this list includes the provisions of section 92(7), "The Establishment, Maintenance, and Management of Hospitals, Asylums, Charities, and Eleemosynary Institutions in and for the Province, other than Marine Hospitals."[49] Court decisions have interpreted this clause as assigning jurisdiction to provincial governments for almost all of the health care system. The federal government is given limited jurisdiction over health matters that have a national dimension or that raise issues of public morality and safety. This division of power undoubtedly arose because, at the time of Confederation, health and health services were generally considered private matters between care providers and individuals and their families. Public involvement was minimal, often as a last resort, and managed by charitable, religious, and municipal organizations. There was no inkling that health care would become among the most costly of government activities.

In the early part of the twentieth century, health services continued to be seen largely as a private matter, with individuals purchasing services from private providers. Governments concentrated mainly on public health, including sanitation and disease control, although provincial governments occasionally adopted a public role in delivery. Saskatchewan was the first province to allow its municipalities to levy taxes to pay for municipally provided physician and hospital services, while Newfoundland (not yet part of Canada) introduced a Cottage Hospital and Medical Care Plan in 1934 to deliver services to individuals living in isolated fishing outports. Nonetheless, such early government health care initiatives as existed were primarily directed at financing the private provision of care. For example, in 1915, Ontario's Workmen's Compensation Plan provided injured workers with cash compensation for lost wages as well as necessary medical and rehabilitation services. As a rule, both the financing and the delivery of health services were primarily private responsibilities.

Historical events then began producing a shift toward a more expansive view of social values related to health. The massive social and economic dislocation of the Great Depression showed that events beyond the control of individuals could profoundly affect the individual's ability to obtain needed health services. The experiences of the Second World War, including the revelation that many men could not be recruited into the armed forces because of poor health, revealed the costs to both individuals and the country as a whole of inadequate access to health services.

The 1942 Marsh Report argued that the Canadian government had a moral responsibility to provide citizens with a basic level of social services and income support. These ideas, along with the central themes of Keynesian economics, suggested that governments could stabilize economic cycles and stimulate growth by expanding their social and economic roles. Government's expanded industrial and economic role during the war also suggested that the public sector could effectively and efficiently produce goods and services that the private sector had been unable to accomplish. It began to be argued that government involvement would provide greater public access to needed health services and would thus benefit individuals (who received the services), providers (who were guaranteed to be paid for them), and society as a whole (through a more healthy population). It was believed that total health spending would eventually level off as Canadians became healthier.

The expansion of the role of the Canadian government in the health field after the Second World War marked a fundamental shift in social and political values, which must be understood as the context for current debates about the public-private mix in the health system.

After the demise of federal proposals for a national health insurance system because of failure to reach agreement with the provinces over funding arrangements, a number of private, physician-sponsored plans emerged, which even at their peak in the mid-1960s (10.6 million people covered in 1965) protected less than half of Canada's population. In 1947, Saskatchewan became the first Canadian province to introduce universal hospital insurance; less comprehensive plans were introduced by British Columbia in 1949 and Alberta in 1950. These provincial developments culminated with the passage of the federal Hospital Insurance and Diagnostic Services Act.[50] Under this act, the federal government agreed to share the costs of hospital care and diagnostic services with any province that established an insurance program complying with the national conditions. All provinces had established such programs by the beginning of 1961.

In 1962, Saskatchewan once again took the initiative and introduced an insurance plan covering the physician portion of medically necessary services. The leaders of the medical profession resisted public financing, preferring that medical insurance be provided through a series of private plans, with the government subsidizing (in whole or in part) the premiums for people who could not afford to pay. The clash led to a month-long doctors' strike and an eventual compromise. The provincial government asserted its authority to be the sole insurer, but physicians retained their right to practice privately outside the plan and to extra-bill their patients for insured services beyond the fee levels paid by the provincial plan. However, no insurance coverage was allowed for such extra-billing, which clearly constrained the ability of physicians to exploit the policy. (Given an adequate physician supply and the absence of collusion, there would be little reason for patients to pay extra for services that could be obtained "free" from physicians participating in the public insurance plan.)

The introduction in 1966 of the federal Medical Care Act[51] was the catalyst for the establishment and funding of similar medical insurance plans in each of the provinces. As had been the case for hospital insurance, the act provided public financing but did little to change how health resources were allocated or delivered. Medicare institutionalized the prevailing fee-for-service payment system for physicians, retained professional fee schedules negotiated under the private plans, and did little to threaten the continuity of physician control over the content and conditions of medical work, including the work of other health professions. By 1971, all provinces had complying plans: universal hospital and medical insurance was available to all Canadians.

This mixed financing model has proven unstable on two fronts: cost sharing within the public sector, and extra-billing at the interface between public and private.

The cost-shared programs were seen as too open ended and inflexible; they were replaced in 1977 by Established Programs Financing.[52] Established Programs Financing disconnected federal contributions from actual provincial expenditures, funding the provinces through a per capita block grant composed of tax points plus a residual cash transfer. The cash transfer was based on the 1975–1976 base year expenditure and was to be increased on the basis of GNP growth, although subsequent federal budgets altered the formula. The cash portion gave the federal government the ability to enforce the national standards by threatening to withhold funds; the reduction in the cash portion as Ottawa attempted to improve its own financial situation by curbing transfer payments thus threatened to remove any federal ability to enforce national standards.[53]

In 1996, Established Programs Financing was combined with another source of federal funds, the Canada Assistance Plan, which had financed not only income support (welfare) but also many means-tested social programs with health components (e.g., care for the disabled), to form the Canada Health and Social Transfer. Although the total transfers have been severely reduced and the national standards for the former Canada Assistance Plan programs weakened, the current version of the Canada Health and

Social Transfer does guarantee a floor amount intended to preserve the ability to enforce national standards for medicare. (Whether this transfer arrangement will be maintained by future governments cannot be known.)

The second source of instability was the coexistence of extra-billing and universal insurance, which meant that a floor price existed and that no one could be priced out of the market. Economists soon recognized that this mixed system lacked powerful mechanisms to constrain costs. Others wondered whether additional direct charges to patients undermined the security and equity that were the basis of medicare. This tension led to the establishment of a second Royal Commission under Justice Emmet Hall; its report reaffirmed the principles of medicare and criticized direct charges to patients for insured services. After additional political disputes, the federal government passed the Canada Health Act (CHA),[54] which imposed financial penalties on provinces permitting such charges. In consequence, extra-billing and user fees as defined by the CHA largely disappeared.[55] Ontario physicians reacted in 1986 by staging a 25-day strike, arguing that being forced to accept a publicly insured fee schedule as full payment for their services in effect transformed them into public employees and eroded their economic and clinical freedom.[56] The argument was unsuccessful; it also showed little awareness of the distinction between public financing of clinical activities and public delivery of services. Indeed, as Tuohy has noted, Canadian physicians have managed to preserve far more clinical autonomy than U.S. physicians, who are reimbursed by private insurance plans within managed care settings.[57]

Current Legislative and Regulatory Framework

The current legal foundation of Canada's national health care system is thus primarily based on two statutes: the Canada Health and Social Transfer and the Canada Health Act (CHA). The Canada Health and Social Transfer is the vehicle through which funds are transferred from the federal government to provinces in support of hospital and medical insurance programs defined by the Canada Health Act, as well as for postsecondary education and the programs formerly funded under the Canada Assistance Plan.

The Canada Health Act

The CHA outlines the federal-provincial cost-sharing agreement on health care. Under its terms, the provincial governments receive full federal payments only if they comply with the requirements and criteria established in the CHA. The result is that this cost-sharing program gives the federal government influence within areas of primarily provincial jurisdiction. The process used to attain desired ends requires cooperation between federal and provincial jurisdiction and has been described as "cooperative federalism."[58]

The CHA includes five program criteria, which draw on the criteria established under the federal Hospital Insurance and Diagnostic Services Act and the Medical Care Act. To receive full federal funding, provincial plans must comply with five federal conditions:
- universality
- accessibility
- comprehensiveness
- portability
- public administration.

Section 10 of the CHA specifies, "In order to satisfy the criterion respecting universality, the health care insurance plan of a province must entitle one hundred per cent of the insured persons of the province to the insured health services provided for by the plan on uniform terms and conditions." The act's definition of "accessibility" includes the requirement that the health care insurance plan of a province "must provide for insured health services on uniform terms and conditions and on a basis that does not impede or preclude, either directly or indirectly whether by charges made to insured persons or otherwise, reasonable access to those services by insured persons." The law thus not does require *equal* access, and does not define what constitutes "reasonable."

At first glance, the CHA appears to take a broad definition of health. Section 3 declares "that the primary objective of Canadian health care policy is to protect, promote and restore the physical and mental well-being of residents of Canada and to facilitate reasonable access to health services without financial or other barriers." However, the operational definitions within the act are far more narrow.

Section 9 of the CHA states, "In order to satisfy the criterion respecting comprehensiveness, the health care insurance plan of a province must insure all insured health services provided by hospitals, medical practitioners or dentists, and where the law of the province so permits, similar or additional services rendered by other health care practitioners." This restriction to care provided in hospitals and by doctors is becoming increasingly obsolete. Technology has allowed much care to be provided in community or home settings and to be delivered by nonphysicians. These trends have led to creeping deinsurance, or what the Canadian Medical Association has termed "passive privatization." Relevant definitions in section 2 of the CHA include the following:

> "Insured health services" means hospital services, physician services and surgical-dental services provided to insured persons, but does not include any health services that a person is entitled to and eligible for under any other Act of Parliament or under any Act of the legislature of a province that relates to workers' or workmen's compensation;

"hospital" includes any facility or portion thereof that provides hospital care, including acute, rehabilitative or chronic care, but does not include

(a) a hospital or institution primarily for the mentally disordered, or

(b) a facility or portion thereof that provides nursing home intermediate care service or adult residential care service, or comparable services for children;

"hospital services" means any of the following services provided to in-patients or out-patients at a hospital, if the services are medically necessary for the purpose of maintaining health, preventing disease or diagnosing or treating an injury, illness or disability, namely

a) accommodation and meals at the standard or public ward level and preferred accommodation if medically required,

b) nursing service,

c) laboratory, radiological and other diagnostic procedures, together with the necessary interpretations,

d) drugs, biologicals and related preparations when administered in the hospital,

e) use of operating room, case room and anaesthetic facilities, including necessary equipment and supplies,

f) medical and surgical equipment and supplies,

g) use of radiotherapy facilities,

h) use of physiotherapy facilities, and

i) services provided by persons who receive remuneration therefor from the hospital, but does not include services that are excluded by the regulations;

"surgical-dental services" means any medically or dentally required surgical-dental procedures performed by a dentist in a hospital, where a hospital is required for the proper performance of the procedures.

Section 18 of the act defines extra-billing as "the billing for an insured health service rendered to an insured person by a medical practitioner or a dentist in an amount in addition to any amount paid or to be paid for that service by the health care insurance plan of a province," and user charges as "any charge for an insured health service that is authorized or permitted by a provincial health care insurance plan that is not payable, directly or indirectly, by a provincial health care insurance plan, but does not include any charge imposed by extra-billing."

Because health care is under provincial jurisdiction, the federal government has no direct power to direct how insurance plans are run. Nonetheless, many ambiguities remain about the reach of the federal spending power; it does appear that Ottawa can attach strings to its financial aid. Accordingly, the CHA specified that the federal government could withhold or deduct cash transfer payments from any province that did not comply with the five federal conditions, albeit after consultation with the offending province. Although judgements about compliance with some of the conditions are discretionary, there is an automatic requirement of dollar-for-dollar reductions in the federal cash contributions for extra-billing or user charges. However, the terms of the act establish obligations between governments only. There is no provision for individual redress.

Implications for private funding of medically necessary services – The CHA is a mechanism designed to partially defray the costs incurred by the provinces in providing a publicly administered, comprehensive, universal, portable, and accessible health care system without extra-billing or user charges. It dictates the conditions that must be met for the provinces to receive federal cash transfers under the Canada Health and Social Transfer. The CHA does not directly regulate health care providers. There is nothing in the CHA to prevent private insurers from supplementing provincial insurance plans by insuring services not covered by the provincial plans. Accordingly, the CHA does not preclude or prohibit the provision of private health services in Canada, because this issue is under provincial jurisdiction. Assuming the federal government chose to use the discretionary enforcement mechanism, such charges would, at most, disentitle the province that allows such practices from receiving its full cash transfer.

In a recent publication, the Canadian Bar Association described the current debate over the role of private health care services in Canada as rooted in two differing interpretations of the CHA.[59] Under what is referred to as the single-tier interpretation, the act is seen as supporting a national system of insured health services composed of a set of provincial and territorial health care systems, all of which satisfy the principles of the CHA. This system was created to ensure that all Canadians, regardless of financial means or province of residence, would have reasonable access to a wide range of high-quality health care services based on medical need rather than on ability to pay.

Alternatively, the two-tier interpretation holds that the publicly financed health care system is only a means of ensuring a basic level of health care services. Under this interpretation, the CHA was not intended to prevent a parallel system of privately funded health care, as long as this parallel system does not undermine the public system. Private facilities providing insured health care services would therefore be permissible, as long as there is still reasonable access to public facilities. The federal government has adopted the one-tier interpretation, but is losing its ability to enforce it as the cash portion of federal transfers diminishes. As noted in the section "Frameworks for Making Decisions," some provinces are leaning toward a two-tier interpretation. The resolution of this dispute will clearly have major effects on the future of medicare.

Canadian Charter of Rights and Freedoms

A second set of potential legal constraints on health policy arises from the Charter of Rights and Freedoms. Three sets of issues are involved. In general, there have been few court tests on these questions, so the following discussion remains largely speculative.

First, do providers have a protected right to sell their services?

A 1989 decision of the Supreme Court of Canada held that the Charter's section 7 provision for the right to life, liberty, and security of the person protects only the rights of human beings and not of corporate and other artificial entities.[60] The court also held that property-related rights or economic rights of a corporate or commercial nature are not entitled to constitutional protection. The courts have consistently held that purely economic rights are not covered by section 7.[61] The courts have considered and rejected the application of section 7 to such matters as the right to market wine kits in grocery stores,[62] the right to do business with the government,[63] the right of the aluminum industry to compete in the soft-drink can business,[64] the right to hold a liquor licence,[65] the right to be free from compensation orders made by human rights commissions,[66] and the right to be free from administration fees charged by government.[67] By extension, there would not appear to be any constitutional protection for organizations wishing to provide private health care services. Recently, the Ontario government's omnibus legislation has given considerable power to the province to regulate which services are covered, including the power to bring formerly private clinics in under the Independent Health Facilities Act (where they would be subject to government regulation).[68] The answer to the first question would thus appear to be "no, providers do not have a protected right to sell their services." Although courts have shown more sympathy to claims by professionals that the right to "pursue a calling or profession for which we are qualified, and to move freely throughout the realm for that purpose" is a fundamental liberty,[69] they have been divided on that issue.[70] They do appear to agree that the purely commercial aspects of a profession are not covered. For example, a Manitoba doctor who challenged reductions in hospital insurance payments for "overservicing" was told by the Manitoba courts that such payments were not protected by section 7.[71]

Second, do individuals have a constitutional right to purchase health services on the private market, regardless of the provisions of the CHA? If they do, is it a general right, or is it restricted to situations in which government cannot provide adequate, timely care?

It is difficult to imagine how individuals could successfully argue that section 7 protected a right to purchase private health care, particularly if medically necessary services were being adequately provided by a provincial health care insurance plan. Section 1 of the Charter states that Charter rights are guaranteed "subject only to such reasonable limits prescribed by law as can be demonstrably justified in a free and democratic society." To justify any possible restrictions on the section 7 right of an individual to purchase private health care services, the government could plausibly argue that continuing a single-payer system is required to protect the integrity of the existing Canadian health care system.

Third, do individuals have a constitutional right to receive publicly financed treatment, or, more narrowly, do nondiscrimination provisions mean that such services, if provided, must be allocated in ways that satisfy the courts?

It appears unlikely that individuals could use legal remedies to force governments to provide and fund particular services. However, certain mechanisms for allocating services that are publicly financed may not stand legal scrutiny if they are seen to violate prohibitions against discrimination. For example, if assistive devices are provided without charge to some but not all residents of Ontario, is it a violation of equality rights? A recent Ontario Court of Appeal ruling invalidated an age limit for provincial funding of assistive devices (in this case, visual aids were subsidized only for those 18 and under) on the grounds that this constituted age discrimination.[72] Should future court decisions accept this line of argument, it may force governments to make "all or none" decisions, unless clear and legally defensible criteria for specifying who can benefit from particular programs are implemented.

Should health care services not be adequately provided for, there may indeed be a legal case; an individual or group could argue that section 7 covers not only the right to medically necessary services, but extends to a right to be able to obtain such services privately when the government cannot or is not willing to provide adequate services. In such a situation a court would likely agree that persons should not be denied access to medically necessary health care services. It is unlikely that the government could justify a violation of these rights under section 1 of the Charter. A court would be unlikely to support a government denying an individual access to medically necessary services that are not being effectively provided by the government because of a lack of funding, a lack of cooperation between the federal and provincial governments, or deliberate intentions.[73] In *R. v. Oakes*, the Supreme Court of Canada held that, to successfully invoke section 1, the government must demonstrate that its objectives are sufficiently important to warrant overriding a constitutionally protected right, and that its chosen means are reasonable and demonstrably justified.[74] The governmental measures must be rationally connected to their purpose, must impair the rights or freedoms as little as possible and must be proportionate, insofar as their effects on the protected right are concerned, to the governmental objectives pursued. To successfully justify limiting access to health care, a government would arguably have to demonstrate not only that it was under financial pressure, but also that, in allocating its reduced resources, it had reallocated funds to sectors of greater importance than health care and had done so in an equitable manner.[75]

Because there is no definition of medically necessary services in the CHA, there is nothing to prevent considerable variation in which services are funded from province to province (and, by extension, which services are provided from region to region should service delivery be so devolved). While there are national standards in the CHA as well as the Charter, relevant terms that would ensure homogeneity and define the minimum standard implied by "reasonable access" have not been defined. In practice, there is a fair degree of consistency among provinces in terms of the range of services covered under physician and hospital services.

From a legal perspective, any provincial government may choose to allow private health care. The CHA does not regulate health care providers directly, but simply dictates the terms on which cash transfers to the provinces will occur. On a practical level, the provision of federal funds has been an effective means of prohibiting private health care for publicly insured services. Provinces with health care systems that violate principles of the Canada Health Act therefore are not only subject to potential federal financial penalties under the act, but may also be subject to Charter challenge by individuals denied care. Because the Charter supersedes the CHA, it is possible that court decisions might invalidate the public administration condition if it is seen as overly limiting private sector alternatives should the public sector prove itself unable to provide adequate care. Although this argument is an exceedingly speculative one, as no such litigation appears imminent, one could divide the hypothetical situations under which the publicly funded system denies care to an individual as follows:

There are unlikely to be legal ramifications if

- the government provides global funding to an organization (e.g., a hospital), which in turn limits what care they provide (there is probably no legal recourse against such hospital rationing decisions if they are made in good faith)
- the government directly specifies which services will be covered (e.g., in a fee schedule), but no one receives the service from the publicly funded service (the service is uninsured and falls outside the scope of the CHA)
- although some get the service (e.g., on the basis of "appropriateness"), such care is clearly inappropriate for the individual refused care.

Legal challenges therefore would appear to be possible only when the individual is deemed less appropriate than others, but might still benefit. One issue is whether the individual can purchase the specific care outside the publicly funded health care system. Clearly, the only barriers to purchasing care outside Canada are financial ones. However, the public administration condition and provincial legislation may indeed prohibit the purchase of such care within the country. Hypothetically, courts might then choose to distinguish the reasons why the individual had been assigned a low priority for care. If the reason was that the person is at high risk, it is not impossible that courts would rule that Charter issues of life and security of the person apply and that the individual should not be prohibited from seeking care. In contrast, preferences for more rapid treatment for low-risk individuals seem less likely to evoke such arguments. In any event, as noted, such a case could arise only from the potential care recipient, since there appears to be no legal basis for a provider to argue for a Charter-protected right to sell those services. Certainly, the Ontario government's omnibus legislation seems to adopt the premise that government can control the availability, location, and price of insured services offered within the province.[76]

Provincial and International Legislation and Regulations

Provinces are also bound by their own legislation and regulations. For example, all but four Canadian provinces explicitly prohibit private insurance for services that are insured by the provincial health plans. This provision would need to be changed if a different financing mechanism were deemed wise. Most provinces have laws or regulations that specify what services are financed and which copayments and deductibles are allowed for home care, long-term care, drug benefits, assistive devices, ambulance services, physiotherapy, and so on. Some of these services (e.g., physiotherapy, chiropractic, etc.) may constitute "partially insured services," giving rise to questions about the extent to which private insurance will be permitted.

Ontario's Bill 26 amended the provincial Health Insurance Act to introduce authority for "nil" payments;[77] this mechanism classifies a service as insured (thereby prohibiting it from being privately insured) but also precludes physicians from charging insured patients for the service. The examples given by the government to justify when such a provision might be employed appear relatively benign (e.g., "where a regulation provides that the payment for the simultaneous excision of a number of lesions is $X for the removal of 'up to 5 lesions' and nil thereafter, the removal of the 6th lesion remains insured but the insured patient cannot be charged for the service."[78] Nonetheless, this mechanism has the potential to make certain services unavailable (abortion?), and it is speculative whether a court would find such measures justifiable.

Provincial programs set up under their own legislation can subsequently be changed by any provincial government willing to take the political consequences. Other interesting dilemmas are likely to arise as regional reforms progress; for example, will the concept of portability be seen to extend across regions within a province? In the absence of federal terms and conditions, there will be relatively few constraints on provincial governments in determining how best to provide health care services for their populations. (It must be noted that British Columbia has moved to legislate the five CHA principles at the provincial level.)

Although beyond the scope of this paper, there are also questions about what implications, if any, the North American Free Trade Agreement (NAFTA) might have on the funding of health services. The thrust of such international trade agreements as NAFTA and the General Agreement on Trade in Services is to prohibit discrimination against "foreign" signatories to the treaty. U.S. and Mexican providers should therefore have the right to "enter an area and compete, without discrimination" with Canadian providers.[79] Annex II to NAFTA spells out that "Canada reserves the right to adopt or maintain any measure with respect to the provision of public law enforcement and correction services, and the following services to the extent that they are social services established or maintained for a public purpose: income security or insurance, social security or insurance, social welfare, public education, public training, health and child care." There has been some controversy about whether annex II will be given a broad or narrow interpretation; in particular, it is not clear what degree of government funding or regulation would be sufficient to establish that the service is being provided for a public purpose rather than on a commercial basis. Accordingly, there has been controversy about whether the particular services included under this provision should be spelled out.

Under some interpretations of NAFTA's antimonopoly rules, once a service is provided in both the public and private sectors, it can never be recaptured exclusively by the public sector. However, an agreement between Canada, the United States, and Mexico in March 1996 has clarified that parties need not list specific measures under annex II and may introduce new NAFTA-inconsistent measures in the health sector. Even if NAFTA did restrict the ability to limit those who deliver care, this would not affect financing or allocation. As noted, international evidence suggests that properly regulated private delivery can indeed be compatible with a high-quality, publicly financed system. If regulatory and monitoring authority is in place to guarantee that the services delivered are of high quality and delivered only when appropriate and at an affordable total cost, the question of whether such care is delivered by nonprofit or for-profit organizations, or by Canadian or foreign concerns, would appear to be an economic policy issue rather than a health issue.

NAFTA concerns thus offer one more reason for governments to act quickly to ensure that the door is not opened for an unwanted influx of private clinics operating outside medicare. Such an influx might erode cost control and quality—prohibitions which would appear justifiable on their own merits whether such companies are American or homegrown.

THE CASE OF CANADA: SELECTED DATA ON THE EXTENT OF THE PUBLIC-PRIVATE MIX

Medicare has become one of the defining features of Canada. It is often cited as the major difference between us and our neighbour to the south. Rachlis and Kushner cite evidence from Gallup polls indicating that 96 percent of Canadians prefer our system to the one in the United States and that public confidence in the quality of care in our system is up from 71 percent in 1991 to 89 percent in 1993.[80] The March/June 1995 *Canada Health Monitor* reports that support for each of the five principles of the CHA has once again risen, after a decline between 1992 and 1994 of between 8 percent and 15 percent. Currently, support for the five principles stands at 89 percent for universality, 82 percent for accessibility, 81 percent for portability, 80 percent for comprehensiveness, and 64 percent for public administration. Most Canadians (71 percent) believe in a role for the federal government in maintaining national principles, and a slim majority (56 percent) support the federal withholding of funds for uncooperative provinces. Although most Canadians are not in favour of user fees, especially physician extra-billing, support for user fees does come from high-income earners and the young.[81]

Financing

The Canadian health care system has both public and private elements. As Evans points out, Canada does not have socialized medicine, but does have "socialized insurance."[82]

As noted, the CHA requires that provinces pay for all medically necessary inpatient acute hospital care, institutional chronic care (but not the accommodations component), and the physicians' services component of ambulatory or outpatient care.[83] Although provinces are not required to cover other services, they can and do cover a number of services in other sectors (e.g., ambulance services, home care), with considerable inter-provincial variation, including in the existence and extent of user fees. Private funding is largely restricted to the noninsured sectors (e.g., dentistry, pre-scription drugs outside hospitals, long-term care, and preferred accom-modation) as well as most additional costs incurred if treatment is sought outside the province (these costs can be particularly onerous for people obtaining treatment south of the border). Some provinces finance some of these supplementary services (e.g., drugs) for particular population groups (e.g., social assistance recipients or the elderly). For example, Saskatchewan funds 75 percent of special care home services and has a layered safety net for prescription drugs, with full public funding for palliative care drugs and sliding scales of copayments for other products and people.

Obtaining and interpreting data about health financing in Canada can be complex. Several series can be examined: total health spending, total public spending for health, total provincial spending for health, total private spending for health, and health spending by particular sectors (e.g., workers' compensation, private health insurance).

Total Health Spending

The following data on total health spending were collected by various government agencies and collated by Health Canada.[84] Useful summaries were prepared from these and other data by the Canadian Medical Association.[85]

The charts in figure 2 illustrate where the money comes from—that is, the percentage distribution of national health expenditures by source. It is notable that the proportion coming from private sources has increased from 23.8 percent in 1984 to 28.2 percent in 1994. Supporting details about percentages and the dollar totals by sector between 1975 and 1994 are listed in table 4.

Figure 2

Distribution (%) of national health expenditures by sector of finance, Canada, 1984 and 1994

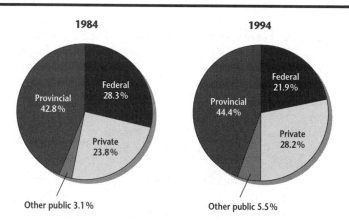

The charts in figure 3 illustrate where the money is spent—that is, the distribution among major categories. Hospitals continue to be the largest cost centre but constitute a smaller portion of a larger pie, having dropped from 42 percent of total health spending in 1984 to 37.3 percent a decade later. Supporting details are listed in table 5.

Table 4

Total health expenditures by sector of finance, Canada, 1975–1994

Year	Federal, direct (%)	Provincial expenditures, federal transfers (%)	Provincial expenditures, provincial funds (%)	Municipal expenditures (%)	Workers' comp. (%)	Private expenses (%)	Total (million $)
1975	3.2	27.7	43.4	1.1	1.0	23.6	12,254.8
1976	3.1	28.3	43.6	1.1	1.0	22.9	14,099.0
1977	3.1	30.1	41.6	1.1	1.0	23.2	15,497.6
1978	2.8	31.2	40.2	1.0	1.0	23.7	17,168.8
1979	2.7	31.6	39.4	1.5	1.0	23.9	19,288.5
1980	2.6	30.7	39.9	1.6	0.9	24.3	22,398.4
1981	2.6	29.0	41.5	1.8	1.1	23.9	26,441.5
1982	2.8	27.9	43.2	1.5	1.0	23.6	30,910.1
1983	2.9	28.0	43.6	1.3	0.9	23.3	34,165.1
1984	3.0	28.3	42.8	1.1	0.9	23.8	36,810.4
1985	2.9	28.1	42.2	1.5	1.0	24.3	40,038.2
1986	2.9	27.6	42.4	1.6	0.8	24.7	43,554.4
1987	2.9	27.1	42.7	1.6	0.8	24.9	47,023.6
1988	3.0	26.4	43.0	1.4	0.8	25.3	51,050.9
1989	3.1	25.6	43.7	1.4	0.8	25.4	56,234.7
1990	3.3	24.2	44.8	1.4	0.8	25.4	61,041.6
1991	3.4	22.8	46.3	1.3	0.9	25.4	66,290.3
1992	3.4	22.1	46.5	1.3	0.8	25.9	70,032.1
1993	3.5	21.9	45.7	1.2	0.8	26.9	71,775.3
1994	3.6	21.9	44.4	1.2	0.8	28.2	72,462.6

Source: Health Canada, *National Health Expenditures in Canada 1975–1994, Full Report* (Ottawa: Health Canada, Policy and Consultation Branch, January 1996), tables 2A and 2C.

Figure 3

Distribution (%) of national health expenditures by category, Canada, 1984 and 1994

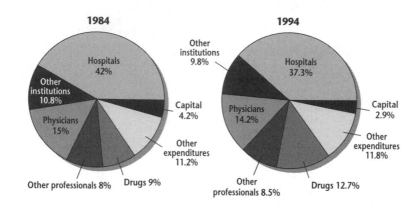

Total Public Spending for Health

Since 1972, public expenditures on health care have averaged about 75 percent of total expenditures, which is lower than the OECD average. However, there is a trend toward increasing private sector financing. In 1975, public expenditures represented 76.4 percent of total expenditures. In 1994, they made up 71.8 percent of total expenditures. Provincial health expenditures in 1994 declined by 1.98 percent from the previous year, while private expenditures grew by 5.8 percent,[86] implying that cost shifting is occurring.

Public spending comes largely from general revenues. Although provinces and territories have occasionally financed a portion of their expenditures through health premiums, these so-called premiums really constituted disguised and politically sellable taxes whose yield simply went into general revenues—coverage was not contingent on premium payment, the premiums were never risk rated and the amount spent by the provinces was not linked to how much revenue was raised from premium sources. One example was Ontario's Employer's Health Tax, subsequently repealed by the current Conservative government. Even in those few provinces using them, premiums never accounted for more than about one-third of provincial health care spending.[87] Other sources of revenue used to finance health care have included income taxes, corporate taxes, payroll taxes, sales taxes, property taxes, special excise taxes, lotteries, licences, permits, fees, and certificates. Some of these sources are aimed at health expenditures, most are not.[88]

Details about federal transfers are listed in table 6. In 1993, Established Programs Financing accounted for 96.2 percent of total federal health care funding, and Canada Assistance Plan for 3.6 percent (the remaining

Table 5

Total health expenditures by category of expenditure, Canada, 1975–1994

Year	Hospitals (%)	Other institutions (%)	MDs (%)	Other professionals (%)	Drugs (%)	Capital (%)	Other expenditures (%)	Total (million $)
1975	45.0	9.2	15.0	7.4	8.8	4.4	10.3	12,254.8
1976	45.4	9.7	14.7	7.5	8.5	3.9	10.4	14,099.0
1977	44.1	10.2	14.7	8.0	8.4	3.6	10.9	15,497.6
1978	43.3	10.8	14.9	8.3	8.4	3.9	10.3	17,168.8
1979	42.4	11.2	14.8	8.5	8.6	4.1	10.4	19,288.5
1980	41.9	11.3	14.7	8.5	8.4	4.7	10.5	22,398.4
1981	42.1	10.9	14.5	8.3	8.8	4.6	10.9	26,441.5
1982	42.8	10.8	14.3	8.1	8.5	4.7	10.7	30,910.1
1983	42.6	10.8	14.8	8.0	8.6	4.4	10.7	34,165.1
1984	42.0	10.6	15.0	8.0	9.0	4.2	11.2	36,810.4
1985	40.9	10.2	15.1	8.3	9.5	4.6	11.5	40,038.2
1986	40.7	9.3	15.3	8.3	10.1	4.7	11.5	43,554.4
1987	40.6	9.2	15.6	8.4	10.4	4.4	11.4	47,023.6
1988	40.1	9.2	15.6	8.4	10.8	4.0	11.9	51,050.9
1989	39.8	9.1	15.1	8.5	11.1	3.9	12.6	55,234.7
1990	39.1	9.4	15.2	8.5	11.3	3.7	12.9	61,041.6
1991	38.8	9.5	15.4	8.5	11.6	3.2	13.0	66,290.3
1992	38.2	9.8	14.9	8.4	12.1	3.3	13.3	70,032.1
1993	37.3	9.8	14.4	8.4	12.3	3.2	14.0	71,775.3
1994	37.3	9.8	14.2	8.5	12.7	2.9	14.6	72,462.6

Source: Health Canada, *National Health Expenditures in Canada 1975–1994, Full Report* (Ottawa: Health Canada, Policy and Consultation Branch, January 1996), tables 4A and 4C.

0.2 percent consisted of health payments to the territories by Indian and Northern Affairs Canada).

During the 1980s, the federal government unilaterally amended the Established Programs Financing arrangements a number of times to limit the funding to provinces; the effect of this measure was to increase the proportion of total public health spending covered by the provinces from their own sources of revenue. In addition, Canada Assistance Plan payments to the non-equalization-receiving provinces (Alberta, British Columbia, and Ontario) were capped to no more than an annual increase of 5 percent. From 1979 to 1994, federal transfers as a portion of total health expenditures fell from 31.6 percent to 21.9 percent. This decrease was largely offset by increases in provincial funding and private funding.[89]

The CHA requires provincial plans to cover only medically necessary services, but it does not define "medically necessary." Each provincial and territorial government establishes which services are medically necessary by including or excluding them from their list of insured health services. Historically, the term has meant services provided in hospitals or by physicians. As a result, there is no requirement that provincial plans cover the services of other health providers outside hospital care, nor does the federal government contribution take such care into account. Because continuing developments in technology and drugs are shifting much care outside hospitals, an increasing number of services are not covered by the public plans.

Total Provincial Spending for Health

Provincial health spending comes from general revenues; therefore, any attempt to break down the sources of funding is arbitrary. Details about the proportional breakdown of provincial spending are given in table 7. Again, hospitals are clearly the largest cost centre, but they have been shrinking as a proportion of total provincial health spending, dropping from 56.3 percent of spending in 1975 to 48.4 percent in 1994. This reduction is largely due to a combination of cost containment measures and cost shifting as care moved to the community (e.g., more day surgery, reduced length of stay). Expenditures on physicians stayed roughly the same, ranging from 20.4 percent in 1975 to 20.9 percent in 1994, having peaked in 1987 and in 1988, and again in 1991 at 21.8 percent. The single largest growth area in provincial spending was in expenditures on drugs, which is one of the most market-oriented sectors.[90]

Hospitals receive most of their operating funding from provincial governments, usually as a prospective global budget (although some experimentation with case mix–based funding is under way in some provinces). However, as the fiscal capacity of provincial governments shrinks, hospitals have been looking for alternative methods of financing their programs. Citing Pink and Hudson,[91] Adams and colleagues[92] categorize alternative

Table 6

Federal health transfers by type of transfer, Canada, 1975–1994

Year	Established Program Financing			Canada Assistance Plan				Total (million $)
	Insured health services tax (%)	Insured health services cash (%)	Extended health care (%)	Extended health care (%)	Other health care (%)	Health resource funds (%)	Payments to territories (%)	
1975	0.0	92.4	0.0	5.7	1.1	0.7	0.1	3,389.6
1976	0.0	91.5	0.0	6.6	1.2	0.6	0.1	3,983.8
1977	33.8	54.1	7.5	2.9	1.1	0.5	0.1	4,660.4
1978	43.0	44.0	9.4	1.7	1.0	0.7	0.1	5,364.0
1979	43.2	44.3	9.3	1.8	1.0	0.3	0.1	6,102.5
1980	44.6	43.3	9.2	1.5	1.0	0.2	0.1	6,865.8
1981	45.6	43.0	9.3	1.0	0.9	0.1	0.1	7,674.8
1982	45.5	43.0	9.3	1.0	0.9	0.0	0.1	8,627.7
1983	42.9	45.6	9.4	1.0	1.1	–	0.1	9,575.3
1984	42.2	46.1	9.3	1.0	1.1	–	0.2	10,429.0
1985	42.8	45.4	9.3	0.9	1.4	–	0.2	11,249.9
1986	44.1	44.2	9.3	0.9	1.3	–	0.2	12,004.6
1987	46.5	41.7	9.3	0.8	1.4	–	0.2	12,729.4
1988	48.3	39.7	9.3	0.9	1.6	–	0.2	13,495.9
1989	49.8	38.1	9.3	1.0	1.7	–	0.2	14,370.4
1990	50.8	37.0	9.3	0.7	2.0	–	0.2	14,774.4
1991	49.9	37.5	9.4	0.6	2.4	–	0.2	15,116.1
1992	48.4	38.4	9.4	0.8	2.7	–	0.2	15,450.9
1993	48.6	38.2	9.4	0.9	2.8	–	0.3	15,684.4
1994	50.0	36.8	9.4	0.9	2.7	–	0.2	15,862.4

Source: Health Canada, *National Health Expenditures in Canada 1975–1994, Full Report* (Ottawa: Health Canada, Policy and Consultation Branch, January 1996), tables 12A and 12C.

Table 7

Provincial government health expenditures by category, Canada, 1975–1994

Year	Hospitals (%)	Other institutions (%)	MDs (%)	Other professions (%)	Drugs (%)	Capital (%)	Other expenditures (%)	Total (million $)
1975	56.3	9.1	20.4	1.4	1.6	3.8	7.4	8,710.4
1976	56.6	9.8	19.7	1.4	1.9	3.0	7.6	10,131.2
1977	55.1	10.6	19.9	1.5	2.2	2.8	8.1	11,103.3
1978	53.7	11.1	20.2	1.6	2.5	3.1	7.7	12,271.1
1979	52.7	11.5	20.1	1.9	2.6	3.3	7.9	13,697.0
1980	52.4	11.5	20.1	2.0	2.7	3.2	8.1	15,795.6
1981	52.3	11.5	19.8	2.3	2.8	3.1	8.3	18,657.7
1982	52.7	11.3	19.5	2.0	2.9	3.7	8.0	21,968.0
1983	52.1	11.2	20.0	1.9	3.1	3.9	7.8	24,456.4
1984	51.4	11.0	20.5	1.9	3.4	3.8	8.0	26,182.9
1985	50.6	10.7	20.8	1.9	3.7	3.8	8.5	28,146.9
1986	50.7	9.6	21.3	1.9	4.0	3.8	8.6	30,488.4
1987	50.7	9.4	21.8	1.8	4.2	3.4	8.6	32,823.7
1988	50.6	9.6	21.8	1.8	4.5	2.9	8.8	35,455.0
1989	50.4	9.6	21.3	1.8	4.7	3.0	9.2	38,955.0
1990	49.8	9.6	21.4	1.8	5.0	2.8	9.5	42,097.1
1991	49.3	9.7	21.8	1.8	5.3	2.6	9.6	45,819.6
1992	48.8	10.1	21.2	1.7	5.6	2.6	10.1	48,008.4
1993	48.6	10.1	20.8	1.5	5.6	2.7	10.7	48,511.8
1994	48.4	10.1	20.9	1.4	5.7	2.3	11.3	48,039.2

Source: Health Canada, *National Health Expenditures in Canada 1975–1994, Full Report* (Ottawa: Health Canada, Policy and Consultation Branch, January 1996), tables 7A and 7C.

revenue-generating activities as clinical and diagnostic insured services sold to the uninsured, clinical and diagnostic noninsured services, hotel services (televisions, phones), retail outlets (gift shops, cafeterias), administration (contract management), and finance (sale and leaseback). The revenue raised by these activities remains small.

Capital costs are not cost shared under the CHA, and provinces vary in how they fund capital expenditures. The capital proportion of total spending has been decreasing. Most provinces attempt to regulate capital, not least because capital purchases have long-term implications for operating budgets. Costs are often shared with municipal governments, privately raised funds, or both.[93]

Most physicians work as independent practitioners on a fee-for-service basis with a high degree of autonomy. Patients have been free to choose their own physicians, although some provincial fee schedules have provided disincentives for direct referral to specialists without going through a general practitioner as gatekeeper.

Fee schedules for physicians on fee for service are negotiated between provincial governments and medical associations. The focus of negotiations is the overall percentage increase to the existing schedule. Medical associations generally determine the fee allocation among types of physicians. The fee schedule in each province is binding on all physicians, and technically physicians cannot bill their patients above these rates. Since the introduction of the CHA in 1984, the federal government has deducted an equivalent amount from the cash portion of the federal transfer as a penalty for provinces that charge or allow providers to charge patients for services covered under the public plan. Physicians are free to bill patients directly for noninsured services.

Information on health spending per capita by province in 1994 is graphically illustrated in figure 4. Differences are becoming substantial—whereas the Canadian average was $2,478, Nova Scotia spent $2,231, and British Columbia $2,631. (We have omitted expenditures in the territories, which are not precisely comparable.) However, the information in figure 5 reveals that health expenditures as a proportion of provincial or territorial gross domestic product (GDP) are a greater burden to the poorer provinces. Although the Canadian average was 9.7 percent, the lowest spending province (Nova Scotia) devoted 11.3 percent of GDP, and the highest spender (British Columbia) 9.7 percent. Indeed, the least burden on the provincial economy (7.9 percent) occurred in Alberta, and the highest (13.5 percent) in Newfoundland.

These findings suggest that the current federal policy of reducing federal transfers and increasing provincial power is indeed likely to have considerable long-term impact. A weaker federal role is likely to further increase the gap among provinces in what they can afford, and may even call into question the ability of the poorer provinces to sustain existing programs.

Figure 4

Per capita total health expenditure by province, 1994

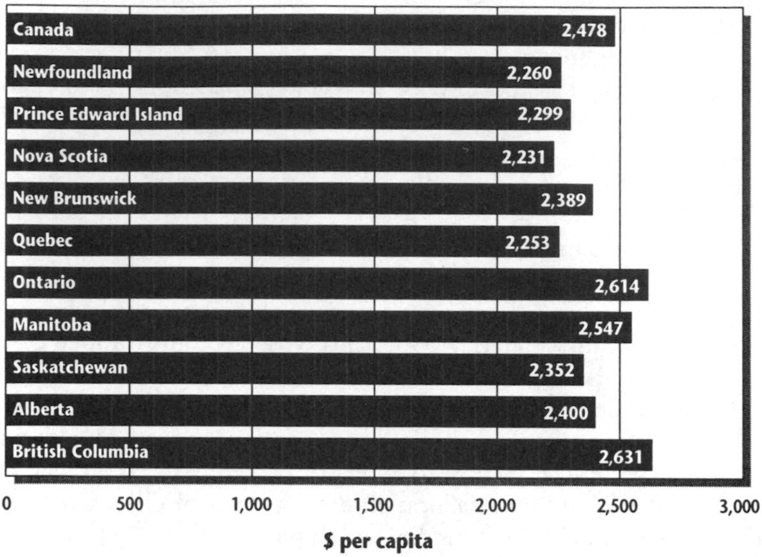

Province	$ per capita
Canada	2,478
Newfoundland	2,260
Prince Edward Island	2,299
Nova Scotia	2,231
New Brunswick	2,389
Quebec	2,253
Ontario	2,614
Manitoba	2,547
Saskatchewan	2,352
Alberta	2,400
British Columbia	2,631

$ per capita

Source: Health Canada, *National Health Expenditures in Canada 1975–1994, Full Report* (Ottawa: Health Canada, Policy and Consultation Branch, January 1996), table 15B.

Total Private Spending for Health

Health Canada's statistics on private health expenditures include various uninsured and privately insured health services. Their estimate of private expenditures reflects the residual that remains after calculating the difference between total health spending estimates and the sum of provincial and other public sectors. Although better data are being gathered, most provinces do not yet have good data about private spending (either the amount or where it was being spent).

In private sector health spending, expenditures in almost all categories, including physicians, went down between 1975 and 1994. The exceptions are expenditures on hospitals, which increased from 10.9 percent to 13.7 percent, and the "other expenditures" category, which includes out-of-country premiums, which increased from 13.1 percent to 15.9 percent.[94]

We contacted every province and territory to seek data on private financing; none was able to provide such information. Not surprisingly, the smaller provinces had a better sense of the magnitude (which was small). None of the provinces appeared to believe that documenting the private role was of high priority. Neither were governments monitoring what happened once services were deinsured. (What, for example, happened to

Figure 5

Health expenditures as a percentage of provincial GNP, 1994

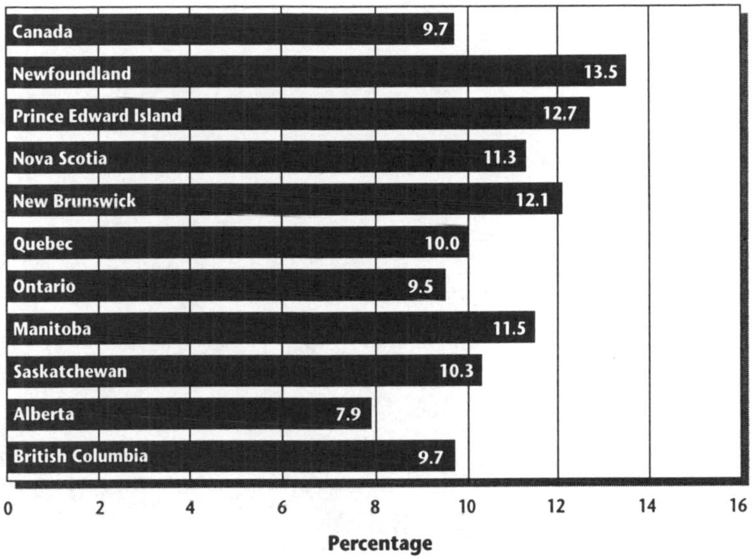

Source: Health Canada, *National Health Expenditures in Canada 1975–1994, Full Report* (Ottawa: Health Canada, Policy and Consultation Branch, January 1996), table 27.

the rates and costs of eye examinations in provinces where these were deinsured?)

Particularly in view of the belief that private spending was a way of relieving the pressure on the public purse, it is of some interest to examine the data. We used OECD data for Canada from 1971 to 1993 to correlate the percentage of GDP devoted to total health expenditures against the percentage of health spending coming from public sources; the correlation was −0.664, with a slope to the regression line of −0.49, revealing that lower shares of health spending coming from public sources are associated with higher shares of GDP being devoted to the health sector (figure 6). Although correlation is not causation, this evidence again suggests that private funding is less economically efficient. At minimum, it does suggest that increasing private spending is unlikely to achieve cost control.

Health Spending by Particular Sectors

Workers' compensation – Trends in workers' compensation–paid health expenditures by category from 1975 to 1994 indicate that although hospital expenditures increased from 74.9 million to 206.9 million, the hospital

Figure 6

Health spending as a percentage of GDP vs. private spending

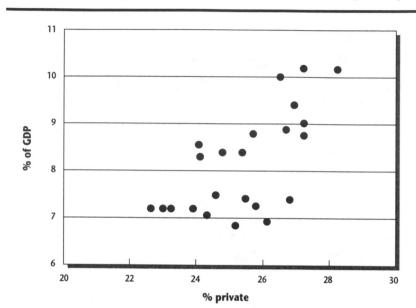

proportion of total spending decreased from 61.9 percent to 35.8 percent (table 8). Physician services went mildly down from 23.8 percent to 21.0 percent of spending. The big increase came in other professionals (from 7.2 percent to 17.7 percent), on drugs (from 1.6 percent to 6.9 percent), and other expenditures (from 5.4 percent to 18.5 percent).[95]

Private health insurance – As an indication of the growth of the private insurance industry, the Canadian Life and Health Insurance Association (the association of private for-profit life and health insurance companies) claims that total health insurance premiums in Canada of all insurance companies during 1993 was $6 billion, 86 percent of which was from group insurance contracts with employers, unions, or other sponsoring organizations. Group premiums grew from $1.6 billion in 1980 to $5.1 billion in 1993, and premiums for individually purchased contracts grew from $221 million to $876 million. According to the association, total assets at the end of 1993 were over four times those at the end of 1980, reflecting the rapid expansion of the private insurance industry.[96]

The costs of supplementary benefits to employers in Ontario alone is considerable: 30 large employers (with 350,000 employees) estimated that they would pay about $1 billion in 1995 through employee benefits and the employer health tax, and reported that the amount had increased by nearly $100 million since 1994. As noted earlier, the employer health tax is

Table 8

Workers' compensation health expenditures by category, Canada, 1975–1994

Year	Hospitals (%)	Other institutions (%)	MDs (%)	Other professions (%)	Drugs (%)	Capital (%)	Other expenditures (%)	Total (million $)
1975	61.9	0.1	23.8	7.2	1.6	–	5.4	121.1
1976	61.1	0.1	23.4	7.4	1.6	–	6.4	141.9
1977	60.6	0.1	23.2	8.1	1.6	–	6.4	153.1
1978	61.6	0.1	22.1	8.1	1.6	–	6.6	173.8
1979	58.8	0.1	23.7	8.7	1.7	–	7.1	184.9
1980	53.5	0.0	24.2	9.2	2.0	–	11.1	211.0
1981	52.8	0.1	23.2	8.6	2.1	–	13.2	289.0
1982	54.6	0.1	18.4	7.4	2.5	–	17.1	300.2
1983	53.5	0.1	18.4	7.3	2.9	–	17.9	310.5
1984	56.3	0.1	18.9	6.9	3.2	–	14.7	339.3
1985	53.9	0.1	23.4	6.9	3.2	–	12.5	388.8
1986	53.9	0.1	21.2	8.6	4.1	–	12.1	369.0
1987	52.0	0.1	20.6	9.8	4.6	–	13.0	385.5
1988	49.8	0.1	21.2	10.6	4.9	–	13.5	427.7
1989	49.3	0.1	20.3	11.5	5.0	–	13.8	453.3
1990	44.0	0.1	21.1	13.7	5.4	–	15.7	510.8
1991	40.7	0.1	18.6	17.7	5.8	–	17.0	569.8
1992	37.6	0.1	19.8	18.5	6.4	–	17.6	592.6
1993	36.0	0.1	20.9	17.6	7.0	–	18.4	578.4
1994	35.8	0.1	21.0	17.7	6.9	–	18.5	578.1

Source: Health Canada, *National Health Expenditures in Canada 1975–1994, Full Report* (Ottawa: Health Canada, Policy and Consultation Branch, January 1996), tables 9A and 9C.

merely another source of general revenue rather than an example of cost shifting; however, the employer group did report that between 1990 and 1994, the cost of providing health and dental benefits had increased by 74 percent (at a time when general inflation was 9 percent). Thus, the extent to which overall costs are controlled (rather than shifted) by this financing model is dubious; the large employers have requested that the Ontario government consult with industry to find savings through greater efficiency rather than through continuation of the cost-shifting approach.[97]

The Canadian Life and Health Insurance Association estimated that, in 1994, over 20 million Canadians were covered through supplementary group health and dental plans.[98]

The public-private mix for 1992 is summarized by subcategory in table 9.

Delivery

Delivery in Canada is predominantly private, consisting largely of self-employed physicians, nonprofit community and teaching hospitals, and a mixture of for-profit and not-for-profit clinics and other providers. Until the recent regional reforms in many provinces, most Canadian hospitals were owned by voluntary organizations, municipal or provincial authorities, or religious orders and were governed by voluntary boards of trustees. In many provinces, these voluntary boards have been subsumed into regional boards appointed by provincial governments or elected by local voters. Fewer than 5 percent of hospitals are privately owned; these largely provide long-term care or elective procedures and often receive public funding.

Allocation

The Canadian health care system is administered by the provincial and territorial governments. Allocation to hospitals has been organized around planned command-and-control models (e.g., global budgets to provide particular service mixes). Allocation to physicians and other fee-for-service providers (e.g., walk-in clinics, physiotherapists, etc.) is based on a market allocation model, which reimburses providers as a function of the volume and mix of services they deliver. Although most provinces have now imposed caps, distribution of funds among physicians still retains market elements, as capitation models also represent market-based allocations (with the advantage of capping the total amount to be allocated). At present, physician fees in most provinces are negotiated between medical associations and provincial governments. The managed care models introduce a corporate gatekeeper between patient and provider; all such plans present issues of potential risk selection.

Table 9

Health expenditures by subcategory of expenditure, Canada, 1992

Subcategory	Public sector (million $)	Private sector (million $)	Public %	Private %	Total (million $)
Hospitals	24,369.1	2,408.9	91.0	9.0	26,778.0
Other institutions	4,944.2	1,889.9	72.3	27.7	6,834.1
Physicians/psychologists	10,368.7	95.2	99.1	0.9	10,464.0
Other professionals:	965.7	4,947.2	16.3	83.7	5,912.9
– dentists/denturists	326.8	4,269.8	7.1	92.9	4,596.6
Other:	638.9	677.4	48.5	51.5	1,316.3
– chiropractors	198.2	–			
– optometrists/orthooists	205.6	–			
– podiatrists	18.7	–			
– osteopaths/naturopaths	2.4	–			
– private duty nurses	4.5	–			
– physiotherapists	209.4	–			
Drugs:	2,862.6	5,589.0	33.9	66.1	8,451.6
– prescribed	2,862.6	3,187.5	47.3	52.7	6,050.1
– nonprescribed	0.0	1,122.7	0.0	100.0	1,122.7
– health personnel supplies	0.0	1,278.8	0.0	100.0	1,278.8

Table 9 (cont.)

Subcategory	Public sector (million $)	Private sector (million $)	Public %	Private %	Total (million $)
Capital	**1,721.4**	**557.1**	**75.5**	**24.5**	**2,278.5**
Other expenditures	**6,646.2**	**2,666.8**	**71.4**	**28.6**	**9,313.0**
– home care	915.6	–			
– ambulance	783.2	–			
– eyeglasses	18.1	1,295.3	1.4	98.6	1,313.4
– hearing aids	11.9	–			
– health appliances	294.0	–			
– unspecified services	216.9	–			
– prepayment administration	416.3	808.2	34.0	66.0	1,224.5
– public health	3,280.5	–			
– health research	463.8	264.2	63.7	36.3	728.0
– miscellaneous health care	245.8	–			
– other private health care	–	299.2			
All categories	**51,877.9**	**18,154.1**	**74.1**	**25.9**	**70,032.0**

Source: Health Canada, *National Health Expenditures in Canada 1975–1994, Full Report* (Ottawa: Health Canada, Policy and Consultation Branch, January 1996), table 13A.

Note: Bolded rows represent totals; nonbolded rows give further detail by subdivisions of indicated categories.

CASE STUDIES OF SOME EXPERIENCES WITH DIFFERENT MODELS

In this section, we describe a few examples of the public-private mix that illustrate the working of particular models.

Hospitals

Hospitals in Canada have operated under delivery model IV (predominantly private delivery, but heavily regulated by the public sector) and received their budgets through command-and-control planned allocation, although with comparatively few performance expectations. As discussed in the section "The Case of Canada," they are the largest single cost centre in the Canadian health care system, amounting to 37 percent of total health expenditures in 1994. Most policymakers agree that Canada has tended to rely too heavily on acute hospital care, in large part because of the incentives inherent in what was required to be covered by medicare.[99] International comparison indicates, for example, that Canada has tended to make relatively high use of hospital beds. As of 1989, Canada had 6.7 inpatient beds per 1,000 population, compared to 6.4 for the United States and 4.8 for the United Kingdom; for acute care hospital beds the ratios were 4.3 per 1,000 in Canada, 3.6 in the United States, and 2.8 in the United Kingdom.[100] More recently, this ratio has been dropping rapidly.

A number of systemic problems exist in Canada's hospital sector. Many arise from technological innovations, which have meant considerable changes in what hospitals do. New technologies have shifted how care is delivered; conditions may be treated by drugs rather than by surgery, or minimally invasive technologies may enable care to be delivered on an outpatient basis. In consequence, lengths of stay have decreased considerably, with much surgery now being performed on a day surgery basis (as much as 70 to 80 percent in some hospitals). It must be recognized that these replacements (e.g., drugs, home nursing) are not necessarily defined as insured services under the CHA, meaning that provincial governments have an increasing ability to shift the costs of care away from the public plan. For example, almost no surgical dental services are now performed in hospital, making relatively meaningless the provision that such services must be insured under the CHA if performed in a hospital. Technological changes have also meant that patients who are in hospital tend to be sicker and hence more expensive to treat.

Some provinces have attempted to encourage the shift from institution-based services to community-based services by developing publicly funded home care services Although the shift of care to the community is widely thought to produce net savings, the evidence is not clear. Certain factors, such as the need to include travel time for providers, tend to reduce productivity and hence increase costs. Many people may be treated at home who would never have been institutionalized.[101] Nonetheless, these models may achieve longer-term savings if provinces do not have to build new institutions and pay for their upkeep. Other savings can be illusory, such as savings arising because community agencies pay lower wages, particularly if reallocation then forces an equalization of wage rates. To the extent that the shift to the community represents privatization by attrition or abandonment of groups in need, costs are shifted rather than controlled.

A clear example of shifting is reliance on private insurance and out-of-pocket payments if community services are not covered under the public plan (such as the Extramural Hospital, or "the hospital in the home," in New Brunswick). A more debatable one is the replacement of paid workers (e.g., nurses) by unpaid workers (often family members). A classic example of how not to shift care to the community was the deinstitutionalization of mental health patients without the establishment of adequate community services; considerable misery resulted, and some mental health costs ended up being shifted to correctional services.

Another reform that attempted to optimize the use of community-based services was the establishment of single points of entry for long-term care services. Ontario's proposed multiservice agency (MSA) model for long-term care reform (which referred largely to home-based nursing and support services) was almost unique in the current climate, in that it proposed to replace private delivery with quasi-public delivery, while in effect deinsuring the requirement to finance these services by moving them beyond the ambit of the CHA.[102] Implementation of the MSA model was halted by Ontario's current Conservative government—perhaps fortunately, since the models reviewed in this paper suggest that those reforms were likely to increase total costs, decrease access to needed services, or both.

People concerned about the issues of population health and the determinants of health stress that medical care is not the most important determinant of the health status of the population, and that it may be more cost effective to concentrate marginal resources on programs outside the traditional health system (e.g., nutrition, road safety, antitobacco measures, etc.).[103] Even within medical care, however, as care has shifted to the community, resources have not always followed. Most provinces note the problem of "silos" or "stovepipes," terms used to refer to funding arrangements that make it difficult to shift funds from one organization (or set of activities) to another. Regional reforms are a common method of dealing with this issue; a global budget for hospital and community-based services enables regional boards to shift resources to achieve maximum health benefits. These reforms are often unpopular, with many local people still desiring to maintain strong hospitals, but have been strongly pushed by provincial governments and by health reformers. As noted in the section "Frameworks for Making Decisions," such global budgets also have the potential to ease implementation of alternative methods for determining medical necessity.

Simultaneously, other factors have increased pressure on hospital budgets. For example, many provinces have sought to raise the wages of hospital workers, many of whom are women, on the grounds that they were relatively poorly paid in the years before medicare. Also, expensive technology must be accommodated within relatively constrained budgets. In addition, the hospitals built during the boom years after the introduction of hospital insurance are reaching the stage where considerable capital resources are needed to maintain them. Meeting these needs while attempting to constrain the resources given to the hospital sector has led to the recognition that "business as usual" is a prescription for mediocrity. Many institutional administrators feel that they are suffering "death by a thousand cuts" and are concerned that quality of care and timely access may be jeopardized.

It is well recognized that similar technological and financial trends have meant that most industrialized countries face the problem of reducing what was a considerable overcapacity of hospitals and hospital beds. Nonetheless, downsizing the sector has been resisted everywhere. People are proud of the facilities they have built, and hospital workers not unreasonably wish to retain their jobs. A number of mechanisms have been employed to attempt to reduce excess capacity, ranging from market forces (e.g., purchaser-provider splits) to planning directives. These have not always been effective.

Ontario has provided an extreme example. Over the last several decades, downsizing pressures had led to the closure of thousands of hospital beds in the province, but almost no change in the number of hospitals. Politicians have been frightened off by the fierce reactions to an attempt by Progressive Conservative Health Minister Frank Miller to reduce the number of hospitals in the 1970s, which led to his being pelted with snowballs, the minority government risking being thrown out of office, and a court case—which the government lost—ruling that government did not have the power under its existing legislation to close hospitals.[104] Since then, in many communities that only need one hospital, Catholic and lay hospitals across the street from one other have battled over programs. An attempt at a voluntary merger between Women's College Hospital and The Toronto Hospital led to a revolt by the medical staff and a portion of the hospital board of the first institution, and resulted in the resignation of the hospital CEO and the replacement of the promerger forces on the board.[105] Potentially surplus hospitals with poor physical plants have nonetheless succeeded in exerting political pressure to get government funds to rebuild. Other hospitals have run deficits and been bailed out by the Ontario government. More recently, the government did enforce its fiscal targets, but in large part through mechanisms that cut services (by forcing people to take unpaid days off) without solving structural issues, and with little attention to how the costs "saved" by the so-called social contract would be absorbed once it expired. There is already concern that the quality of services is declining and anecdotal suggestions that waiting lists for certain procedures with high marginal costs (e.g., hip replacements) are growing to unacceptable proportions in some jurisdictions. Many administrators have expressed uncertainty about how they can maintain quality while absorbing the additional cuts that the province will impose to meet its fiscal targets. In 1996, the Ontario government included within its omnibus legislation provisions to give the Minister the power to close hospitals if Cabinet decided that closure was in the public interest,[106] and delegated this authority to a newly formed Health Services Restructuring Committee; the extent of implementation, however, is still unclear. In contrast, Quebec and Alberta have undertaken extensive restructuring of hospital care; the ultimate effects in these provinces have not yet been evaluated.

Financial pressures faced by provincial governments, the disproportionate share of hospital expenditures in health budgets, and recognition of imbalances in the continuum of care have been the major drivers of change in the hospital sector. As governments seek to encourage more efficient hospital operations and shift care from expensive acute care beds to less expensive levels of care, they have taken on greater involvement in the management and planning of the hospital system. Although resources in the past were allocated within a command-and-control model, the degree of state involvement was limited in large part to deciding the overall amount to spend on hospital care each year. Indeed, by the mid-1980s, most provinces had replaced line-by-line hospital budgeting with global budgets to increase hospital flexibility and planning capability, achieving cost control through enforcement of global limits. Over time, there has been a change from this loose command-and-control model, with many provincial governments becoming more activist and using such levers as altered hospital reimbursement systems, mandated hospital closings and mergers, and reallocation of resources from institutional to community-based care.

Deber and colleagues concluded that while all the above reforms have not been evaluated for effectiveness, there are areas of concern resulting from the shift from institutions to the community:

- This shift often represents a shift in allocation model from globally capped and well-controlled budgets (such as exist for hospital services) to volume-driven expenditures.
- Cost shifting to multiple payers may further undermine cost control.[107] One advantage of regional envelope models is that they can, in theory, apply the same global budget controls as have been applied within the hospital sector to a wider array of services.

Private Clinics

In the past, the existence of private clinics represented an example of the private sector financing specialized or elective services, while the public sector retained sole responsibility for paying for a comprehensive mix of services.

The growth in private facilities can be seen as movement toward a model wherein the private sector has the potential to compete alongside the public sector as one of many providers of health services.

As noted in the section "The Case of Canada," more than 28 percent of total health care spending now comes from private sources. This spending has been largely concentrated on such items as drugs, nonphysician providers, cosmetic surgery, some types of eye surgery, long-term care, and dental care. Although historically the people who could afford it always had the option of seeking publicly insured services from other countries or even from private clinics in Canada, the existence of high-quality "free" services coupled with the requirement that all additional costs be met by out-of-pocket payments by patients meant that there was little market. However, there is an increasing trend to seek care in the private sector for services traditionally covered by medicare, either as privatization by attrition is reflected in waiting lists or as governments refuse to buy as much of the latest technology as doctors and patients desire. Hence, it is becoming more common for patients to seek care for surgery to repair a torn shoulder or have a magnetic resonance imaging (MRI) scan at a private clinic, even though these procedures are insured and available in public hospitals.

The definition of what constitutes a private clinic and how many exist in Canada is disputed; one estimate suggests that there are as many as 300. Until recently these facilities have focused on offering care for such simple procedures and treatments as abortions, in vitro fertilization, or laser eye surgery. However, there are initiatives to build small private hospitals or stand-alone surgicentres to provide more complex treatments such as gallbladder operations, hip and knee replacements, and even emergency services. For services not covered by provincial insurance programs, patients must pay the full cost out of their own pockets. For covered services, doctors bill the provincial plan and patients are required to pay an extra facility fee, which can range from $200 to $1,300.[108] This latter practice has been deemed counter to the Canada Health Act and the federal government has reduced transfer payments to provinces who allow this to continue.

A disquieting trend is for hospitals that do not have the budget to fully operate their expensive equipment to make "surplus" capacity available for a fee, even if there are waiting lists for such care. In Toronto, St. Michael's Hospital has allowed individuals to jump the queue for MRIs by booking through a private insurance company. The Mineral Springs Hospital in Banff is negotiating an arrangement with a U.S. preferred provider organization for ambulatory care surgery, whereby U.S. patients can combine a trip to a Banff hotel with minor orthopedic procedures. The hospital justifies the arrangement as the only way to retain an orthopedic surgeon in an area where the budgets allocated by the regional health authority would otherwise not be adequate to maintain the service. Cardston Hospital in Alberta is actively marketing a stomach stapling service to U.S. patients.

Typical of the new breed of private clinics are the two MRI facilities operating in British Columbia.[109] The incentive to start these clinics has arisen from the provincial government's curb on technology acquisition among public sector providers. Although more MRI machines are scheduled to be acquired, Canada has one machine per 700,000 to 800,000 people, while in the United States the figure is one per 90,000 people. Although the number of machines is less important than the number of procedures, some B.C. patients were travelling for testing across the border to nearby Washington state. MRI clinics can cost between one and three million dollars to set up, but the returns to investors can go as high as 60 percent of equity investment. In 1995, the B.C. private clinics were charging about $750 for producing an MRI image along with a radiologist's interpretation. This fee allowed them to underprice neighbouring U.S. facilities that were charging about Can$1,600, not including the cost that cross-border patients would have to incur for travel and accommodation, or any fluctuations in currency exchange rates.

To Canadian consumers, the attractions of private health services are that they often allow patients to avoid waiting in line for several months for a service in already hard-pressed public sector facilities, they often boast state-of-the-art equipment, and they often place a greater emphasis on customer comfort and convenience. The main incentive for entrepreneurs to invest in private facilities is the opportunity to break into the $72 billion health care industry and accrue favourable rates of return. In addition, a number of clinics have been set up by members of the medical profession who are dissatisfied with their access to privileges or facilities in public institutions. For example, the development of surgicentres has been driven by sharp reductions in surgeons' operating room privileges for non-emergency and elective cases as hospitals attempt to streamline their operations and cut costs.

The issues surrounding the competition between private and publicly financed services highlights issues surrounding the long-term sustainability of the public system, the quality of privately delivered care, and the consequences on overall health care cost containment.

Three main issues arise from offering preferential access to "paying customers." First, such clients are usually highly subsidized by the public system. Costing is rarely complete, and charges are often based on the marginal cost of adding an additional patient rather than on the full expense of maintaining the service (including training). In addition, the private clients often incur costs to the public system (labs, follow-up visits, etc.), including the medical costs of any resulting complications. The potential of public costs can be particularly problematic for risky or experimental procedures (e.g., stomach stapling); the Consumers Association of Canada (Alberta) has estimated that the hidden costs of such services include the additional malpractice premiums that must be paid by all physicians.[110]

Second, not all provinces have mechanisms in place to ensure quality of care in private facilities. (Ontario's Independent Health Facilities Act does ensure such a legislative framework.) This issue is transitional—there is no reason why an accreditation process similar to that employed by hospitals cannot be established—but is also one that may require action in some jurisdictions.

Third, and crucially, there is a high risk that a private alternative could pull resources away from publicly insured services and thus impoverish them. For example, physicians may choose to spend more time with private patients, allowing waiting lists for "free" care to grow. The limited information available suggests that these fears have some grounding in reality. A study of access to cataract surgery by the Consumers Association of Canada (Alberta) found that the waiting list for patients whose ophthalmologists performed surgery only in the public sector was an average of two to six weeks.[111] Longer waiting periods of up to 18 months for "free" surgery were encountered only by patients of ophthalmologists having a dual practice; payment of a facility fee decreased the wait by about two to four weeks. However, in one clinic, if a referring physician had performed the necessary tests, surgery could be performed on the same day as the initial clinic assessment.

These results suggest that the waiting list issue pointed to by advocates of private clinics may in part be artificial, since the lists appear to arise only if a second tier is permitted. However, the results also raise a number of questions. What mechanisms exist to moderate the inherent conflict of interest of clinics claiming that procedures are "needed" in order to increase revenues? The Manitoba Centre for Health Policy and Evaluation examined cataract surgery in Manitoba, where there are three private clinics. Between 1990–91 and 1994–95, there was rapid expansion in both the public sector (from 3,556 procedures to 5,222) and the private sector (from 284 to 692 procedures), suggesting that the private sector growth could not be explained by cutbacks or rationing within the publicly funded sector. The Centre also noted that patients using private clinics had to pay as much as $1,270—about twice the estimated cost of a public hospital procedure—and that at least one-third of the Manitobans paying for their cataract surgery in 1993–94 were from Winnipeg's low-income neighbourhoods, raising equity concerns in addition to concerns about increased costs.[112]

The well-known variation in surgical rates across jurisdictions leads to some concern, especially if there are incentives to overservice. Although there is no way to determine the "correct" rate, the figures in table 10 indicate that the rate of cataract surgeries for residents of Alberta—where the renowned private Gimbel eye clinic is situated—is considerably higher than the rate in other provinces. The extent to which private clinics meet otherwise unmet demand, as opposed to helping generate demand, is therefore unclear.

Another key issue is whether the existence of a privately financed alternative will allow the public sector to "off-load," assigning fewer resources to such care and thus creating a self-fulfilling prophecy of shortages. The United States again provides a cautionary example—25 percent of physicians simply refuse to treat Medicaid patients, while two-thirds of the remainder limit the number they will treat. Accordingly, patients in the U.S. public tier may not have access to willing care providers.[113] The use of privately financed clinics has often been justified in terms that apply only to private delivery (i.e., that such clinics are more innovative). This line of argument leads to confusion—there is no reason why such clinics cannot exist within the publicly financed system, should government decide that they are of sufficiently high priority. If there are indeed shortages of medically required services, the response presumably should be to reallocate resources to ensure that high-quality, timely care is available when needed. As this report notes, the evidence suggests that piecemeal adoption of multiple financing options comes at a fairly high cost—increased health spending, decreased equity, and higher employer burden.

Physician Services

Physician care is predominantly a case of the private delivery of publicly financed services, heavily regulated by the public sector. Until recently, resources for most physician services in Canada had been distributed within a pure market allocation model, with physician earnings depending on the volume and mix of patients seen, and payment on the basis of a negotiated fee schedule.

As noted, market allocation models are relatively weak at cost control. For a number of reasons, including the shifting of care to the community, a growth in physician supply and minimal controls over utilization, the use of medical services over the past 20 years has grown faster than either the population or the gross domestic product. From 1980 to 1991, there was a 95 percent increase in net physician incomes.[114] Although no one knows what the "right" number of physicians is, Canada's ratio of 1.9 physicians per 1,000 people was higher than the ratio in Japan (1.57) or the United Kingdom (1.37). In consequence, there have been a number of efforts to alter physician training and practice patterns, including attempts to reduce the supply of physicians.[115] A number of these efforts have represented a change in which allocation model is employed, moving from the market end of the continuum toward more of a command-and-control planned allocation model. Such measures have included capping the overall resources allocated for physician services and changing reimbursement mechanisms.

Throughout most of the 1980s, all provinces but Quebec financed medical care on an open-ended basis. Since then, caps on earnings have been negotiated by some provinces for physicians individually, or for all billing physicians

Table 10

Interprovincial comparison of number of cataract surgeries provided by all specialties per 1,000 covered population,[a] 1983–1991

Province	1982–1983	1983–1984	1984–1985	1985–1986	1986–1987[b]	1987–1988[b]	1988–1989	1989–1990	1990–1991[b]	Average annual % change, 1982–1983 to 1990–1991
Newfoundland	1.88	2.53	2.57	3.85	6.05	7.97	9.17	10.20	9.57	22.72
Prince Edward I.	4.04	4.40	6.31	8.18	n/a	n/a	6.86	5.42	n/a	n.a.
Nova Scotia	6.00	5.79	6.63	7.98	9.18	9.42	11.05	12.05	12.69	10.03
New Brunswick	6.19	5.58	6.74	6.21	7.26	7.97	10.00	11.05	11.60	8.17
Quebec	4.95	6.12	6.50	6.72	7.55	6.12	7.27	6.36	10.55	9.92
Ontario	6.07	6.85	7.80	6.76	9.71	10.65	11.62	12.51	13.16	10.13
Manitoba	8.38	7.17	7.81	6.19	10.12	10.69	10.72	11.74	11.34	7.50
Saskatchewan	5.21	5.79	6.62	6.99	7.20	7.38	9.97	14.05	15.64	14.91
Alberta	7.10	6.54	9.05	11.10	12.41	13.99	14.64	16.31	21.00	14.36
British Columbia	5.87	6.17	9.60	10.37	11.49	11.95	12.62	14.16	16.34	13.65
Total	5.71	6.76	7.54	8.39	9.35	9.67	10.64	11.84	13.43	11.28

Source: W. Armstrong, 1996. Personal communication.

n/a = not available; n.a. = not applicable.

[a] Covered population = men and women 45 years and over. Rates per 1,000 men and women aged 45 and older were revised using new estimates received from Statistics Canada.

[b] Total excludes Prince Edward Island in 1986–1987, 1987–1988, and 1990–1991.

Notes: 1. The data consist of fee-for-service items that each provincial plan paid to physicians in the respective province for cataract surgeries provided to residents of the province. The data are compiled on a date-of-payment basis. 2. The data include cataract surgeries provided by ophthalmologists, as well as services provided by other specialists. 3. The data exclude services that were provided out of province. 4. For the definition of cataract surgery used in compiling the data for each province, please refer to the document Provincial Cataract Surgery Fee Codes, October 25, 1993, Professional Services, Alberta Health.

collectively, or both.[116] For example, Ontario and British Columbia have introduced caps and clawbacks on physicians earning above a certain income per year. Other provinces have introduced caps on the global budget available for physician services. If aggregate billings exceed this amount, all physicians contribute to a repayment of the amount exceeding the cap. This model has a number of undesirable consequences, including the potential for what is known as a tragedy of the commons,[117] in that providers who voluntarily curb their utilization can nonetheless be penalized if others do not follow suit. In the absence of mechanisms to discipline all participants, these types of formulae present incentives for everyone to try to increase their own share of a capped pie, leading everyone to be worse off. (An analogous situation has led to the virtual destruction of the Atlantic fishery.) Such formulae may also accentuate the underuse of resources noted in the private clinics case (e.g., waiting lists may grow for eye surgery or hip replacement through the publicly financed system because the surgeon has reached his cap). In contrast to strategies such as moving from fee for service to alternative reimbursement methods, such hard caps are blunt instruments, which tend to be unresponsive to clinical need.

Recent policy moves have attempted to control physician numbers and distribution by such mechanisms as a national agreement to cut medical school enrolments by 10 percent, similar cuts to postgraduate training, tighter restrictions on allowing foreign-trained physicians (or even physicians trained in other provinces) to practice or bill fee for service, differential fees to encourage physicians to practice in underserviced areas, and physician resource plans.

Different physician reimbursement mechanisms are also being explored. Unlike many other countries, Canada has relied heavily on fee for service medicine (67.7 percent of physicians billed fee for service for over 90 percent of their practice).[118] The greater use of capitation and salary models is currently being explored in most jurisdictions.

To the extent that such controls attempt to shift delivery from private to public models, the literature suggests that the undesirable effects (decreased client sensitivity) are likely to outweigh the desirable ones. However, the provincial experiments with allocation models are more defensible; they represent more explicit trade-offs between cost control and client responsiveness, for which defining the appropriate balance is not likely to be simple.

Deinsurance of Medical Procedures

As discussed in the section "Frameworks for Making Decisions," one response to difficult economic times has been to deinsure services that need not be included under the provisions of the CHA. For example, a number of provinces have deinsured routine eye examinations. In response to our inquiries, we were told that there has been little attempt to monitor the consequences at the provincial level. However, the Consumers Association of Canada (Alberta) surveyed a convenience sample of 71 optometry (involving 75 optometrists) clinics and 22 ophthalmology clinics between May 8 and May 12, 1995, to assess the impact.[119] Before December 1994, optometrists and ophthalmologists were reimbursed $35.94 by Alberta Health for basic eye examinations. After that date, care moved to the private market. Prices rose an average of $10.76 (29.94 percent) for 74 of the optometrists and $11.20 (31.16 percent) for the 22 ophthalmologists. Waiting times were short—often same day or next day, and rarely more than one week (Wendy Armstrong, personal communication, 1995). Anecdotally, prices also rose in Saskatchewan after eye examinations were de-insured (S. Lewis, personal communication), although we have not yet obtained precise data (we were informed that it has not been monitored by Saskatchewan Health). These findings confirm the suggestions from the literature review that competition and markets for services perceived as necessary appear to increase costs, rather than to constrain them.

Automobile Insurance and Rehabilitative Services in Ontario

No-fault automobile insurance is an example of financing model II(A): mandatory private coverage of services that are not covered in the public provincial plans. The CHA definitions of comprehensiveness are ambiguous about how rehabilitation should be handled, and Ontario has chosen to shift responsibility for much of the rehabilitative care of patients injured in automobile accidents from the Ontario Health Insurance Plan to car insurance premiums. Every individual who wants to drive is required to purchase car insurance from the private insurance industry; premiums are actuarially based and vary considerably according to age, residence, and driving history. Automobile insurance is provided by competing private companies.

Our review of the international evidence suggested that the Ontario financing arrangement would present the problem of risk selection (no insurer would wish to cover those at high risk) and hamper the ability of insurers to use their monopsony power to achieve cost controls. In consequence, one could predict that cost escalation would be greater than in the publicly financed sectors of care. Accordingly, it is of interest to examine whether those theoretical problems have indeed arisen. We obtained information from Jim Daw, who researched an award-winning series of articles,[120] and from the Institute of Work and Health, which has been studying rehabilitation care in Ontario (Terry Sullivan, personal communication).[121]

The previous system left most medical costs within financing model I (public sector as sole financer of a comprehensive mix of services). Automobile insurance claims were expected to cover disability (including loss of income) and property damage. Minor claims were paid by the insurer following their regular processes. Recovery for damages from serious injury depended on the results of lawsuits. Insurers usually settled these lawsuits by negotiating lump sum payments, with the claimant then responsible for purchasing whatever services were appropriate to meet his needs. Only a few services were purchased from private sources.

By the mid-1980s there was perceived to be a crisis because of the steadily increasing automobile insurance premiums and the high costs and uncertainty of using the courts for redress. Courts were making higher awards for economic loss (based on expectations about inflation, rising medical costs, and awards for people's pain and suffering), yet many of those injured collected little or nothing.[122] In 1987, the provincial Liberal government proposed no-fault insurance, immediately capped premium price rises, and appointed Justice Coulter Osborne to report on the issue. Justice Osborne advised that the incentive to sue might be reduced if higher payments were available to all injury victims without the necessity to prove that one or the other party was at fault in an accident. In 1990, the Justice's recommendations were implemented when amendments to the Insurance Act created the Ontario Motorist Protection Plan. The plan was not fully no-fault in that there was only a partial limitation on the right to sue; cases of death or serious injury could still be argued in court. Another provision of the no-fault system appears to have arisen in part from a cost-shifting imperative: insurers faced stiff penalties for late payment and had to pay the cost of resolving disputes through the Ontario Insurance Commission. There was a $2,000 charge to an insurer whenever someone requested an arbitration, and the insurer could be fined up to $100,000 for withholding benefits to claimants and $200,000 for each subsequent offence. Accordingly, there was a disincentive to challenge the merit of claims, which both benefitted claimants and increased the likelihood of fraud. Since insurers can spend up to $50,000 to challenge some claims, it was often more cost effective to settle dubious claims than to contest them. The new plan substantially improved benefits from pre-1990 amounts; under the new plan, payment for medical rehabilitation and care, a wheelchair, and other medical costs could be up to $500,000.

Lawyers, annoyed at being prevented from fighting lawsuits in 90 percent of cases, started testing the definition of what would pass the cutoff or injury threshold for lawsuits, and victims started testing what could be claimed. The no-fault provision led to a flood of injury claims, and dozens of new private rehabilitation clinics were started to serve people who had been in automobile accidents. Weeks after the new insurance system came into being, the New Democratic Party was elected. The NDP further improved benefits, in terms of both the amount to be paid and a widening of the range of no-fault benefits that could be available. The money available for medical expenses and rehabilitation increased from $25,000 to $500,000 in 1990 and to $1 million in 1994; up to $10,000 per month (with no lifetime limit) could be allotted for attendant care for the chronically disabled. Clearly, these measures could relieve the pressure on publicly funded plans (e.g., chronic care, welfare).

The Statutory Accident Benefits Schedule requires automobile insurers to provide supplementary rehabilitation, medical, and attendant care benefits to bona fide accident claimants. Rehabilitation benefits focus mainly on vocational training costs, but can include payment for counselling, case management, and renovation of victims' homes and vehicles if needed because of the nature of their disabilities. Automobile insurers are obliged to pay these benefits only if provincial plans do not completely cover claimants' health care needs; hence, automobile insurers are only second payers after the Ministry of Health. Again, these provisions create an incentive for provincial governments to deinsure care so that costs can be shifted to the private sector.

The availability of these supplementary benefits has spawned a new private sector seeking to serve the needs of potential claimants. Private rehabilitation clinics have become a growth industry. Their advertisements filled 10 pages of the Ontario Insurance Directory in 1993 and 34 pages in 1994. Between 1993 and 1994, accident benefit claims increased by 62 percent (largely driven by increased spending on medical services such as chiropractic, physiotherapy, and acupuncture). In 1994, insurance companies hiked their rates by an average of 11.5 percent. The industry claims losses of $44 million in that year alone. Insurers estimate their total payouts for doctors, therapists, and medications for accident victims in 1994 to be 88 percent higher than in 1993. Medical costs now account for more than 50 percent of the $2.6 billion automobile insurers were estimated to have spent in 1994. The amounts automobile insurers are estimated to have paid for rehabilitation policies from 1991 to mid-1994 are listed in table 11.

The new Ontario government has announced its intention to revise automobile insurance policy

Table 11

Estimates of auto insurers payments for rehabilitation policies, 1991–1994

Claim classification	Claims in year ($)			
	1991	1992	1993	1994 (first half)
Private auto	161,597,523	244,870,324	288,815,597	178,918,020
Commercial vehicle	5,210,038	6,006,688	6,418,054	4,045,578
Motorcycle	5,843,444	6,921,588	5,254,458	3,781,046
Total	172,651,005	257,798,600	300,488,109	186,744,644

Source: Institute for Work and Health, *Rehabilitation Services Inventory and Quality Project: Phase One Report* (Toronto: IWH, 1995).

Travel Health Insurance

Travel health insurance is an example of financing model II(B) (voluntary private coverage of services not covered in the public plan). Our review of the literature suggests that such models are likely to lead to problems with risk selection. Jim Daw of the *Toronto Star* has produced an excellent study of travel health insurance.[123]

Travel health insurance has become an issue because some provincial plans have chosen to reduce their coverage for services. The portability condition of the CHA requires provinces to pay home province rates for necessary out-of-country coverage (elective procedures can be excluded). This condition is clearly inadequate for certain jurisdictions (especially the United States) and leaves insured Canadians who happen to fall ill in the United States with large residual bills (over $2,000 per day is not uncommon). Although Ontario had voluntarily exceeded legal requirements by covering all out-of-country hospital charges for eligible individuals, in 1991 the province chose to shift costs by limiting their payment to a maximum of $100 per day for such costs. In 1995, the Progressive Conservative government chose to comply with the portability requirements of the CHA by increasing this maximum to $400 per day. However, purchase of supplementary travel health insurance has now become a practical necessity—in its absence, an accident outside the home province could lead to financial catastrophe.

In 1994, the Canadian Life and Health Insurance Association fielded 6,700 travel health calls from members of the public. The health plan market for trips longer than 30 days is now worth between $100 and $125 million in premiums to insurers. *Sun Times of Canada,* a paper catering to Canadians travelling to Florida, now produces a comparison report of travel health plans that cover almost 10 tabloid-sized pages. Risk selection ("cherry picking") indeed appears to be occurring. The premiums for health plans offering coverage for six months can vary from $503 for healthy (preferred) travellers to as much as $2,520 for less healthy travellers. Developments in the travel health insurance industry are similar to those reported for U.S. health insurance. Plans vary considerably in comprehensiveness (i.e., what services will not be covered). Many policies exclude or limit coverage for claims related to preexisting conditions. Seniors considered less healthy because they are on medication, have been hospitalized, or have a history of heart, lung, or other functional problems have to pay much higher premiums—if they are even accepted for coverage.

As the demand for travel health insurance has grown, insurers have become more restrictive about whom they accept for coverage and under what conditions. Most insurers now require potential customers to complete health questionnaires, some as long as 21 questions, to screen for preexisting conditions. In 1992, the standard time limit for a preexisting condition to be covered was three months—that is, a person would qualify for coverage if a preexisting condition had not required treatment or a change of medication in the past three months. Now, the time limit has been extended to six months to a year. One consequence is that some people distort information about their preexisting conditions, and insurers have become more aggressive in checking medical records to approve qualification for coverage or before paying claims. Indeed, the snowbird paper *Canada News* reported that 75 percent of readers' disputes with insurers were related to preexisting condition clauses.

Another way insurers attempt to limit their risk on travel health insurance policies is by reducing the comprehensiveness of coverage through exemptions and caveats. These exemptions can include refusing coverage for a second occurrence of a health problem while on holiday, forcing the client to pay the full costs for even large emergency care bills and then be reimbursed later, charging deductibles on every claim rather than the standard one time during a policy's period, making provisions for other insurers to share the cost of claims, forcing clients to call the insurer's assistance line within a certain period or even before receiving medical care in order to be covered, refusing to renew or extend plans if the time away is longer than expected, and refusing to pay for medical services that the insurer judges did not result from a true emergency (or denying charges considered unusual or not customary). Businesses have sprung up to repatriate such patients (e.g., by air ambulance) so that costs of further care can be shifted back to the home province.

Costs, plus the wide variation in how policies handle preexisting condition or exemption clauses, have forced snowbirds to shop widely and wisely in their search for an insurance plan that fits their needs and budget. Indeed the investment in time and resources for plan shopping has been described as "a stressful part-time job for thousands of Canadian seniors."[124] Some find themselves uninsurable. The consequences of being unable to travel outside Canada because of an inability to purchase affordable (or any) health insurance can be viewed as relatively minor, although the senior unable to attend a family function or forced to remain housebound during cold weather may not agree. However, if this model were used more widely, such that necessary care within the province was also encompassed, it appears likely that large proportions of the population—including those most in need of care—would be at high risk of being left out of the resulting insurance market.

Paying for Pharmaceuticals

Payment for pharmaceuticals in Canada is primarily a case of voluntary private coverage of services not covered in the public plan (through extended coverage or top-up insurance). While provincial plans cover drug costs for seniors and welfare recipients, the overwhelming majority of expenditures for drugs originates from private sources. Canada is one of few countries in the OECD that has such a heavy reliance on private sector sources for the financing of drug expenditures. In many cases, employers are induced to offer payment for drugs as part of employment benefit plans.

Nonetheless, although private sector plans have grown tremendously over the years, so too have public sector plans.[125] Indeed, increases in drug expenditures in both the public and the private market have been substantially greater than those for health expenditures as a whole. Prescription drugs alone have increased their contribution to overall health expenditures by 63 percent—from 4.6 percent of total health expenditures in 1980 to 8 percent in 1993. Drug costs have increased as a function of offloading from hospitals, more beneficiaries, more prescriptions per beneficiary, and higher cost per prescription. For public drug plans—which have been shedding beneficiaries, and increasing copayments—the largest cost increases have come from changes in the price of the drugs covered.

When Ontario's plans to introduce user fees for drug benefits come into effect, every province will have instituted some form of cost sharing for groups covered by their drug plans. Governments justify cost sharing on two grounds: as a source of revenue, and to limit overutilization of drugs. However, the plans do not distinguish between necessary and unnecessary use. Attempts have also been made to control what drugs are included on provincial formularies. Private drug plans have focused their cost containment efforts on limiting drug consumption and plan coverage through such strategies as restricting the benefit list, encouraging plan flexibility or allowing employees to opt out of plans altogether, and providing drug education to employees. However, increasing attention is being paid to bulk purchasing and to disease management approaches, which would treat drug costs as part of a balanced care plan.

Given that access to pharmaceuticals in Canada is primarily a result of voluntary private coverage (through extended coverage or top-up insurance) of services not covered in the public plan, there is a potential for uneven coverage. Availability of drug plan coverage (as well as copayments and deductibles) is often tied to a person's location and job situation; the unemployed (if not on welfare), the self-employed, people working for small businesses, and part-time workers often have no drug insurance. Provincial plans usually concentrate on the elderly and people on social assistance.

The fairly rapid increase in payments for health benefits reported by the members of Canadian Life and Health Insurance Association is illustrated by the numbers in table 12.

Table 12

Supplementary health benefit payments by type of benefit ($), 1984–1993

Year	Extended health care	Supplementary hospital	Drug	Dental
1984	442,246,919	24,802,198	12,156,185	529,018,377
1985	503,751,280	33,341,132	14,526,589	565,220,092
1986	565,946,725	42,393,889	15,133,324	616,635,467
1987	651,353,296	45,092,304	15,539,215	648,954,656
1988	805,064,992	36,500,827	20,897,190	690,351,591
1989	834,053,485	37,523,040	23,047,350	748,064,151
1990	958,409,062	37,505,191	18,190,665	820,959,109
1991	982,862,334	40,574,166	17,215,251	856,156,477
1992	1,010,698,001	45,562,488	21,042,539	890,865,955
1993	1,135,615,438	49,325,729	25,511,565	914,926,555
% change	156.78%	98.88%	109.86%	72.95%

Sources: D.E. Angus, L. Auer, J.E. Cloutier, T. Albert, *Sustainable Health Care for Canada: Synthesis Report* (Ottawa: Queen's University–University of Ottawa Economic Projects, 1995); Canadian Life and Health Insurance Association Inc., *Survey of Health Insurance Benefits in Canada*, annual surveys 1975, 1980, 1984–1993.

Private Insurance in Australia

In recent years, Australians have been debating the future of their health care system. The debate has focused on issues similar to those in Canada, but Australia has allowed a greater role for private insurance. A July 1993 working paper by J. Richardson, codirector of the National Centre for Health Program Evaluation, notes that there was a widespread assumption—not grounded in any evidence—that the privatization of public insurance would increase efficiency and that copayments would control costs.[126] Private insurance was also justified as a way of funding expenditures that governments "cannot afford" and as a way of "forcing the wealthy to pay an equitable share." A system therefore evolved in which the national basic scheme promises to provide all beneficial services, with a private second tier available to people wishing to purchase it. It has not been customary for businesses to provide health insurance as a benefit (in part because such costs are not tax deductible) (Carol Kushner, personal communication, December 1995).

An interesting policy development has been the economic difficulties faced by private insurance. As Richardson writes,

Higher premiums plus the economic recession have led to less private health insurance. But as the best risk members are the first to leave, those retaining insurance have a worse risk profile which, in turn, forces a further increase in premiums and a further reduction in the number privately insured. This has resulted in an accelerating decline in insurance, particularly in Victoria.

Private insurance represents an opportunity to shift costs away from public budgets. Accordingly, the economic difficulties outlined by Richardson have been seen as a problem by the Australian government, which has therefore passed a private health insurance reform bill to help support the private insurance industry.[127] An additional complexity is that Australia has a mixed delivery system; without a healthy private insurance industry, the survival of private hospitals was also threatened. According to a May 1995 speech by the then Secretary of the Commonwealth Department of Human Services and Health, the reform bill removed "some of the regulations which have limited the competitiveness and innovation within the industry" and was "intended unashamedly to benefit private health insurance contributors." The previous system did not allow insurers to contract selectively; the reforms attempted to strengthen the ability of private insurers to contract with hospitals and doctors without allowing total selectivity, evidently in the hope that some of any resulting savings could be passed along to consumers and "allow them to take out their insurance cover at a lower cost." Consumer information and complaints procedures are also intended to strengthen the ability of informed consumers to purchase coverage in a free market. However, other reforms limit the new opportunities by restricting the ability to "discriminate" against hospitals, as well as by specifying coverage requirements: "to ensure that patients are protected from the effects of underestimating their risk of contracting some kinds of illness, all health insurance products will include cover for psychiatric, palliative, and rehabilitative care. This will also provide some protection for those private hospitals who specialise in treatment for these types of illnesses." Doctors would be able to contract with private insurers for fee levels above those paid by the public plan. The speech concluded by noting that the private health insurance participation rate was declining and could be rescued only by bringing about a "change in culture ... critical to ensure that those Australians get good value for money from a product of choice."[128]

Clearly, it is too early to see whether these reforms resolve the problems. However, it is noteworthy that, given an adequate, publicly supported, basic level of services and without further government intervention, risk selection rose to the extent that the financial viability of the private insurers was threatened.

EVALUATING THE MODELS: EQUITY, EFFICIENCY, SECURITY, AND LIBERTY

A range of options exists for balancing the public-private mix in the Canadian health system. The issue is not whether the system will be public or private in the future, since few systems operate at either extreme. Rather, the implications of alternative models with varying mixes of the two sectors need to be examined and clarified to understand the push for certain options and the resistance to others.

In any debate over policy, there is a struggle over objectives and the values that underlie them. All policies contain values, whether they are stated explicitly or merely implied. Such frequently invoked objectives as equity, efficiency, liberty, choice, quality, accountability, and empowerment are all rooted in values. Yet the imprecision of these terms often hides conflicting though, at times, equally plausible interpretations of these values, which in turn determine who is included or excluded under a policy, what items will be distributed and how.

In this section, we identify criteria for evaluating the outcomes of different options for adjusting the public-private mix in the Canadian health system. Although these criteria may be categorized and priorized in different ways (see, for example, the evaluation of financial incentives and disincentives by Groupe Secor[129]), we have chosen initially to note two broad categories derived from the field of public administration and to outline how the balance between them has shifted over time in response to changing political and economic circumstances. We then adapt Stone's description of the four general policy goals or values underlying most public policy—equity, efficiency, security, and liberty—and discuss key criteria under these headings.[130] (More specific policy goals—such as client satisfaction, consumer empowerment, accessibility, national coordination, and provincial flexibility—can usually be subsumed under these four general headings.) Finally, we review each of the models we described earlier in terms of the prominence given to some values over others and the various trade-offs among them.

Conceptual Issues and Historical Debate

The field of public administration distinguishes between two broad categories that can be used to evaluate public policy: value issues (which tend to be subjective or qualitative and rarely directly measurable, e.g., equity and liberty) and technical-administrative issues (which are often connected with the costs, efficiency, and effectiveness of different options). Value issues define what decision makers believe should be primarily individual (private) versus collective (public) responsibilities—that is, what individuals should be expected to do for themselves, and what they should expect as a social entitlement. The definition and application of these values are often the focus of intense and ongoing political debate. There are no correct answers, although there may be consensus within particular societies at a given time.

Having determined social goals, it may then be possible to analyze and even measure the extent to which particular policy tools are likely to attain them. Are alternatives workable within the available finances, expertise, human resources, and technology? Will different options produce more of the desired outcome with the same resources? Evidence-based medical practice and practice guidelines aim to maximize the efficiency and cost-effectiveness of clinical decision making but assume that the goals of medical practice have already been determined. At the macrolevel of policy, one may similarly question the relative abilities of the public and private sectors to maximize cost-effectiveness and efficiency.

The central question of public administration, and one at the centre of current public debate on the future of medicare, is how values in these two categories, and the categories themselves, should be weighted and balanced to guide policy decisions. Ideally, policies should address social and political goals (recognizing that support for particular goals may vary across stake-holders and over time) and constitute the best way, technically and adminis-tratively, to achieve those goals.

Balancing Social and Political Values with Technical and Administrative Values

In general, every industrialized country, with the exception of the United States, espouses the principle of universal health coverage for its people as a right of citizenship, rather than as a commodity to be bought and sold in the open market. Historically, principles of universality and equity of access have been the driving forces behind decisions about financing health. These principles have recently been challenged as the general social and economic climate has turned to questions of efficiency and cost-effectiveness. This shift in dominant values has motivated many recent efforts at health system reform in Europe and North America and has brought changes in the ways governments arrange for the financing of health systems.

Canada is one of the few countries in the world that states explicit goals for its health system. As noted in the section "Legislative and Regulatory Framework," the five national standards in the Canada Health Act require that all Canadians have reasonable access to insured services, that such access be transferable across provincial boundaries and that provincial health insurance plans be nonprofit and administered by public agencies. From an evaluative perspective, it is noteworthy that four of the five goals deal primarily with social and political values relating to the rights of Canadians collectively to obtain needed care; only the public administration principle primarily relates to technical and administrative considerations.

Evaluation Criteria

Stone examines the four values—equity, efficiency, liberty, and security—that she believes are most frequently called on in the evaluation of public programs and policies.[131] Defining these values is not simple. For example, social conservatism tends to define equity as the result of a process of fair acquisition, liberty as the freedom to make one's own decisions and to dispose of one's own property, property as an individual creation of one's own actions, and work and productivity as motivated by financial need. Social liberalism, on the other hand, defines equity as a fair share of basic resources, liberty as freedom from dire necessity, property as a social creation, and work and productivity as motivated by security.

As Stone notes, equity and equality are not the same. "Equality usually denotes sameness and uniformity, whereas equity implies distributions that are regarded as fair even though they may contain both equalities and inequalities." The Canadian federal Equalization Program is a good example of using inequalities to achieve equity. The "have" provinces pay a disproportionate amount into the program so that the "have not" provinces can provide an equal level of public services. To understand the sources of the different interpretations of equity, Stone argues that we have to examine three aspects of any distribution of scarce resources: the recipient (i.e., who benefits from a policy program and how beneficiaries are defined), the item (i.e., what benefit is being distributed in the program and how it is defined), and the process (i.e., the social processes by which the distribution of the benefit are determined).

Stone defines efficiency as a comparative idea—"that is, it compares inputs to outputs, expenditures to income, or costs to benefits. No matter which comparison we undertake, we need to know what is to be measured, how it is to be measured, and who is benefiting from the program and who is shouldering the costs." Although efficiency is normally thought of as an objective criterion, the measurement of efficiency contains a large subjective component. For example, are the wages paid to providers viewed as an input (expenditure, cost), or as an output (income, benefit) (e.g., are they considered as a creator of employment)? The benefits attributed to a program may range from the objective and physical to the subjective and psychosocial. Determinations of cost-benefit ratios often depend on which costs and benefits are included, which in turn links back to which goals are being pursued. Different analysts can come up with very different conclusions; one person's efficiency can be seen as another person's waste.

Stone defines liberty as "being able to do as you wish as long as it does not involve harm to others. It is the value where there is the greatest tension between individual will and collective result." In other words, when can society compel people to bear individual costs in order to achieve social benefits? Environmental regulations are usually viewed as a legitimate restriction on individual liberty for the greater good; for example, restrictions on fishing are legislated to protect future fish stock. In the classical liberal tradition, it is believed that government should interfere with individual choice as little as possible and can justify restricting individual behaviour only if the behaviour adversely affects others. This definition is known as a "negative concept of liberty," because it concentrates on the absence of restraint. It is this definition that we use. From this viewpoint, policy issues are usually seen as a choice between protecting the liberty of individuals and preventing harm to others. However, restricting behaviour necessary to prevent one type of harm often results in another type of harm. As a result, questions of liberty often involve questions of equity because they require decisions about who will suffer the harm and whose activities should be restricted.

An alternative conception, termed a positive view of liberty, tends to further confuse liberty and equity. In this view, liberty is defined as the availability of meaningful choice and the capacity to exercise it. This definition accordingly leads to different questions: What kinds of resources (political rights, wealth, knowledge, health) are necessary to allow an individual to exercise effective choice? What role should society take in ensuring that these resources are distributed? The concept of positive liberty reveals the heart of the liberty-equality trade-off. People have different talents, skills and abilities that enable them to secure valued resources and opportunities. To maintain equality, government would have to redistribute resources and opportunities from the haves to the have-nots. This redistribution to achieve equality can be seen as infringing on the liberty of the advantaged.

Stone defines security as "the satisfaction of minimum human needs." The conflict over security usually involves the kinds and level of needs governments should attempt to meet and how to distribute the burdens of making security a collective responsibility. Accordingly, one can debate what is needed and by whom. Different policy prescriptions result if poverty is defined as absolute (e.g., falling below some predefined poverty line) or relative (e.g., falling below a predefined percentile in the income distribution; by definition, relative poverty can never be eradicated). Publicly funded health care can be justified because health is a desired outcome on its own or on the grounds that it produces a healthy and therefore more productive workforce, which allows for a more economically competitive nation. Benefits can also be justified on the basis of communal needs (e.g., dignity, self-esteem), a line of argument that leads to the often heard statement that medicare is precious to Canadians not only because of the physical needs it satisfies, but also because it defines us as a kinder, gentler nation.

The pattern of what are seen to be public needs is one of the defining characteristics of a society. Definitions of medical necessity differ from one country to another, and to some extent from one Canadian province to another. These differences reflect the trade-offs among security, efficiency, and liberty. Again, ideology often enters the debate. For example, some consider security and efficiency to be incompatible, on the grounds that security undermines work motivation and productivity and hinders progress and innovation; some argue that security also undermines liberty because it breeds dependence. In contrast, others maintain that security is essential for liberty, for people are free to make genuine choices only when their basic needs have been met. Debates about the extent to which one is justified in curtailing individual liberty to promote security and derive economic efficiency (e.g., seatbelt or smoking legislation) also boil down to the permissibility of paternalism in a free society.

How do these values relate to the different models of financing, delivery, and allocation outlined in the section "Understanding the Basis for the Current Public-Private Mix of Services"? The complexity of the reform debate often results from the same words being used to mean different things, as well as to different preferences for the trade-offs among these values. To that end, it is perhaps useful to examine the extremes in the models across the three dimensions and highlight the shifts in values as one goes from the public end of the continuum to the private in financing, delivery, and allocation.

Financing

The previously described financing models range from the public sector as the exclusive funder of a comprehensive mix of services, to the public sector having a minimum role with care being largely privately financed. Between these two extremes are a number of models that allow for complementary or parallel public and private plans.

Whenever the state is the sole financer of a comprehensive mix of services in the health system, equity is a dominant value, in that coverage usually includes all residents except perhaps those who have temporary or tenuous ties to the country. To the extent that financing of the public plan is achieved through progressive taxation and pooled risk, the burden is spread throughout the population. As one moves along the public-private continuum to include more private sector involvement, equity decreases; segments of the population (e.g., the unemployed, part-time workers, farmers, etc.) may be left out of the insurance system. Risk selection can mean higher premiums or no coverage at all for people whose risks are likely to be higher. At the extreme, one has the U.S. system, in which over 40 million are uninsured, and even more underinsured for medical costs. Options employing private financing for necessary care thus clearly rank lower on equity criteria.

The evaluation of financing models for the value of security is less clear. The extent to which basic needs for medical services are likely to be satisfied are more related to such issues as comprehensiveness of coverage, ease of access, and portability of benefits. Security for providers is clearly related to allocation mechanisms (e.g., whether there are provisions for fair and guaranteed reimbursement).

Although economic barriers to insured care are removed in public plans, there are still reasons why people do or do not seek care, and inequities in health status are likely to remain. Given the broadly recognized determinants of health, questions arise about the range of social services and the strategies for reducing income disparities that should be included. In theory, such security considerations could be met by either publicly or privately financed plans. In practice, equity considerations may imply differences in security, depending on what level of coverage can be afforded.

From a technical standpoint, continued public support for any plan is likely to be contingent on maintenance of its quality, including the availability of timely, high-quality care whenever it is needed. The mere existence of a private alternative could make it easier for governments to withdraw funds from the public system; that scenario could in turn lead to privatization by attrition—the progressive deterioration of public services and thus, for people who can afford it, greater incentive to flee the public system. Thus, the erosion of public plans affects the security of people who are not in a position to purchase private insurance, and equity in the quality of care provided. A number of indicators can be used to monitor the extent to which patients and providers are seeking to exit from the publicly funded plan (e.g., use of privately funded alternatives, difficulty in staffing the public system, waiting lists, emigration), and to indicate where improvements should be made to sustain a high-quality system.

As we have noted, international and Canadian evidence suggests that exclusive public financing of medically necessary care is the most efficient method. Efficiency is increased through the state's monopsony power over total budgets and over fee and salary negotiations with providers, as well as through reduced administrative costs and the pooling of risks. Proponents of increased private financing argue that an injection of additional private funding into the health system will increase overall levels of funding in the health system, lessen demand on an already overextended public system, and offer both consumers and providers a greater range of choice. In effect, such arguments concede the efficiency of public funding, noting instead that spending will increase (and carefully not commenting about whether the additional spending would purchase additional health benefits).

An additional efficiency consideration is that private plans rarely cover the higher-risk groups unless compelled by regulations. Both international and Canadian evidence suggests that national expenditures on health care as a proportion of gross domestic product are positively correlated with the proportion of private spending: the greater the private share, the greater the total share of national wealth devoted to the health care sector. The case studies have revealed that the cost escalation appears to have been higher in those areas of health care having greater roles for private financing (e.g., drugs, automobile insurance, travel health insurance) than in those with public financing and monopsony control (e.g., hospitals).

From a macroeconomic perspective, it is important to consider the impact of the type of health system financing on a country's economic productivity and competitiveness in world markets. For example, one must consider the extent to which funding for health systems diminishes the money available for other services and programs (e.g., education) that may be crucial to national prosperity. On the other hand, although public expenditure takes from the private economy money that might otherwise be available for other investment or consumption, the efficiencies of publicly financed health insurance relieve employers from having to pay the high costs of privately purchased health benefits for their employees, giving them a competitive advantage over producers in countries that must bear such costs on their payroll (e.g., the United States, Germany, and the Netherlands). Even if these costs are eventually passed on to workers through lower wages, the higher total cost is still a competitive disadvantage. In addition, work-based coverage may increase "job lock," interfering with labour mobility. Indeed, during the Canada-U.S. free trade negotiations, the Americans tried to argue that Canadian medicare was an unfair subsidy to Canadian industry. Current policy initiatives in Germany, and the Netherlands are seeking ways to remove health financing costs from payrolls because of fears that they have become "job killers."

Models that incorporate private sector financing of specialized or elective services alongside a publicly financed, comprehensive array of services are said by their advocates to provide for enhanced consumer and provider choice. Two-tier systems, in which people with the ability to pay can buy their way out, clearly affect equity, particularly if one's place in the queue is determined by ability to pay rather than by need. Patient security is not necessarily sacrificed if services in the public sector remain adequate and of good quality. Flight to the private sector by either providers or patients may threaten the viability of the public system if it is left to deal with a population of higher-risk patients. However, the greatest shortcoming of these models appears to be effectiveness. The Alberta data has demonstrated that private providers often charge more for similar services. In addition, private clinics receive hidden subsidies from the public, including the use of providers trained at public expense and the ability to send patients who incur complications back to the public system. Tax deductibility for private insurance payments also represents a subsidy by other taxpayers, including people who do not receive those benefits.

Contrary to naive economic thinking, our review suggests that public financing for medically necessary services increases both equity and efficiency. The key justification for the mixed financing plans therefore must rest on liberty. Single-source (public) financing restricts the ability of individuals to expend their income as they wish. As a result, private coverage is favoured by supporters of liberty in that people can choose not only the type of coverage they wish, but whether they wish to purchase coverage at all. Private coverage increases individual liberty by removing the subsidization of illness by those currently healthy (which often amounts to subsidy of the poor by the wealthy, and of the old by the young).[132]

Liberty—if defined as consumer choice of provider and care options and provider choice of practice setting, employment status, and method and level of remuneration—is determined more by the delivery and allocation models selected than by the financing model. However, until recently, public sector plans have interfered less in the medical decision making of providers than have private sector plans, largely because of the allocation methods being employed.

To the extent that liberty goals are paramount, policy options with respect to financing might be selected that are inferior on other dimensions. For example, although evidence suggests that public financing is superior when considering equity and efficiency, people with an ideological belief in markets may find these facts irrelevant.

Delivery

The public or private nature of delivery per se is not likely to have major implications for these values, except at the margin. Monopoly providers are seen to be less efficient and innovative; by the same token, public delivery is more likely to ensure service to areas that are not economically efficient to serve (e.g., rural and remote areas). The key weakness of public delivery is individual liberty; providers are not free to choose their type of practice, the payment method, or the amount of income they can earn. To the extent that delivery models force patients to roster, such models may be less responsive to consumer choice. However, economic efficiency can be pursued in either sector.

At the other extreme, models in which the public sector has a minimum role and in which service is largely delivered by private providers maximize liberty as defined in terms of provider and patient choice. However, equity in service provision and security can potentially suffer, the extent depending on the amount of government regulation of the industry, the health professions, and the quality of services. The efficiency of private, for-profit delivery depends on the nature of the services being delivered. The literature suggests that for-profit private sector institutions can provide good value for money when delivering programs with easily measured goals that are monitored and evaluated regularly. Therefore, in some sectors of the health system, such as the housekeeping services for institutions, the for-profit private sector may perform well. However, the for-profit private sector fares less well in delivering programs that have complex goals, such as most health and social services. In these cases, attention to the bottom line may detract from other complex social objectives. Providing services cheaply but without meeting intended goals is not efficient; it is a waste of money. Thus, delivery probably needs to be accompanied by performance expectations to ensure that providers are accountable and goals are met.

One reason that efficiency may increase in private delivery models is that private workers are less likely than public workers to be unionized and therefore are likely to be paid lower wages. In this equation of inputs and outputs, the workforce is seen as an input to health care. However, unions could equally view the employment of their members as an output and could, therefore, argue that efficiency through private sector delivery is bought at the price of equity and security for workers. As noted earlier, this question does not have a correct answer, but it does highlight the importance of clearly defining terms.

Any efficiency gains that may be realized through potential competition between the two sectors may be lessened if the private sector can "cherry pick" the people at lowest risk, leaving its competitors with the higher-risk (and higher-cost) groups. Once again, the subsidy of private sector services through publicly trained providers should be accounted for in any analysis of efficiency.

It must be understood that competition among private and public deliverers does not in itself reduce equity and security. Both privately and publicly delivered care can be publicly funded. However, if public financing is tied to public delivery and private financing to private delivery, as in the United States, the three values of equity, efficiency, and security are diminished, while liberty for those with the ability to pay is enhanced. Delivery models that are predominately private (both institutional and individual providers), but heavily government-regulated, can continue to ensure patient and provider choice while protecting the goals of both equity and security. In situations where public regulation is high, these institutions become quasi-public, mediating structures. Efficiency in these models can be maintained through a single-payer public financing model and an appropriate allocation mechanism.

Allocation

The public-private dimension relates to allocation models to the extent that certain forms of financing and delivery models are more compatible with certain allocation mechanisms. Allocation models vary most in their trade-off between liberty and efficiency; the level of equity and security depends more on the adequacy and quality of the plan than on the particular allocation mechanism chosen. Command-and-control models can provide macrolevel efficiencies through greater cost control exercised by monopsony power over budgets, fees, and even the ability to force closure of institutions. However, this control is often achieved at the expense of patient choice, not only in terms of what services are provided, but also in terms of where they are provided and by whom. In addition, provider security and liberty can be at stake if government uses its monopsony bargaining power to impose budget and fee ceilings, restrict billing privileges and hospital privileges, or micromanage medical decisions.

Pure market allocation mechanisms give more weight to liberty, but may sacrifice cost containment. Mesolevel and microlevel efficiencies can be realized through provider competition and through enhanced levels of institutional innovation. However, macrolevel efficiencies through system-wide cost control efforts are usually sacrificed.

The mixed allocation mechanisms also vary in their likely impact. For example, do providers compete for contracts from purchasing agents, or do they compete for patients? If patients can no longer directly choose their provider, what mechanisms are in place to ensure that the purchasing agents are accountable for their decisions? (At one extreme, elected regional bodies are, in theory, accountable to their community; at the other, for-profit insurance companies are accountable to their stockholders.) Efficiency gains through the competition for contracts or patients in planned markets may also be made at the expense of provider autonomy, as witnessed in many health maintenance organizations in the United States, where care decisions may be based on the desire to achieve microlevel efficiencies as well as on medical grounds.

FRAMEWORKS FOR MAKING DECISIONS ABOUT WHAT SHOULD AND WHAT SHOULD NOT BE INSURED

In any system relying on third-party payment, someone must decide what will be covered and what will not. In this section, we outline a number of approaches that have been used and comment on their perceived adequacy from the viewpoint of various people who must deal with them. We begin with the results of telephone interviews that we conducted with officials in the provincial and territorial governments to assess their views of the approach currently employed in the CHA.

We next briefly outline four alternatives: (1) Oregon's well-publicized attempts to ration what care should be provided to their Medicaid population, (2) the model proposed but not yet implemented in the Netherlands, (3) the four-screen model proposed by Deber and Ross for the Health Action Lobby, and (4) the Canadian Medical Association (CMA) modification of the four-screen model, currently being used by the CMA in an effort to define core and comprehensive services.

Each of the models of health care examined purports to provide a basic benefits package that ensures comprehensive coverage to a particular population. We found it useful to apply the following eight criteria:

- Who is included in the model (*universality*)?
- What is covered (*comprehensiveness*)?

- Is the model sufficiently *flexible* to allow for innovation and change in treatment patterns?
- Does the model recognize *variation* in clinical (expected) benefit and in patient values?
- Is the model able to monitor costs and *outcomes?* Does it set performance expectations?
- What are the model's needs for *information* in terms of procedures covered?
- How easy is the model to *implement?*
- How easy is it to control the *volume* and cost of core services to be provided?

Canada Health Act Model

As noted in previous sections, the CHA requires universal coverage for insured services. The federal government is responsible for determining the amounts of any deductions or withholdings pursuant to the act, including those for extra-billing and user charges.

As part of this study, we conducted a series of telephone interviews with senior officials of all Canadian provinces and territories. We very much appreciate their cooperation. The interview schedule is available on request. Here, we summarize key insights from our respondents.

Adequacy of CHA Definitions of Comprehensiveness

The key observed weakness in the CHA is its definition of comprehensiveness. As noted, advances in technology have allowed services to be delivered outside hospitals and by providers other than physicians. These developments have led the provinces to conclude that the CHA's definition of comprehensiveness is inadequate.

In a desire to cut costs, provinces and territories are attempting to deinsure services, often in consultation with the provincial medical association. One province, in collaboration with its medical association, has gone through the physician fee codes and clustered the insured services into three components, differing in political sensitivity. (An example of a service in the most sensitive category is abortion.) They then set up a review panel of government and physician representatives to examine services that could be cut from each category; the results are to go to the government and then to the medical society, but no formal public involvement is planned. Some provinces are establishing specific dollar targets for savings wrought by deinsuring services (e.g., Ontario and British Columbia). It should be noted that there are few specific fee schedule items whose elimination could give large savings with minimal health consequences, and that the medical services being deinsured are, to date, those perceived as marginal (e.g., Ontario removed facial hair removal and routine circumcision) and for which a private market is likely to remain.

However, provinces are also reducing or eliminating support for services not required under the terms of the CHA. Often, these support a broader definition of health (e.g., assistive devices, eye care, dental care, home support, pharmaceuticals), and their removal can be somewhat at odds with the determinants of health belief that most respondents professed to hold.

Comments from our respondents made it clear that difficult economic times have converted the CHA criteria from a floor to a ceiling. The act requires that particular medically necessary services be insured, but does not preclude coverage of additional services. Nonetheless, the provincial respondents commented that the definitions in the act reduce the opportunity for ancillary services to be covered and argued that the act is inflexible. Our respondents also noted that the concept of "medical necessity" is too vague. Sample comments include the following:

> Core services should represent comprehensiveness; we haven't given a lot of thought to it. We're dealing with a moving target.
>
> I don't know who should decide what is medically necessary. I'd consider the physicians who work in the system, but these groups are filled with self-interest.
>
> Society should decide what's medically necessary through their elected politicians.
>
> That's a tough question. I honestly don't know. Maybe we should tighten up the definition.
>
> Maybe it shouldn't be as rigidly defined as it is now.

All the provincial respondents believed that the government, in collaboration with providers and consumers, should decide the meaning of "comprehensiveness" and what is included under "medically necessary." They all stated that this decision making should use some sort of evidence-based efficacy and benefit analyses of health outcomes, but none of the provinces has made any moves in this direction to date. There is a huge amount of dissatisfaction with the current definitions, which are seen as inflexible, vague, and unresponsive to the changing needs of consumers. Although almost everyone believed that the concept of medical necessity perpetuated a medical model of illness rather than supporting a broad definition of health, no one could identify a useable alternative.

Particularly in the current economic climate, provincial governments appear unwilling to pay for items unless required to do so. Indeed, although most respondents stated that their province employs a broader definition of health than the one implicit under the terms of the CHA, there is little connection between this rhetoric and current funding patterns.

In reaction to federal changes to transfer payments, most provinces argue that if the federal government is reducing its financial role, it should also accept a reduced role in identifying priorities for health expenditures. This argument is often framed in terms of shifting the health care emphasis away from doctors and hospitals to what are presumably more cost-effective modes of care (including prevention).

The process of deinsurance has been relatively opportunistic and ad hoc. Comparatively few decisions have been evidence based or have considered the likely impact of coverage changes on the health of the population. Leapfrogging—the practice of provinces following one another's lead to deinsure services—is very common. Public participation in this process has been minimal, and indeed has not been sought by most provinces.

The federal government remains somewhat involved. The Department of Finance administers transfer payments to provinces. The Health Insurance Directorate is charged with ensuring systematic monitoring of the criteria and conditions as set out in the CHA. Currently, the provincial deputy ministers of health are considering comprehensiveness and trying to define what should be covered.

At this moment, the provinces that are worst off financially are generally covering only those services required by the CHA. The point made by many Atlantic respondents is that there is very little that could be cut without massive public disapproval.

Views of the Private Role

The role of private insurance was seen to be to pay for such extras as out-of-country benefits, but not for basic health services provided by the public sector. User fees were considered to be generally wasteful and ineffective for insured services, but copayments on drugs or user fees for home services or other uninsured services were seen to be acceptable by our respondents. Most stated that they do not want a tiered health system, but that they nonetheless believe one already exists.

The provinces interested in increasing the private role tend to be the most affluent. None of the Atlantic Provinces or northern territories is interested in reducing the public role; their focus instead is on how to finance current services with a smaller budget. These reactions strengthen the inference that the mixed funding models are cost-shifting rather than cost-saving measures and can only exist when there are enough affluent potential customers to allow a parallel market. Respondents from the more affluent provinces saw the efforts of the federal government to limit private involvement as a direct violation of their right to administer their own systems.

Cost was the major issue for all our respondents. There is a strong belief that it is necessary to scale back services today to help the system cope with increasing future demands. The current climate of cost control is leading to the belief that only those services that are "really needed" should be provided by the provincial governments. Privatization is thus seen as a way to move a cost burden away from governments, and hence as an option worth examining. A more restrictive view of the CHA is therefore emerging—that it should be interpreted to mean that no one should be denied access to health care, but not to mean that fees at point of service for some specified services are precluded.

Services That Governments Believe They Should Not Be Paying For

We asked which services our respondents thought that provincial governments should not be paying for. In general, they were uncomfortable with a list-based approach, recognizing that there is a sliding scale of benefit and that it is too easy to "game" any list-based approach. Some of our respondents hoped that changes in allocation procedures could allow the provincial governments greater flexibility. For example, it was suggested that primary physicians should be providing "needed care, not item by item." Some respondents explicitly rejected the Oregon approach, noting, "That didn't work out too well, did it? You end up priorizing everything." One of our respondents argued, "Most people can't connect with morbidity/mortality evidence-based statistics; what might be really important to someone's health is a primary care provider giving comfort, and that is unmeasurable." Clearly, it is easier to delegate to providers and patients the responsibility for deciding what is needed, after instituting a capped allocation system in which there are no financial incentives to overservice.

The difficulties of deinsuring on an item-by-item basis were pointed out by one respondent through the example of gallbladder surgeries, which he believed were performed inappropriately in 30 percent of total cases. He believed that it would be both politically impossible and generally unwise to deinsure all gallbladder surgery, particularly because designating 30 percent as inappropriate meant that 70 percent were appropriate. Also, because there are a large number of procedures on the fee schedule, there are unlikely to be great savings through delisting any individual item. For this reason, deinsurance has tended to happen around the margins of insured services, with physicians cooperating. The metaphor used by one representative was that we require a dimmer switch rather than an on-off switch. For instance, annual physicals have been deinsured in many provinces and territories for segments of the population, with the assent of physicians. However, it is important not to forgo the benefits of health education, health promotion, and early detection, which can occur through the mechanism of such examinations (e.g., following the recommendations of the Canadian Task Force on the Periodic Health Examination). In addition, it is important not to deinsure merely to create an additional private market operating outside cost constraints.

Our respondents noted that deinsuring services tends to be a long, slow, tedious process, particularly as insured services are provided by physicians, whose opinions are sought before any such action is taken.

As mentioned above, the most common pattern is referred to as leapfrogging, or "keeping down with the Jones"—in other words, deinsuring a service once another province takes the lead. The quick succession of deinsuring annual physical examinations is one example; eye care is another.

Although not discussed by our respondents, a number of interesting dilemmas arise. One is how to reconcile the role of primary physician as de facto gatekeeper with the desire to deemphasize physician services and focus on the broader determinants of health. Clearly, this reconciliation will depend on whether there are major changes in the delivery of health services. Another dilemma is whether attempts to allocate resources on the basis of perceived or actual benefit will run afoul of the equality protections of the Charter of Rights and Freedoms, particularly if the reallocation is construed as countenancing discrimination on the basis of age or disability.

In some provinces, these decisions have been delegated to regional health authorities.

Services That Would Ideally Be Insured

All the people we interviewed had a series of comments on the issue of what services would ideally be insured, centering on the narrow range of services that are currently insured and noting the need to get away from the "stovepipe" or "silo" mentality. As one respondent noted, "Insulin might be more medically necessary than a checkup. We have a whole series of anomalies based on providing basic acute crisis care." When patients are being sent home quicker and sicker and are able to be managed in the community as a result of pharmaceutical or technological advances, the deinsurance of the community-based portion of the care episode is a worry for most provinces and territories. The drive to cut costs is leading to ad hoc deinsurance, but it is also leading representatives to wonder why some costs are being borne while others, equally important to health, are not. However, the respondents noted that it is impractical to insure new services in the current economic climate, when other services are being cut.

Respondents from most provinces and territories made the point that their citizens had special requirements for comprehensive health coverage, and that national standards were therefore not fully appropriate. We confess to finding the argument uncompelling. In our view, medical necessity applies to the individual; provinces may differ in the proportions of their residents who need particular services, but not in whether Manitobans need things that people in Prince Edward Island do not. Equalization payments were designed precisely to ensure that Canadians could get similar levels of crucial services, wherever they happened to live, and Canadians strongly believe that health care is one such crucial service.

This question tended to tap into the dissatisfaction surrounding the services covered under the CHA; many of our respondents suggested that if the provinces were left to their own devices without federal conditions and requirements, they could identify which services would be most appropriate to insure for their constituency. The further fragmentation of the Canadian health system and the discrepancies that would likely increase as a result of such a shift did not seem to be a concern.

Processes for Insuring and Deinsuring

Of the respondents interviewed, only those from the territories indicated that the public has more than a nominal role in insuring or deinsuring services. The territories do not have many of the services that their southern counterparts do, and many of the services that they now offer and insure stemmed from grassroots demands. For instance, a segment on the television program *W5* on certain laparoscopic techniques led many residents of the Northwest Territories to lobby the government to provide this service, which it now does. The Yukon government was lobbied by its physicians to deinsure a surgical process for obesity in which excess skin is removed, on the basis of ineffectiveness and lack of medical evidence for the procedure. Both of the territorial respondents stated that public involvement can lead to an overemphasis on the demands of specific special interest groups. If their experiences can be generalized, the assumption underlying current provincial reforms—that planning on the basis of smaller regions will lead to more rational decision making based on the health needs of the population—may not hold up in practice.

Most decisions on insuring or deinsuring services are based on input from a limited number of stakeholders—primarily government and the provincial medical association. Participation by other groups, including affected members of the public, is rarely extensive, though lip service is paid to the concept. Although provinces believe that their processes are effective, the absence of evidence is striking. Neither insurance nor deinsurance decisions are commonly based on evidence, usually because decisions must be made too quickly for such evidence to be obtained. Neither is there systematic monitoring of the impact of coverage decisions (e.g., how has the deinsurance of routine eye care in Saskatchewan and Alberta affected the public and the health system).

A thread that ran through most of the discussions on this issue was that only those services with proven positive health outcomes should be paid for by the government. This notion begs the question of the burden of proof; are interventions effective until proven ineffective, or the other way around? Certainly, patients may not be able to wait until the evidence is clear, and many interventions are not readily susceptible to rigorous evaluation. Because few services are 100 percent ineffective, blanket deinsurance is not seen to be the answer. Accordingly, a scientific basis for determining effectiveness is being sought by most provinces and territories.

Examination of Canada Health Act Model

The current CHA model delegates determination of what medical or hospital services are required to the individual practitioner (usually, the physician), subject to professional judgement and any fiscal limitation imposed by the existence of an appropriate billing number within the fee schedule. Provinces are encouraged to adopt an all-or-nothing approach—either a service is insured for everyone or it is not insured for anyone—which has the difficulty of hindering the ability to target specific high-needs groups within the overall population.

One of the perceived strengths of the CHA model is its ability to keep up with changes in clinical patterns within the acute care setting—new technologies and techniques that are hospital based are easily absorbed into the model. On the other hand, the advent of technologies and drugs that shift care outside the physican-and-hospital sector can have the effect of deinsuring services that were once covered. No reference is made to geographic distribution, except in terms of the principle of accessibility, and no requirements are made for services provided outside hospitals, even if they are identical to inpatient services. Thus, there exists considerable scope for deinsuring outpatient services, particularly if they are not delivered by physicians. Neither public health nor mental health services are formally a part of medicare, which places such preventive services as well-baby clinics, family planning clinics, and community mental health programs in a tenuous position.

The current Canadian model leaves provinces in an ambiguous legal status when determining what procedures are or are not necessary, depending on how the provincial legislation is written. The explicit use of the hospital as the location of insured health services and of the physician as the gate-keeper of service relies on the who and where of service provision in a way that no longer adequately reflects the realities of health care needs nor the mounting fiscal pressures on the public system. There is currently no limitation based on effectiveness and affordability within global budgets, and the result has been an ad hoc deinsurance of services at the margin (even though many of these might be very effective).

One advantage of the current CHA model is that it is quite unambiguous about what must be covered. A disadvantage is that the clear rules both include procedures that are of dubious effectiveness and appropriateness and may omit necessary care delivered outside the physician and hospital sectors.

Oregon Model

The Oregon experiment began with an attempt to rank all potential interventions to determine explicitly what benefits should be publicly financed for the poor.[133] The monumental task of computing cost-effectiveness ratios for all procedures was undertaken, with the ranking process involving individuals, communities, and other interest groups in a debate to priorize a list of health services in terms of their value to society. A massive amount of information was required for the exercise, which included measuring marginal versus average costs and an ethical analysis of the resulting list and its exclusions. Decisions based on the Oregon model amount to judging net benefit of a health care service on its ability to maintain life, be cost effective, restore a person to an absence of disease, and be consistent with community values.

The Oregon model has been commended for its explicit nature, the effort to introduce efficiency criteria and the conscientious involvement of the public, which forced "an articulation of social values and a focus on accountability."[134]

On the other hand, weaknesses with the approach are also evident. One cause of disquiet is that the judgements apply only to the subset of low-income people who are eligible for Medicaid, while the community participants aiding in the ranking were middle-class individuals (many, health professionals) who were unlikely to be bound by the decisions they were making. Another concern relates to the technical complexity of the task; unfortunately, the calculations were not performed correctly, and the resulting numbers proved neither reliable nor valid.[135] A third was the omission of potentially beneficial treatments; the example given by the Canadian Medical Association is the medical or surgical treatment of metastatic cancer of various sites where treatment would not result in greater than 5 percent survival five years after onset.

The debate centering around ethical problems with the model has not run its course, for the informational requirements are very large. In addition, because the model is the result of a snapshot exercise resulting in a static list of insured services, it will encounter difficulty absorbing innovation and changes in clinical practice or treatment patterns. Adding or subtracting procedures will be time consuming and complex. Indeed, the inflexibility of the Oregon model was noted by many of the Canadian government officials interviewed in this research and was the major reason for their belief that the model would be inappropriate as a possible replacement for the current CHA approach.

The Oregon process starkly revealed how little consensus there is about what medical care is appropriate or necessary: a large number of iterations were required to come up with a list and there was very little agreement on specific rankings. To designate a service as necessary, the Oregon list relies on the service's proven effectiveness. This method is not tailored to the needs or desires of individual patients, and it therefore results in a list of services that is both static and disempowering of the patient. There is no mechanism for a flexible approach to new technologies or for a quick response to changes in clinical practice, nor does this model reflect the fact that patients vary in how likely they are to benefit even from effective care.

Netherlands Model

The Netherlands model defines health as the ability to function normally, and then breaks this definition down further into three parts: for the individual, this ability is defined as self-determination and autonomy; the medical professional defines normal as the absence of disease; and the community sees health as allowing every member of society to function normally.

Which definition is applied is based on the level of the decision being made. At the level of the nation (macrolevel), the community approach is emphasized; at the institutional (meso) level, the professional approach rules; and the individual caregiver (microlevel) is guided by the individual approach. The Netherlands model uses a top-down approach, with limits imposed by the macrolevel shaping the parameters of the mesolevel, and the limits defined by the macro- and mesolevels curtailing the scope of the individual approach. The result is that necessary care is defined differently for each group, allowing targeting of specific needs, although overlap is permitted.

The process of defining necessary care in the Netherlands involves four sieves. The first sieve takes out unnecessary care based on a community approach, the second sieve allows only documented effective care to pass through, the third selects on efficiency (as measured by cost-effectiveness or similar methods), and the fourth eliminates care that can be left to individual responsibility. Only care that falls through all four sieves is included in the basic benefit package.

Based on the premise that not all health care services should or can be publicly funded, the Netherlands model recommended that individual rights and professional autonomy be limited in the interests of equity and solidarity in health care. It argues for the appropriate use of waiting lists. It recommends that health care professionals be accountable for the continuity of patient care by making appropriate use of many services that Canada does not consider to be part of comprehensive services, such as community-based psychotherapy, drugs, and physiotherapy.

The Netherlands model recommended a legal description of the rights in the basic package, the legislation of the quality of care for mentally and physically handicapped patients and psychiatric patients, and the promotion of research into the costs and benefits of the health care offered. Other recommendations include a critical review of waiting lists; a setting of priorities; an independent agency with links in the European community to assess new technologies for safety and effectiveness; accountability by professionals, their associations, and other providers by working with insurers and patient organizations and setting up protocols, guidelines, and essential lists for appropriate care; and a process to encourage public discussion to create the social consensus desirable for political decision-making.

The Netherlands model is highly restrictive—it excludes much care that might be beneficial but whose benefits are not yet proven, and it also excludes expensive care, regardless of benefits. The model suggests that such services should be provided elsewhere (and therefore only to those who can afford additional insurance coverage) and as such is not an excellent fit for a universal single-payer system. Particular decisions are also somewhat arbitrary (e.g., the model suggests that sports injuries and admission to homes for the elderly should be included in the basic package).

Four-Screen Model (Deber-Ross)

The four-screen model was developed by Deber and Ross for the Health Action Lobby in reaction to the difficulties with the comprehensiveness definition of the Canada Health Act. The model begins at a microlevel (individual), considering whether to pay for a particular intervention for a particular individual, although implementation is greatly simplified if it is then aggregated to the macrolevel (societal) to determine a global budget, within which specific allocation decisions can be made. (We refer to this variant as the global four-screen model.) Like the Netherlands model, the four-screen model suggests that decisions about coverage should be made as a function of four screens, arranged hierarchically, such that only those interventions passing an earlier screen need be considered at the next stage (table 13).

The first two screens are evidence based. Screen 1 (effectiveness) examines whether the given intervention works. Screen 2 (appropriateness) incorporates information about the risks and benefits to particular individuals, and is therefore individualized to a particular person in a particular setting. An ongoing issue is how to handle uncertainty about the evidence. A number of approaches purporting to be evidence based (including the Netherlands model described above) make the fundamental error of presuming that "proven ineffective" is the same as "not proven effective; since so much of medical practice has not yet been evaluated, this approach would reject most interventions, including many which are likely to be of considerable benefit."[136] Such policies thus tend to be counter-intuitive, and thus unacceptable to providers and the public. It is notable that few attempts to implement such stringent guidelines have been successful. The four-screen model instead suggests that such interventions receive a conditional pass, contingent both on encouraging evaluation such that future decisions can be made on better evidence, and on fully informing decision makers about the extent of evidence supporting the intervention.

Table 13

The four-screen model

Screen	Criteria	Basis for choice: Who is involved?	Additional issues
1. Effectiveness *Does it work?*	*Clinical:* Safety, effectiveness, efficacy, etc.	*Evidence based:* International researchers Professional organizations Providers/institutions	Burden of proof? Quality of evidence?
2. Appropriateness *Is it needed?*	*Clinical:* Expected benefit, given clinical situation	*Evidence based:* Providers/institutions Professional organizations (e.g., guidelines) International researchers	Burden of proof? Extent of benefit?
3. Informed choice *Is it wanted?*	*Personal:* Match between expected outcomes and patient wishes	*Value based:* Patients Providers	Informed patient?
4. Public provision *Should the public pay?*	*Economic/political:* 1. Cost minimization? 2. Can society tolerate denial? 3. Advance knowledge/evaluate pratice?	*Value based:* Citizens Governments	Participation process? Available resources?

The third and fourth screens are based on values. Screen 3 (informed choice) incorporates the view of the recipients of care (as patients, clients, or consumers). The model is not a pure consumer sovereignty approach; people would not be offered choices unless those interventions had passed the first two screens. However, many clinical decisions are toss-ups—offering almost equal chance of success or risk of failure—and patient values and preferences can often determine what would be the optimal choice in such cases. The logic of the four-screen model is that items that do not pass the first three screens should not be paid for by anyone—if something is ineffective, inappropriate, or not wanted, it is difficult to justify why it should be provided at all.

In ideal practice, the key dilemmas would thus arise at screen 4 (public provision). Given that something might benefit an individual, should a third party pay for it? Deber and Ross propose that such decisions should include at least three considerations: cost minimization, social values, and advance knowledge.

Cost Minimization

Is the proposed service the least expensive way of achieving a desired goal? For example, exercise may be beneficial to health, but there are many inexpensive ways of exercising, and therefore health club fees need not be publicly financed. Similarly, providers should be encouraged to deliver care as efficiently as possible (which might include major restructuring of the system of care). This criterion is not equivalent to determination of cost-effectiveness, because it makes no effort to determine whether a particular benefit is worth purchasing; rather, it presents the far weaker requirement that any benefit purchased (of a specified level of quality, timeliness, etc.) be obtained at the lowest possible cost.

Social Values

The four-screen model proposes asking the following question: "If an individual would like to receive an intervention that is likely to benefit him, but cannot afford it, do we as a society find it acceptable that the intervention be withheld from that person?" We propose that a "no" answer implies that we find the procedure medically necessary for that individual. As the literature suggests, single-source financing is preferable under such circumstances, and hence public financing is appropriate for reasons of cost control and avoidance of risk selection. However, if we do find it acceptable to deny such care, the model would not require that it be included in the public plan.

Advance Knowledge

To resolve the future of conditional passes and to ensure progress in the ability to improve health, one might also want to publicly finance the introduction and evaluation of interventions (within the context of research) and thus to improve future decisions.

The Model in Practice

How would the four-screen model work in practice? Consider several examples. Many currently funded treatments would clearly pass. A cardiac bypass would pass screen 1—it can be effective. Screen 2 would further specify the categories of patients for whom benefit would probably outweigh risk. At screen 3, such potential patients would be informed of the alternatives; some would choose less aggressive treatment. Screen 4 might argue that other approaches (e.g., diet) would be more appropriate for some categories of patient, but would recommend public provision for those categories of patients to whom society would not be willing to deny treatment. Other currently funded interventions (e.g., routine X rays) might not pass; screens 2 and 4 might imply that they should be more clearly targeted. Some interventions not currently funded—e.g., insulin for severe diabetics—would probably pass all four screens. Decisions about health promotion and disease prevention efforts would be similarly mixed; exercise classes and alternative therapies with no evidence of effectiveness might not pass, whereas prenatal classes and psychological support for cancer patients might.

The logic of the four-screen model would thus give a role for private financing for a limited subset of items.

The same logic, however, presents difficulties for private insurance. At first glance, it is not clear why anyone would want to pay for interventions that were ineffective, inappropriate, or unwanted. There could be a niche market for luxury care that failed the cost minimization or social values tests. However, such interventions are very likely to give rise to issues of moral hazard among potential customers. For example, insurance companies are unwilling to insure cosmetic surgery, knowing that the biggest market would be among the people most likely to use it.

In practice, difficulties may instead arise at screen 2, appropriateness. The four-screen model assumes that the publicly financed system would provide all needed care and that such care would be accessible, timely, and of high quality. Should this assumption not be true, there would be pressure to allow individuals to buy their way up the queue. The availability of a private alternative would in turn present ethical dilemmas for providers. This screen is based on expert judgement, but nonetheless would rarely be clear cut. Accordingly, there would be economic incentives to give a lower priority for publicly financed care to people willing or able to pay for private treatment.

This issue has been less noticeable within hospitals: although global budgeting requires that priorities be set, one does not worry that a patient turned away from an intensive care unit will be induced to attend the private unit down the street. However, community-based care has fewer barriers to entry; accordingly, implementation would have to include mechanisms to minimize the opportunity for this kind of "gaming." Fortunately, a number of such controls exist. First, and most importantly, a strong control is the professionalism of providers, who wish to ensure high-quality care for their patients. Under this model, it would be important to reinforce these ethical standards by reimbursement mechanisms that do not provide perverse incentives; for example, physician payment arrangements should be neutral with respect to clinical judgement, and payment arrangements should not encourage churning a high volume of patients regardless of clinical appropriateness. Current provisions to prohibit clinicians from practicing both within and outside the publicly financed system for necessary care might need some modification, but should remain largely intact.

Finally, mechanisms would need to be in place to ensure that financing bodies provided adequate funding to cover the service mix and volume deemed necessary. This model does not see a role for private insurance to provide necessary care that was unavailable due to the inadequacy of the public system; if a nation is too poor to afford care within the available public financing, it is difficult to see how it can afford the higher bills to provide such care through the private sector, unless it is specifically envisioned that only a handful of people able to benefit will in fact receive the intervention.

The global four-screen model might be implemented relatively simply. First, one would compute, using the best available epidemiological data (e.g., incidence and prevalence of conditions for which a particular intervention would be effective and appropriate, and estimates of the proportion of people with that condition who would wish to receive the intervention), an estimate of the mix and volume of interventions that would pass all four screens for a defined population. Next, one would establish a global budget that would be sufficient to provide those services. If the sum were out of line with available resources and sufficient economies could not be achieved through reforming delivery models, the expectations (especially at screen 4) would have to be revisited. Once the budget was determined, providers and patients, in partnership, would make the microallocation decisions. Feedback mechanisms would be established to determine where better data was needed for future budget setting, how best to obtain such data, and how to incorporate the results into future decision making. The approach would be continuous, but one would not need to gather evidence about all procedures; one could begin with procedures having the greatest impact and progress incrementally, using best-guess data, for the remainder.

In effect, the global four-screen model expands the concept of a hospital global budget to include the wider array of health-related interventions funded from the public purse, allowing internal reallocations by providers to provide the needed care as efficiently as possible. The regional budgets now being tried across Canada are one—but not the only— way of achieving this goal; populations need not be defined geographically, and the critical mass for different interventions may vary. The four-screen approach merely suggests that budgets be established within which providers would be expected to provide a particular volume and mix of services to a particular population. Accountability mechanisms would ensure that the needed care was indeed being delivered in a high-quality, timely manner. This approach would probably not require the reopening of the Canada Health Act, assuming that provincial and regional governments are willing to maintain the spirit of the act within the broader range of services to be provided (i.e., take advantage of the "practitioner" definition of the act, and consider clinics to be the equivalent of hospitals).

CMA Core and Comprehensiveness Project

The four-screen model was one of those considered by the Canadian Medical Association (CMA) for their Core and Comprehensiveness Project. This ambitious effort has been a laudable attempt to see whether an organized process can be used to make coverage decisions and gives some guidance about the growing pains inherent in any attempt to use such a model.

The designers of the CMA process believed that the four-screen model places too much emphasis on the microlevel and, by not being specific about how such decisions would be aggregated, relies too much on top-down planning. Their modified model therefore includes questions that look explicitly at the macro- and mesolevels, as well. They commented that decision making occurs in the system at all levels: What seems to be an acceptable decision at the macrolevel may not be deliverable at the meso-level and may not be appropriate for the patient or practitioner at the micro-level. For these reasons, they broke the model down into three levels of decision making. The CMA framework sees the screens as encompassing three content dimensions: quality of care, ethics, and economics. It also considers the perspectives of three stakeholder groups: patients, providers, and payers. In an effort to be comprehensive, the guide to using the CMA model includes 11 questions about quality (5 macro, 3 meso, 3 macro), 19 about ethics, and 18 about economics.

The model was first employed to make recommendations about three clinical issues: prostate-specific antigen screening, gastroplasty, and the annual physical examination. A comprehensive literature review of the evidence about these interventions was commissioned,[137] and a committee then met to try to apply the CMA model.

Although in general the process appeared to work quite well, a number of practical problems arose. For example, clinicians at the microlevel reportedly found the model to be "unwieldy, unhelpful and not applicable to their decision-making processes," largely because it seemed to ignore the realities of the current practice of "defensive medicine," wherein a patient's demand for insured health service may be acceded to, regardless of expected benefit. (To the extent that a more rational process would attempt to eliminate defensive medicine, of course, this aspect may be an advantage rather than a disadvantage of the model.)

Examination of Four-Screen Model and CMA Approaches

Concrete examples make it clear that there are some fundamental differences between what is covered by the CHA and what would pass the four-screen model. For example, many pharmaceuticals (e.g., insulin for diabetics) would probably be included under the four-screen model, whereas many marginal physician services would probably not be. We do not pretend that such decisions would be simple—for example, new reproductive technologies would probably not pass screen 4 (if for no other reason than a belief by many taxpayers that people who cannot afford the procedure probably cannot afford a child), yet there are strong proponents for these procedures.

The major difference of the four-screen model from the CHA approach is the ability to tailor coverage (using screens 2 and 3) rather than making all-or-nothing decisions. That ability, in turn, implies that significant changes would have to be made in other parts of the health care system. For example, fee-for-service systems require a fee schedule. It is unclear whether court decisions will permit tailored fees—services are usually covered or not covered. In contrast, the global four-screen model could be used by planners to estimate how many times each procedure would likely be needed in a defined population and thus to determine a global budget. Providers and patients could then determine the precise allocations within the organization. The funder would have performance expectations (which would have to be enforced by accountability mechanisms and recourse for patients dissatisfied with allocation decisions), but the organization would have the flexibility to allocate resources within those expectations. The evidence requirements are also lower than for Oregon-style models, since evaluation could be staged to concentrate first on the areas where evidence is most needed.

The global four-screen model was designed to operate at the microlevel, but to be capable of aggregation. In other words, there would be no list of procedures that would be covered; rather, the global budget would be set on an epidemiological prediction that, for a given population, there should be approximately X hip replacements, Y cases of diabetes, and Z patients with high blood pressure. Individual clinical decisions would thus be made within the provider organization by patient and provider. New therapies could be substituted as long as they stayed within the budget; if necessary, an extra hip replacement could be performed by diverting resources from other services. Performance expectations would be set and monitored by the financing organization, but no micromanagement would be performed.

The CMA model resembles the four-screen model in terms of flexibility. Patient values and clinical benefit are evaluated at all three levels of the model in the same way as is in the four-screen model at the macrolevel. From the limited evaluation of the CMA model that we are aware of, the model has most problems at the microlevel, where physicians evidently feel unable to deny to the patient access to insured health services, regardless of anticipated benefit. The CMA model also resembles the four-screen model in that it relies heavily on evidence for decision making, but with a looser evaluation of effectiveness than the Netherlands model, because in many instances the information required to evaluate a potentially useful health care service is inadequate. At each level in the CMA model, the efficacy and appropriateness of the health care service is evaluated according to the quality of the available evidence and its capacity to be generalized.

The impact on comprehensiveness of the CMA model is difficult to analyze, because of disturbing questions related to private insurance and a lack of attention paid to continuity of care outside physician-as-provider models. Whereas the Netherlands model explicitly states that physicians have an obligation to ensure effective continuity of care through appropriate health services such as physiotherapy or community mental health, there is no such explicit demand in the CMA model.

Summary of Models

The characteristics of the approaches examined are summarized in table 14.

Although the global four-screen model has not yet been tested, we believe that it (or an adaptation) has the most potential to improve resource allocation at the microlevel. However, it does presuppose reforms in allocation, reimbursement, and the organization of health care delivery. In contrast, the other models appear to assume a continuation of current patterns of physician reimbursement, and to allow a larger place for private payment for services. For example, the CMA model explicitly asks whether private insurers are willing to insure a core health service, without grounding this question in a consideration of under which circumstances (if at all) this insurance would be justifiable. However, our analysis has led to the conclusion that the concept of a needed service that is privately insured poses both economic and ethical difficulties.

Table 14

Summary of model characteristics

Criterion	Model					
	CHA	Oregon	Netherlands	Global four screen	CMA	
Who is included (*universality*)?	All	The poor	All	All	All	
What is covered (*comprehensiveness*)?	P, h	List	List	Needed care	Core services	
Is it sufficiently *flexible* to allow for innovation and change in treatment patterns?	No	No	Maybe	Yes	Yes	
Does it recognize *variation* in clinical (expected) benefit and in patient values?	Maybe	No	No	Yes	Yes	
Is it able to monitor costs and *outcomes*?	Yes	Yes	Yes	Yes	Yes	
Does it set performance expectations?	No	No	No	Maybe	Maybe	
Does it deny potentially beneficial care?	No	Yes	Yes	Maybe	Maybe	
What are its needs for *information* in terms of procedures covered?	Low	High	High	High	High	
Is the model simple to *implement*?	Yes	Med.	Med.	Med.	Med.	
How easy is it to control the *volume* and cost of "core" services to be provided?	Low (p) High (h)	Low	Med.	High	Med.	

p = physicians.

h = hospitals.

POLICY IMPLICATIONS AND RECOMMENDATIONS

A number of combinations of public and private financing are feasible within advanced industrialized countries. This document has presented a conceptual framework and a review of selected activity. We conclude with a risky step—indicating what our preferred model would be, in the full recognition that this model reflects our own values and biases.

Recommendations

Recommendation 1 – Public Financing for Medically Required Services

Adams and colleagues[138] discuss the various financing mechanisms used in Canada and summarize their effects on health policy, in particular on the policy objectives of equity, utilization and cost containment, economic competitiveness, public acceptability, and economic efficiency. They conclude that the more pluralist mechanisms (i.e., those that move away from single sources of financing) tend to have negative effects on the policy objectives of equity and efficiency. France and the United States have clear examples of health systems with high levels of cost sharing, and both countries are currently coping with increases in the volume of physician services and escalating health care expenditures. The United States spends the greatest amount of money on health care in the world, and France spends among the highest amounts in Europe. Both countries have focused more on cost shifting than on cost containment.

As discussed earlier, a more pluralistic array of funding sources gives rise to two key policy dilemmas. First, it is easier to shift costs than it is to cut them. There is a tendency for each payer to attempt to avoid clients likely to generate high costs. As Evans has noted, "Private insurance for the whole population is impossible in a competitive market, because insurers cannot cover the poor and the ill and remain competitive."[139] Systems using multiple competing insurers then run into the ethical dilemma of cherry picking or cream skimming. Insurance companies try to shift costly patients over to other (frequently public) insurers, while retaining the youngest and least costly patients for themselves.

Second, monopsony (or single purchaser) bargaining power over providers is harder to achieve in multiple-payer systems. If public policy agrees that individuals should not be denied services that they need but cannot pay for, no one can be priced out of the market. Under such circumstances, no pure market can be said to exist, and alternative measures may be required to achieve cost control, which the evidence suggests are easier to accomplish in a single-payer system.

We conclude that single-source, public (or heavily regulated private) financing of medically necessary services coupled with private sector delivery seems to be the optimal model for health systems in terms of maintaining equity while increasing cost-effectiveness. The lesson is that it is inadvisable to reform health systems by privatizing financing for medically required services. Our reading of the international evidence suggests that these policy directions may seem to have short-run political benefits, but will prove to be unwise in the long run. Our review also suggests the need for greater attention to allocation mechanisms and greater consideration of what incentive structures will exist for payers, providers, and patients.

This recommendation is perhaps the least controversial—the evidence strongly supports the advantages of continuing to maintain public financing, and indeed the European reforms do not challenge this approach. We would accordingly reject any models that encourage the more affluent to opt out by purchasing private coverage for insured services, particularly if this purchasing were seen as necessary because timely and appropriate care was not available within the publicly funded system.

Acceptance that medically required services should be publicly financed would require modification of Canada's current system in two directions. First, many services now being offered are of dubious value to many recipients. Greater attention to the appropriateness of care may help prune such marginal activities. There is also a great potential in educating patients; shared decision-making experiments suggest that few patients are likely to desire unnecessary care. We are cautious about the scope of placing such pruned services into a privately financed supplementary system—unnecessary care should not be worth purchasing at any cost. Necessary care is likely to be purchased by those who can afford it; as Evans has noted, market assumptions do not apply well to these issues. Deinsurance of valuable services thus raises equity issues in denying care to people who cannot afford to pay, and efficiency issues inherent in any moves to a multiple-payer system. Instead, we suggest the probable need to reexamine methods of provider remuneration to ensure that reimbursement is independent of clinical judgement and that clinicians are not penalized financially for not providing marginal care. Deinsurance of services not seen as potentially beneficial yields fewer dilemmas, as long as information provisions ensure that patients are aware of the facts. Models in which patients are informed by their providers that there are uninsured services that might benefit them, but that are available only at a price, are generally dubious in our view.

Second, some medically necessary services do not fall under the requirements of the Canada Health Act. Some provincial governments have taken steps to insure such care (e.g., catastrophic drug insurance plans); these steps should be encouraged.

Recommendation 2 – Mixed (Largely Private Not-for-Profit) Delivery

Our recommendation for mixed but largely private delivery is also fairly uncontroversial, and it should be noted that countries that had employed public delivery are now tending to privatize it. There is, and should be, a major public role in regulating providers to ensure that their services are of high quality; such activities can be delegated to mediating structures (e.g., professional colleges), but must operate in the public interest. We therefore reject the "no public role" delivery models for services that could present harm to the public if delivered inappropriately. We also reject, in general, models of public provision, on the grounds that they are likely to be less sensitive to client needs.

Equity criteria would presumably reject stigmatizing delivery models (e.g., social safety net). Assuming the ability to deliver high-quality services to people requiring them, and to deliver them efficiently, a wide array of models would be appropriate. In general, however, we suspect that the best combination is likely to be competing private deliverers (many if not most being not-for-profit if the goals are complex and difficult to define).

However, it appears important to have strong performance expectations. At a minimum, it is reasonable to expect that providers deliver high-quality, timely care to people who need it at an affordable price. At least anecdotally, situations are emerging in which unacceptable waiting lists are arising. To the extent that such problems arise from underfinancing, payers must scrutinize how resources are employed and redeploy them as necessary. To the extent that such problems arise from poor management or perverse incentives (e.g., to underuse expensive resources), allocation mechanisms should ensure that providers are responsive and accountable.

This recommendation implies, however, that the resources must be adequate to ensure that all medically necessary services can be provided in a timely manner, that resources are sufficient to maintain high quality and that providers obtain reasonable reimbursement for their activities. We share the widely held belief that, with appropriate restructuring of the delivery system (which may imply fewer providers being paid by the health care system) and careful attention to allocation mechanisms, Canada has sufficient resources to accomplish these goals.

Recommendation 3 – Public Competition Allocation

Although a number of models are possible, the precise combinations required to both achieve cost control and maintain sufficient liberty for patients and providers are not yet established. We are nonetheless cautious about either extreme on the allocation continuum. Overly planned models may achieve equity, but so infringe on liberty as to lose public support. Managed competition models pursue efficiency, but may present threats to equity, security (if risk selection occurs), and liberty. Market allocation models without spending caps threaten efficiency. We suspect that investigation of the best models will consume the attention of health planners for the next decade. Perhaps the highest value, then, will be flexibility, so that modifications can be made as the inevitable problems arise.

At least two observations can be made. First, it is important that allocation models avoid incentives for risk selection; models encouraging competition among integrated delivery systems by paying each a capitated age-adjusted and sex-adjusted sum may present such problems, particularly given the current inability to risk-adjust such payments fully and accurately. Second, the increasing visibility of privately financed options for medically necessary services, despite fairly clear evidence of their undesirability, suggests three cautions:

- The existing allocation system may not have sufficient performance expectations to ensure that existing providers give high-quality, timely care when it is needed. Perverse incentives may lead to underutilization of existing resources (e.g., machines, operating rooms, physicians) and artificially lengthened waiting lists.
- The existing allocation system does not give sufficient attention to monitoring outcomes.
- Government has incentives to off-load costs, even if off-loading threatens the system.

We do not believe that many Canadians would wish to purchase care privately if high-quality care were accessible in a timely manner. We believe that the evidence suggests that people find choice far more important in the context of delivery.

Recommendation 4 – Client-Sensitive Determination of Medical Necessity (No Lists)

Our review of the Canada Health Act has suggested that the current definitions of medical necessity are no longer adequate, having been overtaken by technology. In addition, list-based approaches tend to be rigid and inflexible. Therefore, our final recommendation suggests the need to recognize that people vary widely both in what care would be appropriate for them and in what care they would wish to receive. We suggest that an approach similar to the global four-screen model, which incorporates evidence about effectiveness and appropriateness, the values held by patients and the public about what care they wish to receive and how they wish resources to be used, has considerable potential to lead to wiser use of public medicare dollars.

This recommendation has a downside—it is clearly easier to implement a list indicating what is covered and what is not, even if decisions at the margin may be irrational and suboptimal (i.e., covering unnecessary and inappropriate care, omitting crucial services). We believe that systems can be designed to minimize the possibility of "gaming," although no system is immune to problems. The global four-screen model relies heavily—perhaps too heavily—on the professionalism and goodwill of providers, patients, and funders. It suggests that people should forgo the opportunity to seek care outside the publicly financed system; this suggestion in turn implies that they can obtain what they need inside the system. It suggests that providers forgo the opportunity to earn additional income beyond what the publicly financed system is willing to provide; again, this suggestion implies fair treatment of providers and sensible reimbursement systems without perverse incentives. It suggests that government spend the resources necessary to achieve high-quality, timely care and forgo the political temptation of cost shifting.

It is often said that Canadians value their health care system; maintaining a workable model will give us the opportunity to prove this.

Acknowledgements

This report could not have been completed without assistance from a wide assortment of people, to whom we offer our grateful thanks:

- *the National Forum on Health, especially Marcel Saulnier and the members of the "Striking a Balance" working group—Steven Lewis, Bob Evans, Bill Blundell, Richard Cashin, André-Pierre Contandriopoulos and Tom Noseworthy*
- *the Task Force on the Financing and Delivery of Health Care, especially George Connell and Vicky Wooten (An earlier version of the sections "Understanding the Basis for the Current Public-Private Mix of Services" and "Legislative and Regulatory Framework" was prepared for their report; we appreciate their willingness to let us adapt it.)*
- *Jim Daw, Toronto Star, who gave us access to his excellent reporting about automobile insurance and travel health insurance*
- *Wendy Armstrong, Consumers Association of Canada (Alberta), who gave us access to their research and her considerable knowledge*
- *Carol Kushner, Toronto, and Dr. S. Duckett for information about Australia, and helpful conversations*
- *William Tholl, Mary Colbran-Smith, Owen Adams, Dr. David Walters, Margo Rowan, and other staffers at the Canadian Medical Association for sharing their work on the Core and Comprehensiveness Project*
- *Eleanor Ross, Tina Smith, and Gilbert Sharpe for helpful suggestions*
- *all of our interviewees and sources in the provincial governments, many of whom have asked to remain nameless, who were patient and who helped provide data*
- *Ann Pendleton for exemplary research assistance, and Christina Lopez and Florinda Cesario for secretarial skill and excellent chart making.*

Raisa Deber *is a professor of health policy in the Department of Health Administration at the University of Toronto. She holds a Ph.D. in political science from the Massachusetts Institute of Technology. She has written, taught, and consulted on many aspects of Canadian health policy. Her current research focuses on the public-private mix, implications of purchase models for specialized services, shared decision making, and patient empowerment.*

ENDNOTES

1. *The Public and Private Financing of Canada's Health System,* discussion paper. (National Forum on Health, 1995).

2. A. BLOMQVIST. Sound advice: Prescription for health care reform in Canada. *C.D. Howe Institute Commentary,* 58 (1994): 1–20; A. BLOMQVIST and D. M. BROWN, eds., *Limits to Care: Reforming Canada's Health System in an Age of Restraint.* (Toronto (ON): C.D. Howe Institute, 1994).

3. P. STARR. The meaning of privatization. In *Privatization and the Welfare State,* eds. S. B. KAMERMAN and A. J. KAHN. (Princeton (NJ): Princeton University Press, 1989), 15–48.

4. R. B. SALTMAN. *The Public-Private Mix in Financing and Producing Health Services.* mimeo report prepared for the World Bank, February, 1995.

5. M. OLSON. *The Logic of Collective Action: Public Goods and the Theory of Groups.* (Cambridge (MA): Harvard University Press, 1965).

6. R. B. DEBER. Philosophical underpinnings of Canada's health care system. *Can-US Outlook,* 2(4) (1991): 20–45; L.A. PAL. *Public Policy Analysis: An Introduction,* 2nd ed. (Scarborough (ON): Nelson Canada, 1992).

7. M. JÉRÔME-FORGET, J. WHITE and J. M. WIENER, Eds. *Health Care Reform Through Internal Markets: Experience and Proposals.* (Ottawa (ON): The Institute for Research on Public Policy/The Brookings Institution, 1995).

8. STARR 1989.

9. M. BENDICK Jr. Privatizing the delivery of social welfare services: An ideal to be taken seriously. In *Privatization and the Welfare State,* eds. S. B. KAMERMAN and A. J. KAHN. (Princeton (NJ): Princeton University Press, 1989), 97–120.

10. CANADIAN MEDICAL ASSOCIATION WORKING GROUP ON HEALTH SYSTEM FINANCING IN CANADA. *Toward a New Consensus on Health Care Financing in Canada,* discussion paper prepared by the Working Group on Health System Financing in Canada (Ottawa: Canadian Medical Association, July 1993).

11. D. E. OSBORNE and T. GAEBLER. *Reinventing Government: How the Entrepreneurial Spirit Is Transforming the Public Sector* (Reading (MA): Addison-Wesley Publications, 1992).

12. SALTMAN 1995.

13. OSBORNE and GAEBLER 1992.

14. O. ADAMS, L. CURRY and R. B. DEBER. *Public and Private Health Care Financing: Literature Review and Description: Volumes 1 and 2* (Ottawa (ON): Curry Adams & Associates, 1992); BLOMQVIST and BROWN 1994; R.G. EVANS, *Strained Mercy: The Economics of Canadian Health Care* (Toronto (ON): Butterworths & Co., 1984).

15. R. B. DEBER, N. KRAETSCHMER and J. IRVINE. What role do patients wish to play in treatment decision making? *Archives of Internal Medicine* 156 (1996), 1414–1120.

16. R. B. DEBER. The patient-physician partnership: Changing roles, and the desire for information. *CMAJ* 151(2), (1994), 171–176; R. B. Deber. The patient-physician partnership: Decision making, problem solving, and the desire to participate. *CMAJ* 151(4), (1994), 423–427.

17. EVANS 1984.

18. ADAMS, CURRY, and DEBER 1992.

19. R. B. DEBER, E. ROSS and M. CATZ. *Comprehensiveness in Health Care.* (Ottawa (ON): Health Action Lobby, 1993).

20. B. ABEL-SMITH. *Cost Containment and New Priorities in Health Care.* (Brookfield: Avebury Books, 1992); B. ABEL-SMITH, *The Escalation of Health Care Costs: How Did We Get There?,* High-Level Conference on Health Care Reform, OECD, Paris, November 17–18, 1994; ADAMS, CURRY, and DEBER 1992; R. B. DEBER, O. ADAMS, L. CURRY. International healthcare systems: Models of financing and reimbursement. In *Proceedings of the Fifth Canadian Conference on Health Economics,* ed. J.A. BOAN. (Regina: Canadian Plains Research Centre, 1994), 76-91; J. FRENK. Dimensions of health system reform. *Health Policy* 27 (1994), 19–34; B. M. KLECZKOWSKI, M. I. ROEMER and A. VAN DER WERFF. *National Health Systems and Their Reorientation Towards Health for All—Guidance for Policy Making.* Public Health Papers no. 77 (Geneva: World Health Organization, 1984); ORGANIZATION FOR ECONOMIC CO-OPERATION AND DEVELOPMENT. *Financing and Delivering Health Care: A Comparative Analysis of OECD Countries.* (Paris: OECD, 1987); OECD. *Health Care Systems in Transition: The Search for Efficiency.* (Paris: OECD, 1990); OECD. *The Reform of Health Care: A Comparative Analysis of Seven OECD Countries.* (Paris: OECD, 1992); OECD, *The Reform of Health Care Systems: A Review of Seventeen OECD Countries.* (Paris: OECD, 1994); M. PFAFF. Differences in health care spending across countries: Statistical evidence. *J Health Polit Policy Law* 15(1) (1990), 1–67; M. I. ROEMER. The public/ private mix of health sector financing: International implications. *Public Health Reviews* 12(2) (1984), 119–130; R. B. SALTMAN. A conceptual overview of recent health care reforms. *European Journal of Public Health* 4 (1994), 287–293.

21. R.B. DEBER, A.P. WILLIAMS, P. BARANEK and K. DUVALKO. *Report to the Task Force on the Funding and Delivery of Medical Care in Ontario: The Public-Private Mix in Health Care.* (Task Force on the Funding and Delivery of Medical Care in Ontario, Government of Ontario, July 1995).

22. SALTMAN 1995.

23. J. APPLEBY. *Financing Health Care in the 1990s* (Philadelphia (PA): Open University Press, 1992).

24. CANADIAN MEDICAL ASSOCIATION WORKING GROUP ON HEALTH SYSTEM FINANCING IN CANADA 1993.

25. OECD 1987.

26. G.B. DOERN and R. W. PHIDD, *Canadian Public Policy: Ideas, Structure, Process,* 2nd ed. (Toronto (ON): Nelson Canada, 1992).

27. M. L. BARER, V. BHATIA, G. L. STODDART and R. G. EVANS. *The Remarkable Tenacity of User Charges: A Concise History of the Participation, Positions, and Rationales of Canadian Interest Groups in the Debate Over "Direct Patient Participation" in Health*

Care Financing. (Ontario Premier's Council on Health, Well-Being and Social Justice, June 1994); V. BHATIA, G. L. STODDART, M. L. BARER and R. G. EVANS. *User Charges in Health Care: A Bibliography.* (Ontario Premier's Council on Health, Well-Being and Social Justice, June 1994); DEBER, ADAMS, and CURRY 1994; R. G. EVANS, M. L. BARER and G. L. STODDART. *Charging Peter to Pay Paul: Accounting for the Financial Effects of User Charges.* (Ontario Premier's Council on Health, Well-Being and Social Justice, June 1994); R. G. EVANS, M. L. BARER, G. L. STODDART and V. BHATIA. *Who Are the Zombie Masters, and What Do They Want?* (Ontario Premier's Council on Health, Well-Being and Social Justice, June 1994); R. G. EVANS, M. L. BARER, G. L. STODDART and V. BHATIA. *It's Not the Money, It's the Principle: Why User Charges for Some Services and Not Others?* (Ontario Premier's Council on Health, Well-Being and Social Justice, June 1994); U. E. REINHARDT. Can we learn health care lessons from Germany? *Internist* 32(5), (1991), 6–9; SALTMAN 1995; G. L. STODDART, M. L. BARER and R. G. EVANS. *User Charges, Snares and Delusions: Another Look at the Literature.* (Ontario Premier's Council on Health, Well-Being and Social Justice, June 1994); G. L. STODDART, M. L. BARER, R. G. EVANS and V. BHATIA. *Why Not User Charges? The Real Issues* (Premier's Council on Health, Well-Being and Social Justice, Toronto, September 1993).

28. D. U. HIMMELSTEIN and S. WOOLHANDLER. Cost without benefit: Administrative waste in U.S. health care. *New England Journal of Medicine* 314(7) (1986), 441–445; S. WOOLHANDLER, D. U. HIMMELSTEIN and J. P. LEWONTIN. Administrative costs in U.S. hospitals. *New England Journal of Medicine* 329(6) (1993), 400–403.

29. R. FEIN. *Medical Care, Medical Costs: The Search for a Health Insurance Policy* (Cambridge (MA): Harvard University Press, 1986).

30. DEBER, ADAMS, and CURRY 1994.

31. FRENK 1994.

32. OECD 1987.

33. CMA Working Group on Health System Financing in Canada 1993; SALTMAN 1995.

34. DEBER, ROSS, and CATZ 1993.

35. OECD 1992; OECD 1994.

36. CANADIAN LIFE AND HEALTH INSURANCE ASSOCIATION INC. *The Canadian Life and Health Insurance Industry and the Health Reform Process* (Canadian Life and Health Insurance Association Inc., July 1994).

37. M. G. TAYLOR, *Health Insurance and Canadian Public Policy: The Seven Decisions that Created the Canadian Health Insurance System* (Montréal (QC): McGill-Queen's University Press, 1978).

38. ABEL-SMITH 1992; ABEL-SMITH 1994; OECD 1992; OECD 1994.

39. K. JUDGE. Value for money in the British residential care industry. In *Public and Private Health Services: Complementarities and Conflict,* eds. A.J. CULYER and B. JONSSON. (Oxford: Basil Blackwell, 1986), 200–218.

40. M. KNAPP. The relative cost-effectiveness of public, voluntary and private providers of residential child care. In *Public and Private Health Services: Complementarities and Conflict,* eds. A.J. CULYER and B. JONSSON. (Oxford: Basil Blackwell, 1986), 171–199.

41. BENDICK 1989.

42. SALTMAN 1995.

43. R. B. SALTMAN and C. VON OTTER. *Planned Markets and Public Competition: Strategic Reform in Northern European Health Systems.* (Philadelphia (PA): Open University Press, 1992).

44. JÉRÔME-FORGET, WHITE, and WIENER 1995; SALTMAN and VON OTTER 1992.

45. R. B. SALTMAN and C. VON OTTER. Public competition versus mixed markets: An analytic comparison. *Health Policy* 11(1) (1989), 43–55.

46. SALTMAN and VON OTTER 1992; R. B. SALTMAN and C. VON OTTER, Eds. *Implementing Planned Markets in Health Care: Balancing Social and Economic Responsibility.* (Philadelphia (PA): Open University Press, 1995).

47. J. DIXON and H. GLENNESTER. What do we know about fundholding in general practice? *BMJ* 311(7007) (1995), 727–730; R. PETCHEY. General practitioner fundholding: Weighing the evidence. *Lancet* 356(8983) (1995)), 1139–1142.

48. TAYLOR 1978.

49. GOVERNMENT OF GREAT BRITAIN, *British North America Act (Constitution Act),* (Victoria: Government of Great Britain 1867), 30–31.

50. GOVERNMENT OF CANADA, *Hospital Insurance and Diagnostic Services Act,* Statutes of Canada, 1957, c. 28, s. 1.

51. GOVERNMENT OF CANADA (1966–67), *Medical Care Act.* Statutes of Canada, c. 64, s.1.

52. GOVERNMENT OF CANADA, *Federal-Provincial Fiscal Arrangements and Federal Post-Secondary Education and Health Contributions Act,* Revised Statutes of Canada, 1985, c. F-8.

53. R. B. DEBER, *Regulatory and Administrative Options for Canada's Health Care System.* Background paper prepared for The Health Action Lobby, October 8, 1991; M. RACHLIS and C. KUSHNER. *Strong Medicine: How to Save Canada's Health Care System.* (Toronto: Harper Collins Publishers Ltd., 1994).

54. GOVERNMENT OF CANADA, *Canada Health Act, Bill C-3,* Statutes of Canada, 1984 (R.S.C. 1985, c. 6; R.S.C. 1989, c. C-6).

55. S. HEIBER and R. B. DEBER. Banning extra-billing in Canada: Just what the doctor didn't order. *Canadian Public Policy* 13(1) (1987), 62–74.

56. H. M. STEVENSON, A. P. WILLIAMS and E. VAYDA. Medical politics and Canadian Medicare: Professional response to the Canada Health Act. *Milbank Q* 66(1) (1988), 65–104.

57. C. J. TUOHY. Medicine and the State in Canada: The extra-billing issue in perspective. *Canadian Journal of Political Science* 21(2) (1988), 267–296.

58. W. R. LEDERMAN, *Continuing Canadian Constitutional Dilemmas: Essays on the Constitutional History, Public Law and Federal System of Canada* (Toronto (ON): Butterworths, 1981).

59. CANADIAN BAR ASSOCIATION TASK FORCE ON HEALTH CARE, *What's Law Got To Do With It? Health Care Reform in Canada* (Ottawa (ON): Canadian Bar Association, 1994).

60. *Irwin Toy v. Quebec,* [1989] 1 S.C.R., 927.

61. *Re Gershman Produce Co. Ltd. and Motor Transport Board,* [1985] 22 D.L.R. (4th) 528; *Smith, Kline & French Laboratories Ltd. et al. v. Attorney General of Canada,* [1985] 24 D.L.R. (4th) 321.

62. *Re Homemade Winecrafts (Canada) Ltd. and Attorney General of British Columbia et al.,* [1986] 26 D.L.R. (4th) 468.

63. *Home Orderly Services Ltd. et al. v. Government of Manitoba,* [1986] 32 D.L.R. (4th) 755.

64. *Aluminum Co. of Canada Ltd. and The Queen in Right of Ontario; Dofasco Inc. Intervenor,* [1986] 29 D.L.R. (4th) 583.

65. *Re R.V.P. Enterprises Ltd. and Minister of Consumer and Corporate Affairs,* [1987] 37 D.L.R. (4th) 148.

66. *Re Pasqua Hospital and Harmatiuk,* [1987] 42 D.L.R. (4th) 134.

67. *Re Snell and Workers' Compensation Board of British Columbia,* [1987] 42 D.L.R. (4th) 160.

68. GOVERNMENT OF ONTARIO, *Savings and Restructuring Act, 1996,* Bill 26, Statutes of Ontario, 1996, c.1.

69. *Re Mia and Medical Services Commission of British Columbia,* [1985] 17 D.L.R. (4th) 385.

70. *Re Branigan and Yukon Medical Council et al.,* [1986] 26 D.L.R. (4th) 268, at 278; *Charboneau et al. v. College of Physicians and Surgeons of Ontario,* [1985] 22 D.L.R. (4th) 303; *Re Wilson and Medical Services Commission,* [1987] 36 D.L.R. (4th) 31 (British Columbia Supreme Court); *Wilson v. British Columbia (Medical Services Commission),* [1988] 53 D.R.L. (4th) 171.

71. *Re Isabey and Manitoba Health Services Commission et al.,* [1985] 22 D.L.R. 503 (Manitoba Queen's Bench); *Re Isabey and Manitoba Health Services Commission et al.,* [1986] 28 D.R.L. (4th) 735 (Manitoba Court of Appeal).

72. *O.H.R.C. v. Ontario,* [1994] 19 O.R. (3d) 387 (C.A.).

73. CANADIAN BAR ASSOCIATION TASK FORCE ON HEALTH CARE 1994.

74. *R. v. Oakes,* [1986] 1 S.C.R. 103.

75. CANADIAN BAR ASSOCIATION TASK FORCE ON HEALTH CARE 1994.

76. STATUTES OF ONTARIO 1996.

77. STATUTES OF ONTARIO 1996.

78. G. SHARPE, *Driving Ontario's Health Care Revolution.* Paper presented at Insight Conference, Sutton Place Hotel, Toronto, February 28, 1996.

79. B. P. SCHWARTZ, *In the Matter of: NAFTA Reservations in the Areas of Health Care.* Opinion prepared by B. P. SCHWARTZ for Buchwald Asper Gallagher Henteleff, Barristers and Attorneys-at-Law, Winnipeg (MB), 1996.

80. RACHLIS and KUSHNER 1994.

81. E. BERGER, *Canada Health Monitor Survey no. 11* (Ottawa (ON): Price Waterhouse Survey Research Centre, 1994); E. BERGER, *Canada Health Monitor Survey no. 12* (Ottawa (ON): Price Waterhouse Survey Research Centre, 1995).

82. R. G. EVANS. Canada: The real issues. *J Health Polit Policy Law* 17(4) (1992), 739–762.

83. STATUTES OF CANADA 1984.

84. HEALTH CANADA. *National Health Expenditures in Canada 1975–1994, Full Report.* (Ottawa (ON): Health Canada, Policy and Consultation Branch, January 1996).

85. CANADIAN MEDICAL ASSOCIATION. *Health Facts.* (Ottawa (ON): Canadian Medical Association, May 1995).

86. HEALTH CANADA 1996.

87. OECD 1994.

88. ADAMS, CURRY, and DEBER 1992; CMA WORKING GROUP ON HEALTH SYSTEM FINANCING IN CANADA 1993; HEALTH CANADA 1996.

89. HEALTH CANADA 1996.

90. HEALTH CANADA 1996.

91. G. H. PINK and S. K. HUDSON. Sale and leaseback by Canadian hospitals: Theory and practice. *Healthcare Management Forum* 1(3) (1988), 16–23.

92. ADAMS, CURRY, and DEBER, 1992.

93. R. B. DEBER, G.,G. THOMPSON and P. LEATT. Technology acquisition in Canada: Control in a regulated market. *Int J Technol Assess Health Care* 4(2) (1988), 185–206; R. B. DEBER, M. WIKTOROWICZ, P. LEATT and F. CHAMPAGNE. Technology acquisition in Canadian hospitals: How is it done, and where is the information coming from? *Healthcare Management Forum* 7(4) (1994), 18–27; R. B. DEBER, M. WIKTOROWICZ, P. LEATT and F. CHAMPAGNE. Technology acquisition in Canadian hospitals: How are we doing? *Healthcare Management Forum* 8(2) (1995), 23–28.

94. HEALTH CANADA 1996.

95. HEALTH CANADA 1996.

96. CANADIAN LIFE AND HEALTH INSURANCE ASSOCIATION INC. *Canadian Life and Health Insurance Facts.* (Toronto (ON): Canadian Life and Health Insurance Association Inc., 1994).

97. M. GIBB-CLARK. Ontario employers' group seeks input on health care: Trying to ensure costs cut, not just shifted. *Globe and Mail,* July 20, 1995, B5.

98. CALU/LUAC Task Force on Health Care, *Employer-Paid Health Benefits.* Report submitted to the House of Commons Standing Committee on Finance, November, 1994.

99. D. E. ANGUS, L. AUER, J. E. CLOUTIER and T. ALBERT. *Sustainable Health Care for Canada: Synthesis Report* (Ottawa: Queen's–University of Ottawa Economic Projects, 1995).

100. CMA 1995.

101. W. G. WEISSERT. Cost-effectiveness of home care. In *Restructuring Canada's Health Services System: How Do We Get There from Here?* eds. R. B. DEBER and G. G. THOMPSON. (Toronto (ON): University of Toronto Press, 1992), 89–98.

102. R. B. DEBER and A. P. WILLIAMS. Policy, payment and participation: Long-term care reform in Ontario. *Canadian Journal on Aging* 14(2) (1995), 294–318.

103. R. G. EVANS, M. L. BARER, and T. R. MARMOR, Eds. *Why Are Some People Healthy and Others Not: The Determinants of Health of Populations.* (New York: Aldine de Gruyter, 1994).

104. R. B. DEBER, Ed. *Case Studies in Canadian Health Policy and Management,* volume 1 (Ottawa (ON): Canadian Hospital Association Press, 1992).

105. A. HOLT, A. NEUFELD and R. B. DEBER. The merger that wasn't: Lessons for senior administrators. *Healthcare Management Forum* 6(4) (1993), 33–37.

106. STATUTES OF ONTARIO 1996.

107. R. B. DEBER, S. L. MHATRE and G. R. BAKER. A review of provincial initiatives. In *Limits to Care: Reforming Canada's Health System in an Age of Restraint,* eds. A. BLOMQVIST and D. M. BROWN (Toronto (ON): C.D. Howe Institute, 1994), 91–124.

108. D. JONES. Surgery on demand. *Globe and Mail Report on Business,* November 1995, 82–90.

109. JONES 1995.

110. CONSUMERS' ASSOCIATION OF CANADA. *Current Access to Cataract Surgery in Alberta.* (Edmonton (AB): Consumers' Association of Canada, Alberta Branch, 1994).

111. CONSUMERS' ASSOCIATION OF CANADA 1994.

112. MANITOBA CENTRE FOR HEALTH POLICY AND EVALUATION. "Eye to eye," *Centre Piece,* 1996.

113. S. D. WATSON. Medicaid physician participation: Patients, poverty, and physician self-interest. *Am J Law Med* 21(2–3) (1995).

114. CMA 1995.

115. M. L. BARER, and G. L. STODDART. *Toward Integrated Medical Resource Policies for Canada.* Report prepared for the Federal/Provincial/Territorial Conference of Deputy Ministers of Health, June, 1991.

116. J. LOMAS, C. FOOKS, T. H. RICE, and R. J. LABELLE. Paying physicians in Canada: Minding our Ps and Qs. *Health Affairs* 8(1) (1989), 80–102.

117. G. HARDIN. The tragedy of the commons. *Science* 162 (1968), 1243–1248.

118. CMA 1995.

119. CONSUMERS' ASSOCIATION OF CANADA 1994.

120. J. DAW. Pain in the neck: Under the hood of Auto Insurance (first of five parts). *Toronto Star,* May 13, 1995, C1, C3; J. DAW. Fakers and frauds: Under the hood of auto insurance (second of five parts). *Toronto Star,* May 14, 1995, D1, D3; J. DAW. A second opinion: Under the hood of auto insurance (third of five parts). *Toronto Star,* May 15, 1995, C1, C3; J. DAW. Does Quebec have the answer: Under the hood of auto insurance (fourth of five parts). *Toronto Star,* May 16, 1995, D1, D9; J. DAW. Taming the beast: Under the hood of auto insurance (last of five parts). *Toronto Star,* May 17, 1995, C1, C3.

121. INSTITUTE FOR WORK AND HEALTH. *Rehabilitation Services Inventory and Quality Project: Phase One Report.*(Toronto (ON): IWH, July 6, 1995).

122. P. C. COYTE, D. N. DEWEES and M..J. TREBILCOCK. Medical malpractice—The Canadian experience. *New England Journal of Medicine* 324 (1991), 89–93.

123. J. DAW. A blizzard of choices. *Toronto Star,* October 14, 1995, E1, E3; J. DAW. Check your health coverage next trip. *Toronto Star,* October 15, 1995, E8.

124. DAW, October 15, 1995.

125. ANGUS, AUER, CLOUTIER and ALBERT 1995; Brogan Consulting Inc., *Pharmaceutical Purchasing in Canada: Implications for the National Pharmaceutical Strategy.* Unpublished manuscript, Brogan Consulting Inc., 1995; CANADIAN LIFE AND HEALTH INSURANCE ASSOCIATION INC., *Survey of Health Insurance Benefits in Canada.* Annual surveys, 1975, 1980, 1984–1993; The facts on escalating drug plan costs. *Group Health Care Management* Special Edition 3(1) (1995), 1–27.

126. J. RICHARDSON. *Medicare: Where Are We? Where Are We Going?* National Centre for Health Program Evaluation, Working Paper 31, July 1993.

127. S. J. DUCKETT. Opening Address to 1995 Australian Private Hospitals Association Casemix Conference. Melbourne, Australia, May, 1995.

128. DUCKETT 1995.

129. A.-P. CONTANDRIOPOULOS, F. CHAMPAGNE, J.-L. DENIS, et al. *Financial Incentives/ Disincentives in Canada's Health System: Executive Summary.* Presented by Groupe Secor, Gris-Université de Montréal, to Health Canada, March, 1996.

130. D. A. STONE, *Policy Paradox: The Art of Political Decision Making* (W.W. Norton and Company, 1996).

131. STONE 1988.

132. D. A. STONE. The struggle for the soul of health insurance. *J Health Polit Policy Law* 18(2) (1993), 287–317.

133. L. D. BROWN. The national politics of Oregon's Rationing Plan. *Health Affairs* 10(2) (1991), 28–51; C. J. DOUGHERTY. The proposal will deny services to the poor: The Oregon Act is ethically flawed. *Health Program* 71(9) (1990), 21, 28–32; D. M. EDDY. Clinical decision making: From theory to practice. What care is "essential"? What services are "basic"? *JAMA* 265(6) (1991), 782, 786–788; D. M. EDDY. Clinical decision making: From theory to practice. Oregon's methods. Did cost-effectiveness analysis fail? *JAMA* 266(15) (1991), 2135–2141; D. M. EDDY. Clinical decision making: From theory to practice. Oregon's plan. Should it be approved? *JAMA* 266(17) (1991), 2439–2445; D. C. HADORN. Setting health care priorities in Oregon: Cost-effectiveness meets the rule of rescue. *JAMA* 265(17), 1991, 2218–2125; J. A. KITZHABER and M. GIBSON. The crisis in health care: The Oregon plan as a strategy for change. *Stanford Law and Policy Review* 1991, 64–72; R. KLEIN. Warning signals from Oregon. *BMJ* 304(6840) (1992), 1457–1458; H. D. KLEVIT, A. C. BATES, T. CASTANARES, P. KIRK, P. R. SIPES-METZLER and R. WOPAT. Prioritization of health care services: A progress report by the Oregon Health Services Commission. *Archives of Internal Medicine* 151 (1991), 912–916; R. STEINBROOK and B. LO. The Oregon Medicaid Demonstration Project: Will it provide adequate medical care? *New England Journal*

of Medicine 326(5) (1992), 340–344; J. E. WENNBERG. Outcomes research, cost containment, and fear of health care rationing. *New England Journal of Medicine* 323(17) (1990), 1202–1204.

134. DOUGHERTY 1990.

135. T. O. TENGS, G. MEYER, J. E. SIEGEL, J. S. PLISKIN, J. D. GRAHAM and M. C. WEINSTEIN. Oregon's Medicaid ranking and cost-effectiveness. *Medical Decision Making* 16(2) (1996), 99–107.

136. R. B. DEBER. Translating technology assessment into policy: Conceptual issues and tough choices. *Int J Technol Assess Health Care* 8(1) (1992), 131–137.

137. R. B. DEBER, M. M. COHEN, and S. MERCER. *Literature Review and Report on Three Medical Services.* (Ottawa (ON): Canadian Medical Association, April 1995).

138. ADAMS, CURRY, and DEBER 1992.

139. R. G. EVANS. "We'll take care of it for you": Health care in the Canadian community. *Daedelus* 117(4) (1989), 155–189.

Integrated Models

International Trends and Implications for Canada

JOHN MARRIOTT, M.P.A. AND ANN L. MABLE, B.A.

Management Consulting Partnership of Marriott Mable

SUMMARY

This paper attempts to set the groundwork for discussion of the future evolution of integrated models in the Canadian health care system. Historically, much of the discussion of the Canadian system has focused exclusively on the total system in global terms or on the evolution of one sector without addressing the implications for other sectors in the system.

There is one thing critical to understanding and appreciating the utility of this paper—the need for a grasp of multidimensional factors to discuss the organizational principles and features towards which Canada's system should evolve and to support the discussion based on observations drawn from what other countries are doing. These factors cover a variety of overlapping and interrelated concepts, theories and practices, spanning a range including (but not limited to) health care, social services, organizational behaviour, business notions of "markets," fiduciary responsibilities, and financial management. These in turn are experienced and observed from the perspectives of various stakeholders—patients, governments, and health care providers—which together comprise the health care "industry."

To cover such ground adequately within the parameters of this exercise is the task this paper sets out to accomplish. The hope is at least to provide a prima facie *case for reform in Canada, based on existing recent trends. The paper presupposes some familiarity with the Canadian and international health care environment, and covers a lot of ground without expansive background or detailed discussion.*

The harnessing of the interrelated subject matter, like the harnessing of integrated organizations to meet health care goals, requires thoughtful attention and sufficient time to achieve an optimum appreciation. As proved elsewhere, the results are worth it.

TABLE OF CONTENTS

Introduction 551

Overviews of Systems in Selected Countries 558

   Overview of the Health System of the United Kingdom 559

   Overview of the Health System of the Netherlands 573

   Overview of the Health System of New Zealand 583

   Overview of the Health System of the United States 594

Overview of the Canadian Health System and Models 609

   Background 609

   Macroenvironment 610

   Provincial Overview 612

   Summary of Features of Emerging Models—Canada 625

Key Features of Integrated Models 626

   Patterns of Change 626

   Stages of Organizational Reconfiguration 628

   Implications of the Change to Integrated Models 630

   Comments Regarding Implementation 637

   Protection against Self-Enrichment and Sector Bias 637

   The "Primacy" of Primary Care 639

Key Features of Integrated Models in the Canadian Context 640

   Selected System Objectives 641

   Distinguishing Features 642

   Additional Government Support 652

   Discussion 653

   Summary of Features of Integrated Models—Canada 660

Evaluation of Integrated Models 662

   Response to Objectives 663

International and Canadian Perspectives on Evaluation 664

Selected Functions to Monitor and Evaluate 667

The Evaluation/Evidence Excuse 668

Conclusions and Observations 669

Bibliography 673

LIST OF FIGURES

Figure 1   Context: The delivery system environment 554

Figure 2   Horizontal and vertical integration 556, 615

Figure 3   Consolidation of health authorities in
the United Kingdom. 565

Figure 4   U.K. Transformation: DHA and FSHA merged. DHA
geographic purchaser. Providers now independent
contractors 566

Figure 5   Transformation of Sickness Fund organizations from
geographic monopsonies to competing roster-based
national purchasers 574

Figure 6   New Zealand transformation 586

Figure 7   Example of purchaser/provider HMO model within
mixed private and public funding in the United States 603

Figure 8   Devolved local authority 617

Figure 9   Local health board 619

Figure 10 Comprehensive Health Organization (CHO) 620

Figure 11 A CHO health system 621

Figure 12 Fundholder vs. Integrated Purchaser/Provider Model 655

LIST OF TABLES

Table 1   Population served, by type of coverage 599

Table 2   Provincial models of integration 614

INTRODUCTION

> When we began to plan Medicare, we pointed out that it would be in two phases. The first phase would be to remove the financial barrier between those giving the service and those receiving it. The second phase would be to reorganize and revamp the whole delivery system—and of course, that's the big item. That's the thing we haven't done yet.
>
> Tommy Douglas, former premier of Saskatchewan, 1982.

The organization of health services planning, allocation, funding, and delivery is undergoing profound change around the world and in Canada, as governments attempt to enhance the efficiency and effectiveness of their health systems. Despite obvious cultural, geographic and other distinctions, societies in general have been facing an array of similar issues related to health care, including rising costs, fragmentation and lack of coordination, and reductions in efficiency and effectiveness. The world is now experiencing a wave of reform, producing dramatic and subtle changes from which lessons may be derived for Canada—or indeed, which reaffirm characteristics in which Canada exemplifies the ideal.

Major trends and features of the present wave of reform are emerging, such as the importance of *integration* of resources. Most systems, whether privately or publicly funded, are producing models of integration—by design, or in response to evolving pressures. Increasingly important are *vertically integrated models* of planning, purchasing and providing services, with built-in mechanisms for *checks and balances.* There has been a reaffirmation of the significance of *primary care* and the importance of the role of *physicians as gatekeepers* to the larger system. Such knowledge facilitates Canadian efforts to evolve the system toward its ideal—the highest and best levels of performance. The chief historical reform of the Canadian health system took place in the 1960s, with the introduction of a single-payer system of universal medical insurance (commonly, though not officially, called *medicare*). Organizational models for providers remained essentially the same as they were prior to medicare. And while much recent change has focused on financial controls, recognition of the impact of the system's *organizational* design on its effectiveness lagged behind, as reinforced by the Douglas quotation at the beginning of this section. This final task—to reevaluate and reform the organizational components and interrelationships in the system—is now evolving at different rates across Canada.

The organizational reforms of countries reviewed for this paper represent recent initiatives—mostly in the 1990s—and should be considered work in progress. An apparent absence of information in strategic areas may be due in part to changes so recent as to preclude adequate time to refine, evaluate and/or document. In addition, systems are often "fine-tuned" immediately as issues arise. This further inhibits assessment of performance, in that circumstances do not stabilize long enough for a thorough review of their implications. Important attributes may be missed in the rush to examine particular characteristics. To date, much of the literature on these reforms has focused on broad policy and/or systemwide elements of countries' health systems, with much of the discussion falling into one or more of four predominant streams:

- attempts to understand the broad trends associated with the rubric of large-scale, systemic adjustments such as decentralization, deconcentration, devolution, and regionalization;
- attempts to understand performance to date in terms of economic efficiency, effectiveness and outcomes, and to assess the impact of changes on performance, primarily with particular goals in mind, such as reduction of waiting lists;
- early speculation on adjustments to existing reform policy or elements of it, to improve the potential of the reform to achieve stated goals and objectives;
- analysis and discussion of the interfaces among patients, providers, (physicians, other caregivers, hospitals and other institutions, and programs) and government.

Furthermore, much of the focus has been repeatedly on the same subsectors such as hospitals and doctors, without giving due or appropriately weighted consideration to the *many* other factors, practitioners, and procedures involved in *caring for health*.

What appears to have been generally missing is an approach to understanding present and emerging integrated models in the delivery system, from the perspective of *organizational or structural design*. For the purpose of this exercise, "model" refers to an interrelated set of elements—functions and/or organizations—which together establish a paradigm for delivery of a given set of services. How these elements are organized—how they interact, how decisions are made, what authority or autonomy they do or do not possess—all have implications for the appropriateness, the cost, the quality, and other aspects of the end product: service.

This paper will focus primarily on identifying and describing *pivotal* attributes of select current and emerging international and Canadian organizational models of planning, purchasing and providing health services, for populations whether defined by geography or roster. For all models identified, the review will take into account the macrocontext within which they operate, and those elements of the larger system that are necessary for defining particular models, to complete the inventory of critical structural and systems interrelationships. Such key attributes will be considered in terms of how they position and support the model in its planning, allocation and delivery, and serve as indicators for evaluation.

The purpose of this study is to contribute to an improved understanding of the constituent elements of new and emerging integrated models and, based on this, to outline the key organizational principles and features which should guide the future evolution of Canada's health care system. Implementation of these principles and features in part, would produce a range of options of partially integrated models. When implemented in full, the result would be a fully vertically integrated organizational model. This review will attempt to show how "modules" of services may be added to a primary care "base," in gradual development toward a fully vertically integrated model. While scope and timing of this exercise dictate only a *prima facie* consideration, the inquiry attempts to discern significant underlying structures, processes, and lessons for efficiency and effectiveness of the *Canadian environment*.

To begin the process, it is necessary to consider three major sources of contextual pressures, which together constitute the environment within which models operate, and which exert contrasting and conflicting influences on organizational design and operations (figure 1).

Microenvironment – The discrete interface(s) between individuals/ populations and providers. This comprises the environment wherein patient (consumer/client) and population (size and demographics) needs and demands, in conjunction with system responsiveness (timeliness, quantity, and appropriateness) and quality of services (or lack thereof), lead to satisfaction (or dissatisfaction) of patients and/or population. As well, assessments are made of "achievement" or "failure" in responding to individual and population needs. It is the definition of population need and its rationalization with demand that defines the profile of health resources required to respond. Together, these factors begin to define parameters of the "market" environment for integrated models in the delivery system.

Macroenvironment – The legal and social framework of health services set by purchasers of services (governments and/or employers, depending on the country), encompassing legislation, negotiated benefits, sources of funds, and goals of the system. Together, these establish health system "rules"—the broad health policy and organizational parameters for the total health system—in order to:

- establish defining principles and standards for the system;
- define core benefits funded by the health plan, quantity and distribution of funds;
- regulate providers and provider/purchaser relationships;
- regulate citizen entitlement regarding access to benefits, providers, and funding support.

Figure 1

Context: The delivery system environment

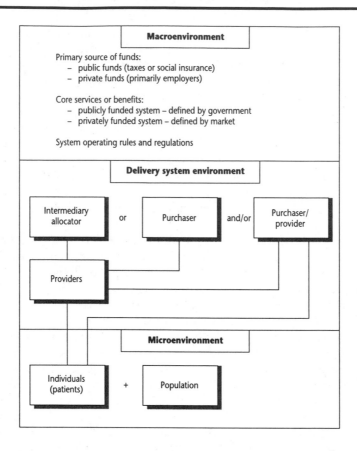

The delivery system environment: This is the "zone" where most reform has been targeted. Within the delivery system, discrete organizations receive public or private funding to plan, allocate budgets, and purchase and/or provide health services for the population. In some systems, provider sectors have historically received direct funding allocations from government, with or without an intermediary authority through which funds were channelled. Reform in these systems has changed direct allocation of provider budgets to "purchasing" (contracting for) provider services. Regardless of the extent or absence of regulation, the introduction of purchasing into the system has activated certain internal dynamics which appear to motivate or propel organizations "naturally" toward survival, efficiency, effectiveness or other, less successful ends. Critical relationships and interactions at this level are

influenced by both competitive behaviour and collaboration. These characteristics, in turn, influence movement toward varying levels of *integration*—
consolidating or merging of resources.

This is demonstrated in examples of either *horizontal* integration—
consolidating or merging a range of similar entities within one sector into
one organization, for example operating several hospitals under one board;
or *vertical* integration—consolidating or merging of different interdependent
sectors under one organization, such as an organization composed of hospitals, primary care, physicians, home care, and long-term care services (figure 2).

There is a somewhat rigid view of a vertically integrated health organization as a single entity that "owns" and manages the various health sector
components, and which administers an "amalgamized" version of their preexisting funding. A more expansive and flexible version exists. For example,
a corporation or other organization may be *exclusively responsible* for most
or all health services for a defined population, and receive all the associated
funding. It is left up to the organization to determine whether it directly
owns a given component of health services, or elects to purchase those services
from an external provider. This autonomy is an essential ingredient of the
predominant emerging examples of vertical integration, "purchaser/provider"
models, which are now challenging the efficacy of separate all-purchaser or
all-provider models.

This autonomous, vertically integrated "purchaser/provider" model is
now evolving in many countries and putting strong pressure on the preexisting "exclusive–government purchaser" or "exclusive-provider" arrangements. In highly regulated environments such as the United Kingdom and
New Zealand, successful purchaser/providers benefit from the support and
encouragement of government. Even in the very open market system of the
United States, indemnity plans are being challenged by HMOs. Besides
autonomy, rostering (requiring patients/consumers to register with the
practice of their preferred physician), and capitation are critical
organizational dimensions that support and strengthen the organization's
potential for effectiveness and efficiency.

To identify the important features, this review of models at the delivery
system level will consider the following attributes:

- organizational structure;
- responsibility and accountability to government, society, and the
  population and individuals served;
- governance, management, and administration;
- gunding and financial management;
- organizational and financial relationships with providers and with
  citizens (as patients, consumers, and members);
- service/program profile (primary care physicians, specialist physicians,
  other providers, home care, drugs, diagnostic and hospital services, long-
  term care facilities, and other programs).

Figure 2

Horizontal and vertical integration

	Nursing home	Nursing home	Nursing home	Nursing home	Nursing home	Nursing home	Nursing home
	Home care	Home care	Home care	Home care	Home care	Home care	Home care
1.	Hospital	Hospital	Hospital	Hospital	Hospital	Hospital	Hospital
	Specialists	Specialists	Specialists	Specialists	Specialists	Specialists	Specialists
	General practitioners	General practitioners	General practitioners	General practitioners	General practitioners	General practitioners	General practitioners
	Practitioners	Practitioners	Practitioners	Practitioners	Practitioners	Practitioners	Practitioners
							2.

1. Horizontal integration—example of one organization owning several hospitals.
2. Vertical integration—example of one organization owning all components of the delivery system.

Note: 2. Also illustrates a single organization with integrated responsibility and funding for "all" the service sectors in the health system, where the organization exercises the option of owning or contracting any component of service delivery.

The market-like dynamics of the delivery system environment complete the set of pressures and influences that define organizational models, their interrelationships, and their ultimate viability. The review of other countries will explore the critical dynamics and key features of exclusive-purchaser, purchaser/provider and exclusive-provider models, and will examine their move toward integration. Primary emphasis is placed upon those with purchasing authority, as they appear to generate a higher degree of integration of responsibility for all benefits, funding, and services. In summary, an improved understanding—of models of planning, purchasing and provision of services, the contextual elements that guide, position and support the models, their relationship to governments, other sectors, the individuals, and public that they serve—is a prime objective of this paper.

The countries selected for review are the United Kingdom, the Netherlands, New Zealand, and the United States—a group which includes several publicly funded systems similar to Canada's (with notable dissimilarity from each other) and one predominantly privately funded, open market system. Although the systems of the United Kingdom and the Netherlands have quite different histories, to a certain extent they serve as proxies for similar reforms elsewhere in Europe. New Zealand's pattern is not dissimilar, but is notable for its greater tolerance for pluralism. The United Kingdom, the Netherlands, and New Zealand have strong influential central governments; the United States and Canada have federal governments with strong states or provinces. The strong centrally directed governments have enacted quite strident national reforms in comparison with more decentralized systems. The United States was chosen because it faces issues similar to the others, does have a publicly funded sector (contrary to general understanding), and due to the nature of its privately funded market system, is a laboratory for the independent development and refinement of organizational models. This review will consider the relative importance and role of primary care and general practitioners (GPs) in each environment. In the process, we try to determine whether similar organizational trends and critical elements are evolving in spite of major national variances, with parameters which may be applicable to Canada.

In addressing the Canadian environment, it is not the intent of this exercise to conduct a detailed, province-by-province review of reforms; rather it is to identify generic characteristics for comparison. Because attributes of provincial reforms are somewhat similar, a summary overview will be presented along with several generic models, representing key features in current Canadian reform. A review of emerging Canadian thinking regarding primary care will be included.

The ultimate goal of this exercise is to identify key organizational principles and features contained in models used in other countries, as well as emerging Canadian models and thinking. The discussion will also identify important supporting elements necessary in the larger context, to drive and support critical structural and systems interrelationships. Key attributes will be considered in terms of how they position and support organizational models of planning, purchasing, and/or provision of services. In addition, the presentation will attempt to establish how health sector components might be added to an existing primary care base, to facilitate a gradual development toward a fully vertically integrated model. It will explore steps to implement such models in the system.

The next section presents overviews of selected countries, followed by a presentation of the Canadian situation and evolving generic models in the section "Overview of the Canadian Health System and Models." The section "Key Features of Integrated Models" identifies key features of integrated models, and the section "Key Features of Integrated Models in the Canadian Context" considers how these features might take shape in the Canadian context. A summary of guidelines for internal and external evaluation of integrated organizations follows in the section "Evaluation of Integrated Models." The final section will summarize conclusions and observations.

OVERVIEWS OF SYSTEMS IN SELECTED COUNTRIES

This section begins the exercise of identifying and describing key attributes of several countries' models of planning, purchasing, and providing health services. Such key attributes will be considered in terms of how they position and support the model in the delivery system and serve as indicators for evaluation. Brief backgrounds of the countries' prereform health systems and summaries of the current systems will orient each subsection, followed by a discussion of important purchaser, purchaser/provider, and delivery models.

Several of the countries have historically had fairly rigid, highly regulated systems, often with direct state management of hospitals and community services. In many cases, one or more layers of regional authority were interposed as intermediary structures between the central government and the providers and patients. These agencies exercise their delegated authority to allocate budgets to and, in some cases directly manage, hospitals, community care, and other services as well as provide remuneration to general practitioners and other physicians. The United Kingdom, the Netherlands, and New Zealand reflect this prereform profile. For the most part, they remain publicly funded (through general taxation or compulsory social insurance), but all exhibit variations of private funding. The U.S. system demonstrates an immensely pluralistic environment, with variations on both publicly and privately funded models of care. In all of these nations, organizational reform has been a response to pressures originating both within and outside the system.

The countries reviewed for this exercise are the United Kingdom, the Netherlands, New Zealand, and the United States. The discussion of the Canadian context and generic models for comparison is presented in the section "Overview of the Canadian Health System and Models."

Overview of the Health System of the United Kingdom

Background

Prior to the most recent reform in 1990–1991, the organization of the National Health Service (NHS) was a public, vertically integrated health system (hospital services, for example, were provided directly by the local health authority), funded through general tax revenues and national insurance payments from employers and employees. Structurally, there were two levels of authorities: the Regional Health Authority (RHA) and the District Health Authority (DHA). RHAs were responsible for supplying some regional services and employing senior hospital doctors and for funding of district health authorities (DHAs), which provided health services and ran the hospitals and community care programs (OECD 1992; Klein 1995). General practitioners, on the other hand, were "contractors" of the NHS. Their number and distribution were controlled by the family health service authorities (FHSAs), which have now been merged with the DHAs. (Hatcher 1996).

Several issues gave rise to the demand for reform. First, there was increasing recognition that establishment of an integrated public health system under a single bureaucratic agency does not, in and of itself, necessarily result in equal treatment and equal access. In addition, there were concerns that the system was too rigid, inhibited free consumer choice, and was becoming complacent and unresponsive (Glennerster et al. 1994). In addition, funding was attached to facilities and providers rather than to the population and their needs. Specialists ("consultants" in the British terminology) defined "need" in their facilities with their accomplishments marked by professional recognition rather than achievement of best use of resources. Prior to the late 1980s, there was little incentive to improve efficiency or rectify the prevalent lack of financial and management information, which made performance review a doubtful exercise (Bradshaw and Bradshaw 1994). As noted in an OECD review, *Internal Markets in the Making* (OECD 1995):

> The motivation for the reforms centred on the belief that an alternative system could be devised that retained the advantages of the NHS—universal coverage and effective cost control—while expanding consumer choice and reducing supply-side inefficiencies. With the reforms, the government aimed to preserve free, or almost free, access to health care and to keep tax-

based finance, but to use competition between providers of both hospital and clinical services to improve health and increase consumer satisfaction within a tight budget. In short, it wanted to squeeze more out of the system.

After 1991, the reform transformed district health authorities into purchasers. In addition, individual GPs could opt to administer funds for purchase of a limited range of health care services for their patients from providers. GPs who selected this option would be known as GP Fundholders. Hospitals and community services were given autonomy to run their own operations and to compete for contracts with DHAs and GP Fundholders. In this system, money was to follow the patient or consumer, rather than continue to be attached to the provider. The old system based on hierarchical bureaucratic control was replaced by one based on elements of competition between providers (Klein 1995). Organizational features which were preserved are described below.

The Macroenvironment: The National Health Service (NHS)

Benefits

Although there is no explicit itemization of services which should be funded by the NHS, the organization is guided by the principles initially articulated in the Beveridge Report of 1942 and refined in subsequent legislation. The Beveridge Report called for a comprehensive, universally available, publicly funded system of health care. According to Hatcher, "comprehensive" meant medical treatment on the basis of need, regardless of the ability to pay, provided both in the home and in hospital by general practitioners, specialists, dentists, opticians, nurses and midwives, and was to include the provision of medical appliances and rehabilitation services (Hatcher 1996). Subsequent legislation called for a health service dedicated to prevention, diagnosis, and treatment of illness. Within the system the consumer had a right to access the service—but it was the professional provider who determined what treatment was appropriate (Klein 1995).

Funding

Funds for the system are primarily derived from general tax revenues and national insurance payments from employers and employees. In 1993, 84.2 percent came out of general tax revenues and 12.2 percent from National Insurance Scheme employee and employer compulsory contributions. The remaining 3.6 percent came from payments by patients, including statutory charges for such items as prescriptions and dental treatment, and hospital charges for discretionary private services (Hatcher 1996).

Funds were allocated to RHAs on a weighted capitation basis, and they in turn funded DHAs through a modified capitation formula (Bundred 1996). Prior to the conversion to purchasing, DHAs were responsible for running and funding health services only within their districts. The fact that some consumers entered their territory to access health services, and others left their territory to access services in neighbouring districts meant that the DHA had to continually adjust the capitation funding. They had to add money to the district's capitation funding to account for the estimated population entering from elsewhere, and subtract money for those estimated to be leaving to access services elsewhere.

The conversion of DHAs from *operators* of health facilities and programs to *purchasers* of services, with, more importantly, the right to purchase from *any* provider, whether in or outside their district, eliminated the need to add or subtract funding to adjust for cross-boundary flows. The population to be served by a given DHA is identified through census data, and funds are now allocated through a capitation formula weighted by age, sex, health risk factors of the population, and geographical cost differences. The cost differences recognize historical funding patterns. The long-term commitment is to reduce the adjustment for historical expenditure patterns, to move to a more purely weighted capitation formula that will adjust for factors beyond age and gender, to include proxies for need (e.g. standardized mortality ratios or SMRs, and deprivation factors such as the number of single mothers, etc.). This incremental pace of adjustment recognizes that stabilization time is required to gradually alter referral and utilization patterns.

Citizen Coverage/Entitlement

Full universality is accorded to all residents of the United Kingdom as well as the right to purchase private insurance or pay directly for services in the privately funded system. An estimated 8 percent of total expenditures for health in 1992/93 went to private hospitals and specialists (Hatcher 1996). While residents can register with only one GP at a time, they may change GPs at any time. This "right of exit" existed prior to reform; however, the requirement that individuals notify the GP of their decision to leave has now been dropped.

Principles and Regulation

The reform transformed the NHS from a vertically integrated public model (a bureaucracy which had funding and ran service programs), to a "public contractor" or *purchaser*. It no longer provides services nor allocates budgets; instead, it only negotiates contracts. The single-payer system was preserved along with universal access for consumers. Reform also brought with it a commitment to the principles of freedom and choice for both physicians and patients. Physicians are allowed to practice in the private sector as well as in the NHS, and patients have the right to choose their physician as well as to receive and pay for physician services outside the NHS. In essence, the objectives of the reform could be summarized as increased efficiency in resource use, a balance among primary, secondary and tertiary care, extended patient choice, and heightened responsiveness to consumers (Ham and Brommels 1994).

The NHS in England is responsible for health policy development and implementation. National guidance regulations have been developed in a number of areas. For example, there is a national target for a maximum waiting time of 26 weeks, with 90 percent of patients waiting for no more than 13 weeks for a first clinic appointment with a hospital specialist after referral from a GP. Following specialist referral, the target maximum waiting time for admission for elective inpatient care is 12 months (Hatcher 1996).

The current strategic direction of the NHS is to become "primary care–led." This means that the locus of decision making should be as close to patients as possible, and positions general practitioners as the coordinators of care (Ham 1995). To achieve this, the NHS encourages the development of GP Fundholders, and beyond this, the provision of a wider range of services in the primary care setting, to include diagnostics, specialists' clinics, and the employment of such staff as dieticians, physiotherapists, and counsellors. The gatekeeper role of the GP, in conjunction with a primary care team, complete the foundation of "primary care–led" services.

Four *structural* elements of "managed care" are integral to the NHS. These include:

- limited consumer choice of a GP;
- control of access to secondary care by GP gatekeepers;
- selective contracting by purchasers (i.e., negotiate contracts with select providers based on cost, quality, availability, and accessibility);
- the use of financial incentives for GP practices.

Two complementary *functional* elements of managed care—quality and utilization management—are relatively underdeveloped (Hatcher 1995).

Information Systems and Evaluation

The NHS stresses the importance of information systems, which are evolving along a number of fronts. At the national level, a central database for drug prescriptions identifies the physician and pharmacist, and includes information on hospital/specialist encounter information. This information is compiled, analyzed, and distributed to DHAs, hospital trusts[1], and other providers. At the DHA level, information on GP practice activity is built up from profiles of roster information (e.g., age, sex, and address of all

---

1. Under the reformed system, hospitals are organized into trusts. This arrangement is explained in more detail later in this section.

rostered members). At the purchaser/provider level, the contracting activity of the DHAs and GP Fundholders is providing information which is improving in response to demand for better data for planning, monitoring, and education.

This information forms the foundation for evaluation of the system by the NHS, purchasers (DHAs and GP Fundholders), and providers. Evaluation will also include assessment of how well the total system (or DHA region) achieved health and system targets or priorities set at the NHS and DHA, such as reduction in the incidence of a disease or establishment of required services in a particular area. As well, contracts increasingly specify expectations regarding outcome and quality, and require provision of evidence-based services. This is expected to contribute positively to continued system improvement in management of the system, quality, and evaluation.

The Delivery System

Organizational Structure

Organizational reform is evolving as initiatives to refine the system are implemented. Regional health authorities have, for all intents and purposes, been abolished and replaced by eight regional offices of the NHS. The new mandate of these offices is to monitor and regulate. They report directly to the NHS Executive for implementation of national health policy and for development of education, research, and public health (Hatcher 1996).

A number of factors led to the abolishment of the RHAs. In the early stages of reform, RHAs had the job of regulating the new purchaser/provider market and were responsible for the regional strategy for tertiary care; but conflict developed in two areas. One was the desire of the NHS to increase central control and to decrease the size and complexity of the bureaucracy. Secondly, the new purchasing role of DHAs began to affect hospital viability. Some RHAs used "top-sliced" money (funds withheld from transfers to DHAs to fund other parts of the system), to prop up tertiary hospitals that were experiencing difficulty in making the transition to the new environment. According to a confidential source, "Many of these tertiary hospitals were in fact functioning as expensive secondary hospitals, because they were unable to distinguish between tertiary and secondary care and failing to deal with the increasing shift of the balance of care away from hospital-based medicine towards primary care." In any case, this activity by the RHAs was perceived as conflicting with evolving market forces. In addition, as GP Fundholders took over more and more of the purchasing function, DHAs increased their role in the areas of needs assessment, establishing priorities, and monitoring. As a result, the monitoring, regulating and priority-setting functions were being handled more and more by the central NHS and the DHAs. While RHAs have been phased out, the number of DHAs has been reduced by more than half (225 to 100), increasing their population base accordingly (Hatcher 1996).

Another structure being phased out is the family health services authorities (FSHAs). The FSHAs were responsible, among other things, for approving the establishment of GP practices, pharmacies and dental practices. The plan called for the merger of FSHAs with their corresponding DHAs. Beginning with "voluntary" mergers, this national shift was required by statute to be complete by April 1, 1996 (Bundred 1996). The policy of "voluntary" movement was also applied to hospitals and community organizations in their transformation to semiautonomous self-governing hospitals and community trusts (figures 3 and 4).

Purchasers

There are presently two purchaser models in the United Kingdom: the district health authorities (DHAs) and the GP Fundholders.

DHAs are the predominant budgeters and fundholders in the system at this stage. They receive their funding from the NHS through a capitation formula, weighted for population factors including age and sex and regional expenditure factors. The population used for calculating the capitation for a DHA is defined based on census data. DHAs are responsible for purchasing services for the total district population. At this stage of evolution, DHAs are monopsonists (the sole purchasers) of many hospitals' services, although this is already being challenged by GP Fundholders (OECD 1995).

DHAs are not restricted to contracting within their district, which means that they are free to contract for hospital services in or outside their districts. This simplifies their capitation funding, as adjustments are no longer required for cross-boundary movement of consumers to access services. And as mentioned, DHAs have been merged to reduce the number of districts from 250 to approximately 100. The typical population served by a DHA now ranges from 500,000 to 1 million. DHAs are responsible for population needs assessment and based on this, subsequent purchase of appropriate services. Although most of the population is registered with a GP, not all are; and the NHS/DHA responsibility is for *all the population, registered or not* (Hatcher 1996). Each DHA has a director of public health who assesses health needs and evaluates the cost-effectiveness of various services. This closely integrated relationship has resulted in increasing emphasis on purchasing for health improvement, as well as for health services (Ham and Brommels 1994).

DHA boards have 11 members. The chair and five of the members are appointed by the NHS from outside the executive staff of the DHA, who comprise the remaining five board members. Community health councils link the DHA with the community. It is the job of these structures to bring

Figure 3
Consolidation of health authorities in the United Kingdom

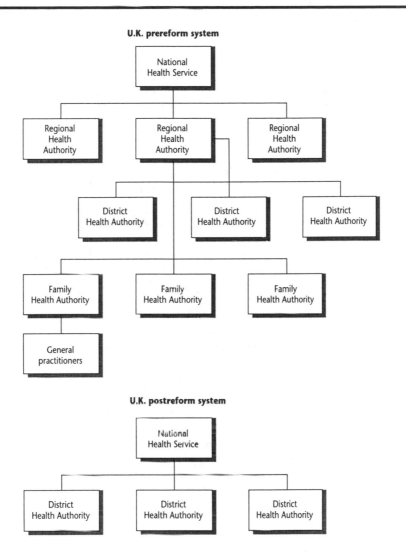

the community perspective to the DHA and to facilitate effective DHA-community communication. They also assist in bringing complaints to the attention of the DHA.

GP Fundholders are the other purchasing organization in the NHS. To date, their mandate includes drugs, specialist services, hospital services, and community services. All GPs, fundholders or not, function as independent contractors and are paid a mixture of capitation and other allowances. GP

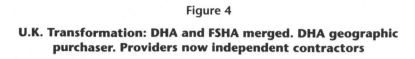

Figure 4

U.K. Transformation: DHA and FSHA merged. DHA geographic purchaser. Providers now independent contractors

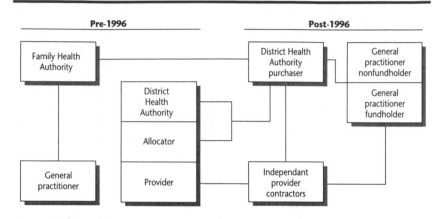

Note: Independent provider contractors includes diagnostics, specialists, hospitals, and community care

Fundholders also have access to "top-sliced" funding (out of the capitation allotment to DHAs) for the purpose of contracting for specialist, hospital, and community trust services. Such funding is based on historical use, and is not yet capitated. This funding will be described in more detail under the *providers* section later in this report, which will present additional financial and other factors, pertinent to the GP Fundholder status.

GP Fundholders can negotiate a one-time payment to buy computers, and a "flat" fund to pay for administrative or other nonprofessional staff to support the increased complexity of contracting for hospital and other services (Hatcher 1996). They also negotiate a budget to pay for other professional staff such as nurses and physiotherapists, as well as a budget for drugs. GP Fundholders and DHAs split the cost of such staff (GP Fundholder 30 percent and DHA 70 percent), and also negotiate a budget for specialists. Many GP Fundholders are establishing specialist clinics at their practice locations. Depending on the type of GP Fundholder, they may also assume responsibility for negotiating contracts with hospital and community trusts which must include community nursing and home care (other than custodial).

None of these funds, or any surpluses derived from them, may be used to pay GPs in the GP Fundholder practice. However, savings in one sector may be applied to another—for example, funds originally intended for drugs may instead go toward hospital services. Savings may also be applied to purchase of supplies such as equipment, materials, or furnishings, if their purpose is improvement of patient care services or enhancement of service responsiveness to their rostered patients.

Improvements ascribed to the introduction of GP Fundholder practices have included more informative and prompt discharge letters, faster response to GP enquiries, and improved access to physiotherapy, inpatient care, and specialists' clinics (Dixon and Glennerster 1995). If successful in improving the quality and range of services offered (but not by changing prices), GP Fundholders may attract more patients to their rosters and thus increase the revenue they derive from capitation (Maynard 1994; OECD 1995). Conversely, patients/consumers in a poorly managed practice may exercise their "right of exit" and move to another practice.

GP Fundholders have also been able to demonstrate improved access to hospital services for their patients, for reasons which include more effective contracting and increasing responsiveness by hospitals to attract GP Fundholder contracts. Because patients of GP Fundholders may enjoy improved hospital access over patients in nonfundholding practices, some commentators have made references to a system of "two-tiered health" (Dixon and Glennerster 1995). However, this situation may simply reflect the early stages of transition in the system, during which such inconsistencies occur before stabilization (e.g., hospitals may need to review their consistency of allowing access); or may reflect another transition for the system to make over time (that Fundholders' practices embody advantages and will predominate). Despite this sort of evolving development, these are all services within the publicly funded health system.

All consumers except children, pregnant mothers, the elderly, and people on social security pay a flat fee for prescription drugs with the NHS paying the pharmacist any remainder. The NHS keeps track of all prescriptions and expenses, and provides the relevant information to GP Fundholders with whom it has negotiated a budget for drug expenditures. If the expenditure is less than the budgeted amount, the GP Fundholder practice—like other potential purchasers—may transfer the "surplus" to other services. There is evidence that GP Fundholder practices have slowed the rate of increases in drug costs, when compared to nonfundholding general practices. For example, prescription costs increased 8 percent among GP Fundholders in 1992–1993, compared to a national increase of 12 percent (OECD 1992).

There is also growing evidence that GP Fundholders are more discerning than nonfundholding GPs, in their referrals to specialists and hospitals. In the Wirral district, for example, a recent review showed a significantly lower standardized admission ratio (SAR) for hysterectomies among patients of GP Fundholders (SAR 93.75) than for those of nonfundholding GPs (101.94) (Bundred 1996).

There are three types of GP Fundholders:

Total Fundholders, who purchase all community health services, including staff, drugs, diagnostic tests and community trust services, along with all hospital services for their rostered population. The DHA is not responsible for purchasing any health services for these people (Department of Health 1994). Initially 50 practices adopted this arrangement in the pilot stages; there are now approximately 100 practices involved, with significant rosters.

*Standard Fundholders,*who may purchase most services. Only hospital services are restricted, with Standard Fundholders limited to purchase of elective and outpatient procedures, and a few high-cost procedures such as heart transplant and renal dialysis procedures costing less than the equivalent of $12,000. All other hospital services are purchased by the DHA. To qualify for this arrangement, GP Fundholders must have a roster of at least 5,000 (a reduction from the original entry limit of 11,000).

Community Fundholders, who may purchase all but hospital services. These are purchased by the DHA. Community GP Fundholders must have a roster of at least 3,000.

As of April 1995, approximately 40 percent of the population were rostered with GP Fundholders in England. In an interesting example of horizontal integration, many of the GP Fundholders have created "multi-funds" to link their organizations and pool administrative resources. Several of these multifund groups have total rosters of approximately 200,000 (Maynard 1994). This results, in some cases, in settings that appear to be "miniauthorities" within primary care (Ham and Shapiro 1996).

In one district, all of the GPs are GP Fundholders. This may signal a future trend, and the need to address the role of the DHAs in a world where they may no longer be involved in contracting. One future role would be for DHAs to take a role in public health and needs assessment, including the establishment of special health targets. Another result could be increased pressure to establish full capitation for GP Fundholders.

Other contemporary trends include the increasing popularity of team practice which includes both GPs and specialists, and the accompanying emergence of "integrated care pathways" (Bundred 1996).

DHA and GP Fundholder Purchasing

Initially, contracts between purchasers (DHAs and GP Fundholders) and providers (such as hospitals) tended to be block contracts. Over time, contracts began to specify cost and volume, and to add "quality" specifications such as clinical protocols, maximum waiting times, and maximum times for issuance of discharge notes. The latest trend is to find ways to ensure that evidence-based decision making is taken into account in contractual arrangements. In addition, DHAs and GP Fundholders can threaten to exercise the "right of exit" on behalf of consumers, to choose to move a contract from one provider to another (OECD 1995). These measures have encouraged hospitals to implement quality improvements, utilization reviews, and other measures to make their services more efficient and effective. The "price" a hospital quotes for a service in negotiations is supposed to represent actual cost. In addition, hospitals are expected to achieve a 6 percent return on capital assets in their contracts. While contracts are often for particular services, they can also be for an integrated care package to cover an episode of illness. There is greater potential for this to lead to a more efficient skill mix and expanded treatment location options, creating incentives for suppliers to analyze the costs and benefits of vertical integration (Maynard 1994).

The move to contracting has also spurred the development of improved data systems, with increasing transparency of the system and public visibility of information related to performance quality. While the number of people on waiting lists increased after 1991, the time spent waiting for admission fell sharply for those having to wait at all, from an average of 7.6 months in April 1991 to 4.8 months in December 1993 (Klein 1995; OECD 1995). There has also been an increase in sensitivity to consumers, with the introduction of good business practices and incentives. For example, appointment scheduling is becoming more sophisticated, and consumer satisfaction is being tested.

Providers System

GPs tend to be independent contractors organized in both solo practices and groups. They are funded through a combination of capitation and fee for service, plus a budget for administrative costs. There is increasingly strong encouragement to form group practice to the extent that only about 10 percent of GPs are still in solo practices. All GPs have contracts with the DHA/FHSA. Payment sources are mixed, with 60 percent of general practitioners' incomes derived from capitation for their rostered patients and allowances (e.g., for seniority, practice in a rural area, employing assistants, etc.). They also receive fees per item of service for night visits, contraceptive services, and health promotion clinics (approximately $100 per clinic session), among other services (Kristiansen and Mooney 1993). Together, this income is meant to cover general medical services, with a contingency that GPs must provide 24-hour access to their services, and home visits where warranted.

In addition, GPs are paid to achieve specified targets such as immunization (approximately $1,200 per year if 70 percent of children in the relevant population are immunized, $3,600 per year if 90 percent are immunized). Similarly, incentives are paid for coverage of identified target populations. For example, GPs who provide pap smears to 50 percent of the eligible women in their roster receive $1,500 a year; this rises to $4,500 for 80 percent coverage (Kristiansen and Mooney 1993). Additional payments are made for health promotion, childhood development, management of patients with cardio-vascular disease, asthma and diabetes, and for providing services to lower socioeconomic populations. GPs are the gatekeepers of the system, and all access to specialist, community, and hospital services is via GP referral—although they do not yet enjoy admitting privileges. Further, all GPs must provide information on their rostered (registered) population, including the age/sex profile, the number of patient visits, and "billing" information on services such as immunizations and pap smears.

Specialists (or consultants) were historically paid directly by the NHS according to a standardized package of remuneration and increases. With reform, they now have contracts with hospital and community trusts as well as with GP Fundholders. The standardized remuneration is still prevalent, although this may change as the trusts are being given the freedom to negotiate this aspect of their contractual arrangements.

Hospitals have been transformed into semi-autonomous "trusts." They have autonomy of operations, which now compete with other hospitals and newly evolving integrated entities and organizations for contracts with DHAs and GP Fundholders. Like DHAs, the new trusts have 11-member corporate boards. The CEO, the medical director and directors of finance, nursing, and one other senior executive automatically become members of the board. The chair and the remaining five members (who are not employees), are appointed by government from the outside, and are typically chosen for their business or community expertise. Technically, hospital trusts have freedom to innovate; however, they face a number of constraints on their activity due to the imposition of performance targets and rules about prior approval for capital borrowing and asset disposal. The hospital trusts appoint their own CEO, hire staff and doctors, and own and sell property. With their new autonomy and requirement to compete for contracts, they have moved from a position of *budget* dependency to one of *revenue* dependency. In this new environment, trusts are able to retain surpluses, but are required to submit encounter information (e.g. admission, discharge, diagnosis, treatment provided, etc.).

Community services programs are now referred to as community trusts. Like hospital trusts, they are semiautonomous organizations with a corporate board. They are responsible for a variety of services, including community nursing provided by specialist nurses called "health visitors," other nurses, chiropodists, dentists, psychiatrists, and physiotherapists. They are not responsible for the homemaking component of home care.

Long-term care funding has largely been transferred out of the NHS to local government social services departments. Within this environment, responsibility for long-term care includes nursing homes and residential care homes (mostly privately owned) as well as nonclinical home care. Health services required by the residents of these facilities are covered by the appropriate DHA or GP Fundholder.

Trend toward Provider Integration

The degree of integration of entities, has been a notable trend in the United Kingdom. This includes both horizontal integration, such as amalgamations of physicians with other physicians or hospital trusts with other hospital trusts, and vertical integration by which different sectors of the health system such as hospitals, communities, and specialists affiliate under a single organization. One major reason for this occurring is the strategic decisions of entities to form integrated organizations in order to secure contracts with DHAs and GP Fundholders. Another is to avoid closure through rationalization and merger with trusts and physician services.

Summary of Features of Emerging Models—United Kingdom

Purchasing Models

There are two models for purchasing:
- district health authorities;
- GP Fundholders.

Key Features

District health authorities:
- Have an appointed board.
- Are responsible for all core services and benefits.
- Are responsible for planning and monitoring activities such as needs assessments, priority setting, determination of resource requirements.
- Have a client population which is identified through the census, involving no consumer choice. Population per DHA ranges from 500,000 to 1 million.
- Are funded by weighted capitation.
- Do not directly provide services.
- Purchase services for their assigned population, except for those services purchased by GP Fundholders.
- Have a jurisdiction which is geographically defined, but may purchase services from providers in any DHA jurisdiction.

GP Fundholders:
- Are independent contractors, primarily in group practice.
- Are responsible for provision of GP and primary care services including provision of a multidisciplinary team. Are responsible for negotiating contracts for purchase of drugs, community services, and specialist services. Depending on the type of fundholding arrangement, they may be responsible for the purchase of some or all hospital services.
- Patients are identified through rostering, who have the right to join the practice of their choice and exit it at will.

- They operate in competition with other GP Fundholders and non-fundholding practitioners to attract and hold the rostered population.
- Are funded for provision of GP/primary care services through a combination of capitation and other incentive and specified funding.
- Are funded through the DHA for purchase of drug, community, specialist, and hospital services. These funds are not part of a GP's remuneration. Currently they are based on historical expenditure, but the plan is to move to capitation in the future.
- Capitation funding follows the rostered individual, not the GP practice.

Government Regulation and Direction

The system provides for:
- a regulated market environment;
- capitation funding which follows the patient;
- unique identification of population;
- a single-payer system with tax-derived central fund for comprehensive health services;
- an emphasis on primary care, exemplified by an increasing amount of service controlled by and in that sector and also by the growing presence of GP Fundholders as major purchasers in the system;
- needs assessments and needs-based planning to establish national and regional priorities and health goals;
- increasing emphasis on quality, evidence, and outcomes in the contracting environment.

Other Integration

Both horizontal and vertical integration is taking place to create efficiencies and attract and hold contracts.

Role of Primary Care and the GP

- Emphasis on primary care development and coordination of the system.
- Primary care is provided by multidisciplinary teams.
- The GP is the gatekeeper to secondary and acute care.

Other Trends

There is some evidence that the DHA purchasing role is diminishing in the face of GP Fundholder purchasing (now covering approximately 50 percent of the population). This may ultimately result in DHAs withdrawing from purchasing over time and placing more emphasis on the assessments of need, establishment of priorities, evaluation and monitoring, and the fine-tuning of capitation funding.

Overview of the Health System of the Netherlands

Background

Various organizational reforms have taken place in the Netherlands since the Second World War. An early one was the transformation of health plan monopolies—nongovernmental, not-for-profit public insurance organizations called Sickness Funds. Originally organized around religious and political affiliations, they were converted into *geographically* defined monopolies. Attempts to control costs in the 1970s and 1980s led to a number of government legislative and regulatory controls, an example being capped global budgets for hospitals, implemented in 1983. This has been described as a period when "tight and detailed central regulation of prices, volume and capacity had been superimposed on an essentially private system of provision and a mixed system of finance" (OECD 1992).

Pressure for further reform continued, influenced by factors such as the uncoordinated financing of health care, lack of free choice between different Sickness Fund organizations, and few or lack of incentives for consumers, insurers, or providers to act efficiently. For example, there were no incentives for consumers to restrain demand, or for the Sickness Fund organizations to select efficient providers. In part, this was because Sickness Funds were obligated to enter into contracts with *any* local provider wishing to provide services to its members. This constrained them to a role of "passive funders of care rather than active, cost-effective purchasers of services" (OECD 1992). In addition, highly centralized government regulation was seen as complex, costly, rigid, and working against progress.

A new wave of reform transformed the Sickness Funds from geographic monopolies into organizations which could compete across the country to roster (register) eligible consumers (figure 5). This has been characterized as a move from government-regulated cartels to government-regulated competition among insurers and providers. Concepts of "markets" and "incentives" were and continue to be integral to reform, despite a subsequent political shift to the left in Holland, resulting in "lighter" terminology such as "shared responsibility between parties, consumer choice and decentralization" (van de Ven and Schut 1994). The market-based concepts have shaped what Bultman calls a "health care system with market incentives" and are still in place, integral to reform (Bultman 1996).

While other schemes of reform had been envisioned, such as an earlier proposed amalgamation of the various private and government macro-insurance schemes (referred to as the "Dekker reforms"), they were not incorporated. Nonetheless, there is a move to ensure that private insurers offer a standard package with the same benefits as the public health insurance. This will be discussed later in the presentation of the macrosystem.

Figure 5

Transformation of Sickness Fund organizations from geographic monopsonies to competing roster-based national purchasers

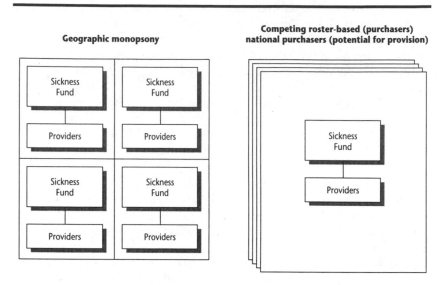

The majority of the Dutch population is supported by public funding for health services. The funding is derived primarily from social insurance rather than taxes. According to Maarse, the "main characteristics of social health insurance are: social solidarity; universal access; compulsory membership; payroll taxes with employer-employee split; and implementation by Sickness Funds" (Maarse 1994). Private health insurance covers the bulk of the remaining population. This basic funding profile has remained essentially the same.

The Macroenvironment

Benefits and Funding

At the macrolevel, the Netherlands has achieved its version of a universal health system based on a blend of public and private health insurance to cover everyone. High-cost services are provided through one public plan for everyone, while the remainder are all covered under a minimum comprehensive set of benefits for "ordinary" health coverage in the public and private health plans. Most of the population here is covered under public health plans. Focused primarily on the public sector, the aggregate effect of both public insurance plans is a comprehensive set of health benefits, which unlike that in many other countries, also covers illness or injury that occurs in the workplace.

There are four insurance schemes at the macrolevel within the Netherlands. They are:

- universal insurance for the entire population under the Exceptional Medical Expenses Act (known as the AWBZ);
- scheme for provincial and municipal government employees;
- private insurance;
- standard health insurance under the Health Insurance Act (known as the ZFW).

The Exceptional Medical Expenses Act (the AWBZ) covers the entire population against serious medical risk. Initially, this insurance was meant to cover exceptional costs associated with long-term care or high-cost treatment, where the costs cannot be borne by individuals or adequately covered by private insurance. Over the years, however, the scope of the act has been extended to cover a number of items that are neither long-term nor expensive. It was the original intent under reform to inevitably extend the benefits of all insurance schemes under this one plan for everyone, but this did not happen (Ministry of Health, Welfare and Sport 1995). Benefits include coverage for hospital stay beginning after the first 325 days in hospital, long-term care in nursing homes and homes and hostels for the physically disabled, psychiatric care in hospitals and other settings, care of the mentally handicapped, and home nursing care.

Until recently, funding for the AWBZ was covered by government funds coupled with percentage and flat-rate contributions. Insured persons are liable to pay contributions. People who do not receive wages or a salary, but who are liable for tax and social security contributions, are issued with an assessment for percentage contributions, while employed individuals have contributions deducted from their earnings and paid to the tax authorities by their employer. Beginning on January 1, 1992, a flat-rate contribution was also levied, in an amount determined by the insurers themselves. This flat-rate contribution was abolished on January 1, 1995 for children under the age of 18, and for the remaining population effective January 1, 1996 (Ministry of Health, Welfare and Sport 1995; Bultman 1996). Until recently, the government insurance plans, private insurance plans, or Sickness Funds with which an individual was registered assumed the responsibility for administering the AWBZ. Since January 1, 1996, the budgeting of private insurers for AWBZ ended (Bultman 1996).

The remaining "normal" or standard medical expenses are covered by one of three types of insurance plans: government plans, private plans, and standard health insurance under the Health Insurance Act. As described below, whether one is covered by public or private insurance depends on one's income and whether one is employed in the public service.

The *Civil Servants Scheme for Provincial and Municipal Government* covers 5 percent of the population, with compensation for health care costs reimbursed by employers as part of their general "labour contract." The employees pay no contribution.

Private insurance plans are purchased by individuals whose earnings exceed the maximum income threshold for standard health insurance. Private insurance covers approximately 40 percent of the population. Long-term plans call for increasing harmonization of the private and standard insurance plans over time. This is likely to be accomplished through a harmonizing of a standard package of benefits as a threshold of coverage. It should also be noted that anyone can take out supplementary insurance for services beyond the basic coverage. Private insurance organizations are obliged to accept everyone who no longer falls under the public scheme (Groenewegen 1994).

Standard health insurance under the Health Insurance Act is compulsory for everyone who receives social security benefits or who earns below a defined statutory ceiling (currently 57,700 guilders). A person earning more than this amount must leave the plan and purchase private health insurance. Entitlement for coverage is based primarily on residency, not nationality, although there is provision for Dutch nationals working outside the country. In order to obtain coverage, individuals must register with one of the competing Sickness Fund organizations.

Funding for standard health insurance is based on payments by insured individuals. One payment is based on the percentage of income which is paid into the central fund. The current income-dependent rate is set at 7 percent of income with the employer paying 1.65 percent and the employee 5.35 percent (Bultman 1996). The other payment is a flat rate determined by and paid directly to the Sickness Fund organization. Sickness Funds may charge a flat rate which is less than the statutory maximum. Once a flat fee is determined, the Sickness Funds must charge that same rate to all of its enrollees who choose the same insurance package (van de Ven and Schut 1994). The central funds are transferred to the Sickness Funds on the basis of capitation which is weighted by age, sex, a disability index (i.e., the number of people who get allowances under the Disability Act), and region (e.g., big cities or rural). Since 1 January 1996, the Sickness Funds are only budgeted for the variable costs of hospitals. The fixed costs are reimbursed from the central fund (Bultman 1996).

This insurance scheme covers all medical and surgical treatment; obstetric care; dental care for children and preventive care for adults; inpatient and outpatient hospital care (hospital admission for up to 365 days, plus psychiatric care not covered by the Exceptional Medical Expenses plan); ambulance; maternity care; haemodialysis, and other special programs. There are no copayments for GP services or user charges for hospital services. There are, however, a number of additional charges, such as for drugs, assistive devices (e.g., orthopaedic shoes, hearing aids), and for nursing home care.

One feature of all Dutch health insurance schemes is that they all "provide coverage not only for sickness and maternity, but also for the health care costs due to industrial injury and occupational disease" (Brasker and van Uchelen 1995).

Principles and Regulation

It is the job of the Health Insurance Council, an independent administrative body, to oversee elements of the insurance system. It oversees the implementation of both the Exceptional Medical Expenses Act and the Health Insurance Act. It also advises the Minister of Health on the approval of new Sickness Fund organization's, based on the statutes of the organization, the degree to which the rostered members relate to the board and the organization's potential to perform in accordance with expectations. The Health Insurance Council administers the central funds, dividing them among the various Sickness Fund organizations using a capitation formula, and it monitors expenses. Finally, in response to requests or at its own initiative, the Health Insurance Council advises government on matters of social insurance and health care provided in that context (Bultman 1995).

To support its monitoring and planning mission, the Health Insurance Council receives aggregated data from Sickness Funds about the "production" of providers, such as GP activity, all referrals to specialists and hospital care, and prescriptions. It uses this information in annual evaluations of Sickness Fund organization performance, keeping track of patterns of expenditure against services for rostered members, auditing expenditures against defined benefits or core services, and auditing the roster as the foundation for capitation. The council also has the authority to review the performance of a Sickness Fund organization at any time in response to any signals of "bad performance," and if necessary to appoint a temporary director (Bultman 1996).

The Central Agency for Health Care Tariffs (known as the COTG) is a "quasi"-nongovernmental body that is responsible for developing policy guidelines on tariffs (e.g., for specialists and hospitals), reviewing and approving rate proposals, providing advice to the Minister of Health on policy associated with establishment of rates, and providing arbitration in case of conflicts during rate negotiations. A recent attempt to maintain central control on rising costs while encouraging competition has involved the introduction of maximum tariffs that "allow" the provider to charge less than the maximum.

The government also licenses hospitals for specialty services. Using this mechanism, the number of sites offering highly specialised services are controlled centrally, as are the tariffs for funding. Control over the number of sites is particularly important to ensure that there is a sufficient volume of work at each site to maintain quality, while ensuring that there are sufficient number of these sites to support adequate access. Cost is controlled through tariff maxima or imposed tariffs.

It is the government's intention to bring the Health Insurance Act, the government's public servants' plan and private insurance plans closer together. The vision is to have a more integrated health insurance system defined at the macrolevel to "guarantee a high standard of accessible and affordable insurance for all" (Ministry of Health, Welfare and Sport 1995). To achieve this goal, complementary insurance packages are envisioned to cover three distinct areas (Ministry of Health, Welfare and Sport 1995):

- "Uninsurable risks"—that is, long-term or costly care, covered under the Exceptional Medical Expenses plan.
- "Ordinary" care, which will ultimately be covered under a statutorily defined package of benefits. These will be the same for the public servants' plan, the Health Insurance Act, and private insurance packages.
- "Supplementary" insurance that falls outside statutory control, which people may purchase if they wish.

The criteria used to determine which services would be included in the ordinary or basic insurance are that the care provided must be necessary, effective, and efficient and cannot be left to individual responsibility (Holland 1992). In addition to the focus on insurance plans, the government is investigating ways to create more incentives for GPs and for primary care in general to take on a bigger role in the provision and coordination of services.

Delivery System

The primary organization of the publicly funded system is the Sickness Fund. Once geographic monopolies, these organizations now compete to sign up populations across the country. Individuals register with a Sickness Fund organization of their choice, normally for a period of two years. A person may conceivably change Sickness Fund organizations every two years. Registered individuals receive a certificate as proof of entitlement to services (Ministry of Health, Welfare and Sport 1995). Registering with a given Sickness Fund automatically confers on that organization the responsibility to administer the benefits of both the Health Insurance Act and the Exceptional Medical Expenses Act. Registration is deemed to begin as of the date upon which the individual signs up. Sickness Funds are not allowed to select registrants against risk (Groenewegen 1994).

Elements of managed care "tools," as employed by American health maintenance organizations, can be seen throughout the Dutch system. For example, all individuals registered with a given Sickness Fund are also obligated to select and register (roster) with a GP chosen from those under contract with the Sickness Fund. The same is true for selecting and registering with a pharmacist.

Sickness Fund revenue is based on risk-adjusted capitation from the central fund in addition to flat-rate premiums paid on a monthly basis by the enrollees. Sickness Fund organizations are not-for-profit corporate structures, with historical roots of either "foundations" or "mutualities" (mutual benefit organizations or societies). Board structure varies. There is no guarantee of participation of the insured in the board; rather, the Sickness Fund must ensure that the insured have a reasonable influence on the organization—usually through advisory committees or similar mechanisms (Bultman 1996).

Many Sickness Fund and private insurance organizations have merged. Reasons for this include a desire to market supplementary insurance (they offer not only health insurance, but also all other types of insurance, such as damage, life, etc. Some also offer commercial banking activities—"all-finance concept"). A more important reason is to introduce business-oriented skills aimed at stimulation of more effective performance in the new environment of competing for populations and contracting with providers. Given these new demands, "administration-oriented chief executives who go into [early] retirement are replaced by entrepreneurial, market-oriented managers. The service to their members is being improved, such as better opening hours and mobile offices" (van de Ven and Schut 1994).

The number of Sickness Fund organizations has decreased dramatically over the past few years, as organizations merge to better position themselves to succeed in the new and evolving environment. The size of the Sickness Fund organizations, as determined by the number of registered consumers, ranges from 30,000 to 1.2 million registered members (Bultman 1996).

Sickness Fund organizations assess the needs of their registered population, and based on a corresponding assessment of health resource requirements to meet this need, negotiate contracts with providers. In this sense, the Netherlands has a purchaser/provider split. However, even under the current system a Sickness Fund organization has the potential to own a provider practice or institution, if a special case is made and specific authorization obtained from the Health Insurance Council (Bultman 1996).

Any provider meeting quality standards may offer services. Contracts vary by Sickness Fund, provider, the types of care required, and conditions or specifications that must be met. For example, a referral from a GP is needed for reimbursement of a specialist. Generally, GPs are paid by capitation and pharmacists and specialists by fee for service, while hospitals negotiate a global budget with the Sickness Funds and other insurers (Sonneveldt 1994; Bultman 1996). Sickness Funds cannot innovate to the same extent as fully vertically integrated organizations in other national jurisdictions, in terms of planning and negotiating the purchase of all health services for its population. State regulation still plays a major part in imposing payment rates, providing guidelines, and arbitrating any breakdown in negotiating agreements. For example, the COTG may impose tariffs or fees, if negotiations between the National Association of Specialists and the national associations for the Sickness Funds and private insurers do not reach agreement.

Effort being made to strengthen the role of primary care includes introduction of payment incentives to reward treatment of target populations—for example, diabetics—in the GP's office. GPs already function as gatekeepers. A referral letter from the GP is required to access specialist and hospital services, in addition to written approval from the Sickness Fund for hospital admissions. The GP also receives funding to participate with pharmacists in pharmaco-therapeutic meetings, to update education on drugs and prescribing, and for continuing education in general.

Hospital contracts are established on the basis of collective bargaining with all the Sickness Funds and other insurers who use or plan to use that hospital's services (as opposed to the hospital pursuing individual contracts with each Sickness Fund organization). The insurer with the largest block of required work takes the lead for the insurers. Essentially, the contracts are negotiated on the expected volumes of different services required for the next year, using an established tariff for each service as the foundation for establishing the overall global budget.

Maximum tariffs are established by the COTG as a guideline. This allows a hospital to compete with other hospitals by using a lower tariff to negotiate its global budget. Once the global budget is established, the hospital is not rigidly required to provide the precise type and quantity of services negotiated; "mixing and matching" is appropriate to the actual evolving demand from the Sickness Funds and private insurers. A hospital's cash flow is based on charging a *per diem* rate for each service, plus fees for specific services not otherwise covered, such as the use of surgical suites. The hospital is free to determine which approach it will take for different services. Ultimately, it is expected to live within the predetermined total budget, absorbing the cost of services when the volume of work or demand is greater than anticipated. As insurance against unforeseen conditions, the hospital may receive approval to reopen negotiations if special circumstances warrant it (Bultman 1996).

There has been concern about the potential conflict of incentives between paying specialists on a fee-for-service basis, and negotiating a global budget for the hospital. One recommendation has been to include funding for specialists within the hospital contract. There are approximately 13 experiments under way to include funding for specialists within the hospital contract, involving approximately 1,600 medical specialists. Current plans are to introduce a new law in 1997–1998 to require this integration. The expectation is that incorporating hospitals and specialists' funding could lead to further innovation in contracting (Bultman 1996).

Sickness Funds are also demonstrating innovation in their business practices. As van de Ven and Schut (1994) explain,

For example, Sickness Funds have broken the price cartel of providers of some medical devices. Subsequently, prices went down by a quarter to a third. Insurers are developing mail order firms as an alternative distribution method of pharmaceuticals. All kinds of electronic data interchange (EDI) projects are being developed, aimed at better cooperation among providers and a more efficient cooperation between providers and insurers.

Sickness Funds require providers to submit information. GPs submit aggregate information on all prescriptions and referrals to specialists, as well as encounter information from specialists and hospitals. With this information, the Sickness Fund is able to monitor and manage the care of individual registered members as well as develop profiles of physician activity. Aggregate information is submitted to the Health Insurance Council.

Providers

GPs are independent contractors who are free to open a practice wherever they choose. As of 1992, half of all GPs worked in groups or community health centres (OECD 1992). Patients must select and register with a physician from among those who have a contract with their Sickness Fund. At this stage, private insurance patients can go to any GP they choose. GPs in the Netherlands have a higher average list size—2,300 inhabitants per GP—than their counterparts in Denmark, Belgium, Italy, or France (van der Zee and Hutten 1995). As gatekeepers, they control access to specialists, paramedics, and hospital services. They receive capitation from the Sickness Funds and fee for service for privately insured and funded services. They also receive funding for continuing education as previously mentioned. While it is possible in principle for individual GPs to hire other health care providers, they generally apply their capitation funding to an administrative assistant who makes appointments, does simple laboratory tests, and so on. In contrast, some GPs work in neighbourhood health centres where nurses, social workers, midwives, physiotherapists, and other practitioners work as independent providers or employees of the centre.

Generally speaking, specialists are linked to hospitals and are remunerated primarily on a fee-for-service basis. Their fees are negotiated centrally with the National Association of Health Insurance and the National Association of Medical Specialists (Maarse 1995). As mentioned previously, there is a move toward integrating specialist remuneration and overall hospital funding.

Hospitals are primarily private, nonprofit, voluntary institutions. "Most former public hospitals (which were owned by local governments) have been transformed into private entities." (Maarse 1995). For-profit hospitals are prohibited in the Netherlands, although this does not rule out the nonprofit facilities earning surplus revenues.

The association of GPs has developed some 50 protocols for frequently occurring medical complaints. Specialists are organizing quality assurance site visits in hospitals. Dentists are developing protocols. All associations of medical professionals are discussing or developing a system of reregistration (for example, every 5 years) or certification (van de Ven and Schut 1994). For GPs, such a system is already in place.

Summary of Features of Emerging Models—The Netherlands

Purchasing Model

Sickness Funds are the only purchasing model in the publicly funded health system in the Netherlands.

Key Features

Sickness Fund organizations:
- Are not-for-profit corporations.
- Have corporate boards.
- Bear responsibility for all core services and benefits.
- Have a rostered population, in which individuals have the right to join and exit the Sickness Fund organization.
- Are funded by weighted capitation.
- Assess and plan for population need; and determine required resources.
- Purchase an appropriate array of health services from providers. (At this stage an "all-purchaser model"; there are no barriers to a Sickness Fund organization owning a provider practice or institution to provide some services if they can make a case for it with authorities.)
- Compete with each other to attract and hold their rostered populations throughout the country (no imposed geographic constraints).

Government Regulation and Direction

The system:
- Is a regulated health system with market elements.
- Operates under a degree of regulatory constraint on the market elements which is still fairly prominent. For example, there are constraints on innovation in business development and in organizational and contractual relationships. There has been evidence of movement toward further fine-tuning to support some freeing up of options, such as allowing for blended hospital/specialist contracts.
- Is funded by weighted capitation.
- Requires rostering of the population.
- Provides government-established core services and benefits.

Other Integration

There has been some effort toward horizontal and vertical integration among hospitals and other providers to better position themselves to attract and hold contracts.

Role of Primary Care and the GP

- The GP is the gatekeeper to secondary and acute care.
- The government is looking for ways to encourage GP practices to take on more services and a stronger role in coordination.

Overview of the Health System of New Zealand

Background

New Zealand underwent a phase of reform in its health system in the 1980s. Fourteen geographically defined area health boards were created, partly through the merger of hospital boards and district public health units. Each board was responsible for purchase and provision of secondary care for a population ranging between 35,000 and 900,000. Primary care was essentially separate and was funded, in part, through public funding on a fee-for-service basis. Individuals also paid a copayment to the GP. Overall, the system was a mix of private and public funding and service delivery. Approximately 80 percent of expenditures came from public funds derived from general taxation. Area health boards were funded through a population-based formula weighted for age, sex, mortality, and fertility.

Despite reform efforts, a number of problems were summarized in the Minister of Health's "Green and White Paper" of 1991:
- Waiting times for hospital care were too long. For example, some patients waited more than a year for pain-relieving surgery.
- There was concern about conflict of interest in purchasing by area health boards. For example, there were incentives for boards to buy their own services rather than contract with the most cost-effective or appropriate provider.
- Funding of the system was fragmented, with secondary care funded on an adjusted population basis, while primary care was sustained through a bizarre mixture of subsidies.
- There were problems with access, with some evidence that the poor were not going to doctors due to user charges.
- The lack of assistance for doctors in making decisions; for example, primary medical benefits were set at varying levels and differences between levels were illogical.

- A lack of consumer control (e.g., people want more say in how their health care is delivered). It was felt there was too little consultation, and too little opportunity for local involvement in the delivery of health services. Further, health services were seen as not sufficiently responsive to consumers' changing needs.
- The system was perceived to suffer from a lack of fairness. It was intended that the system treat people fairly, guaranteeing all New Zealanders reasonable access to an adequate and affordable range, level, and quality of service (Upton 1991).

Other identified problems included a loss of innovation in the bureaucracy, disincentives for hospitals to treat patients for fear of going over budget, the copayments required by GPs which could lead patients to use hospital services instead, and local political pressure on area health boards which might inappropriately influence decisions (Borren and Maynard 1994). In addition, some groups—in particular the Maori community—wanted to run their own systems through HMO-type models, providing or purchasing their own health care and innovating in accordance with their own sense of priorities.

Overall, the government felt that the system was too centralized, rigid, and unresponsive to change. In July 1993, elements of competition and choice were introduced with the establishment of four regional health authorities (RHAs). The government's objective was to separate purchaser and provider functions, and to integrate responsibility for purchase of both primary and secondary care. Prior to this, primary care and secondary/ acute care had been handled separately with the secondary/acute care handled under the area health boards (Scott 1994). RHAs are funded on a weighted capitation basis.

The 14 area health boards were converted to 23 crown health enterprises (CHEs) to compete with each other for contracts with the RHAs. A standard package of core benefits was to be introduced in part that competing purchasers would provide a comparable comprehensive package and could not define the package in such a way that only healthy people could enroll. The government also intended that other "purchasers" or budget/fundholders would evolve to compete with RHAs for purchasing, and to present greater choice for consumers in selecting their budget-holding/purchasing organizations. Despite the vision, the initial intent of this policy of growing budget/fundholding models, which are sharing or assuming the purchasing role for rostered populations

The Macroenvironment

Benefits

All New Zealanders are entitled to health benefits; however, two important features of the system should be highlighted. One is that benefits paid for GP consultations and prescription drugs is a *subsidy* given to providers as partial payment for service, rather than a complete payment. Individuals with incomes below a certain level are provided with "community service cards" entitling them to a higher "subsidy" health services. In addition, those who have chronic conditions which require frequent services are issued with "high-use" cards which guarantee higher GP subsidies, no charge for hospital services, and reduced prescription charges (Scott 1994; Shipley 1996).

The 23 newly converted crown health enterprises are primarily hospital organizations which negotiate contracts with purchasers in a new system based on separation of purchasing and service provision. The four regional health authorities (RHAs) were created to purchase health services defined by the government. The initial plans were to allow for other "insurers or purchasing organizations" to evolve in competition with RHAs to provide consumers with greater choice and to enhance contestability in the system. This aspect of the initial reform has not yet been implemented, although, as will be presented later, there are a number of moves to extend purchasing authority to newly evolving integrated provider organizations, and to develop "managed care" organizations (figure 6).

The Ministry of Health monitors RHA purchasing, provides advice to RHAs on the services they are to purchase, and sets principles which must be observed in making these purchasing decisions. The principles are (Shipley 1996):
- equity (fair access to services);
- effectiveness (services which result in improved health);
- efficiency (the best value for money);
- safety (protection of consumers from avoidable harm);
- acceptability (that people are informed, have choice, and that treatment is culturally appropriate);
- risk management (minimization of purchasers' financial and service risks).

The government defines which core services it will fund, based on advice from the Core Services Committee. The government publishes detailed purchasing guidelines for RHAs covering each of the benefit areas, including dental and diagnostic as well as primary, secondary, and tertiary services. New Zealand has developed geographic criteria to fulfil the principles and goals of *equity of access* to services, as opposed to equal outcomes (Scott 1994). The health services as defined in 1996 purchasing requirements for RHAs include the following:

Figure 6

New Zealand transformation

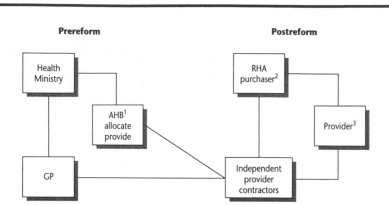

1. Area health boards (AHBs) converted from small geographic public integrated models to crown enterprises as independent provider contractors (primarily hospital) along with GPs and other providers
2. Creation of large geographic purchaser—Regional Health Authority (RHA)
3. Development of purchaser/providers (e.g. GP Fundholders and HMO-type organizations).

- *Public health services* – all those traditional services ensuring the safety of food, water and so on, as well as preventive programs such as immunization and health promotion to encourage healthy choices by individuals and groups concerning nutrition and use of tobacco, alcohol, and drugs.
- *Primary care services* – the services of general practitioners (GPs), accident and emergency treatment, well-child and adolescent care, and family planning services. Government geographic and financial access criteria for primary care services require RHAs to ensure that primary care service is available within 30 minutes of travelling time for 90 percent of the population within their areas, and within three hours for 99 percent. People are not charged for selected services including cervical screening, well-child services, vaccinations on the National Immunization Schedule and primary care for sexually transmitted diseases. The payment for GP services is a subsidy; physicians may charge extra. The subsidy is paid by RHAs to GPs for all children and for all persons who have community service or high-use health cards.
- *Primary diagnostic, therapeutic and support services* – laboratory diagnostic services such as blood tests, diagnostic imaging services such as ultrasound, prescription medicines, and other pharmaceutical and support services. All of these services are usually available by referral from a GP, and a part charge to the individual applies.

- *Pregnancy and childbirth services* – the services of midwives, GPs and specialists, along with the required facilities for the provision of each of these services. Women have access to at least one of these providers free of charge. Appropriate facilities for normal birth are available to at least 90 percent of women of childbearing age within 90 minutes of travel.
- *Dental services* – preventive, educational, and restorative dental services for preschool, primary, and intermediate school children and adolescents are provided free of charge throughout the country. Emergency dental services are subsidized for low-income adults.
- *Secondary and tertiary medical and surgical services* – services are provided on an outpatient, day-patient or inpatient basis and usually require referral from a primary service provider. Hospital inpatient services are provided free of charge, and day-patient and outpatient services are also available free of charge after the first five visits per family per year. Community services card holders and high-use health card holders use outpatient and day-patient services free of charge. Day-patient and out-patient visits can be charged for up to a maximum of $31 per visit for adults ($16 for children) who are not community services card holders or high-use health card holders.
- *Mental health services* – services to treat or support mental health or substance use disorders. There are no charges for inpatient, day-patient, or outpatient mental health services provided by crown health enterprises (CHEs).
- *Disability support services* – including needs assessment, service coordination, personal care, household management, caregiver support, rehabilitation and habilitation, information provision, environmental support, residential, and continuing care services. These services are purchased and coordinated by RHAs for people with intellectual, physical, sensory, psychiatric, or age-related disability.
- *Cervical screening* – purchased from locally managed cervical screening services, which serve women in their defined geographical areas.

Funding

Funds for the health system are derived from general taxation. One of the features of the 1991 health care reform was the consolidation of primary and secondary care funding under single purchasers—the RHAs (Scott 1994). RHAs receive per capita funding to purchase the required health services for their population. The capitation formula is adjusted for population size, age, sex, ethnicity (e.g., Maori), urban/rural mix, and other socioeconomic factors. Funding is adjusted upward from year to year to allow for demographic growth. There are no automatic adjustments to health funding for inflation, technology, or demand pressures; however, the government has made a number of discrete decisions to increase health funding in recent years in response to demand in technology pressures.

The Core Services Committee provides independent advice to government "on the kinds and relative priorities of personal health services and disability support services that should be publicly funded" (Edgar 1995). The committee uses four criteria to determine which services should have priority for public funding (Edgar 1995):

- Benefit or effectiveness of the service (does it do more good than harm?).
- Value for money or cost-effectiveness (is the service sufficiently effective to justify the cost especially if an equally effective but cheaper alternative is available?).
- Fairness in access and use of the resource (is this the best way to use the resource or should it be used for someone else or at some other time?).
- Consistency with community values (are these the services most valued by communities?).

An interesting footnote is that the requirement for provision of defined core services was seen as a safeguard in the event that competing purchasers evolved in New Zealand. "The establishment of a core ensures that competing purchasers cannot define packages of services in such a way that only healthy people enroll (i.e., risk selection or cream skimming), or in ways that make it difficult for enrollees to make an informed comparison of different health plans" (Cumming 1994). The package has been defined in broad general terms in the service obligations to RHAs. The Core Services Committee is working to define explicit clinical criteria and the priority people have for access to those services. (Edgar 1996).

Information and Evaluation

As a result of work spearheaded by the Core Services Committee, the government is supporting the development of evidence-based guidelines and needs assessment procedures, in order to ration access fairly and improve quality. It is also supporting the development and implementation of information technology. The Ministry of Health has access to a growing database to support its monitoring and benchmarking of RHA performance, as well as other elements of the health system.

RHAs all have performance contracts with the Minister. The Ministry sets out requirements for RHAs each year. Based on this, each RHA plans its purchase of services and negotiates an agreement with the Minister to establish the services to be purchased, and for the funding to be made available to the RHA. The Ministry then develops quarterly and annual reports based on the performance of each RHA based on detailed reporting of activity and expenditures submitted by the RHA to the Ministry.

At the provider level, GPs submit claims information for the fee-for-service subsidies they receive (for over 50 percent of the population). Many physicians are moving into independent practitioner associations and other budget/fundholding practices that are moving to capitation funding. They submit patient roll data and information pertinent to performance and quality of service as required by their contracts. Claims information is also submitted for pharmacy prescriptions and laboratory services.

Contracts with CHEs are monitored by RHAs and evaluated in terms of the specifications of the contract. All hospital discharge information from CHEs is provided to the National Information Services section of the Ministry. The government's "ownership" of shareholder interest in CHEs is monitored by a separate agency: the Crown Company Monitoring and Advisory Unit.

Delivery Environment

Purchasers

The four RHAs serve populations that range from some 680,000 to just over 1 million in 1991 (Upton 1991). They are incorporated bodies, and their boards are required by law to make all operating decisions. The board comprises seven directors appointed by the Minister for a three-year period, but they are eligible for reappointment. Directors are chosen on the basis of their ability to determine, within broad general service obligations, the best range and mix of services to meet the health needs of the people in their region, and to establish purchase agreements for quality, effective services at the best price, and to consult with their communities in performing their functions (Edgar 1996). Within this framework, RHAs are accountable to the Minister of Health and receive integrated capitation funding. They are responsible for the purchase of health, disability, and public health services for their populations. Personal health services focus on the delivery of health care to individuals. The disability services purchased include services which improve or maintain independence. Public health includes disease prevention, health promotion, and health protection services.

RHA purchasing is influenced by government guidelines, including the principles for purchase decisions previously presented. They are also guided by government health gain priorities or targets to be achieved. Presently, the priorities are in the areas of child health, Maori health, mental health, and improved physical environment. The New Zealand Ministry of Health (1995) has summarized several ways in which RHAs are seeking to improve the contracting process:

- using longer-term contracts;
- arranging for contracts for specific services to be negotiated at different times of the year, so that the contracting pressure on RHAs and providers is less concentrated;

- more widespread use of simple contracts or memoranda of understanding for low-cost contracts that cover small levels of services;
- combining some related services into single contracts instead of purchasing them separately—this has already happened in some area of disability support and is currently being proposed for maternity care; and
- splitting block contracts into discrete elements—for example, a long-term contract with one provider for access to a hospital facility could be coupled with separate and more flexible contracts with a range of professional teams to deliver services using the facility (this would allow greater choice for consumers, even where there is room for only one hospital in an area.

Budget/Fundholding (Purchaser/Provider Blends)

Other "purchasers" are evolving in the New Zealand health system. General practices and other integrated health organizations are receiving additional funding to purchase services other than those they provide themselves. In the current lexicon of the New Zealand Ministry of Health, they are referred to as "subpurchasers" because the RHAs act as the instrument of government policy and they currently retain legal accountability for the services they contract with the "purchasers" to subcontract for. This evolution is the result of government policy which stipulates that:

> To allow purchasing to be more responsive to people's needs and preferences, more organizations will play a purchasing role in the future. Purchasers will also actively use the contracting process to make services more equitable and effective, and will make greater use of contestability. At the same time they will be sensitive to the need for providers to share information and work together more collaboratively (New Zealand Ministry of Health 1995).

This represents an incremental move toward vertical integration of responsibility for GP organizations and other evolving organizational structures similar to HMOs.

For example, RHAs have implemented "budgetholding" for pharmaceutical and diagnostic laboratory testing with a number of GP practices. Under this arrangement, a GP practice receives a budget for subsidizing these services for its patients. Any savings realized this way can then be invested in the delivery of further health care (Shipley 1996). Budget-holding organizations may also receive funding for secondary services or mental health services. Most budgets are based on historical expenditure, although RHAs are exploring approaches to capitation. All budgetholder agreements are for a defined set of services and for an identified population. RHAs monitor these operations to ensure that there is no cost shifting and that the needs of the identified population are being met. They may also enter "joint-venture" arrangements with providers to collaborate in planning and monitoring specific services for an identified population.

This direction demonstrates the motivation toward increased integration and coordination of services to include, ultimately, all aspects of the health system under single, vertically integrated organizations, responsible for an identified population, capable of implementing managed care. The government is supporting the development of managed care and managed care organizations to deliver it for a number of reasons, as summarized by the Ministry of Health:

> By clearly defining the population and services for which an organization is responsible, managed care encourages providers to be more responsive to consumer needs and preferences. These arrangements make it easier for providers to co-ordinate services and monitor outcomes for their consumers. They also give providers an incentive to use health promotion, illness prevention and early intervention to keep people well and independent (New Zealand Ministry of Health 1995).

A variety of integrated models are being assessed in pilot projects, most of them focusing on primary health care services and primary referred services. Nearly 40 percent of GPs already belong to independent practitioner associations (IPAs) or other groups/networks that have assumed some degree of responsibility for budgets for laboratory tests and prescriptions that their consumers use. Savings may be maintained to improve and increase other services, or to reduce or waive user charges.

Other more specialized integrated organizations are developing, including Maori-run health organizations. In addition to primary care, it is anticipated that these integrated organizations will assume responsibility for secondary care in the future (New Zealand Ministry of Health 1995). In all cases, it is government direction that primary and community services will be the focus of coordinated care. From this base, it is anticipated that functional and organizational linkages will be built with CHEs and other secondary care providers.

The government has recognized the importance of consumer registration (rostering) with a managed care organization and is actively encouraging this direction. Organizations must update their registers for capitation or budgetholding purposes every three months. They have already developed a number of "safeguards" including the following (New Zealand Ministry of Health 1995):

- People must be able to choose which provider they register with.
- People must be able to change the provider they register with, when and if they choose to do so.

- Providers must accept anyone who applies to register with them (within the limits of their capacity to take on additional customers); in particular, they must not discriminate against people with a high potential need for services.

Providers

Primary health service providers include GPs, dentists, district and community nurses, pharmacists, and midwives.

GPs represent a substantial primary care expenditure (prescription drugs prescribed by GPs comprise the largest category of expenditure). GPs are self-employed and operate on a fee-for-service basis. Government subsidies are paid to GPs through the General Medical Subsidy (GMS), through the Maternity Benefit Schedule (MBS), and through pharmaceutical subsidies and laboratory diagnostic services payments. "The GMS is paid to GPs for all visits by children and adult Community Services Card holders" (Shipley 1996). The level of the GMS ranges from $15 for children without community service cards to $25 for children aged less than five years with community service cards. RHAs are also exploring capitation payments to GPs. Under capitation arrangements, the GP practice receives a single annual payment (instead of individual GMS payments), calculated according to the number and demographic profile of people enrolled with the practice.

Maternity benefits are a significant area of primary health care expenditure. Increases in the 1990s can be largely attributed to the Nurses Amendment Act of 1990, which enabled midwives to access the Maternity Benefits Schedule. A new Maternity Payment Schedule introduces a number of modules of care for the second trimester, the third trimester, labour and birth, and for services following birth. The schedule introduces a nationally consistent package that is accessible by independent practitioners, CHEs, and other providers. It is designed to clarify roles and required competencies, and to minimize duplication in the provision of services by GPs and midwives.

Other professional groups receiving substantial direct government funding through RHAs for the provision of health and disability support services are dentists, pharmacists, midwives, radiologists, and physio-therapists. The majority of medical specialists work in crown health enterprises (CHEs) on a salaried basis. Many specialists work part time in a CHE and part time in private practice (private pay sector). A very small number are entirely in private practice.

Crown health enterprises (CHEs) were created on the abolition of area health boards. There are a total of 23 CHEs operating 44 hospitals. "CHEs are publicly owned companies which are expected to compete with other providers and win contracts from RHAs by working in an effective and efficient manner" (Shipley 1996). CHEs may earn and keep surpluses to replace buildings or equipment, or to develop new facilities. Any surplus over and above that needed to maintain or upgrade its facilities and services is to be returned to the government. The government returns these funds to the health system, to be used for the purchase of more health services (New Zealand Ministry of Health 1995).

In summary, in New Zealand, there is a fair amount of movement in the direction of organizational innovation, and both horizontal and vertical integration. As in other jurisdictions, much of this is motivated by the need or desire to better position providers to secure contracts. As well, much integration has been taking place for the purpose of developing purchaser organizations.

Summary of Features of Emerging Models—New Zealand

Purchasing Models

There are several evolving purchasers in the New Zealand system. The dominant purchasers are the four regional health authorities (RHAs). In addition, GP Fundholders and other integrated HMO-like organizations are emerging in the system.

Key Features

RHAs:
- Are government-owned bodies with appointed boards.
- Are responsible for all core services and benefits.
- Carry out planning and monitoring, including needs assessments and determination of required resources.
- Serve a population identified through the census; no consumer choice is involved. Population per RHA ranges from 600,000 to just over 1 million.
- Are funded by weighted capitation.
- Purchase, but do not provide, services for their population. They are now entering into contracts to transfer purchasing, entering joint-purchasing agreements with integrated GP and other integrated provider/purchaser organizations.
- Have a geographically defined jurisdiction.

Other (GP budgetholders and other integrated models):
- Plan for and provide services within their organizations, and purchase those services they have contracted for with the RHA. Potential exists for total purchasers to evolve.
- Have patients who are identified through roster. Patients have the right to join and exit.
- Are moving toward capitation funding for their organizations.
- Compete with other GPs and vertically integrated organizations to attract and hold the rostered population.

Government Regulation and Direction

The government provides for:
- a regulated market environment;
- capitation funding;
- unique identification of population, with a move toward rostering for new purchaser/provider models;
- monitoring and evaluation of performance;
- establishment of core services and benefits.

Other Integration

Both horizontal and vertical integration have occurred in an effort to attract and hold contracts.

Role of Primary Care and the GP

- The GP is the gatekeeper to secondary and acute care.
- GP networks and other organizations are being developed to participate in purchasing secondary and acute care.

Overview of the Health System of the United States

Background

Privately funded health insurance has been and remains dominant in the U.S. health system. However, a widely held perception that this represents most of the *health expenditure* is incorrect. Publicly funded health care through Medicare and Medicaid now constitutes approximately 44 percent of total expenditure.

The historical roots of the traditional indemnity health insurance plans in the United States can be found in the life and accident insurance companies which wrote health insurance policies at the turn of the century. These were primarily loss-of-income policies and benefits for a limited number of diseases. By the 1930s, there was broad agreement on the need for some form of health insurance to alleviate the unpredictable and uneven incidence of health costs. A major issue raised at that time was whether the financing of health insurance should be private or public, although circumstances were already evolving to move society toward private sources of funding.

The 1930s and 1940s witnessed a rapid expansion of private health insurance. A substantial part of this growth was due to restrictions on direct wage increases during World War II, which led to the establishment of health insurance—primarily group insurance—as a fringe benefit at many companies. Its continued growth was supported by a number of factors after the war. Employee benefits, which had evolved (with help from court rulings) as a normal part of labour/management bargaining, were not subject to taxes; thus a dollar's worth of health insurance benefit was worth more than an after-tax dollar spent on health services. In general, the growth of population and prosperity throughout the 1950s catalyzed further rapid expansion.

By the mid-1960s, however, it was evident that there were still vulnerable populations not covered by health insurance, primarily the elderly and the poor who remained, in general, outside the employment-based insurance system. Concern about this led to a major initiative in Congress to establish government funding for health insurance. In 1965, President Lyndon Johnson inaugurated the Medicare program for people over 65 and the Medicaid program for low-income people. Coincidentally, this was the same period that Canada was putting the finishing touches on its universal health insurance program, primarily providing hospital and physician services for all Canadians.

Population growth, coupled with the introduction of health insurance and other postwar initiatives, led to a number of changes in the health system in the United States. To meet anticipated shortages of physicians, Congress allocated federal funds to train more. The Hill-Burton Act stimulated the construction of new hospitals. Hospitals and expanded medical training facilities began to turn out more specialists, motivated in part by the perceived status and greater income potential of specialization. Family physicians were beginning to lose, both in terms of status and in terms of their diminishing numbers in the system.

By the 1960s, specialists outnumbered primary care doctors for the first time. In the 1970s, inflation, higher technology, Medicare, and Medicaid all contributed to greatly increasing health care costs, and by the 1980s acute concern had emerged about the sheer number of physicians in the system and the growing imbalance between general practitioners and specialists. Within a 30-year period there had been dramatic changes in the types and methods of services offered, the kinds of treatable conditions encountered, and the kinds of outcomes which could be achieved. Associated with these changes were major increases in both utilization and costs. "National health expenditures in 1994 were more than 25 times those of 1960" (Prospective Payment Assessment Commission 1995; cited in Marriott 1996).

The United States represents probably the most complex organizational milieu of all the countries reviewed in this paper. Funding is still predominantly private (accounting for approximately 56 percent of expenditures in 1993), although the share of public funding through Medicare and Medicaid has been growing. The proportion of public health expenditures on health rose from 42 percent in 1980 to 44 percent in 1993 (Prospective Payment Assessment Commission 1995). Rising costs are identified as one of the most critical pressures facing the U.S. health care system today, together with wide variation among the population in accessibility to the health system due principally to modes of payment for services. In response, the United States has undergone major structural change in the financing and delivery of care, and presently continues its reevaluation. To date, these reforms have resulted in a declining share of the health insurance market for traditional indemnity insurance plans (i.e., plans that pay providers fee for service), and an increased market share for health maintenance organizations (HMOs) and others capable of managing a full spectrum of services and costs through care coordination or by employing managed care techniques.

The Macroenvironment

Benefits

Private Insurance

Most plans provide coverage for physician and hospital services, and for home care following hospitalization to allow recovery in a less costly environment. However, most do not provide home care or long-term care for chronic conditions or for the elderly (OECD 1994). The profile of benefits of different insurance plans vary in terms of what services are covered and whether patients must make a copayment for the services that are covered. It has been estimated that 55 million Americans with private insurance are underinsured—that is they have no limits to out-of-pocket expenses and risk being impoverished should they experience a costly illness (OECD 1994).

Public Programs—Medicare and Medicaid

Medicare consists of two plans. The Hospital Insurance (HI) plan, known as "Plan A," covers hospital inpatient services, skilled nursing facilities if related to a hospital stay and linked to provision of nursing and rehabilitation services, and home care including part-time skilled nursing, physical therapy, or rehabilitation care if required. Plan A for hospital is automatic without payment of any premium for those who are eligible.

"Plan B" is Supplementary Medical Insurance (SMI). It is optional for those who have Plan A, although almost all who are eligible for Plan A elect to enrol in Plan B and pay the required monthly premium. Plan B coverage includes physicians, clinical laboratory tests, durable medical equipment, flu vaccinations, drugs which cannot be self-administered (except certain anticancer drugs), most supplies, diagnostic tests, some other therapy, services, ambulance services, certain other health care services and blood, which are not provided under Plan A. Medicare does not normally cover the costs associated with long-term care, dental care including dentures, prescription drugs, hearing aids, or eyeglasses unless they were part of a "coordinated care plan" (managed care plan or HMO). Medicare beneficiaries are eligible to enroll in a prepaid, coordinated managed care plan— most of which are HMOs—if they are enrolled in both Plan A and B and continue to pay their Plan B premiums (United States: Health Care Financing Administration 1994).

Medicaid covers both acute and long-term care services. While programs vary from state to state, they all must offer a number of basic services including inpatient and outpatient hospital services, physician services, nursing facility services, laboratory and X-ray services as well as a number of other programs. Federal funding is also provided if states elect to provide other approved services including optometrists' services and eyeglasses.

Funding

Funding is derived from a combination of private and public sources. Private funding represents most of the funding profile, and is the only option for most of the working population and their families. It is derived predominantly from policies bought by individuals and/or their employers. Employers form the largest source of funding for private insurance, followed by trade unions and individuals. Those who cannot afford insurance, but have income higher than the threshold for public funding or are not entitled to special assistance, must self-fund—that is, pay as they go, or go without. Many go without, and many with minimal insurance levels are still considered underinsured.

Public funding is organized through the Medicare and Medicaid programs, as follows:

- Medicare's funding for Plan A (Hospital Insurance) is derived from a tax on individuals' employment earnings. Enrollees in Plan B (Supplementary Medical Insurance) pay a monthly premium which is currently set by government at $46.10 for 1995. Additional funding is derived from the general revenues of the federal government (United States: Health Care Financing and Administration 1994).
- The Medicaid program is financed jointly by the federal and state governments through matching funds. Federal cost sharing varies from state to state, with the federal share required to be not less than 50 percent nor more than 83 percent. Payment is based on a federal formula that compares the state's average per capita income level with the national income average. The average federal share among all states in 1993 was 57.5 percent with 11 of the wealthier states receiving 50 percent and Mississippi receiving 79.0 percent (United States: Health Care Financing and Administration 1994).

Method of Transfer

There are two forms of transfer for Medicare: fee for service and capitation. Fee-for-service claims for Plans A and B are processed by organizations or agencies (called intermediaries or carriers) that contract to serve locally as fiscal agents between providers and the federal government. HMOs under Medicare are paid a capitated (per-person) amount for each beneficiary, adjusted to reflect the individual's age, sex, Medicaid status, institution-alization and employer-based coverage. The base rate for these programs is 95 percent of the average Medicare fee-for-service program payments. The managed care plans assume the financial risk for all the covered services used by the Medicare beneficiary.

A variety of payment arrangements are used for Medicaid. Most states are attempting to control costs through the implementation of prospective payment systems such as case-based reimbursement of hospital services and fee schedules for physicians. Capitation of HMO and other managed care models is on the increase.

Citizen Coverage/Entitlement

There is no standard entitlement to private health insurance, other than the right to purchase it if one can afford it. Most policyholders obtained their health insurance as an employment benefit—although this varies by employer. Many small employers, for example, do not provide health insurance for their employees. A recent estimate is that 50 million are without health insurance (United States: HCFA Office of the Actuary 1995–96). This group includes those who would "self-insure" (pay as they go), or go without.

Medicare is the government health insurance program established initially for those 65 and over. In addition, the program now covers persons who are entitled to disability benefits for 24 months or more; persons with end-stage renal disease requiring dialysis or kidney transplant, and certain otherwise noncovered persons who elect to buy into the Medicare program. Medicare covers 95 percent of the aged population plus many of the disabled persons who are on Social Security.

Medicaid is the largest health insurance program, providing medical and other health-related services to 36 million of America's poorest people. Not all the poor are eligible, however, due to varying income and eligibility standards.

The most recent estimates of population served, by type of coverage, from the Health Care Financing Administration Office of the Actuary are indicated in table 1.

Table 1

Population served, by type of coverage

Type	Number of persons
Private health insurance (obtained in or outside of the workplace)	155 million
Medicare—national health insurance for the elderly	37 million
Medicaid—federal/state health insurance for persons with low incomes	36 million
Uninsured population	50 million

Source: United States: HCFA Office of the Actuary 1995–96.

Principles and Regulation

While the public programs of Medicare and Medicaid are centrally defined and regulated, the U.S. approach to private insurance relies much less on regulation and more on competition among private funders, budget or fund-holding organizations (HMOs and other insurance/delivery plans), and delivery organizations (individual providers, networks, and integrated models). While the market remains relatively unregulated, what does serve as de facto policy with this competitive model, is strong encouragement of "managed care" approaches to cost control and to address quality of services.

Information Systems and Evaluation

In general, the private health insurance system operates in a highly decen tralized, even fragmented environment. Nonetheless, excellent integrated information systems are developing within given integrated managed care organizations like HMOs. Databases are maintained on the patients (age, gender, address, etc.), participating providers, expenses by encounter and episodes of care, and satisfaction surveys for rostered members and providers with whom the organization has working or contractual links. This information is also being incorporated into electronic health records. Many organizations are developing and implementing quality profiles and targets as well as health intelligence into their systems, to assist individual providers with decision making and to support population-based planning, outcomes measurement, prevention and health promotion programming.

An accreditation process for the industry is under development by the National Committee for Quality Assurance (NCQA). The NCQA evaluates managed care organizations in quality assurance, medical records, utilization management, credentialing of health providers, and commitment to rostered members' rights. They are also involved in the continuing development of quality and performance "report cards" to provide comparable information on various aspects of the accessibility and quality of care. Some examples of performance measures are (United States: NCQA 1993):

- measures of how effectively health plans provide preventive services to their enrolled populations (e.g., rates for mammography and childhood immunization);
- measures of health plan effectiveness in providing prenatal care (e.g., infant birthweights, numbers of first-trimester visits among pregnant clients);
- measures of health plan management of chronic conditions (e.g., hospital admission rate for asthmatic patients, proportion of diabetics receiving annual referrals for routine eye care);
- measures of patient health status and outcomes following surgery (e.g., patient functional outcomes following hip replacement);
- measures of patient satisfaction (e.g., enrollee satisfaction with care).

The Health Care Financing Administration (HCFA), part of the Department of Health and Human Services, provides oversight of HMOs in the system. They have access to much of the data referred to above and the information required in the contractual relationship. HMOs which participate in the Medicare market usually also participate in the private one, and in the accreditation processes mentioned above. The HMO Act requires that an HMO meet standards in the following areas (United States: Health Care Financing Administration, Operations and Oversight Team 1995):

- provision of basic and supplemental health services;
- fiscally sound operation;
- satisfactory administrative and managerial arrangements;
- enrollment procedures;
- consumer representation on the board of directors;
- member grievance procedures;
- an ongoing quality assurance program;
- health education services;
- continuing education for health professionals;
- procedures for reporting statistics and other information.

In addition to its own activity in monitoring and evaluating contracted HMOs and providers, the federal government provides funding for peer review organizations (PROs) in each state, made up of practicing doctors and other health professionals. The PROs are charged with the responsibility to monitor the care given to Medicare patients. They have the authority to decide whether the care given to patients is reasonable, necessary, provided in the most appropriate setting, and meets the standards of quality generally accepted by the medical profession. In addition, they review enrollee complaints and work with hospitals and doctors to promote the most effective care in treating disease and injury (United States: Health Care Financing Administration 1995).

Delivery System

Purchaser/Insurance Plans

The highly complex, mixed organizational environment in the United States is evolving daily. Even within categories and subcategories of insurance plans, there are variations in ownership, governance, administration, and organizational design. Indemnity and HMO or other managed care insurance companies are purchasers of services—in this function, they are the counterpart to the Sickness Fund organizations or budgetholders in other countries. Indemnity health insurance plans tend to be all-purchaser models, paying providers on a fee-for-service basis for services rendered to policyholders. Traditional indemnity insurance plans with complete separation of purchaser and provider dominated the market well into the 1980s.

Growing concern about increasing costs persuaded more primary purchasers (i.e., those who pay premiums including individuals, employers, and Medicare/Medicaid) to use lower-cost, high-quality care plans such as those provided by HMOs and other "managed care" plans which integrate funding with service delivery. The resulting transition has now persuaded even indemnity insurance plans to employ some managed care techniques to control costs, such as benefits design and utilization management, although they remain essentially a fee-for-service environment.

Managed Care

Iglehart (1992) defines managed care as a system that integrates the financing and delivery of appropriate medical care by means of the following features:
   contracts with selected physicians and hospitals that furnish a comprehensive set of health care;
- services to members, usually for a predetermined monthly premium;
- utilization and quality controls that contracting providers agree to accept;
- financial incentives for patients to use the providers and facilities associated with the plan;
- assumption of financial risk by doctors.

Only HMOs and "open-ended" HMOs (POSs, see below) incorporate all these elements in their model. What is missing from this definition is the fact that HMOs own, employ, or contract with more than just physicians and hospitals. Their linkages extend to all practitioners, other institutions such as nursing homes (primarily for short-term stay), home care, and pharmaceuticals.

Various forms of health plans are referred to under the rubric of "managed care." They include health maintenance organizations (HMOs), Point of Service (POS) plans, and preferred provider organizations (PPOs). There are variations, with even more acronyms within and between these basic plan types. To varying degrees, these models are purchaser/provider blends in that they provide some services directly and purchase others services from providers or provider organizations, based on self-determined standards of care and cost.

HMOs are managed care plans that integrate financing (health insurance) and delivery of a comprehensive set of health care services to an enrolled population. HMOs may contract with, directly employ, or—in the case of clinics and hospitals—own participating health care providers (figure 7). Usually, enrolled members choose from among these providers and make limited copayments. Providers may be paid by the HMO through capitation, salary, *per diem*, or fee-for-service rates, determined through negotiation.

There are four major types of HMOs: staff, group, network, and Independent Practice Association (IPA) models. This typology primarily reflects how HMOs relate to physicians:

- In the *staff model,* services are provided at one or more locations by physicians who are salaried employees of the HMO. In this model, physicians practice solely within the HMO.
- In the *group model,* the HMO contracts with a single physician group to provide health services at one or more locations. The usual form of payment in this system is capitation, with the group assuming responsibility for distributing funds to individual physicians in a variety of ways including blended approaches (e.g., salary plus prorated fee for service and other financial incentives). Physicians under this model typically do not provide services outside the HMO enrollment.
- In the *network model,* the HMO contracts for service with two or more independent physician groups (single or multispecialty). The usual form of reimbursement of the groups is a fixed monthly fee per enrollee—a form of capitation—with the respective groups determining how these funds will be distributed to the individual physicians within each group. In addition, physicians may be free to provide services to patients who are not HMO-enrolled members.
- In the *independent practice* model, the HMO contracts directly with physicians in independent practice, or with associations of independent physicians—for example, multispecialty group practices. Solo or single-specialty practices tend to predominate. Physicians practice in their own offices and the HMOs negotiate a per capita rate, a flat retainer, or a negotiated fee-for-service rate. By virtue of their independent status, these physicians also maintain practices outside of HMO enrollment.

Even this typology is breaking down, as more and more HMOs evolve as "mixed models" combining any or all of the approaches listed above. Such factors as particular populations, geographic markets, and mode of organization into divisions and subsidiaries contribute to further variation. Specialty HMOs, such as social health maintenance organizations (SHMOs),

Figure 7

**Example of purchaser/provider HMO model within mixed private
and public funding in the United States**

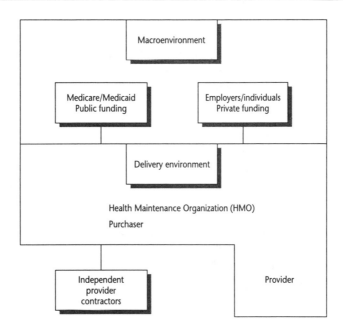

are also evolving, pooling capitation and other sources of funds to provide
acute and some long-term care services to their enrolled Medicare members.

The Point of Service (POS) plan can be defined as a health plan whereby
a network or panel of physicians is available to patients at a lower cost.
Patients must be referred to one of the network physicians, hospitals, or
other services by a primary care physician. They may also consult physicians
outside the network for an additional out-of-pocket sum. This type of plan
is often called an "open-ended" HMO, although not all POSs are part of
an HMO. In some respects, the Primary Care Case Management (PCCM)
model employed by Medicaid is similar to this structure: Medicaid contracts
with a physician to manage and coordinate the care of assigned beneficiaries.
In this model, all services must be authorized by the gatekeeper physician.
The services are then paid for on a fee-for-service basis by Medicaid.

Other practitioners have historically tended and continue to be employees of HMOs or of provider organizations (typically physicians or
hospitals) which contract with HMOs to provide services. As well, HMOs
own or contract with hospitals and diagnostic, laboratory, and home care

services in order to offer a full complement of services to its enrollees. Access to these services is through a primary care doctor who serves as gatekeeper, or the entry point, to the HMO services.

A Preferred Provider Organization (PPO) is a health insurance plan with a network or panel of providers, whose services are available to patients at lower cost than the services of providers outside of the network. Patients may self-refer to any network or panel provider at any time. Even this model is spinning off variations. The Exclusive Provider Organization (EPO) is simply a PPO where enrolled members must pay the entire cost of consulting nonaffiliated providers. Unlike HMO and POS models, there is no primary care gatekeeper.

A fundamental concept of HMOs is the integration of financing and service delivery to enrolled individuals (i.e., the roster). This integration is the foundation of tools and techniques used in varying degrees by all forms of managed care plans to improve service quality and accountability while controlling costs. Integration affects the design of benefits, the selection and payment of providers, and the management of utilization. Incentives and disincentives are used to influence the behaviour of providers, to motivate enrolled individuals to use participating providers, and to encourage compliance with plan procedures.

In the design of benefits, plans seek to influence the costs of providing the service as well as the characteristics of potential enrollees. All HMOs, for example, cover primary care visits and preventive services such as childhood immunization. In contrast, coverage for mental health is often restricted in some form by all health plans to a maximum number of visits per year (Prospective Payment Assessment Commission 1995). Plans also seek to influence the use of covered services through cost sharing.

Physicians are selected based on their credentials, their practice characteristics, and their "fit" with the organizational mission, philosophy, and structure of the HMO. A balance must be struck between the price of the provider and his acceptability to purchasers, enrollees and, to some extent, other providers already in the organization. In addition, the managed care organization must take into account the cost of the provider (e.g., the amount the provider will charge), and the level and appropriateness of the services provided, and there must be a balance between the cost and accessibility of services. In this environment, the HMO strives to achieve lower costs by limiting the number of providers, while being responsive to enrolled members' preferences for accessibility to providers. The HMO carefully reviews a provider's credentials, accreditation, and reputation, and selection of hospitals is influenced by their reputation and by the ability of the plan to negotiate acceptable inpatient rates (prices) to manage hospital utilization, and also by the reputation a hospital has among the plan's physicians.

Payment to providers by HMOs varies with the type of plan, the type of provider, the geographic market area, and the funder (employer or public funder). In all cases, the HMO assumes financial risk (i.e., the potential to make or lose money). Physicians in HMOs may be reimbursed through salary, fee-for-service, or capitation arrangements. This framework allows for potential to negotiate and implement a number of other approaches such as performance-related incentives, a blend of salary and prorated fee for service, bonuses for achievement of utilization targets, or the withholding of portions of payment until these targets are met.

Managed care organizations are contracting with more primary care physicians and fewer specialists than currently serve the general population, in an effort to contain unnecessary cost associated with specialty services which could be handled by GPs. Many managed care plans are offering primary care doctors substantially higher starting incomes than was the case only a few years ago to encourage practice at this level (Iglehart 1994).

Per diem payment remains the most common approach to paying hospitals. Other options include fee for service, discounted rates, capitation, and paying according to specific diagnoses (using diagnostic related groups [DRGs], explained below).

In the *per diem* approach, the hospital accepts a fixed daily rate from the HMO based on aggregate average resource use. The result is a strong incentive for the hospital to control costs. They can lose money in at least two ways: when the average per diem costs for a given patient are higher than the agreed-to rate or when the average length of stay is shorter than that used to calculate the per diem (this is due to the fact that hospital costs tend to be lower for each successive day a patient spends in hospital). The managed care plans and hospitals may also explore other options to modify risk for both parties, including negotiating separate rates for different types of hospital services, for example, surgical or intensive care. They may also negotiate a higher per diem for the first day of stay.

Fee-for-service arrangements represent the next most common approach to paying for hospital services. In this relationship, the hospital seeks to keep charges high enough to minimize its risks, while the HMO seeks to save money by contracting with lower-cost hospitals.

The next most common type of inpatient hospital reimbursement relates payment to treatment for a specific diagnosis. The HMO contracts to reimburse the hospital based on the Medicare prospective payment system, using diagnostic related groups (DRGs). HMOs assume the risk that patients will need services, while the hospital assumes the risk associated with the cost of the entire hospital stay. Capitation arrangements may also be pursued where the hospital receives a fixed monthly amount per member for inpatient care. The per-member amount may be adjusted to reflect characteristics of the enrolled population. All of the above reflect arrangements being *contracted for* by an HMO. Where an HMO *owns* a hospital, it simply establishes a budget for inpatient care (Prospective Payment Assessment Commission 1995). Hospital outpatient services tend to fall into two categories: discounted charges or bundled charges where a single rate is established for a group of procedures (Prospective Payment Assessment Commission 1995).

Utilization management refers to the tracking of cost and service quality from entry to exit in episodes of illness and associated health system encounters. All HMOs have developed policies to influence access and use of services by enrolled members. Traditional HMOs restrict access to their panel of primary care physicians, who in turn must refer patients to a specialist or specialty services. Physician practice patterns within managed care plans are influenced through a variety of clinical rules, including quality assurance procedures, treatment protocols or algorithms, regulations, administrative constraints, practice guidelines, and utilization review (Iglehart 1994).

HMOs also control utilization through case management and service (and coverage) authorization. Case management for high-cost cases seeks to manage service use across all health care settings. In this environment, the case managers spend significant time with the patient. Service (and coverage) authorization is used to control access and use of services. Pre-certification, concurrent, or retrospective review may be used. Under pre-certification review, the plan requires advance notification of required services. With this approach, the plan can alert its staff to set case management to monitor, arrange for cost-efficient diagnostics prior to admission, and prepare for the claim. Under concurrent review, the plan monitors and limits the length of stay and participates in the discharge planning of the patient. Retrospective review helps determine accuracy and gather data on patterns of care by specific providers (Prospective Payment Assessment Commission 1995).

Providers

HMOs and other managed care plans are providers of health services, in addition to their role in insurance, budget- or fundholding. With the exception of the indemnity insurance plans, the managed care plans are purchaser/provider blends in that they both purchase and deliver services. In terms of the direct involvement in delivery, HMOs represent the most integrated in terms of extension of their approach to include employment or ownership, as well as contracting with providers. They are vertically integrated in terms of their responsibility for health benefits, which define the "products" or services of the organization and control of the associated funding to provide these services to their enrolled client base. Their benefits profile is increasing, with the entry of pharmaceuticals into the managed care environment.

Other Provider Reorganization

In parallel with the trend set by HMOs and their funders, physicians, hospitals and other providers are moving toward restructuring and integration at an unprecedented rate. Some are integrating functionally through networks of physicians; others organizationally, through mergers or buyouts of hospitals by physicians or physician organizations by hospitals. Others integrated horizontally encompassing primary care or more comprehensive physician networks. Hospitals are merging with other hospitals or working out linkages—"joint ventures"—with them, and physicians and hospitals are forming physician-hospital organizations (PHOs). Many of these changes are being made in an effort to target specific local markets and secure contracts with HMOs and other insurers. In this context, vertical integration is seen as the best way to provide a broad continuum of care, including primary care, acute, subacute, and postacute care.

Some delivery organizations extend their integration to include budget-holding or insurance functions, competing directly with established HMOs and other managed care plans for contracts with employers and government (Medicare and Medicaid). In one such example, large multispecialty group practices operate their own managed care plans, deriving over half their revenue from these sources (Iglehart 1994).

The Henry Ford Health System (HFHS) is one example of a fully vertically integrated delivery system combined with the insurance system. As described by the Prospective Payment Assessment Commission (1995),

> The HFHS system includes a tertiary care hospital, two community hospitals, 37 ambulatory care facilities, two group practices totalling nearly 1,000 physicians, a mental health facility, a chemical dependency treatment centre, and two nursing homes. It also includes various home health services, pharmacies, and dialysis services. The system has its own HMO (the Health Alliance Plan) and is involved in numerous community improvement initiatives.

In conclusion, there is no one model for ownership and governance of service delivery organizations, which may be proprietary, partnerships, private for-profit, or not-for-profit.

Summary of Key Features of Emerging Models—United States

Purchasing Models

There are a variety of purchasing models in the United States, and new permutations of organizational constructs are continually evolving. The all-purchasing model—indemnity insurance—is losing ground to managed care models that blend provision of care with purchase of services from providers through contracts. Although they vary greatly in their definition of physicians' services, benefits and access, all vie for contracts with other providers such as hospitals. Examples of primary managed care models are:

- Preferred provider organizations (PPOs), which provide access to a network or panel of physicians whose services are available at lower cost to members.
- Health maintenance organizations (HMOs), the original and most-developed approach to managed care. Organizational variants include:
  - staff model (physicians are salaried employees)
  - group model (the HMO holds a contract with single physician group)
  - network model (the HMO contracts with multiple physician groups)
  - IPA (the HMO contracts with independent physician associations)
  - mixed model (a blend of the four standard types)

Key Features

HMOs:

- Have a variety of forms of ownership and governance ranging from private for-profit to not-for-profit organizations, including member cooperatives.
- Are responsible for all benefits defined within the contract with employers (i.e., no standard core set of benefits) or in compliance with core services as defined under Medicare and Medicaid for rostered members within these programs.
- Plan for need, required resources, and monitoring.
- Serve a rostered population. The choices and rights available to patients differ in the private and public environments. In the private sphere, the patient is usually "locked in" for one year. The HMO may represent the only "health plan" offered by an employer or primary funder. In the public Medicare sphere, members are not "locked in" and may change HMOs any time.
- Are funded for a rostered population. In the publicly funded environment, there is very explicit weighted capitation.
- Purchase required services from providers or provide it themselves. This flexibility leaves the organization free to determine the most appropriate organizational and financial relationship with providers.
- Provide access to secondary care and coordinate other services through a GP gatekeeper.
- Compete with other managed care organizations to attract employer groups or to directly sign up and keep individuals who qualify for Medicare/Medicaid.

Government Regulation and Direction

- The health care system is primarily private, supplemented by Medicare and Medicaid programs for the elderly and poor. Government legislation and regulation define standards for managed care organizations competing to provide publicly funded services.
- Government is committed to maintenance of free-market competition.
- Government is committed to the principle of managed care.
- Government has defined no "national" core services or benefits for the total population, only for those who qualify for Medicare or Medicaid.
- The HMO Act defines basic standards for federal recognition.
- Government provides capitation funding for Medicare.
- No principles of "universality" or "equitable access" to services based principally on employment and/or the ability to pay.

Other Integration

There has been very active development of horizontally and vertically integrated health organizations in the United States. The primary motivation has been to capture local and special markets and to attract and hold contracts. Integration is seen as one way to improve efficiencies, coordination, quality, and offer comprehensive services to HMO purchasers, who are in turn responding to government and employer pressures to control costs while maintaining quality.

Role of Primary Care and the GP

HMOs place an emphasis on primary care and on the GP as the gatekeeper to secondary and acute care. This is a cornerstone of the managed care approach. Otherwise, people in the United States are more likely than those in other countries to seek direct access to a specialist.

OVERVIEW OF THE CANADIAN HEALTH SYSTEM AND MODELS

Background

One of the primary distinctions of the Canadian health care system as compared to other countries, is that the constitutional authority for the organization and delivery of health care rests with the *provinces*, whereas other predominantly public systems are well within the jurisdiction of their federal or national governments. In Canada, the federal government contributes funding from tax revenues to support provincial health insurance plans, and retains the right to attach conditions to the transfer of those funds to provinces. The primary transfer vehicles are the Canada Health and Social Transfer (CHST) and the Canada Health Act (CHA). The CHA defines the minimum benefits (physician and hospital services) that provincial health plans must provide, mandates a commitment to five principles (universality, accessibility, comprehensiveness, portability, and public administration), and sets conditions that there must not be extra-billing or user charges in order for a province to receive its full CHST transfer.

What is important to remember in the Canadian context is that these conditions apply only to *physician and hospital* services—and to some dental surgery performed in a hospital. Under the Canada Health Act an "insured health service" means hospital, physician and surgical-dental services provided to an insured person, but does not include any health services that a person is entitled to and eligible for under any other act of Parliament or any provincial act relating to workers' or workmen's compensation. However, each province may define other areas as "insured."

In this environment, it is the *provincial* health system that is the logical counterpoint to the national health systems of other countries. This means that regardless of the federal role in funding and setting conditions, any substantive adjustment to health care service delivery systems must be enacted at and by the provincial level. For this reason, the majority of this paper's discussion will primarily deal with the provincial level. An overview of the macroprovincial environment will be followed by a brief summary of organizational reforms. Given the subtle differences reflected in structural reforms, the review will then discuss four distinctive generic *organizational* configurations representative of the evolving models of integration: horizontal, partial, and full vertical integration:

1. Horizontal integration of provider (hospital) organizations;
2. Devolved, local authority structures;
3. Local health provider boards; and
4. Roster-driven, fully vertically integrated, independent health care organizations.

A summary of primary care models presently being discussed in the Canadian environment completes the section.

Macroenvironment

At the provincial level, health insurance acts and other legislation define what each of the health plans will pay for and under what conditions. In addition to physicians and hospitals, this includes the services of other health practitioners, home care, long-term care institutions, drugs, and other programs. Many provinces have extended their funding umbrella to provide a fairly inclusive and comprehensive "birth to death" or "wellness to illness" health system. However, this coverage varies somewhat from province to province.

Funds are derived from federal transfers and provincial taxes. The collection of premiums has been used by some provinces to supplement tax revenues for building a central health fund or budget. Provinces tend to allocate funds to various sectors according to unique sets of rules: for example, physicians' services may be paid through a fee-for-service arrangement, hospital services through global budgets, and assistive devices through a percentage subsidy. Historically, funding has been distributed from the provincial government's central health budget directly to individual and institutional providers. This "monopsony" or single-payer funding has resulted in the development of large central bureaucracies to administer and manage each separate system (often referred to as stovepipes). There were no intermediary purchasers, budget fundholders, or vertically integrated models of health planning and delivery.

With the phasing in of universal health insurance programs in the 1960s, evolution at the provincial level involved recognizing and developing funding rules for preexisting structures such as proprietary fee-for-service physicians and not-for-profit hospital corporations, and funding them according to unique rules for each. The gradual development and inclusion of other areas such as drug programs and home care followed this pattern. Each area was dealt with in isolation and specific rules of funding and regulations were devised for each. The health data "system" consisted of information received by the central provincial Ministry of Health, and was primarily related to required reporting from each of the sectors or program areas, including fee-for-service claims, encounters for capitated practices, hospital activity reports, and budgets.

A number of persistent problems were identified by the provinces including lack of coordination, fragmentation, overemphasis on the institutional sector at the expense of the community, and the need for greater cost control and for local planning and input.[2] In response, a number of organizational trends have emerged. Most provinces and observers of the system have classified these models under the functional heading of "regionalization," although when examined in more detail, the models actually present a variety of different structural or organizational forms in each province. Generally speaking, however, the models are geographically defined. The newer organizations either allocate budgets to providers or blend the budgeting and service provision functions within themselves.

As stated at the outset, this paper will not include an extensive discussion of decentralization, devolution, deconcentration, and other dimensions of regionalization. However, this perspective will be used in so far as it clarifies organizational design. If the experience of many other jurisdictions holds true in Canada, many of the models being implemented today will ultimately be considered as transitional, and may well evolve from fixed geographic models to more flexible roster-based models.

---

2. A more detailed summary of system objectives to correct such issues is presented in the section "Key Features of Integrated Models in the Canadian Context."

Provincial Overview

This section summarizes the provincial organizational reforms from which generic models will be derived. All provinces, to varying degrees, are exploring approaches to integration of services. Most are pursuing this through the development of similar forms of geographically based change, in short variations on *regions* and *regional boards*. They fall roughly into three patterns:
- division of a province into regions;
- regions further subdivided into subregions with district boards; and
- regions organized in terms of two major subsectors. Institutional (hospitals) and community services, which may overlap geographically.

In addition, several provinces have examined—and at least one is actively considering—a nongeographically oriented, roster-based organizational model more in keeping with the trends observed in other countries.

Selected organizational characteristics in each province are given below (Canada: Health Canada. Provincial Health System Reform in Canada 1996):

- *Alberta* – Seventeen regional health authorities, responsible for planning, resource allocation, and managing health services within capped budgets.
- *British Columbia* – Two levels of regions. Twenty regional health boards plan and coordinate health services at the regional level, lead planning in capital projects, administer a regional health budget, allocate funds to community health councils, and facilitate collaboration among provincial ministries on regional health issues. Eighty community health councils identify local health priorities, plan, coordinate and manage local health services (including hospitals), ensure access to core services, and ensure core services meet provincial standards.
- *Manitoba* – Ten geographic areas approved for planning and delivery of community services.
- *New Brunswick* – Eight regional hospital corporations, responsible for planning and resource allocation for hospital services and physician resources at the regional level. A ninth corporation has been established for the Extramural Hospital, which offers home services.
- *Newfoundland* – Two separate parallel regional structures. Four regional community health boards coordinate, manage, and deliver community-based services in health promotion, health protection, continuing care, mental health, and alcohol and drug dependency. Eight regional health institutional boards oversee care in hospitals and nursing homes.
- *Nova Scotia* – Two levels of regions. Four regional health boards coordinate and allocate regional health resources, evaluate programs, operate and manage hospitals, develop regional health human resources plans, and establish community health boards. The community health boards plan and allocate resources and coordinate all primary care services,

including mental health, home care, long-term care, public health, and addiction services in their area.

- *Ontario* – No current development of regional governance structures. District health councils still serve as planning advisory bodies. The emphasis has been on community-based service delivery and sectoral reform, such as hospital restructuring and rationalization and operational planning for cancer care through six regional cancer care networks. Vertical integration is being pursued through development of comprehensive health organizations—roster-based organizations funded through capitation, which incorporate the funding and responsibilities of all institutional and community-based services.
- *Prince Edward Island* – Five regional boards for health and social/community services, which plan, allocate resources, and deliver services in the following areas: community mental health, hospitals, long-term care, physicians' services, seniors' homes, home care, addictions, public health nursing, dental care, housing, child and family services, social assistance, correctional and probational services, and youth centres.
- *Quebec* – Seventeen regional health boards plan and allocate resources for health, social services, and community health organizations.
- *Saskatchewan* – Thirty district health boards in southern Saskatchewan, together with local health boards in the northern area of the province, conduct needs assessments, develop district health plans, develop community health centres, integrate, coordinate, and manage health services at the district level, and ensure services meet provincial guidelines and standards.

Emerging Generic Provincial Models of Integration

Although varied, reforms in all the provinces can be distilled to a set of four distinct generic models of horizontal, partial, or full vertical integration (table 2).

These models provide a frame of reference for comparison to the international models reviewed, and demonstrate the extent to which key elements of vertically integrated and primary care–based models already exist in our health system.

Model 1—Horizontal Integration of Provider (Hospital) Organizations

Horizontal integration (figure 2) has primarily occurred in the hospital sector, and at two levels of magnitude. The first kind of integration has been the result of local area rationalization and mergers of area hospitals taking place in both large metropolitan areas and smaller communities. The other is a *provincewide* "regionalization," accompanied by the horizontal integration (or consolidation) of all the hospitals within a region into a

Table 2

Provincial models of integration

Horizontal:	1. Integrated provider (hospital) organizations
Partial vertical:	2. Devolved, local authority structures
	3. Local health provider boards
Full vertical:	4. Roster-driven, fully vertically integrated independent health care organizations

single corporation, with multiple hospital divisions or sites. Key features include:

- A single board replaces preexisting boards, which are merged to form a single new hospital corporation.
- Previously separate budgets are amalgamated into one central budget for the total organization.
- The consolidated single organization runs all hospitals in the area/region.
- The organization designates area/regional medical staff, oversees medical credentialing, and approves privileges for physicians.
- The organization coordinates and ensures effective and efficient use of resources throughout its area/region.

This type of consolidation is done for a variety of reasons. It can produce cost efficiencies, reduce duplication of effort, encourage consistency of practices across regions/provinces, better focus planning and procedures for service delivery, and ultimately to streamline and simplify the "total organization"—for patients, providers and taxpayers—to better respond to community health care needs. The regional hospital organizations in New Brunswick provide an example of horizontal (sectoral) integration.

Vertical Integration

Partial vertical integration is present in systematic provincewide effort to merge various programs under a single health organization board. It is also found at a smaller scale at local levels. These models of vertical integration are *partial,* since none include the full scheme of health services and funding and most, if not all, exclude physicians, who tend to have separate individual and group arrangements with government. A fully vertically integrated organization would include responsibility for all services as well as the funding to deliver them.

The government transfers funds to the new organizations through a global budget or "envelope," which combines the preexisting budgets associated with the providers and programs for which the organization is assuming responsibility. Most existing models are exploring or implementing

Figure 2

Horizontal and vertical integration

Nursing home	Nursing home	Nursing home	Nursing home	Nursing home	Nursing home	
Home care	Home care	Home care	Home care	Home care	Home care	
Hospital	Hospital	Hospital	Hospital	Hospital	Hospital	
Specialists	Specialists	Specialists	Specialists	Specialists	Specialists	
General practitioners	General practitioners	General practitioners	General practitioners	General practitioners	General practitioners	
Practitioners	Practitioners	Practitioners	Practitioners	Practitioners	Practitioners	

1.

2.

1. Horizontal integration—example of one organization owning several hospitals.

2. Vertical integration—example of one organization owning all components of the delivery system.

Note: 2. Also illustrates a single organization with integrated responsibility and funding for "all" the service sectors in the health system, where the organization exercises the option of owning or contracting any component of service delivery.

capitation funding to ensure greater equity of distribution, including weighting on the basis of age and gender. All contemplate an adjustment for need; however, there has been no consensus on the approach to take. Many look at mortality-based "proxies" for need such as standard mortality ratios (SMRs). Others explore deprivation factors such as income levels, or socioeconomic factors such as the number of single mothers. Regional differentials are also considered in the weighting of capitation formulae.

Another kind of consideration is how capitation is applied to a situation. Whether it is being used to fund an organization which, in turn, funds providers of care with responsibility for an area within specific geographic boundaries; or funds an organization that will assume responsibility for all health costs on a provincial or greater scale for the population it has a relationship with, determines different variables, values, exposures, and risks encompassed in a capitation formula. All but one of the evolving or contemplated vertically integrated models in Canada are predicated on a *geographic* basis— that is, responsibility for the health of a population within a geographic area and the funding of specifically identified health providers that exist within the geographic boundary. The discussion below will present two such examples.

Model 2—The Devolved, Local Authority Structure

In this model, some of the authority of the Ministry of Health is transferred to a local, public, geographically defined authority (figure 8). It constitutes a partial vertically integrated regional quasi-governmental entity, similar to a school board. Key features include:

- The authority replaces the central government as funder for the local health providers within its geographical jurisdiction. However, in most instances, responsibility tends to exclude physician services as well as specialized programs and institutions.
- The authority is a separate entity from the providers in its region. The hospitals and other providers are intact with their own boards and administration or are in a subregion.
- The authority assesses the health service needs of the population in its region as part of its planning process, and, based on this plan, allocates budgets to subregions and/or providers.
- In allocation of provider budgets, the authority does not negotiate unique service or institution contracts. It is not a contracting body.
- Funding is initially based on local amalgamated budgets or envelopes of funds. The ultimate objective is population-based capitation funding linked to the cost of services within the region.
- There is no registration or rostering of the population within the geographic boundaries of the regional organization.

Figure 8

Devolved local authority

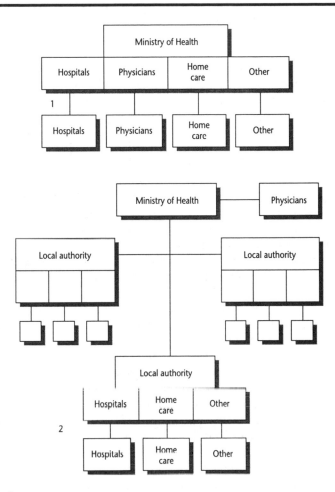

1. Prior system.
2. Transfer of responsibility to geographically defined devolved local authorities along with funds for providers (excluding physicians at this stage of development).

- The authority may actively encourage development of primary care centres.

The regional health boards in British Columbia provide an example of this model.

Model 3—The Local Health Provider Board

This is usually the result of government-sponsored mergers of local hospitals and other programs with, to a lesser degree, subsequent agreements with any local providers who were not merged within the geographic area at the outset (figure 9). Key features include:

- A single board replaces the preexisting boards of the hospitals and other institutions and program agencies merged to form the new single organization, which maintains multiple institutional and program divisions or sites.
- The previously separate budgets are amalgamated under the central board.
- Funding is initially based on local amalgamated budgets or envelopes of funds. The ultimate objective is population-based capitation funding linked to the cost of services within the region.
- Budget allocation is an "internal" exercise. Budgets are defined and assigned to subsidiary hospitals, long-term care, and other divisions by the central board or administration. Those who run the various merged institutions and programs are employees of the integrated organization.
- Responsibility for health services is limited to those preexisting services that are merged or organizationally and financially linked to the health board.
- Assesses the health service needs of the population in its region to determine appropriate allocation of its resources and coordination with other providers not within the district board's jurisdiction (e.g., physicians).
- Generally, geographic areas are defined either by the province or by the local population and providers. This approach tends to be provincewide in application, but in one or more jurisdictions, communities are exploring this type of amalgamation on their own, operating within a pluralistic environment, with no guarantee that it will be replicated provincially. Some are considering both mergers and functional linkages to achieve their goals.
- There is no registration or rostering of the population within the geographic boundaries served by the regional organization.
- The local health provider board may actively encourage development of primary care centres.

District health boards in Saskatchewan represent an example of this model.

Models 2 and 3 represent partial integration in that not all sectors of the health system are incorporated. While they generally assume responsibility for defining the health needs of their population, they are not organizationally or financially responsible for services or sectors outside their geographic area, for physicians' services, or for specialized diagnostic or institutional services accessed outside their geographic area. These models

Figure 9

Local health board

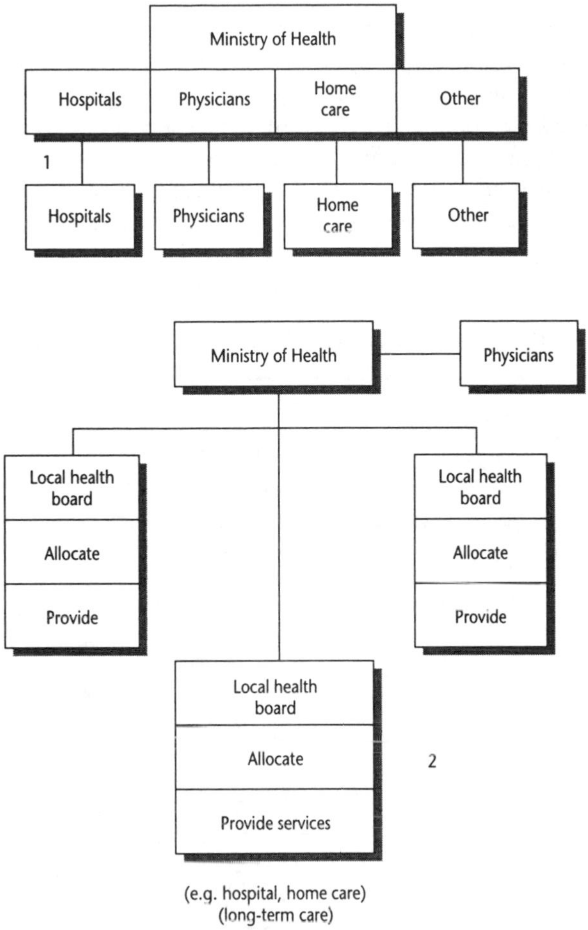

```
Ministry of Health
Hospitals | Physicians | Home care | Other

1

Hospitals | Physicians | Home care | Other


Ministry of Health — Physicians

Local health board        Local health board
Allocate                  Allocate
Provide                   Provide

Local health board
Allocate            2
Provide services
```

(e.g. hospital, home care)
(long-term care)

1. Prior system.
2. Transfer integrated budget to geographically defined single partially vertically integrated organizations, responsible for direct provision of select services (usually excluding physicians).

also must address issues associated with the potential conflict inherent in defining the health needs of the population, funding providers to meet those needs within their geographic areas, and dealing with cross-boundary flows of patients.

Model 4—Roster-Driven, Fully Vertically Integrated, Independent Organization

This model incorporates fundamental features of the health care system, combining and extending them to cover a full spectrum of responsibilities, services, and funding for all services for its population (figures 10 and 11). Important distinctions include that it is an independent, nongovernment corporate organization that serves a registered (rostered) population, rather than a defined geographic area. It is fully vertically integrated in that it has responsibility for funding and delivery (by provision or purchase) of all provincially insured or funded services. Selected other key features of this model are summarized below:

Figure 10

Comprehensive Health Organization (CHO)

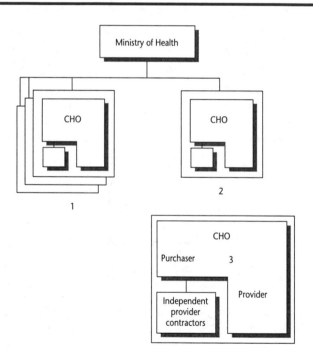

1 and 2. Transfer of weighted capitation for "all" services to roster-based CHO.

2. Demonstrates potential for rural, First Nations, or special population who choose to roster and start their own—may result in a natural geographic monopoly.

3. CHO purchases or provides required services based on the most appropriate organizational relationship with providers.

Figure 11

A CHO health system

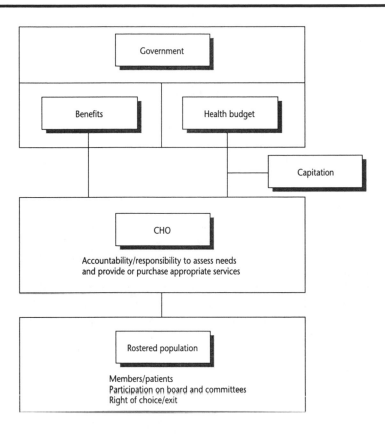

- The organization is a not-for-profit corporation similar to most hospitals. It has a board, an administrative structure, and bylaws which set a framework of commitment to principles and standards of health care.
- There are no imposed geographic boundaries within a province.
- Registered individuals have their health numbers linked to the organization they choose. The rostered population could be any portion of the general population, as well as specifically defined groups which elects to roster together, such as First Nations, ethnic minorities, or populations with special health needs such as HIV/AIDS.
- The organization is responsible for all core services—that is, the defined benefits and services normally funded by the central government.
- Primary care is emphasized to encourage a team approach to services and to make the best use of the most appropriate provider for a given need of a rostered member.

- The organization has the responsibility and the autonomy to provide or to purchase the required services to meet the assessed needs of its rostered population. This means there is no imposed prescription for organizational or financial relationships with providers. The organization could opt to remain an all-purchaser model, simply negotiating contracts with all providers. It could also explore the possibilities of hiring providers or merging on a local basis in order to directly provide services to its rostered members.
- Capitation funding is provided on a provincial scale for all services, so that the organization can assume financial responsibility for its rostered members no matter where they access services within—or possibly even outside—the province.
- The organization must maintain a comprehensive information system, recording and tracking all encounters—episodes of care or service—in the system.
- Organizational design flexibility—autonomy gives it the flexibility it needs to determine the most appropriate organizational and financial relationships with providers, and to "fit" the organization to the needs of its defined population (e.g., to consider special rural or urban requirements).

A fully vertically integrated system of comprehensive health organizations (CHOs) is now being implemented in Ontario, with models developing and/or launching in several communities at this time. Saskatchewan has already reviewed a similar model, and it is under consideration in British Columbia and Quebec (where a variant on the CHO is referred to as OSIS).

Primary Care

Most recently, discussions of organizational reform have focused on the emerging emphasis being placed on primary care organizations. This has included recognition of their potential as an essential module in the development of fully vertically integrated health organizations. Primary care has been defined in a variety of ways, including:

> That level of care where the health system is entered and basic services received and where all health services are mobilized and coordinated (Andreopoulos 1974).

> Primary Health Care is essential health care made universally accessible to individuals and families in the community by means acceptable to them, through their full participation and at a cost that the community and country can afford … It forms an integral part of the country's health care system of which it is the nucleus … It is the first level of contact of individuals, the family and community with the national health system

bringing health care as close as possible to where people live and work and constitutes the first element of a continuing health care process ... Primary Health Care addresses the main health problems in the community, providing promotive, preventative, curative, supportive and rehabilitative services accordingly (World Health Organization 1978).

Primary medical care consists of the first-contact assessment of a patient and the provision of continuing care for a wide range of health concerns. Primary medical care includes the diagnosis, treatment and management of health problems; prevention and health promotion; and ongoing support, with family and community intervention where needed (Canadian Medical Association 1994).

Primary Care Models

A number of organizations are proposing primary care models for Canada, which generally combine the services of GPs plus other primary care practitioners. Key proposals currently under active consideration in various jurisdictions include reports by the Federal/Provincial/Territorial Advisory Committee on Health Services (i.e., the Kilshaw or Victoria Report), the College of Family Physicians of Canada, the Ontario Medical Association, the Ontario Association of Health Centres, and the Ontario College of Family Physicians. While the notion of primary care has long held a position of importance in the system, the present drive to create new models has led to new emphasis on primary care organizations as the first point of entry to the health system. They improve the accessibility, quality and coordination of services, and increase the responsiveness and overall integration of the health system. Key elements of primary care models include:

- *Organization of GPs* – Explicit or implicit in all the proposed models is strong encouragement for the development of GPs working in a *group* environment, either as a group model, or within a primary care organization, or as a network of solo practices. While not always present or clear in some of the proposals, most imply some recognition that the primary care model may be part of another organization, or develop into a fully integrated model responsible for the purchase or the delivery of community, secondary, and acute care for its population.
- *Multidisciplinary team* – All models promote or endorse a multidisciplinary team of caregivers including GPs and others such as nurse-practitioners, counsellors, and nutritionists. Within this context, most support the GP as the gatekeeper to coordinate access to secondary and acute care. At the same time, some of the proposals make allowance for more direct access to other practitioners within the team.
- *Patient registration or rostering* – There is growing recognition of the benefits of patient registration or rostering with a primary care organization, or one which contains the primary care model.

- *Funding* – Most of the models support, in one form or another, population-based or capitation funding for the primary care practice or organization. There is growing recognition that capitation simply defines a cash flow that has specificity to a registered population and does not in any way imply how individual practitioners are to be paid. Most recognize the flexibility to explore a number of payment approaches with the funds derived from the cash flow. These can include blended approaches that recognize base salaries, the potential to preserve fee for service in toto or on a prorated basis, with other performance- or incentive-based funding in the mixture. The recognition that a variety of financial arrangements can be developed in innovative ways, could eventually lead to better understanding of opportunities implicit in fully vertically integrated capitation funding for all health services, for a rostered population.
- *Core services, including health promotion and prevention* – Core services in the primary care environment include health promotion, sickness prevention, diagnosis and treatment of illness, urgent care, 24-hour accessibility, and management of chronic illness. The existence of a set of core services encourages consistency of standards across the system, influencing consistency amongst providers, and enhances reliability for consumers.
- *Records and data* – There is growing recognition that use of a rostering system yields high-quality, specific information which, if well maintained, could provide greater certainty of data for costing. Further, a centralized electronic health record can contribute nonpersonalized aggregate data to regional, provincial or national systems, which can feed back practical and useful information to all primary care organizations throughout the system.
- *"Fundholding" and capitation potential* – A number of the proposed models have envisioned that primary care organizations could acquire responsibility for additional core services and benefits such as drugs, specialists' services, hospitals and home care, and that capitation funding could enable them to negotiate contracts for these services. This would move these organizations further in the direction of vertical integration.[3]

All provinces and territories are participating in the review and development of appropriate primary care models for Canada.

---

3. Sources for the "Primary Care" section include: Association of Ontario Health Centres 1995; Birch et al. 1994; Canadian Medical Association 1994; College of Family Physicians of Canada 1995; Federal/Provincial/Territorial Advisory Committee on Health Services 1995; Forster et al. 1994; Ontario College of Family Physicians, March 1995; Ontario Medical Association 1996.

Summary of Features of Emerging Models—Canada

Purchasing Models

At this stage of development, two purchasing models are being contemplated:
- the fully vertically integrated comprehensive health organization (CHO) model;
- GP/primary care organizations, should they be granted extra capitation for purchasing.

Key Features

A roster-driven fully vertically integrated independent organization (CHO):
- Is a not-for-profit corporation.
- Is funded by weighted capitation.
- Serves a population of rostered individuals who have the right of choice to join or exit. Should an individual move to another organization, the relevant funding also moves.
- Has 50 percent representation of rostered members on its elected or appointed board and major committees.
- Is responsible for all core services and benefits defined by the provincial health plan.
- Plans for population need, resource requirements and monitors and evaluates performance.
- Provides or purchases required services. Flexibility is preserved to pursue and refine the most appropriate organizational and financial relationship with providers. It may own some provider capacity within the organization, or negotiate a variety of contracts with outside providers.

A GP/primary care organization with purchasing authority:
- Is a private practice or corporate structure (e.g., Community Health Centre or CHC).
- Has a board if a corporate structure (community health centres or some health service organizations in Ontario).
- Is responsible for GP and primary care and for any additional approved core services (e.g., drugs, hospital, specialists).

Government Regulation and Direction

Governments are:
- Publicly funded single payer.
- Exploring capitation for funding all or parts of the health system.
- Exploring vertical integration through regionalization initiatives and CHOs (active discussion and implementation).
- Emphasizing primary care in current policy discussions.

Other Integration

Other evolving forms of integration include:

- Various forms of geographically defined vertically and horizontally integrated models, similar to integrated public models in that they provide services (except most physicians' services) but do not "purchase" them.
- Emerging horizontal and vertical integration, both functional arrangements and organizational merging, primarily involving hospitals alone or with others. These are under consideration or proceeding on a localized basis in some areas.

Role of Primary Care and the GP

There is a strong policy thrust toward development of primary care models.

KEY FEATURES OF INTEGRATED MODELS

The purpose of this section is to highlight key features and summarize significant trends and attributes of the system reconfiguration in the countries reviewed; in particular, those which involved variations of integrated models. The paragraphs below discuss and interpret a number of the implications of these features, in light of the future of Canada's health system. Other points on the primacy of primary care are noted for consideration.

Patterns of Change

The reforms to date have resulted in trends and patterns of reconfiguration which have fundamentally changed historic practices and structures, creating new momentum in the system. This, in turn, is spawning new roles, responsibilities, and perspectives for health care systems. Most importantly, these new patterns have motivated what appear to be more appropriate mechanisms to deal with the operation of health care systems, achieving better results while protecting their social integrity. Features such as *integration, purchasing, capitation funding, rostering of populations, competitive and collaborative behaviour* all contribute to the evolution, which is characterized by more comprehensive responsibilities and a new mix of public and private dynamics. The features combine and interrelate, operating as building blocks upon which new organizational constructs are formed. With respect to organizational structures, in summary, geographically based models are in transition, and all countries have developed some form of roster-based, vertically integrated organizational models.

Integration appears to be one of the most important attributes and trends of recent reform. The Gage Canadian Dictionary (1983) expresses its meanings as unifying, bringing together elements into a whole, to make them available to all. It is both a *means* and an *end* in reform, happening by design and naturally as driven by other factors. Integration of health care resources is a major and growing influence in all the countries reviewed; it is multidimensional in that it involves a convergence of health care, policy, organizational design, business practices, ethics, and systemic thinking which appear to be reenergizing participants at all levels. As a strategy, vertical integration has been adapted from industry and management practices as a management tool to enhance productivity, accountability, and quality control. It often occurs in response to regulatory, economic and market pressures, all of which are manifest in Canada and the other systems reviewed. Ultimately, better integration of services, funding, and responsibility should benefit the patient/consumer by improving the overall quality and continuity of services provided by the health system, and it should benefit the taxpayer by making the system more efficient and cost effective.

Purchasing has emerged as a significant function, creating new momentum in health care systems. It involves *negotiating* specific contracts with providers, setting out responsibilities and payment, as opposed to a system which simply allocates funds in accordance with prescribed (regulated) rules. While this was always part of the U.S. system, it is evolving in the other countries and represents a new policy direction on its own, introducing greater autonomy with business and microeconomic behaviour into the system, challenging prior practices. Implicit in purchasing is acknowledgement of a price or value of services, and the need for efficacy of practice to achieve set targets. The underlying dynamics of contracting mandate and motivate desired goals of the system, such as increased attention to patients, pricing and costs; autonomy with responsibility and accountability; increased responsiveness in all relationships; and a service orientation, which, properly balanced, establish the conditions for a more dynamic, adaptive system. The introduction of greater freedom encourages an orientation toward change and innovation in serving members, and in the development of new organizational and financial relationships between and among purchasers and providers (Marriott 1993–1994).

At the same time, purchasing requirements also serve as a catalyst for further integration, as illustrated by evolving provider strategies in response to a purchasing environment. Providers as independent contractors integrate their services as a strategy to attract and hold contracts with purchasers. This has taken a variety of forms. Some merged with their direct competitors (e.g., hospitals with hospitals) to form horizontally integrated organizations. Some horizontally integrated organizations are localized within a geographic area, while others are networked throughout a region, province, or country to attract their share of their specialized market. Others are pursuing vertical integration to expand services. Some involve only physicians and hospitals (e.g., physician/hospital organizations [PHOs] in the United States), while others are attempting to build "total" provider organizations. In addition to the physician and hospital component, these include community care, diagnostic, and other services under one organizational umbrella. The strategy here is to attract and serve a greater portion of the market area and to provide "one-stop shopping" to purchasers and patients. This represents only one area of provider activity spurred by the evolution to a purchasing environment. A more significant systemic driver in these reforms is the movement to purchaser/provider organizations discussed below.

Stages of Organizational Reconfiguration

The following paragraphs summarize three notable developmental stages of organizational reconfiguration in the countries reviewed, all of which spawned models which evolved toward a higher degree of integration of functions and funding, resulting in the emergence of vertically integrated models, with funding and responsibility for rostered populations.

Stage 1

Transition from large geographic authorities which control funding, allocation, and provision of services to a "purchaser/provider split." Geographic authorities lose service provision to independent providers; funding responsibility is moved from an allocation to purchasing function.

Implications – Funds follow patients; capitation funding is based on population census data.

In the United Kingdom and New Zealand, the government has done away with geographically defined public entities which controlled funding, allocation, and service provision. These were regional or local government (or quasi-government) authorities or boards, responsible for allocating funds within their organizations for the direct provision of services, which they also controlled. These were replaced by, or had their role changed to, that of geographically defined purchasers, which negotiate contracts with independent providers (DHAs in England and RHAs in New Zealand). The authorities no longer had a role in the provision of services. The concept is expanded somewhat in the United Kingdom in that purchaser authorities (DHAs) are not obligated to purchase care only from providers within their geographic area, but can purchase from any provider in England.

DHAs and RHAs receive their funding through *capitation* based on population census data (not an explicit registered population). They, in turn, negotiate contracts with independent providers who deliver services. This has been defined as the "purchaser/provider" split. There were many reasons for moving in this direction, including to counteract lack of responsiveness, long waiting lists, limited choice, and the tendency of the administrative systems "to become bureaucratic and insensitive to the public" which leads to consumers' dissatisfaction (Chernichovsky 1995).

Stage 2

Transition from geographic purchasers to roster-based purchasers

Implications – Funds follow patients; capitation is based on specific populations registered with providers (notion of rostering)

The notion of *rostering* or registration of patients with specific provider and/or purchaser organizations emerges as the next important trend and element. The purchaser/provider split was already present in the Netherlands, in the form of geographically defined Sickness Fund organizations. The Netherlands had experienced problems not unlike those raised with geographically defined public authority or board models in the United Kingdom and New Zealand. In response, the Netherlands transformed the function of its Sickness Fund organizations from geographic monopsonists (single payer within a defined geographic area), to roster-based models competing with other Sickness Fund organizations across the country to register (roster) and serve (hold on to) patients.

Stage 3

Transition to roster-based purchaser/provider blends

Implications – The assumption of purchasing responsibility by independent providers stimulates a move away from geographic structures to those based on registered or rostered populations.

In the United Kingdom and New Zealand, roster-based provider models are assuming purchasing responsibility, as illustrated by GP Fundholders in the United Kingdom, and GP as well as HMO-type models in New Zealand. GP Fundholders are evolving toward fundholding practices in the United Kingdom, whereas in New Zealand, a variety of GP-led and other integrated managed care organizations are developing population rosters in a move toward capitation funding and assumption of responsibility to purchase care as well as provide it.

What characterizes this phase of change is emerging sanctioned *competitive behaviour* amongst roster-based, purchaser/provider models (GP Fundholders and HMO-type organizations) to compete with the district and regional health authorities. This competitive behaviour is enhanced by the move from *budget dependency* of the former regime, to *revenue dependency* of the new entities, establishing a new environment and culture as well as new motivations and incentives. These developments are provoking interesting questions about continuing responsibility for purchasing by the large regional health authorities. What remains clear is the significance of the role of these authorities in providing an independent regional assessment of population health needs, and establishing priorities and health goals based on those needs.

In some countries private for-profit entities are allowed to bid within publicly funded environments. Although not included in the group of countries documented in this exercise, Sweden's move to competitive contracting, for example, demonstrates an example of public and private entity competition in a predominantly publicly funded environment. A study comparing the quality of services between a privately managed health care centre and three publicly managed centres serving similar populations demonstrated that the services of the private centre met government specifications measures and provided quality of care as well as the publicly managed centres. The private centre accomplished this through more flexible management practices, higher workloads coupled with higher pay for staff, and costs that were 10 to 48 percent lower than the publicly managed centres (Hansagi, Calltorp, and Andreseasson 1993; Marriott and Mable 1994). This illustrates an opportunity to open up service delivery to a wider array of participants under appropriate conditions.

What is demonstrated by review of other countries, is that evolution of health care organizations from *control-oriented* geographic authority models toward *service-oriented* independent, vertically integrated models, produces beneficial results in the delivery of health care services for a variety of reasons. The combined characteristics of a roster-based, vertically integrated purchaser/provider entity with responsibility and funding for the services it delivers create a more dynamic, continuously adapting organizational construct for the delivery of health care services. The key is *integrated responsibility*, which is not necessarily directive as to how an entity must organize itself to purchase or provide services.

These types of features have emerged consistently across varying national environments. Existing and evolving examples, such as HMOs in the United States, Total GP Fundholders in the United Kingdom, GP and other managed care models in New Zealand, Sickness Funds in the Netherlands, and CHOs in Canada all indicate the potential to operate more comprehensively and effectively (benefitting from economies of scale), and to adapt more readily to changes in population needs or other systemic factors. This observation is not isolated to the countries examined in this paper: many other countries are on a similar track (e.g., Israel with its Sick Fund organizations).

Implications of the Change to Integrated Models

There are extensive implications and potential benefits generated by the implicit dynamics in key features of organizational shifts to roster-based, fully vertically integrated organizational models, which provide and/or purchase health care services. Not the least of these is greater *control,* as expressed by Bundred of the United Kingdom, "With integration of responsibility, and the financial resources for all sectors of the health care in one system, you get control, control and control" (Bundred 1996). This point infers both the accounting sense of *keeping track,* as well as the more commonly known terms of *influence.*

Responsibility for given services and associated funding, plus the immediacy and intimacy of a rostered population, require an organization to face trade-offs, balancing needs within the integrated organization's continuum of health services. Financial and other incentives influence these choices. For example, an avoidance of expenditure in the wellness and primary care sector may lead to higher expenses in secondary and acute care. Conversely, an inappropriate expenditure in secondary and acute care may deny appropriate funding or resources for wellness and primary care. Besides the economic cost of poor choices, the organization may signal poor performance to its rostered members, and therefore, risk losing them (Marriott 1994) and in turn, lowers its profile in the community. Chernichovsky (1995) notes that the emerging dominance of integrated models and reforms as promoting "...system efficiency and consumer satisfaction rather than a particular doctrine. Consequently it denotes efforts to combine the comparative advantages of public systems (equity and social [macro] efficiency) with the comparative advantages of competitive, usually private systems (consumer satisfaction and internal [micro] efficiency) in the provision of care."

The observation has been made that integrated models exemplify a "creative blending or hybridization" of the public-funded environment on one hand with elements of the private entrepreneurial world on the other. Public funding and definition of core services or benefits for all protect the principles of universality (or solidarity) and accessibility. At the same time, introduction of "private sector" style microeconomic behaviour and freedom promote a dynamic environment where organizations can pursue greater responsiveness and quality in serving members, as well as new organizational and financial relationships between and among purchasers and providers (Marriott 1994).

These "market forces" (such as competitive behaviour to attract and keep rostered members with financial and administrative incentives) catalyze the behaviour of roster-based purchaser/provider models, regardless of the extent of regulation in the system. With the exception of the United States, most of the countries reviewed represent regulated environments with market forces and not privately funded markets and competition (Evans and Winter 1995). In the context of the publicly funded environments, *price and benefits* are fixed (by governments). Therefore competitive behaviour is based almost exclusively on *service and quality* to rostered members. Only in the predominantly privately funded systems like the United States is competition also based on price and definition of benefits packages, where they are both allowed to vary and are negotiable (e.g., between HMOs and employers) (Marriott 1993–1994, 1996).

By virtue of responsibility for services and funding, vertically integrated organizations are motivated to improve service coordination for their members throughout the health system. For example, integrated responsibility for all health services provides a powerful incentive to see the "big picture," unlike other providers who focus primarily on their own environment or sector (e.g., nursing, hospita, or laboratory). These organizations must appreciate all sectors of care as well as determine and understand current and projected profiles of need of their rostered population. The understanding of population need is the basis for establishing priorities, and for ascertaining the most appropriate array of health resources required to meet it. This becomes the basis for decisions on providing or negotiating contracts to purchase the required health resources to respond to that need.

Responsibility with funding for services, coupled with autonomy and flexibility to customize organizational and financial arrangements with providers, produces opportunity for innovation in the system and the capacity to do so. Fine-tuning approaches to contracting is evident in all the jurisdictions reviewed, where purchasers are exploring ways to express quality standards, evidence-based outcomes, and services in the specifications of contractual agreements with providers. For example, in New Zealand, multiyear contracts with providers are being explored to match multiyear planning horizons. In the United States, there are countless examples of horizontal and vertical integration of providers for the purpose of better positioning to attract and hold contracts.

From the perspective of public policy, there is a tension between the incentive to improve quality and responsiveness on the one hand and provide equitable access to "standardized" services on the other. Vertically integrated models can use this tension constructively to create more beneficial standards as well as an environment which perpetually strives to ameliorate them.

Publicly funded systems have historically tended to support the notion of equitable access for all to a "minimum" or "same" standard of services. In the old regime, this often led to policy that emphasized consistent "template" approaches to ensure that, at least on paper, no one would receive more than anyone else with the same need. Equity meant the same for all, which produced a "lowest common denominator" approach to health care, and maintained a "minimum" standard of care. The emerging entrepreneurial behaviour of the roster-based integrated model stimulates the development of new approaches and at times, may produce greater variety in service delivery modes. Public protection of minimum standards coupled with the pursuit of new and different ways to do things has been described in Canada as the potential for "positive or progressive inequity." This means that the minimum standard is protected and articulated by the central authority, while entrepreneurial organizations, while committed to never producing less than the minimum standard, are able and permitted to pursue alternative methods which may result ultimately in pushing up those standards.

While this process may result in varying standards as different organizations develop particular areas of expertise (e.g., greater responsiveness or new techniques and efficiencies in clinical treatments), over time, and through assessment by authorities as well as benchmarking with adaptations by other organizations in the system, these initiatives will serve to raise the minimum standards to a higher level for the entire society (Marriott 1993–1994). Organizations can be "safely" encouraged by governments to "compete" in this fashion, with the ultimate goal of raising the threshold of minimum standards of core services. Barr (1990) reinforces this notion, identifying a "…need to encourage technological and organizational advances… dynamic efficiency should be pursued, [and] …there should be a search for technological and organizational advances which raise the productivity of given resources." In summary, common standards, together with entrepreneurial behaviours such as benchmarking and the development of better information systems and communications, can lead to improvements, which will in turn benefit the health care system.

There are areas of the system which require qualifiers with regards to the previous discussion. Certain subsectors of activity, such as highly specialized services which are labour and cost intensive, and which require sufficient volumes of activity for specialists to ensure that quality is maintained and improved, may be better served by a more controlled approach to improvement of standardized services. In such areas, appropriate government intervention may be required—as has been done in the Netherlands—to "license" or regulate the number of these specialized sites to ensure a balance between the required volume of work per site, and to provide adequate access. As in the Dutch model, the regulator could also impose costs of service payments which bear a relationship to the financial needs of the provider, and in this way maintain fairness with no disincentives to the purchaser.

Other equity issues are addressed and protected through the features of rostering and capitation. Weighted capitation funding adjusted for age, gender of rostered members, as well as other factors such as regional variances or proxies for need, provides an equitable cash flow to all integrated organizations serving populations with similar characteristics. This means that, in principle, no organization is receiving more or less funding than another when compared on this basis. With responsibility for the benefits of core services, and assumption of the cost risks implicit in provision of care, there is a strong incentive to provide or purchase care in the most efficient manner possible. If two organizations with relatively similar population characteristics result in one performing better than the other, it is less likely due to "inequity" of funding, than it is to other factors (e.g., less efficient operations which are most likely due to poor management, internal procedures or other elements internal to the organization or its environment). It becomes easier to identify problem areas, formerly attributed to funding "inequity" (the answer may *not* be to throw more money at the problem). This creates greater transparency throughout the system, in that the rules apply more fairly to all, and it becomes more possible to discern inconsistencies as well as top performers.

Universal access and full capitation funding ensure individuals cannot be refused registration (roster) with an organization of choice. As well, freedom of choice means members are free to leave on organization (exercise the right of "exit") to join an organization which better suits their needs. With choice and capitation, funding is, in effect, reoriented from providers and "attached" to consumers and their needs, as reflected by the weighting formula. This means that funding "follows the patient" rather than the organization; and so the exiting member's funding "transfers" with him from the former organization to the new one. The implicit priorities and incentives for organizations, individuals, and governments are many.

In summary, *weighted capitation* represents a significant element in the system, as the fairest way to distribute central funds equitably to integrated organizations and to reorient funding toward patients' needs. A fully vertically integrated organization may be the most effective organizational recipient, because it assumes responsibility for *all* services, matching a single capitation funding for all services. From the government perspective, this represents an administratively more simple and cohesive manner of funding, as compared to the presently segmented "stovepipe" configuration of health care funding in the Canadian environment, prone to inconsistencies and difficulty in tracking and evaluation across the system.

In view of the dynamics in the previous example, it is useful to point out the benefits that can be gained from "artful" balancing of regulation with the necessary autonomy of organizations to operate freely, for the purpose of encouraging appropriate behaviour. In some systems there is potential for inequity when organizations are able to selectively register people who are well and discriminate against those who are less well, or are from a population with a greater propensity for illness. This "cream skimming" is most familiar in the U.S. HMO system, where benefit packages are not centrally determined but negotiated with each of the varied purchasers with which an HMO may deal. HMOs are thus motivated to "select" members according to their negotiated benefit plans, to avoid the higher costs associated with more illness. Centrally defined benefits with capitation mitigate against this, as they obviate the need for "competitive" behaviour in negotiating benefit plans and selecting members, and provide adequate funding (based on the total system) to address the costs of serious illness. Universality with weighted capitation, while perhaps not perfect, better aligns the funding to population needs while protecting access for all. Explicit government regulation against "cream skimming" would also help.

With rostering also comes specificity in documenting important characteristics of individuals, and with that, the potential for the development of superior population data. A database can be compiled from the aggregate of member rosters and other information such as provider rosters, encounter tracking, episodes of care (whether through provision or purchase), satisfaction surveys, outcomes evaluation, and management of contract specifications. All information emanates naturally from the combined activities of integrated organizations. In all the countries reviewed, pressure for further improvement has led to growing sophistication of integrated data systems. The United States is particularly notable for the excellent systems developed in some HMO organizations, as well as the increasing commitment to development and evaluation of data and practices. Vertically integrated organizations can both generate this information and benefit greatly from access to aggregate data, helping them support better medical practice as well as planning for provision and/or purchase of health care services. Central authorities or monitoring agencies already use such information to carry out oversight responsibilities, while researchers, the press, and the general public also benefit. In short, the specificity accorded by rostering populations, encounters, plans, and providers contributes to greater precision and utility of information.

To this end, reporting by all entities operating in a health system becomes critical to the total system. This would be another area where government influence could ensure maintenance and development of a vital resource. For example, in addition to the kind of information discussed above, parameters for consistency and timeliness of reporting would protect the integrity of a provincial or national database. Requirements such as submission of annual plans by organizations would assist monitoring of appropriate operating procedures as well as innovations in the system.

Rostering also presents other opportunities to refine thinking and terminology. In Canada, for example, the notion of "community" is widely used, but is in fact still "fuzzy" and confusing—is it a town, a county, or some other geographically defined territory within which a population lives? "Community" does not have a single consistent definition that is of material use for costing, or for the design and refinement of organizations' responsibilities. With a rostered population, the "individual" becomes the specific and more appropriate major identifier, and the aggregate of individuals— the roster—is the "population" or "community" that the organization serves. Rostered members or enrollees may live in one town or be scattered in many towns or in the country. Regardless, "community" as a term in this context becomes more useful, quantifiable, and meaningful throughout the system.

Another attribute of rostering, as compared to geographically defined entities, is its allowance for optional, improved modes of service delivery within geographic areas. Specifically, population size permitting, several roster-based integrated organizations could operate in the same geographic area, evolving "naturally" as a result of population needs or community preferences and bringing more of the potential benefits of entrepreneurial behaviour into the region. Further, rostered members in rural or northern communities could organize their populations to promote formation of their own specialized organizations. While this could conceivably evolve into what might be considered a geographic monopoly in a given community, that possibility would be offset by the presence in the environment of integrated organizations, all providing "benchmark" information which tends to keep all the entities concerned in line with costs and oriented toward improvement. This has important implications in Canada, where population density varies tremendously across rural and urban areas.

In addition, rostering supports the potential for specifically defined groups to develop their own organizations (e.g., ethnic minorities, people living with HIV/AIDS). For example, First Nations groups could develop and control a roster-based, vertically integrated health organization. In this context, alternative therapies and healing could be blended with traditional Western health care and medicine, and funds used to provide or purchase secondary specialized medical and hospital services. Examples of this approach are demonstrated by Maori health organizations in New Zealand. Such a monopoly can be quite acceptable when supported by the systemic safeguards of rostering for accurate and appropriate data, capitation funding, and practices such as benchmarking to stay in line with typical parameters. Again, good information and reporting would be mandatory under these circumstances.

With a system of integrated organizations there are also opportunities for participation in health services and alliances outside of the mainstream of the publicly funded health system. For example, integrated organizations could provide services funded through private supplementary insurance to which employers contribute for employees such as eyeglasses, drugs, and semiprivate hospital accommodation. Given recent documented success in reducing and improving drug prescribing, it may be expedient to have the integrated organization assume responsibility for private drug plans in addition to the publicly funded benefits, to encourage reduced costs and improved quality for all drugs; or even to provide private supplementary insurance and services itself. These measures can result in lower costs and improved quality for all drug expenditures, as has happened in the Netherlands. And, using another Dutch example, ministries of health in Canada could consider assuming responsibility for work-related illness, injury, and associated compensation (i.e., workers' compensation). Such possibilities are a mere reflection of the range of potential opportunities to be explored.

Comments Regarding Implementation

Implementation may be done all at once or in a series of steps. A general observation is that most of the countries reviewed, excluding the United States, redefined their goals and directions and implemented new models on a national scale. This suggests that countries with strong, centrally directed governments are perhaps better able to accomplish reform (which benefits the entire population consistently) with greater ease than their more decentralized counterparts. These governments appear to have assessed their organizational options, determined whether there was consistent logic in the organizational design and policy goals, and, at least for the major blocks of reform, simply pressed forward. There was no attitude of "waiting to see if the approach had been tried and evaluated elsewhere first": major reform was introduced systemically and comprehensively rather than as tentative "pilots" isolated from the rest of the system. This is not to say that "piloting" and testing have not been part of reform in these countries. It simply reflects that it is difficult or impossible to "pilot" or create microcosms of entire health systems. Instead, major systemic reforms were made all at once, while pilot testing of incremental steps accompanied subsequent evolution and refinement in subsectors. For example, the Netherlands "piloted" the incorporation of specialists into the hospital contracting process, while fundholding and vertically integrated purchaser/provider models are undergoing gradual development in the United Kingdom and New Zealand.

With respect to systems in transition, there appears to have been a corresponding tolerance of pluralistic organizations. This is quite obvious throughout the U.S. system. It is demonstrated in New Zealand, where GP provider/purchaser and vertically integrated managed care corporations are emerging in parallel. Another example is found in the United Kingdom, where development of Total GP Fundholding organizations with responsibility to contract for all health services demonstrates the coexistence of specialized fully vertically integrated organizations and nonfundholding GP practices.

Protection against Self-Enrichment and Sector Bias

When, as in the United Kingdom, a provider is also a fundholder, concerns arise about self-enrichment of providers, or "one-sector bias or control" of an organization. There is an obvious need to mitigate against inappropriate diversion of health care resources from the system or the patients. To ensure, for example, that funds for specialists or hospitals do not end up directly enriching the remuneration of the GP who contracts for these services, the system has developed protective steps via a third-party funding arrangement, which could be described as a "line of credit." District health authorities serve as a third-party payer, transferring funding to the other providers upon delivery of services to the GP's patients.

This extra administrative step outside the GP Fundholder organization (the transferring of the funds by the DHA), may also serve the interest of DHAs by preserving a certain level of authority and jobs. It may also tend to make the integration of other provider "parts" into GP Fundholder organizations less likely, at least at this stage of development. This example suggests that if GP practices or any other single provider moves to fund-holding, rules should be put in place to ensure that the provider is not inappropriately enriched at the expense of the government or the rest of the system, and that the system is not inappropriately enriched at the expense of the patient.

This would not appear to be a concern where the integrated organization has its own accountable and representative board and administration and is not "owned" by any one sector or provider in the health system. Even if the organization itself ends up "owning" or employing various organizations or individuals to increase internal capacity to directly provide services, it is managed by an organization with a mandated systemic perspective. Shared liability and responsibility encourage a greater willingness in these circum-stances to consider transferring full capitation funding to the organization, and to let it work out its provision or purchase options to best serve its rostered population. This makes the process "cleaner" and eliminates the necessity of an offset bureaucracy (such as the DHA in the United Kingdom) between the integrated fundholder model and the providers with which it contracts. It also means that the integrated organization can explore organizational merger or independent development of any part of the health system from within the organization, where it makes sense.

The United Kindgom's "line of credit" solution could be used for provider entities which are developing into fully vertically integrated models, as a way to fund them on a trial basis to handle service outside the typical purview of physician services. This might occur for a period of time during which they must demonstrate competence in contracting for the additional services, after which direct capitation for those services would be added on. Another safeguard to be discussed more fully in the next section is the establish-ment of a corporate/board structure with expanded representation as a vehicle for receiving funding; the services delivered by this structure and the constituency it served would also be expanded. For example, to provide long-term care, a provider organization would expand board representation and management expertise, "earn" the right to provide the new services by demonstrating competence for a test period, during which it would be funded on a line-of-credit basis and after which the organization could receive full capitation for all the services it provides.

The "Primacy" of Primary Care

In all cases reviewed, emphasis has been placed on the importance of primary care and the GP as gatekeeper to the rest of the system. The GP controls access by being the first line of triage before referring patients to secondary services (diagnostics, specialists, hospital, etc.), and serves as a prime participant in the coordination of care. Because GPs are increasingly operating in multidisciplinary primary care environments, the coordination of care may also involve other practitioners. In this context, while a GP may be the exclusive gatekeeper to secondary care, he is *not necessarily the first or exclusive point of entry* to the system for the patient. Rather, in some cases, a patient has direct access to primary care via nurse practitioners or counsellors, and can consult other practitioners (such as nutritionists, social workers, psychologists, or therapists) *who work in conjunction with* the primary care physician. In many jurisdictions, including Canada, primary care is the foundation of community health centres where the principles of multidisciplinary approaches are strongly supported.

The present-day trends in primary care were anticipated by Siegel in 1986:

> Primary care physicians may have new responsibilities for patients' total health care, for appropriate resource allocation, for meeting patients' increasing expectations, and for assuring that patients receive quality health care. Some specialists will experience a shift in roles, including some strengthened responsiveness to the expectations of primary care physicians. Teamwork between primary care physicians and consultative specialists is likely to be promoted by alternative delivery systems, with primary care physicians having increased responsibility for success through managing health care in response to patients' needs. Specialty physicians will be able to concentrate more on their specialty of interest, rather than mixing specialty and primary care.

From the experience of other countries, we know that increased emphasis on primary care results in positive impacts on morbidity and mortality. The increased service orientation of primary care organizations, including the focus and training of practitioners to adopt a holistic view of patients and provide "cradle to grave" (the full spectrum) care, a "wellness attitude" encompassing health promotion and sickness prevention, and practices such as early intervention for diagnosis and treatment. All have a positive impact on health status. Patients seeking consultation are more likely than before to be healthy, and providers function well as gatekeepers, saving money and protecting the rest of system from inappropriate use. Due to such attributes, primary care organizations fit squarely in the scheme as a foundation for the development of integrated models, and provide a natural base for development of a fully integrated model for the Canadian health system.

The upcoming section brings the discussion of key features of integrated organizational models into the Canadian context, considering significant principles and features with respect to the present and future of our health care system.

KEY FEATURES OF INTEGRATED MODELS IN THE CANADIAN CONTEXT

The ultimate purpose of this exercise is to derive the key principles and features which should guide the future evolution of Canada's health system from a critical review of some developments in the countries reviewed and in Canada. The intent of this section is to briefly reconsider the objectives of the Canadian system, to cull a predominant set of principles and features from the broader selection of characteristics of integrated models, and to consider this set of principles and characteristics from the perspective of the Canadian environment and objectives. These key principles and features are then summarized and examined with respect to important attributes and linkages in the Canadian system where there may be a relationship to better performance of integrated organizational models.

The important objectives and principles of the Canadian context are first reviewed, and key features are then identified. These are introduced in terms of the distinguishing, interrelated features which *anchor* the integrated organizational constructs in Canada, and are presented in conjunction with associated features which are integral to successful implementation. Comments are then made regarding potential impacts and benefits, as well as important underpinnings—government regulation and/or operational rules—to support movement towards a greater degree of integration of any or all of these features. Opportunities and constraints of given options are identified where useful to the discussion. The purpose here is not to present an exhaustive examination, but to begin to highlight those characteristics which could be of constructive use to the Canadian system.

The discussion continues with an examination of the present Canadian system, highlighting positive accomplishments and promising trends. The review is completed with a discussion of potential trajectories which could be taken by selected Canadian jurisdictions and organizational models, in keeping with these principles and features. In particular, there appears to be an opportunity to build fully vertically integrated models upon an existing foundation of primary care as a step of transition towards fully integrating these models into the system. In addition, regionally or geographically defined entities now present throughout Canada have incorporated many of the features discussed. Finally, a model of a fully vertically integrated independent health care organization has been developed and is being launched at this time. The section is followed by a brief discussion of evaluation guidelines and criteria geared to integrated models.

Selected System Objectives

The following outline represents a summary of a variety of observations, studies, and commissions which emerged as both a response to issues in the system, as well as to fulfil the common vision of principles expressed by Canadian society and governments (access, comprehensiveness, portability, public administration, and universality). They are roughly organized from the perspectives of individuals, providers, and governments.

Individual Patient or Aggregate Population Needs

- increased emphasis on wellness and sickness prevention;
- empowerment through increased involvement in the system;
- protection of appropriate access to required services;
- enhanced responsiveness by providers;
- increased emphasis on delivery of services in the community and decreased emphasis on hospital and institutional-based services;
- resources which follow the health needs of the population, rather than individual demands for health care;
- appropriate levels of choice.

Purchaser/Provider

- improved or maintained population health;
- appropriate autonomy;
- flexibility, discretion, and choice in a variety of settings including urban and rural environments;
- to stimulate innovations to motivate and reward progress and excellence;
- enhanced responsiveness to patient/consumer needs;
- enhanced efficacy of the health care system;
- improved integration and coordination within and beyond the health system (a "seamless" environment);
- improved efficiency and effectiveness in service delivery;
- opportunity/potential to provide services for private payers within the system (e.g., optometry; workers' compensation; insurance for private hospital rooms; private insurance and corporate health benefits for employees, etc.).

Governments

- fair/equitable distribution of funds to match health needs;
- a health care system based on universality, portability, and accessibility for all Canadians;
- improved continuity of care;

- improved accountability (as opposed to fragmentation of responsibility);
- improved quality, program measurement, and evaluation of outcomes;
- improved cost-effectiveness and predictability of costs;
- macroeconomic efficiency (appropriate fraction of GDP); a structure that contains costs (slow cost increases); to improve Canadian international competitiveness;
- coherence (a simplified system that is easy to comprehend)
- comprehensiveness (all-inclusive for the entire system);
- foster the morale of patients and providers of care; and
- preservation of a relationship between consumers/patients and their local health delivery system characterized by a sense of consumer "ownership" and loyalty (as opposed to alienation).

The review of international and Canadian models of health care service delivery reveals that there is a particular group of features that, when used in various combinations, appears to demonstrate promising present *and future* potential, as well as a consistency with international trends. This group of features "fits" with the Canadian environment and principles, and could serve to stimulate and guide the evolution of the Canadian health care system. The features are particularly useful in that they position the health care system to more effectively address prior issues, and reach the objectives expressed by patients/taxpayers, providers, and governments.

Distinguishing Features

The extent to which Canadian jurisdictions will be able to optimize the potential of vertical integration appears to hinge on a set of predominant and associated features, characterized by integration of *services, funding, and responsibility.* The predominant four characteristics anchor the organizational construct, setting foundational parameters for design and operations. The associated features identify attributes and priorities also essential for carrying out the mission and goals of the organization and system. For the purpose of this discussion, it is assumed that these features are implemented in full, resulting in a fully vertically integrated organization and assume a publicly funded, single-payer system. The identification and discussion follows below.

Predominant Anchoring Features

- *Benefits or core services* – responsibility for all benefits or core services, defined centrally, for the population served;
- *Roster* – responsibility for and accountability to a registered population with specific characteristics and health care needs;

- *Capitation* – the organization is funded by weighted capitation, reflective of the rostered population, for all health service, no matter where provided or accessed in the province or country; and
- *Autonomy to determine organizational and financial arrangements with providers* – freedom to make decisions regarding critical matters "internal" to operation of the organization to best serve its population, such as distribution of funding to care, decisions to provide or purchase and provide services, as well as the development of appropriate organizational and financial relationships with providers and throughout the system, to establish an optimum environment for all participants.

Associated Important Features

- not-for-profit independent corporate organization;
- board of Directors which provides for input and representation reflective of rostered members;
- an obligation to assess and respond to the needs of its individual members and the rostered population as a whole;
- requirement to plan for the most appropriate resources to meet the assessed needs;
- ensure appropriate services through direct provision or purchase of services;
- track and report all encounters and maintain other appropriate health records and data (e.g., roster information, provider profiles, satisfaction surveys);
- emphasis on wellness and primary care with GP as gatekeeper to secondary services and accessible multidisciplinary team for rostered members;
- formal commitment to quality and evaluation as a means of reinforcing the key features and obligations of the organization.

What follows is an examination of the features that make up vertically integrated organizations. The four predominant features are examined in greater detail to clarify what they mean, the minimum rules with which they are associated as defined by government regulation and operational rules, and why they are important. Less detailed comment is provided for the associated elements.

Predominant Features of Vertically Integrated Organizations

- Benefits or core services – responsibility for all benefits or core services, defined centrally, for the population served

Comprehensive benefits or core services include the full array of health programs and services, from primary care to secondary, tertiary and acute care, and from health promotion and sickness prevention to diagnosis and illness treatment.

The minimum rules (government policy) include:

- central definition of benefits on a national basis, for consistency across the system and reliability for individuals. This maintains the "public voice" of government within the system, and also protects the integrity of important principles such as comprehensiveness and portability. Providers could add responsibility for purchase or provision of supplementary benefits and workplace health programs beyond government insured services;
- equal application of benefits to all the population equally;
- emphasis on wellness/primary care, but responsibility for all programs and services defined in the core services or benefits, which means that one sector of care cannot be neglected in favour of another (this is not to say that appropriate substitution is not encouraged);
- must assure the provision of all required services to patients, and demonstrate this for evaluation.

Such minimum parameters set a threshold below which an organization should not fall, and distinct responsibilities allowing for better monitoring and evaluation. The intent is to accomplish the following:

- assure a commitment to accessibility for all patients, and the provision of "all" required services (insured or funded by government);
- centrally defined core benefits maintain the standards and integrity intended for those services, thereby holding these services apart from the entrepreneurial aspect of the organization and protecting them against being diminished by competitive behaviour amongst organizations;
- prevent organizations from escaping responsibility by withholding or providing less core services or benefits, or "laying off costs" to others in the system, once defined as within the core services or benefits.
- having responsibility for all benefits and therefore all programs and services in the health system (i.e., vertical integration of responsibility) which forces more appropriate trade-offs or balancing of services along the continuum of care and increases systemic thinking, promoting coordination of providers, sensitivity to all sectors and services (no one sector dominates), and responsiveness to the population served;
- simplify government responsibility to support, monitor, and evaluate performance by having core benefits distributed across a less fragmented delivery system involving more consistent types of organizations. This would allow government to expand its role to explore better ways to support and enhance improvements in the system.

- **Roster – responsibility for and accountability to a registered population with specific characteristics and health care needs**

Quite simply, citizens register (or roster) with a health organization of their choice, becoming part of its rostered population. Their sociodemographic characteristics as well as health needs are identified and documented in the information system of the organization. By virtue of the greater specificity of information, the organization is more intimately familiar with its population, and can use the information to better tailor programs to its needs.

Minimum rules (government policy) include:
- All citizens must be registered with an organization of their choice;
- Acceptance of all citizens who choose to register with the organization, regardless of their health conditions. No one must be denied the right to join on the basis of health. This protects universality as well as accessibility for the individual; and
- All citizens must be registered with the organization of their choice and have the right to leave ("exit") that organization to join another organization they feel better suits their needs. In addition, the capitation funding attributable to them must also "transfer" with them to the new entity.

Rostering populations to organizations provides an extensive array of benefits, the most important aspect of which is increased precision of data. Specific identification and information records on all individuals and groups served by the organization far exceed the utility of aggregate population census data presently in use. Specific health records contribute to better data systems from which aggregate data on health factors or populations may be extracted to improve planning and evaluation, and to provide a better match between patients and services. Good information allows providers to develop a better understanding of the population they serve, as individuals and in aggregate population groups with special needs.

The precision of rostered population data provides the foundations for more accurate and appropriate calculation of the capitation formula used to fund health organizations. This, in turn, provides an enhanced planning capability for both the organization and governments, promoting better distribution of resources throughout the system. There is an opportunity for enhanced human resource planning, in the development of more precise patient-practitioner needs ratios, to assist in the deployment of practitioners throughout organizations and the larger system.

Single organizations would use individual and aggregated patient health records, encounter information, financial and other data to improve planning for and responding to the needs of both the individuals and the populations they serve. Appropriately aggregated information from all organizations with safeguards to protect confidentiality could be incorporated centrally for ongoing benchmarking and assessment of organizational behaviour and impact throughout the health system.

- **Capitation – the organization is funded by weighted capitation, reflective of the rostered population, for all health services, no matter where provided or accessed in the province or country**

Capitation funding is fundamentally a population-based system of financial allocation from the central health budget. The distribution of funding is directly proportional to the population (roster) of the organization funded. To illustrate it simply, an organization with 10 times the roster of another would receive 10 times as much funding. However, there is general agreement that the need for financial resources is influenced by more than the number of individuals in a roster. Demographic characteristics, such as age and gender, are widely accepted as having an impact on the need for health resources (e.g., more geriatric services and supports for a relatively older population, or more prevention for a younger population).

Other factors are acknowledged as important in a capitation formula to adjust for "need," including *regional variations* in health needs and costs; the use of *mortality* (e.g., standardized mortality ratios (SMRs), acute illness indicators—a relative measure of premature death based on male and female life expectancy, etc.); or *deprivation/health need factors* such as levels of education, car ownership, number of single mothers, and ethnic makeup. There is, however, no final agreement, at this stage of development, as to the most appropriate additional *single or blend of* adjustments. Most countries are employing one or more of these factors in their approaches to capitation. All are including the age and gender weighting. The main point is that this remains, nonetheless, the most equitable or fair approach to distributing the health budget to organizations or models to ensure both "fair share" and some specificity to the relationship between the funding for health resources and the needs of the rostered population served.

Minimum rules (government policy) include:

- the government or system must have a central health fund or budget adequate to fund all the required core services or benefits for the population;
- the governments (provincial and territorial) must commit to capitation funding for the new organizations;
- the capitation formula must be weighted for age and gender at a minimum, with consideration for needs and regional or other factors in the system, in order to maintain specificity in the relationship between the cash flow and the predicted cost of serving the needs of the population; and
- in the context of this model, the capitation must be for *all* health services that could be accessed and provided to roster members anywhere in the province or country.

Capitation brings consistency, equity, and fairness to funding distribution. The same formula is applied to all rosters. When considering roster-based, fully vertically integrated models, no one organization receives more or less money than another, when the sociodemographics of their rostered populations are compared. Any differences in the cash flow will be due to variations in the number, age and gender distribution, regional and geographic locations of members, and the proxies for need applied on a regional basis.

The implications of capitation are summarized below:

- Capitation provides "reasonable" funding in terms of its relationship to the anticipated cost of care for the profile of need of the rostered population.
- Each model receives a "fairer" share of financial resources than it would receive under the historical utilization-based method, which tends to maintain inequitable allocations.
- The capitation method is based on the relative health needs of the population (adjustments for age and gender; adjustments for deprivation/needs and cost). The historical utilization-based and global budget approaches do contain some elements of need, but are also influenced by other factors. Under these other systems, there is little recognition of competing resource demands in relationship to the relative needs of the population served.
- The capitation method is responsive to changes in the size and demographic composition of the model's roster over time. As one organization's roster increases with a relatively older population in comparison to others, it will receive more resources. Historical utilization-based approaches are reticent and slow to respond to change, and tend to perpetuate historical inequities between health organizations.
- The capitation methodology is a systematic process that allocates resources on the basis of observable characteristics of the population and is not heavily affected by "gaming" or political manipulation. Other than occasional discussion of refining the capitation formula, there are few opportunities for interested parties to manipulate the funding system.
- Capitation provides a *variable cash flow*—not a global budget and not an envelope. While this cash flow does not preserve historical financial arrangements (the sum of preexisting budgets for providers), it does promote flexibility to move money to targeted areas in accordance with the plan for need, the profile of demand, and the changes in this profile over time—to the most appropriate provider, with the right service, in the right place, at the right time, for the specific need of the individual rostered member.
- Through capitation, money "follows the patient," encouraging attention to patients' needs with the added incentive of attracting and holding on to rostered members. Simply put, new members increase the cash flow of the organization, while "exiting" members reduce it. Given that there could be more than one organization serving a given geographic area, capitation encourages greater sensitivity and responsiveness to all entities in the system, as well as to the needs of members of the population, who still enjoy the right of choice and exit. If a patient-member chooses to exit an organization, his capitation funding moves

with him to the new one. The implications of this for amelioration of quality and service are many: it stimulates a heightened service orientation as well as the provision of the most appropriate methods of service by providers and organizations. Moreover, the focus is kept on patient care as opposed to building up infrastructure.

- Full financial accountability with full capitation (national or province-wide) for the roster. This represents no "add-on cost" to the system, as all external services can be tracked and charged back to the rostered organization, or through adjustments to its capitation. This guards against leakage, as organizations cannot pass on responsibility and cost to others.

- Capitation offers predictability and simplicity for organizations and governments:
  - organizations: Predictable funding, supports planning, expands potential for multiyear planning
  - governments: Solid forecasting, ease of management, removes need for sector-by-sector negotiations and confrontation with ministers or ministries

- **Autonomy to determine organizational and financial arrangements with providers: freedom to make decisions regarding critical matters "internal" to operation of the organization to best serve its population, such as distribution of funding to care, decisions to provide or purchase and provide services, as well as the development of appropriate organizational and financial relationships with providers and throughout the system, to establish an optimum environment for all participants**

As an entity independent of government, a health organization has the autonomy and freedom to develop the most appropriate operating procedures and organizational and financial relationships with providers, with the ultimate goal of providing the most appropriate services to its rostered population. This autonomy, coupled with the financial capacity to follow through on decisions, has powerful implications for reform throughout the system. Responsibility for a full spectrum of care overlays a total picture of services which must be balanced against population needs, to arrive at appropriate care decisions. Bringing the weight of fiduciary responsibility to negotiating agreements with providers "evens the field" upon which services and responsibilities are negotiated. Assuming equitable capitation funding and a rostered population, the autonomy to make decisions and changes will serve to promote a more refined distribution of funds to needs, and allow for a more dynamic service environment.

Minimum rules (government policy) include:

- the integrated organization must have the right and opportunity to negotiate with providers, as well as pursue the merging of providers and provider organizations within its organization;

- a formal requirement to pursue appropriate contracts with providers where the organization does not have—or prefers not to have—the capacity to provide a service on its own;
- the integrated organization must have the financial and legal freedom to negotiate contracts. To assist the process, the government could establish minimum parameters to serve as guidelines, and/or "default" rules for situations where the two parties fail to achieve an agreement (e.g., funding rates in lieu of an agreed-upon approach);
- the organization must have the freedom to: structure itself within the parameters of protecting the integrity of its health care service mission and goals, as well as its not-for-profit status (for example, specific bylaws could be mandated for this purpose); and to design its organizational setup (management, administrative, financial, human resource procedures) to best respond to the needs of the population it serves. This would allow for variation in different settings; and
- the government may elect to regulate particular specialized services or programs to limit the number and location to appropriate provincial or national requirements. Government could also elect to regulate that certain specialized institutions and services remain autonomous in order to ensure an appropriate number of these services in the province, with the ultimate goal of balancing access with a sufficient volume of work to support continuing expertise and quality. In this case, government may be directive (set guidelines) in the financial arrangements between the health organization and such entities (determine the tariff or cost to be paid) to maintain appropriate volumes of use, expertise and skills of the specialties, or to ensure no disincentive to appropriate use of these services. These parameters do not in any way diminish the direct relationships between organizations and providers. The expectation is still that providers and organizations will negotiate agreements to exchange funds for the provision of services, as well as to obligate the provider to feed back encounter data to the organization, with incentives for performance.

Autonomy of health organizations preserves the freedom with financial capacity to direct their operations in such a way as to enhance the delivery of services appropriate to local conditions. This freedom empowers management to make decisions which promote a better environment for both providers and patients, leading to greater satisfaction of all concerned, in addition to effectiveness and economic viability. The integrated model, by virtue of its nature, cannot be expected to operate in isolation, or to perform without the critical features discussed above. There are other important considerations involved in promoting the highest and best performance of integrated models.

Important Associated Features

In addition to the four anchoring features discussed above, there are a number of other important "underpinnings" of fully vertically integrated organizations, that represent the likely outcome of natural incentives in the reformed system, but should nonetheless be required by government as minimum components and standard operating characteristics. They serve to reinforce appropriate operating parameters and to meet the principles and policy objectives of health reform.

- **Not-for-profit independent corporation organizations**

A not-for-profit independent corporate organizational framework promotes a more responsible and monitorable orientation with a skeletal design specifically focused on a mission to find the most appropriate distribution of resources for health care. Its mission could be embedded in its bylaws, other formal corporate documentation, and operating procedures. Capitation funding serves this overall mission by introducing a more equitable cash flow to the organization, bringing greater support to providers in serving populations with more critical needs. Greater degrees of autonomy with responsibility for services and all associated funding allows for experimentation with optional modes of service delivery and administration to build new relationships and adapt to changing conditions.

A not-for-profit integrated entity may be a more appropriate fit with Canadian principles and objectives than a for-profit organization, at least in the first phases of reform. Within this context, surplus funds resulting from efficiencies in the organization could be redirected to enhance or improve services, quality, or responsiveness elsewhere in the organization. By contrast, in the for-profit environment, the demand for profits from owners (a return for investors) can result in minimizing financial resources being allocated to support the provision and/or quality of services in order to achieve profit for the owners. A not-for-profit environment for the integrated health care organization balances incentives to create surplus with a mandate to redirect it to improved health care.

- **Board of directors which provides for input and representation reflective of the rostered members**

Like any more complex corporate organization, the integrated organization will have an implicit responsibility as well as strong incentives to engage a board and administration reflective of the service it provides and the population it serves to stay abreast of current needs, trends, and costs. Involving representation from among those the organization serves ensures a voice and influence of the patient/consumer population. The option of allowing for provider participation recognizes local decision making to include providers as partners in the organization's governance.

- **An obligation to assess and respond to the needs of its individual members and the rostered population as a whole**

- Requirement to plan for the most appropriate resources to meet the assessed needs
- Ensure appropriate services through direct provision or purchasing of service
- Track and report all encounters and maintain other appropriate health records and data (e.g., roster information, provider profiles, satisfaction surveys)

A formal population needs assessment supports the implementation and refinement of systematic and scientific approaches to assess the profile of need and the development of the best plan to provide the most appropriate array of providers and services to respond to this need. In addition, the commitment to respond to the individual's needs, within the framework of the service needs that would normally be funded within the system, means that no patients would be denied appropriate services because their requirements were unusual or not readily available. Organizational design flexibility allows potential to appropriately "fit" the organization to meet specialized needs of a given population—such as the needs of members of rural communities, whose economies are quite different than urban requirements within a densely populated metropolitan area. Particularly if other organizations are present, competing to attract and keep rostered members.

Funding parameters could require and compel organizations to assess needs responsibly, and to plan and organize the provision of required services. With more direct mutually incentivized relationships among organizations, providers, and rostered populations (acting as both patients and partners in health care), arises the opportunity and responsibility to improve decision making regarding direct provision or contracting for the most appropriate services. In support of these responsibilities, it will track encounters and collect other information to support health records, monitor and evaluate activity, and apply quality measures. Having the rostered membership attached to the health card supports the tracking of use of external providers and negating the cost of that service from the capitation funding. It also means that the role of coordinating advocacy and care is supported no matter where the organization arranges and/or pays for services. Improved communication and reporting of critical information supports development of more useful data systems from which all participants in the system will benefit. Once established, the integrated health care organization's daily operation and administration involves functions consistent with other industries, expanding the potential for benchmarking for new ideas beyond health care organizations.

- Emphasis on wellness and primary care with the GP as the gatekeeper to secondary services and an accessible multidisciplinary team for rostered patients

A commitment to wellness (health promotion and sickness prevention) with more emphasis on primary care and community-based care (and less on institutional care) will give patients more direct access to members of a primary care team including at a minimum a GP, and potentially nurse-practitioners, nutritionists, counsellors, and physiotherapists among other health care professionals. In addition, the GP serves as the gatekeeper in terms of access to medical specialists, hospitals, and other elements of secondary and acute care. These attributes are consistent with current Canadian goals and principles.

- **Formal commitment to quality and evaluation, and through this, reinforcement of the key features and obligations of the organization**

Such a mandate could include procedures which incorporate mechanisms to assure the availability, accessibility, effectiveness and continuity of care, as well as continuous quality improvement. Quality evaluation should take place within a framework which includes: accurate needs assessment; a quality-oriented environment; indicators of quality improvement initiatives; economic evaluation; self-reported health status measurement; and member and provider satisfaction.

A commitment to the provision of encounter information and information related to ensuring that quality standards are met could be a requirement within all contracts to purchase services. This lays the foundation to build an electronic health record that will, in turn, support planning and provide integrated comprehensive information to the physicians and other authorized caregivers in the organization. Like any other health organization already in the system, the organization would be bound by rules of confidentiality.

In general, a more fully integrated organization would be driven and motivated by incentives implicit in its more comprehensive responsibilities, operations and funding, by virtue of vertical integration, to perform better in the present and adapt continuously in the future.

Additional Government Support

In addition to the minimum rules (or government policy) defined under the four key features, government has an important role in developing the system's infrastructure and supporting its integrity by taking the following steps:

- establish health goals and priorities nationally, provincially, and regionally;
- ensure that there is a central fund, and develop and continue to refine a capitation formula, as well as a specific funding pool to serve populations in crisis when catastrophes hit;
- maintain a small central fund to reinforce the achievement of health goals and to respond to the needs of "hard-to-reach" populations (such as street people);

- mandate and support the development of an integrated health information system and participate in the definition of standards;
- must ensure and participate in the appropriate monitoring and formal evaluation, including the assessment of needs and the performance of given models and the system as a whole. This could be further enriched by independent local and regional assessment and projections of need, as well as public audits of performance; and *(if supporting the gradual addition of fundholding and purchasing responsibility for GP/primary care organizations)*
- require that the organizations establish boards and other organizational attributes of the fully integrated organization for consistency of operations, costs, and responsibility across the system (see "Implementation" below).

Discussion

The preceding section elaborated on the key features of vertically integrated organizations which ought to guide the future evolution of Canada's health system. While structural change in the health care sector is difficult in the best of times, and is highly sensitive to the values, culture and politics of the day, there have been a number of positive developments at the provincial and national levels which seem to suggest an evolution which is consistent, or at least potentially consistent, with these key features.

There are at least three areas of promising opportunities for development toward vertically integrated organizations including:
- development from primary care base;
- regionally and geographically defined entities are incorporating in their modelling a number of the key features; and
- implementation of the fully vertically integrated independent health care organizations has already been designed, several communities are under review or development and/or are being launched at this time. These areas of development are summarized below.

Development from Primary Care Base

Recent interest in reforming primary care could well result in the development of independent primary care organizations that receive capitation for their rostered population. Once this is in place, greater integration could be achieved over time by building upon an existing primary care organization's infrastructure. At least one of the proposals for primary care models suggests that this could be accomplished by adding responsibility for specialists, hospital, and other services through additional capitation funding. These additions would also have the potential of introducing the notion of purchasing. There are probably two tracks or trajectories that could be considered in "growing" primary care organizations through incremental steps to complete or full vertical integration of health services responsibility. Each would build on the organizational strength achieved through rostering and capitation. These tracks are summarized below.

Track 1 – GP/Primary Care Organization to Capitated Purchaser-Provider Model

The basic foundation for this model is to receive capitation for services beyond primary care on a staged, incremental basis. Capitation would be added for discrete modules or sectors of care (e.g., drug, specialists, diagnostics, home care). To become a fully mature model, this organization would have to develop the capacity to purchase or provide the additional services (e.g., through employing, or mergers with, other providers).

To move into the provision or purchase of a full array of services outside its historical practice(s), an organization must expand its governance and management structure. If it is not already operating under a not-for-profit corporate structure with a board, it must create one. Governance (the board) and management must reflect representation of both the service sectors it intends to provide, as well as the constituency (rostered population) it will serve. This further broadens the management and operational sensitivity to other areas of practice, to prepare to more appropriately manage funding *in balance with all other services* provided, particularly to guard against problems associated with one-sector bias or control. As well, reporting of aggregate data to a central system, conforming to consistent data standards throughout the province/nation, becomes a mandate. If the organization evolves to include all core health services, it becomes a fully integrated model.

Track 2 – GP/Primary Care Organization to a Purchaser Fundholder, Partial to Full Vertical Integration, with Option to Become Purchaser-Provider

A GP/primary care organization "may be evolved" to become either a partial or a total fundholder. The primary differentiation is that a fundholder in this context is *always only* a purchaser. As a fundholder, an organization does not require a board. Fundholders negotiate contracts for services with providers. To fund delivery of the new services, the government provides a line of credit form of payment directly to providers (as is done with GP Fundholders paid via the DHAs in the United Kingdom). The primary purpose of this method of fund delivery is to ensure that there is no one-sector bias, and that none of these funds form part of the remuneration to GPs.

Fundholding capacity can be developed in stages by adding capitated discrete blocks of program funding (e.g., such as for diagnostic and specialists' services) and associated "line of credit" funding to the organization. The organization must be enabled to "purchase"—that is, to master the skills and data requirements of contracting for services, including defining terms of reference and specifications (defining specific programs and services, expected outcomes, medical, ethical and quality standards, encounter reporting requirements by providers to the organization, monitoring rights of the organization), as well as preparations for contract management (financial and administrative). Fundholders can expand capacity to purchase all core services through the line of credit, to become a total fundholder. They can choose to remain a partial or a fully mature total fundholding organization, but still remain only purchasers.

At any time in their development, fundholders can elect to become capitated purchaser/provider organizations by fulfilling the minimum requirement of corporate/board structure and development of *provider* capacity, as discussed earlier. If a total fundholder elects this route, the organization becomes a fully vertically integrated model (figure 12).

Figure 12

Fundholder vs. Integrated purchaser/provider model

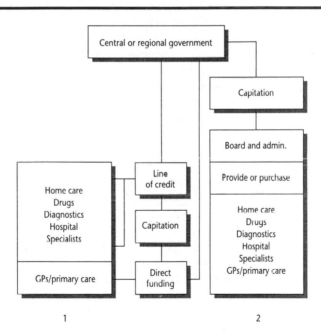

1. GP Fundholder model—no or limited access to money for secondary services—roster based.

2. Roster-based vertically integrated model—full capitation for "all" services.

Regionally or Geographically Defined Organizations

Provincial Modelling Incorporating Some Key Features

Canadian jurisdictions with regionally or geographically defined organizations have incorporated many of the features presented earlier in their current and evolving modelling. Movement toward integration is a component of all of these organizational reform initiatives. In jurisdictions with regional boards for institutions, there is movement toward forms of vertical integration. For example, New Brunswick is developing primary care or community health centres; Newfoundland already includes nursing homes along with hospitals in its regional institutional boards; and other jurisdictions, such as Saskatchewan's district health boards which are not-for-profit corporations, already include either the funding and/or direct "ownership" and therefore management responsibility for multiple sectors of the health system.

Primary or community health centres, home care, long-term care facilities, hospitals, and other programs are now within the board and administrative responsibility of these organizations. This structure serves to broaden the perspective on health and to encourage, if not require, thinking along the health continuum about the most appropriate configuration of resources within their regions to meet the needs of their populations. What is missing in all cases, at this stage of evolution, is physician services (except those in community health centres), and in some cases, tertiary hospital and other specialized services. In addition to the move from organizational fragmentation to integration, the regional structures are engaged in population health planning. Formalization and development of expertise in coordinated, comprehensive planning through needs assessment, and determining the most appropriate set of health resources required to respond to this need is a significant progression in Canadian health reform.

All of the partially vertically integrated models have the potential to move to purchasing models. Regional authorities, such as the regional health boards in British Columbia and Nova Scotia, are better positioned to pursue this approach given their relative separation from direct ownership and management of the health providers in their jurisdictions. However, drawing lessons from the historical progression within the jurisdictions of the countries reviewed suggests that the public integration models of Saskatchewan and Alberta could be transformed by purchaser/provider splits should these jurisdictions elect to move in this direction.

Most of the jurisdictions with partially vertically integrated regional organizations are planning to introduce a more equitable form of funding through capitation. Saskatchewan has already introduced this form of funding. Alberta and British Columbia are currently engaged in developing their own approaches. At this stage of development, the capitation is designed primarily to reflect the cost of the services funded by regional authorities within their regions.

Issue of Cross-Boundary Flows

Associated with this form of capitation funding, is the recognition of the need for a more precise identification of individuals and therefore the population. The current level of organizational development of the regional models (e.g., local authorities and health boards) presents particular challenges in terms of any capitation funding as well as operational responsibility and flexibility. This is a result of standard assumptions that tend to be applied to geographically defined organizations. They are that:

- the organization will assume responsibility for the health of a population that lives within the geographic area; and
- the organization will assume responsibility for the funding of specifically identified health providers that operate within the geographic boundary.

The phrase "within the geographic boundary" is at the core of the challenges. Although "boundary" seems to imply control, in actuality, this characterization sets out parameters of an "open" system containing elements that are difficult to anticipate or control. In theory, the organization is generally capable of assessing a profile of needs for the population it is to serve. However, because the population is not enrolled or rostered in the system, broad census data must be used to "define" the population and to estimate costs, while members of the population still enjoy the right to go elsewhere for services. Thus, "population" is not a fixed element of the equation, and guestimates as to its characteristics and/or associated costs are imprecise at best.

In such an open system, the organization may not have effective influence on the providers (or other health sector elements) within its boundaries, and it certainly does not control providers outside its boundaries. The significance of this is twofold. In terms of accessing services, some of the organization's population will cross the boundary to access services in neighbouring areas, and outside population from neighbouring areas will cross into the organization's geographic area to access providers that the organization is funding. Therefore, some of the service needs the organization projects for its population are accessed elsewhere at no cost to the organization. At the same time, the organization incurs costs serving populations from neighbouring areas. In short, costing becomes unpredictable and more variable.

To adapt to these conditions, the calculation of the capitation funding for the organization has to be continually adjusted by reductions for outflow of population to services elsewhere, and increases for projections of inflow of population accessing services within the organization's boundaries. With such cross-boundary flows it is difficult to anticipate or control the impact upon budgets or effectively monitor services. To improve the situation, the application of population rostering and *full provincial capitation* funding would support greater simplicity and precision in the calculation and management of capitation, and would introduce the potential for better accounting of funds, and greater exchange of information between regional models.

Another challenge for regional entities attempting to achieve a positive reinforcement or improvement of health status of the population within the region, is the absence of physicians (and their associated funding)— and in particular, primary care physicians—are not incorporated into these organizational models. However, the movement to refine the models and to introduce and develop many of the key principles and features positions these models well for further development toward integrated and cost-effective health care systems.

It is also possible to have other forms of roster-based, vertically integrated models that integrate responsibility for only certain sectors of care such as hospital, home care and long-term care institutions, perhaps more appropriately depicted as a primary care model integrated with community services and, potentially, hospital services. Although not the ideal for a variety of reasons (e.g., impact on capitation formula, risk of off-loading responsibility to other sectors/services in the health system, or referring without responsibility or concern for cost), this type of model could serve as one route to creating the foundations for building toward a fully vertically integrated model over time.

Implementation of the Fully Vertically Integrated Model

A model of full integration embodying all of the principles and features discussed has been designed for the Canadian environment. The Comprehensive Health Organization (CHO) was developed in Ontario, and has models developing and/or launching in several communities at the time of this writing. The model has also been reviewed in other provinces such as Saskatchewan, and continues to be examined by other jurisdictions such as British Columbia and Quebec (where a variation on the CHO model is referred to OSIS).

Implementation involves a process of authorization by government of any credible sponsorship which could include physicians (including GP/ primary care organizations), hospital administrators, other health professionals, labour, corporations, community developers, or lay individuals. Any combination of the above sponsors could devise a plan to develop and implement a model. Government approval of the application would be contingent upon demonstration of the following criteria: first and foremost, a fundamental understanding of the model, and its associated requirements; evidence of expertise in governance, management, administration, and finances; a plan to assemble and/or contract with appropriate provider resources; and most important, they must demonstrate the existence and interest of a critical mass of potential roster members. All of the key features and minimum requirements as discussed in the previous section apply to any group proposing to form an organization.

The model can be implemented incrementally, as is taking place presently, or fully, with implementation "all at once," with appropriate government support. A critical element of implementation is the requirement for ongoing commitment by government to establish and support the rules as discussed, in order to provide the foundation upon which the body of work developed to date can be fully constructed. The development effort to date has been sustained continuously through three provincial administrations; it only remains to demonstrate full and public support for the model.

Final Observations

As for the government perspective on transferring capitation funding to any organization, it would make for a cleaner transaction if services and their corresponding funding were always added on to growing organizations in terms of the logical "blocks" of activity which already exist, such as GPs, specialists, hospital services, drugs, long-term care, and home care. In this way, the capitation formula would remain more consistent across the system.

Frustrated reformers have said that horizontal integration does not go far enough, and that primary care is not broad enough. This can be more readily understood from the foregoing. Horizontal integration truly *does not* go far enough by virtue of its function as a consolidating force for similar operations. It does not embody the more powerful vertically "integrative" extent of (appropriately regulated) full responsibility with autonomy for services and funding which *combines* programs and functions to activate the dynamics and incentives implicit in balanced decision making, purchasing, and delivery of health care services throughout the system.

Nor can primary care ever be broad enough in scope to accomplish this alone. Without the more complete perspective of responsibility to serve all of a given population's needs, the balancing effect of more appropriate decision making regarding distribution of funds to patients will not occur to the necessary scale, and inconsistencies of cost and procedure will remain throughout the system.

It is clear that Canada is embarking on an exploration of organizational reform which will fulfil the spirit of the intentions identified at the outset of this paper by individuals such as Tommy Douglas, as the remaining phase of development of the Canadian health care system.

The next section presents an overview of guidelines for internal and external evaluation of integrated organizations as discussed in this presentation.

Summary of Features of Integrated Models—Canada

Key Features (Beginning with the Four Predominant or Differentiating Features)

- Responsibility for all benefits or core services.
- Rostered population.
- Weighted capitation funding.
- Autonomy to determine organizational and financial relationships with providers.
- Not-for-profit, independent corporate organization.
- Board of directors which provides for input and representation in some form by rostered members with some provision for involving providers as appropriate.
- An obligation to assess and respond to the needs of its individual members and the rostered population as a whole.
- Requirement to plan for the most appropriate resources to meet the assessed needs.
- Ensure appropriate services through direct provision or purchase of services.
- Track and report all encounters and maintain other health records and data (e.g., roster information, provider profiles, satisfaction surveys).
- Emphasis on wellness and primary care with the GP as the gatekeeper to secondary services and care provided by an accessible multidisciplinary team for rostered members.
- Formal commitment to quality and evaluation and through this, reinforcement of the key features and obligations of the organization. Their mandate includes that:
  - procedures include mechanisms to assure availability, accessibility, effectiveness, continuity of care, and continuous quality improvement; and
  - quality evaluation take place within a framework which includes: accurate needs assessment; a quality-oriented environment; indicators of quality improvement initiatives; economic evaluation; self-reported health status measurement; and member and provider satisfaction.

Major Elements of Government Policy and Support

- National definition of benefits or core services inclusive of a modern view of health and the health care system, while not being excessively prescriptive. Components of defined core services would include: health promotion; sickness prevention; primary, secondary, and tertiary care (including practitioners, physicians, diagnostic, and hospital services); home care; chronic and long-term care services, and drugs. A discretionary element could be added expressing support for alternatives that benefit or support health, including "cultural" health, that are provided in a coordinated environment, as per the model. Prescriptive elements could be focused on approving new technologies and therapies, and a cautious evidenced-based approach to explicit itemization of treatments and use of technology that are not covered by the publicly funded system, or are banned outright where there is a proven danger to health and life.

- Government guidelines to emphasize a focus on wellness/primary care without diminishing appropriate access to high-quality secondary care where required.
- All citizens must be registered with a primary care organization of their choice, which includes the fully integrated model. In order to facilitate this:
  - Rules must be put in place to ensure acceptance of all citizens who choose to register with an organization, regardless of their health conditions. No one must be denied the right to join on the basis of health. This protects universality as well as accessibility for the individual.
  - All citizens must have the right to choose to register with the organization of their choice and the right to exit that organization to join another organization they feel better suits their needs. In addition, the capitation funding attributable to them must also transfer with them to the new entity.
- The government or system must have a central health fund or budget adequate for funding all the required core services or benefits for the population. In addition, the government should retain a budget to support catastrophic situations, and to support the reinforcement of activities to achieve health goals and to develop approaches to meeting the needs of hard-to-reach populations such as street people.
- The government must commit to capitation funding for the new organizations.
  - The capitation formula must be weighted for age and gender at a minimum, with consideration for other needs and regional factors in the system, in order to maintain specificity in the relationship between the cash flow and the predicted cost of serving the needs of the population.
  - In the context of this model, the capitation must be for *all* health services that could be accessed and provided to roster members anywhere in the province (or country).
- Formal support of the model's autonomy to pursue appropriate organizational and financial relationships with providers, including contracting or direct delivery of service as a result of incorporating or merging providers within the organizational structure.

- Formal requirement to pursue appropriate contracts with providers where the organization does not have—or prefers not to have—the capacity to provide a service on its own.
- In order to assist the process, the government could establish minimum parameters to serve as guidelines, and/or "default" rules for situations where the two parties fail to achieve an agreement.
- The government may elect to regulate particular specialized services or programs in order to limit the number and location to appropriate provincial or national requirements. In this case, government may be directive (set guidelines) in the financial arrangements between the health organization and such entities (e.g., determine the tariff or cost to be paid) to maintain appropriate volumes of use and expertise.

These parameters do not diminish in any way the direct relationships between organizations and providers. The expectation is still that organizations will contract providers to provide services and encounter data back to the organization, and that incentives to perform will be implicit in the contracts.

- Establish health goals and priorities nationally, provincially, and regionally.
- Mandate and support the development of an integrated health information system, and participate in the defining of standards and mandate that annual plans, encounter information, and other pertinent data be reported by the models.
- Must ensure and participate in appropriate monitoring and formal evaluation, including the assessment of need and the performance of the system as a whole, as well as given models.
- *If supporting the gradual addition of fundholding and purchasing for GP/ primary care organizations in addition to the fully integrated model,* require the establishment of boards, nonprofit corporation, and other organizational attributes at critical stages of development.

EVALUATION OF INTEGRATED MODELS

Evaluation of the emerging vertically integrated models will follow some standardized procedures pertinent to all organizations, as well as a more specialized set of criteria specifically geared to its idiosyncrasies. The purpose of this section is to summarize critical guidelines for internal and external review of these models. In general terms, it is clear that evaluation must be approached from the distinct perspectives of key stakeholders such as providers and patients, as well as other major institutional participants (health organizations and governments), to ensure a thorough review of how well the organization responds to issues and addresses objectives of health care such as those discussed earlier.

Because the integrated provider/purchaser organization will necessarily encompass a comprehensive view of the total spectrum of services it provides, its broad perspective on evaluation is not dissimilar from that of government; it is just as concerned about the efficacy and cost-efficiency of service delivery, simply to a lesser degree. The organization needs to understand how it is performing in relation to the rest of the health care system and to similar organizational models. In addition to a broad scope of benchmarking across the health care and other sectors' organizations (to stay on "track"), the organization must continually adapt this information to refine its internal operations; in turn, its evaluation parameters must include more refined measures.

For its part, the government needs to understand how well the new model is performing locally, regionally, provincially and/or nationally in comparison with similar and/or other models in the system, in order to communicate successes and failures and refine regulations and other rules over time. Because the government's role is to guide, support, and monitor ongoing and annual cycles of assessment needs, the establishment of priorities and health goals is necessary. In the pressures of the present environment, scrutiny relative to evaluation is increasing in tandem with increasing transparency of the system to public (and media) observation. Particularly in view of the increased public attention to the health care system, and the potential tangible impact of press coverage, the capacity to effectively evaluate existing and new systems becomes more significant.

Response to Objectives

In the broadest context, governments and organizations can use a list of health system objectives to define evaluation inquiries to be applied to the health system as a whole, as well as to integrated purchaser/provider organizations. The importance of matching evaluation to objectives is that objectives tend to be derived from preexisting issues, observations and/or problems in the system. These provide an excellent starting point, as the objectives are not only valid in terms of performance compared to the old system, but can also be used as a guiding framework to monitor evolving and new systems, to protect against backsliding as new systems evolve. For example, specific data systems and inquiries could be developed to test the accessibility of required services for individuals or population groups distinguished by such categories of population as disease type, ethnicity, geographic region, or specific organization. They could also test the emphasis on community services as opposed to institutional care.

For organizations, questions could be developed to test the impact on health status for the rostered population of these organizations as compared to historical data, and, where a pluralistic environment exists, to compare their success at improving health status with the rest of the health system. Enhanced responsiveness to enrollees' needs could be examined through such measures as mandatory satisfaction surveys. Financial management and accounting procedures could be submitted to rigorous auditing procedures.

For governments, tests could be developed to examine the "fairness" of their distribution of funds and to compare the financial plans and performance of different organizations, as well as their health outcomes in relation to different populations. Macroeconomic efficiency could be assessed in terms of the maintenance and improvement of health in conjunction with control over cost increases.

A simple but critical measure to ensure that evaluation takes place more effectively, and that the commitment to do so is well established at the "grassroots level," could be to include, in the form of required bylaws, mission and/or operating procedures, mandates for provider/purchaser organizations, such as the following:

- Procedures shall include mechanisms to assure availability, accessibility, effectiveness, continuity of care, and continuous quality improvement.
- Quality evaluation shall take place within a framework which includes accurate needs assessment, a quality-oriented environment, indicators of quality improvement initiatives, economic evaluation, self-reported health status measurement, and member and provider satisfaction.

These mandates protect important Canadian principles, as well as functions and responsibilities which will be maintained and documented by organizations to serve as evaluation parameters over time. In the final analysis, the important message is to make a commitment to evaluation *at the outset.* This includes two dimensions: to ensure that the government or appointed agency is prepared to carry out systemic evaluation on an ongoing basis, and to require all provider/purchaser organizations to develop and implement formal quality and evaluation programming at the operational level.

International and Canadian Perspectives on Evaluation

Approaches to and elements of evaluation are evolving in various ways and at different rates in the countries reviewed, and they all demonstrate at least a minimal structure, beginning with the collection of and responsibility for data. In the United Kingdom, the NHS has overall responsibility for establishing national health goals and assessing the overall performance of its system. Drug prescription data and encounter data from the hospital trusts are also included in these assessments. DHAs monitor the activity of providers and GP Fundholders, and contract compliance by providers. GP Fundholders also monitor their contracts with providers and overall performance of their own practices. In both the Netherlands and New Zealand, national agencies do most of the monitoring and evaluation, advising the Minister of Health on performance of organizations, and advising on needed corrective action.

National and regional government structures or offset agencies have been established to conduct evaluation and monitoring of their systems, as well as the operations of models within their systems. National and regional health goals and performance criteria are used to assess the new systems in such terms as their compliance with annual plans, adherence to established terms of reference and rules for the organization, compliance with contracts, and status compared to benchmarks. In addition, much of this same activity is replicated within each of the purchaser/provider organizations.

There have been a number of approaches, as well as *reviews of* approaches to evaluation in Canada. The scope of this paper does not allow for a detailed presentation; instead, it provides a brief summary of key points raised in these reviews in order to stimulate thought and reinforce the importance of this component.

In addition to the obvious requirement for data and monitoring, there are two major functions associated with evaluation: "observation and measurement, as supported by comparisons with criteria, standards and expectations of what are considered as an indication of good performance" (Anderson et al. 1994). Most processes emphasize the importance of establishing the foundations for measurement up front, so that evaluation can assess the extent to which stated goals and objectives have been achieved. For each of the objectives, a set of questions can be constructed and refined over time, and information sources developed to support the evaluation.

A number of the approaches in Canada focused on the criteria of evaluation associated with assessing the implementation of a new model in the system. Several underlying aspects have been identified as important, including the extent to which a community and providers had been prepared for the change, the level of satisfaction and involvement in the process itself, the extent to which stated implementation objectives had been achieved, and the acceptance of transfer of new areas of responsibility to new structures (Premier's Council on Health, Well-Being and Social Justice 1994).

In one focus group sponsored by Health Canada, a number of goals were identified that could be applied to both the implementation of new models as well as ongoing assessment of their performance. In this case, it is clear that assessment of many of these goals, particularly at the early stages, is dependent on a good set of "preimplementation" data—which is not always available. That dependence is evident in the following sample questions from the study:

> *Goal no. 1: Improve or maintain the health of Canadians.* Sample questions: Has the incidence of curable and chronic conditions in the population changed? Has the level of absenteeism at work changed? Has the use of acute care services changed (e.g., number of visits, beds per thousand)?

Goal no. 2: *Ensure the efficacy of the health care system.* Sample questions: Does the new approach address substandard quality and deficiencies? Does the new organization assure the most appropriate resources and evidence-based services are applied in the most effective manner?

Goal no. 3: *Achieve integration and coordination in and beyond the health system.* Sample questions: Is there a change in the number of duplicated services? Are coordinating mechanisms visibly in place? From the rostered member's perspective, is it now easier to get through the system?

Goal no. 4: *Empower Canadians through involvement in health systems management.* Sample questions: Does the new organization provide a shaping role for users of the system? What mechanisms are in place for citizens to participate in the planning of health policies and to make healthy choices for themselves (e.g., participation on the board of governance, advisory committees, etc.)? Do rostered members feel they have enough information to make informed decisions?

Goal no. 5: *Ensure responsivity.* Sample questions: Are there provisions for the rostered members to articulate their needs (e.g., self-reporting surveys)? Are there mechanisms for rostered members to express their satisfaction or dissatisfaction with the performance of the organization (member satisfaction surveys)?

Goal no. 6: *Ensure equity.* Sample question: Are there mechanisms in place to ensure distribution of health services and resources; and access to disadvantaged groups according to need?

Goal no. 7: *Improve cost-effectiveness.* Sample question: To what extent does the organization prevent the unnecessary use of more expensive alternatives which are currently available and make cheaper approaches of equal or greater value available? (Health and Welfare Canada 1993).

There are numerous dimensions and approaches to evaluating the organizations themselves. To begin with, the organizations have to meet core criteria and minimum specifications in order to operate. Examples of these criteria include a mission statement, and minimum requirements that can be used to establish a set of explicit goals, objectives, and evaluation questions on an ongoing basis. Some of these can be defined by a central authority or by the industry; others may be developed by a given corporation to use on its own. One means of setting goals and objectives, and determining evaluation criteria through inquiry is the following Ontario Ministry of Health exercise:

- *Sample mission statement* – To provide and manage integrated health care and all necessary services and support the highest degree of health and independent living possible for our rostered population.

- *Goal no. 1* – Foster health behaviour; self-reliance and independent living for members.
- *Objectives for goal no. 1* – To educate and encourage providers to employ the least intrusive level of care appropriate to support the patient's health, deemphasizing institutional care and emphasizing community-based care wherever possible.
- *Sample question to assess objectives* – Do practice protocols exist which support independence? (information required: protocols, care maps, task lists by profession, information on established professional standards in this area).

In addition, evaluation is an integral part of the annual planning cycle and ongoing management of the organization. Some of the elements of this process might include an assessment of population needs; based on the profile of need, to establish a plan including determining the most appropriate array of health resources, programs, and services to meet the determined need; and implementation of the plan and then evaluation of outcomes (e.g., relationship of utilization pattern to projected patterns, impact on overall and select health status, financial or economic performance etc. (Ontario Ministry of Health 1994).

Another approach could be to develop an evaluation framework which incorporates many or all of the components already discussed, organized along with key functional or operational activities, to construct inquiries from within each of these perspectives. Examples of the key functional or operational activities to be evaluated include: governance, adminstration and coordination; human resource management; member services; provider relations; service delivery and effectiveness; case management; financial management/system cost-effectiveness; information systems; program planning and evaluation, and community well-being (Ontario Ministry of Health 1994; Wanke et al. 1995). Finally, the evaluation of roster-based, vertically integrated models would necessarily ensure that the key features particular to the organization, as summarized below, are rigorously tracked.

Selected Functions to Monitor and Evaluate

- *Integration* – Extent of collaborative behaviour, merging (improvements in procedure, outcomes, costs), tracking, and reporting of successful changes.
- *Organization* – Whether the board is appropriately constructed and maintained, reflective of provider, services, and populations served; whether significant management and operational procedures are reflective of input from patients and providers; relationships with providers, staff, and other organizations.
- *Core services* – Whether there is compliance with a balanced service approach, and the extent of substitution of practitioners or procedures.

- *Capitation* – Whether the weighting adjustment factors are appropriately defined from the roster; the base has been properly established (based on true system costs) by government; there is sufficient funding to cover the costs of care; the capitation is fair to all.
- *Rostering* – Whether the information collected is accurate, the socio-demographics are appropriately characterized and/or prioritized, confidentiality is protected, and special needs are identified and quantified.
- *Purchasing* – Whether contracting procedures are consistent and effective; whether negotiating procedures are appropriate, effective, and in compliance with government parameters; whether decision-making criteria regarding purchasing versus contracting for (e.g., review cost savings, improvements); and whether benchmarking is appropriately implemented across appropriate comparables.
- *Data* – Whether data are accurately collected and appropriate security measures are taken to protect personalized data; whether aggregate data are provided on an accurate and timely basis.
- *Financial* – Whether management procedures for tracking are maintained; whether there is flexibility to redirect funding through appropriate procedure of decision making, and whether proper accounting and reporting procedures are being followed.

Other procedures specific to specialized or individual organizational needs and functions would expand these lists accordingly. The next section completes this exercise, by identifying other considerations important to designing, implementing, and evaluating new models.

The Evaluation/Evidence Excuse

In the past, "the absence of evaluation" has been used as an excuse by entrenched interests throughout the system to block the introduction of new initiatives. As well, in cases where decisions were made to move forward, plans for evaluation in any form were absent, thus undermining the credibility of the endeavour and even the ultimate capacity to assess its success.

The purpose of this part of the exercise was to briefly consider appropriate parameters to evaluate vertically integrated models. While all possible future implications of the effort cannot be foreseen, providing an evaluation framework at the outset not only guides the development of the organization, but also facilitates later assessment of its performance. As seen in the implementation of organizational reform in other countries as well as in Canada, it is the soundness of the organizational and policy design that supports the implementation at the outset. It is also not always required that "pilot projects" be run to test an approach. In fact, full pilots may not be possible in some types of systemic organizational reform. For example, testing the effects of moving hospitals from *budget* dependency to *revenue* dependency, as described previously, would be difficult to test on a local basis without major reconfiguration of the system. Therefore, the absence of specific evidence of "performance" before the opportunity to proceed should not, in this case, be a reason *not* to proceed. That would be a misuse of a legitimate process that should be planned for as an important component of implementing a new initiative, and refined over time.

CONCLUSIONS AND OBSERVATIONS

In keeping with international trends and Canadian objectives, the evolution of Canada's health system should be guided by the following significant principles and features of integrated organizational models:
- responsibility for all centrally defined *core services*;
- responsibility to a population specifically defined through *rostering*;
- a fair share of the provincial health budget derived from provincial *weighted capitation* funding;
- *autonomy* in the development and refinement of organizational and financial relationships with providers.

The Canadian environment appears to have most of the right ingredients in place and the potential for reconfiguration to provide appropriate support for evolution towards these features. The following paragraphs offer comments regarding selected areas of support as well as considerations important to implementation, most of which are directed at governments.

First and foremost, there is a need to promote better understanding of the new terminology of health service organizations among government officials, providers, and citizens. It is essential to overcome inappropriately negative and incomplete understanding and assumptions about the meaning and use of such terms as "market," "competition" and "capitation," and to understand their appropriate application to the health care arena. In the present language of health care, predictable reactions have developed to the use of certain terms when exploring organizational reform. For example, private delivery is confused with private funding—even though private delivery has been and continues to be a major part of our publicly funded, single-payer health system. At times, competition and notions of market are addressed as though they were part of a conspiracy to introduce a private health insurance market—when they may represent extremely useful dynamics for the refinement of our publicly funded system, to improve services. What capitation comprises is often misunderstood; the assumption is often made that capitation is only pertinent to one provider when it has already been used to fund other parts of our health system, and has been demonstrated as a fair and equitable approach to distributing public funds in other publicly funded environments. The important message is that we need to work on increasing understanding of the terminology in its specific application to organizational and health systems reform so that ignorance does not inhibit progress.

There is a corresponding need to reinforce supportive regulation to ensure that important elements of the system such as rostering and integrated information systems become "standard procedure." To facilitate consistent common standards there must be a national definition of comprehensive health benefits or "core services" to protect and maintain reliability for citizens and providers. Appropriate "language" could be developed by governments that is inclusive of a modern view of health and health care systems, while not being excessively prescriptive.

Core services could include, for example, health promotion, sickness prevention, primary, secondary and tertiary care (including practitioners, physicians, diagnostic, and hospital services) and home care, as well as chronic and long-term care services and drugs. In addition, there could be a discretionary element to support "health-benefitting or -supporting" alternatives and cultural healing in a coordinated environment, such as is proposed by vertically integrated organizations. Another area in which constructive influence could be exercised is the approval of new medical and other therapies and technologies. In addition, the public interest would be served by explicit itemization of treatments and parameters regarding use of technology that would *not* be paid for in the publicly funded system, or that should be banned altogether because of the dangers they pose to health.

Government support for rostering individuals with the provider organization of their *choice* is imperative. Equally important is the need to implement and refine full provincial weighted capitation to support equitable distribution of funding to organizations. Weighted capitation for primary care organizations supports incremental growth toward full vertical integration and encourages a more dynamic environment. To accomplish this, provincial ministries of health must commit to reconfiguring presently fragmented "stovepipes" of funding systems to become a more flexible, adaptive system. Concurrently, the implementation of a comprehensive, standardized, integrated information system will support national, provincial, regional and local planning, research and evaluation, while serving as an important management and operational tool for health care organizations throughout the delivery system.

The overall regulatory framework should be one that preserves and protects the public free choice of organizations, along with the autonomy those organizations need to establish their own procedures and develop financial and structural relationships. With autonomy would come the responsibility for organizations to report to government or provincial/national databases, and to make available to the public information such as annual plans, aggregate encounter information, and the results of satisfaction and self-reporting surveys, as well as evaluation studies. Most important, reform of the health system necessitates a reevaluation of and reform within *health ministries* to create healthier bureaucracies, as well as more appropriate alignment with and support for progressive emerging models. For example, introduction of the vertically integrated model brings the potential for innovation in provincial institutions (for example, the merging of workers' compensation functions with the health ministries), making the health system all-inclusive of health issues, prevention, and treatment regardless of place.

With vigorous, positive and enthusiastic support, reform will succeed. There are many physician, practitioner, and institutional leaders in the system who are predisposed to support progressive change. They should be supported and encouraged. Positive and consistent public support is critical to overcoming barriers to any form of integrated model. An adaptation of a comment by Claudia Scott serves as a reminder of the overall mission: "People rather than governments pay for health care. Governments are but the agents of people" (Scott 1994). Introducing and supporting models with a greater service orientation and a more intimate relationship to the population they serve, with strong incentives for responsiveness and advocacy on behalf of these populations, provides a powerful demonstration of the government's commitment to the people.

John Marriott and Ann L. Mable *are partners in the consulting practice of Marriott Mable, providing management advice on health organizations reform and models of integration. They have written and presented widely on the subjects of health system reform and integrated health organizations.*

John Marriott *has served as director of policy and analysis for the National Forum on Health, as founding director of the Health Policy Unit, as well as an assistant professor at Queen's University. He was also the principal architect and founding manager of the Comprehensive Health Organization (CHO) program in Ontario. Other background spans comprehensive health organizations, government, hospital administration, and laboratory services.*

Ann L. Mable *has twenty years experience in the start-up and development of a range of public and private organizations, more recently focused on the health system. She has held numerous executive positions in private sector financial, development and consulting organizations, and roles in the academic environment. As an affiliate of the Queen's Health Policy Unit, she coauthored papers on CHOs and hospital reform, while serving as coordinator of the Centre for Canada-Asia Business Relations at the School of Business.*

Acknowledgements

This paper would not have been possible without the support of many individuals who provided information, advice and in many cases, comments on earlier drafts. In particular, the following individuals deserve special recognition and grateful thanks:

Canada: *David Brindle, Tom Clossen, Michael Decter, Marie Fortier, Vytas Mickevicius, Marcel Saulnier, Hanita Tiefenbach, Eric Vandewall, Dr. Eugene Vayda, and the "Striking a Balance" working group of the National Forum on Health*

United Kingdom: *Dr. Peter Bundred and Peter Hatcher*

Netherlands: *Dr. Jan Bultman*

New Zealand: *Wendy Edgar and Lorraine Hawkins*

United States: *Jon Gabel, Jamie Hadley, Jerry Hicks, Jay Merchant, and James Owen*

BIBLIOGRAPHY

ANDERSON, M., C. BOLTON, K. BRAZIL, J. MARRIOTT, and J. TREMBLETT. 1994. *Quality and Evaluation for the CHO.* Kingston (ON): Queen's University, Queen's Health Policy Unit.

ASSOCIATION OF ONTARIO HEALTH CENTRES. 1995. *Building on Success: A Blueprint For Effective Primary Health Care.*

AVIS, W. S., P. D. DRYSDALE, R. J. GREGG, V. E. NEUFELDT, and M. H. SCARGILL. Eds. 1983. *Gage's Canadian Dictionary.* Toronto (ON): Gage Educational Publishing Company.

BIRCH, S., L. GOLDSMITH, and M. MAKELA. 1994. *Paying the Piper and Calling the Tune: Principles and Prospects for Reforming Physician Payment Methods in Canada.* Hamilton (ON): McMaster University.

BORREN, P., and A. MAYNARD. 1994. The market reform of the New Zealand health care system searching for the Holy Grail in the Antipodes. *Health Policy* 27: 233–252.

BRADSHAW, G., and P. L. BRADSHAW. 1994. Competition and efficiency in health care—the case of the British National Health Service. *Journal of Nursing Management* 2: 31–36.

BRASKER, H.M., and M. VAN UCHELEN. 1995. *Health Insurance in the Netherlands.* 3d ed. Dutch Ministry of Health, Welfare and Sport.

BULTMAN, J. 1995. *Dutch Disease Management.* Lecture given at conference, Disease Management: The European Reality, 23–24 November, London.

_____. 1996. Personal communication.

BUNDRED, P. 1996. Personal communication.

CANADA. Federal/Provincial/Territorial Advisory Committee on Health Services. July 18, 1995. *A Model for the Reorganization of Primary Care and the Introduction of Population-Based Funding— "The Victoria Report."*

_____. Health Canada. 1993. *Planning for Health; Toward Informed Decision Making—Summary of Literature Review and A Proposed Evaluation Framework on Emerging Trends in the Organization and Delivery of Health Care Services.*

_____. Health Canada. 1996. *Provincial Health System Reform in Canada.*

CANADIAN MEDICAL ASSOCIATION. February 1994. *Strengthening the Foundation: The Role of the Physician in Primary Health Care in Canada.*

CHERNICHOVSKY, D. 1995. Health system reforms in industrialized democracites: An emerging paradigm. *The Milbank Quarterly* 73(3): 339–372.

COLLEGE OF FAMILY PHYSICIANS OF CANADA. March 1995. *The Clinical Practice Management Network—Description and Feasibility Phase.*

_____. May 1995. *The Clinical Practice Management Network—Project Summary.*

_____. September 1995. *Managing Change: The Family Medicine Group Practice Model—Green Paper— A Discussion Document on Primary Health Care Reform in Canada.*

CUMMING, J. 1994. Core services and priority setting: The New Zealand Experience. Elsevier Science Ireland Ltd., *Health Policy* 29: 41–60.

DIXON, J., and H. GLENNERSTER. 1995. General practice—What do we know about fundholding in general practice? *British Medical Journal* 311(September).

EDGAR, W. 1995. *Publicly Funded Health and Disability Services—Health Care Priority Setting in New Zealand.* Paper for international seminar on health care priority setting, May, Birmingham, England.

_____. 1996. Personal communication.

EVANS, R. G. 1995. Lessons from Europe on the funding of healthcare. *CHAC Review* (winter): 9–11.

FORSTER, J., W. ROSSER, B. HENNEN, R. MCAULEY, R. WILSON, and M. GROGAN. 1994. New approach to primary medical care: Nine-point plan for family practice service. *Canadian Family Physicians* 40 (September).

GLENNERSTER, H., S. HANCOCK, M. MATSAGANIS, and P. OWENS. 1994. *Implementing GP Fundholding, Wild Card or Winning Hand?* State of Health Series, Open University Press.

GROENEWEGEN, P. P. 1994. The shadow of the future: Institutional change in health care. *Health Affairs* (winter): 137–147.

HAM, C. 1995. *The New NHS: A Guide for Board Members.* Nahat and Health Services Management Centre.

HAM, C., and M. BROMMELS. 1994. Health care reform in the Netherlands, Sweden, and the United Kingdom. *Health Affairs* (winter).

HAM, C., and J. SHAPIRO. 1996. Learning curve. *Health Services Journal* (18 January).

HANSAGI, J., J. CALLTORP, and S. ANDREASSON. 1993 Quality comparisons between privately and publicly managed health care centres in a suburban area of Stockholm, Sweden. *Quality Assurance in Health Care* 4(1): 33–40.

HATCHER, P. 1995. Demystifying managed care. *The University of Birmingham Health Services Management Centre Newsletter* 1 (autumn 3).

_____. 1996. Personal communication.

_____. Forthcoming. U.K. Chapter. In *International Comparative Health Systems—Analysis of Sixteen Countries Health Systems,* 2nd. ed. ed. M.W. RAFFEL. Penn State University Press.

HOLLAND, W. W. 1992. Choices in health care. *Journal of the Royal College of Physicians of London* 26(4).

IGLEHART, J. K. 1992. Health Policy Report—The American Health Care System—Managed care. *The New England Journal of Medicine* 327(10).

_____. 1994. Health Policy Report—Physicians and the growth of managed care. *The New England Journal of Medicine* 331(17).

KLEIN, R. 1995. Big Bang Health Care Reform—Does it work?: The case of Britain's 1991 National Health Service Reforms. *The Milbank Quarterly* 73(3).

KRISTIANSEN, I. S., and G. MOONEY. 1993. Remuneration of GP services: Time for more explicit objectives? A review of the systems in five industrialized countries. *Health Policy* 24: 203–212.

MAARSE, J. A. M. 1994. Lecture, 31 January, Manchester, England.

_____. May 1995. *Hospital Financing in Seven Countries—Hospital Financing in the Netherlands.* Prepared for the Office of Technology Assessment, United States Congress.

MARRIOTT, J. 1993–94. *Health Care System of the Future: Issues in Health Policy.* Course material, School of Policy Studies, Queen's University. Kingston, ON.

MARRIOTT, J. F. 1996. *An Overview of Integrated Health Systems: U.S. HMOs and Canadian CHO Models: What Can Be Learned From the Differences and Similarities?* Paper given at Impulse '96 Conference: The Business of Canada's Health Care Future and its Implications on Managing Care, 1–2 April.

_____. 1996. *U.S. Health System, Managed Care and HMOs.* Conference Board of Canada.

MARRIOTT, J. F., and A. L. MABLE. 1994. *Comprehensive Health Organizations; A New Paradigm for Health Care.* Government and Competitiveness Project Discussion Paper 94–13. Kingston (ON): Queen's University, School of Policy Studies.

MASON, A., and K. MORGAN. 1995. Purchaser-provider: The international dimension. *British Medical Journal* 310 (January): 231–235.

MAYNARD, A. 1994. Can competition enhance efficiency in health care?—Lessons from the reform of the UK National Health Service. *Soc-Sci-Med.* 3a(10): 1438–1445.

NEW ZEALAND. Ministry of Health. 1995. *Advancing Health In New Zealand.*

ONTARIO COLLEGE OF FAMILY PHYSICIANS. 1995. *Bringing the Pieces Together: Planning for Future Health Care—A strategy for primary health care planning.* March.

ONTARIO MEDICAL ASSOCIATION. 1996. *Primary Care Reform: A Strategy for Stability.* Primary Care Reform Physician Advisory Group, Draft 6. February 2.

ONTARIO MINISTRY OF HEALTH. 1994. *CHO Evaluation.* Internal documents.

ORGANIZATION FOR ECONOMIC COOPERATION AND DEVELOPMENT. 1992. *The Reform of Health Care—A Comparative Analysis of Seven OECD Countries.* Paris.

———. 1994. *The Reform of Health Care—A Review of Seventeen OECD Countries.* Paris.

———. 1995. Internal markets in the making—Health systems in Canada, Iceland and the United Kingdom. *Health Policy Studies* 6.

PARKER, A. W., 1974. The dimensions of primary care: Blueprints for change. In *Primary Care: Where Medicine Fails,* ed. ANDREPOULOS, S.

PREMIER'S COUNCIL ON HEALTH, WELL-BEING AND SOCIAL JUSTICE. Task Force on Devolution. 1994. *Framework for Evaluating Devolution.*

PROSPECTIVE PAYMENT ASSESSMENT COMMISSION. 1995. *Medicare and the American Health Care System—Report to the Congress.*

SASKATCHEWAN MINISTRY OF HEALTH. 1992. *A Saskatchewan Vision for Health—A Framework for Change.*

SCOTT, C. D. 1994. Reform of the New Zealand health care system. *Health Policy* 29: 25–40.

SHIPLEY, Hon. J. 1996. *Health Services 1996—Facts on the Purchasing and Provision of Health and Disability Support Services for New Zealanders.* New Zealand Ministry of Health.

SONNEVELDT, Ton. 1994. *On the Role of Government in Health Care—A General Comparison between the Debates on Health Care Reform in the Netherlands and the US.* U.S. Department of Welfare, Health and Cultural Affairs.

Statutes of Canada. 1984. Canada Health Act, Bill C-3.

THE NETHERLANDS. Ministry of Health, Welfare and Sport. January 1, 1995. *Health Insurance in the Netherlands.*

UNITED KINGDOM. Department of Health. 1994. *Developing NHS Purchasing and GP Fundholding— Towards a Primary Care-Led NHS.*

UNITED STATES. DEPARTMENT OF HEALTH AND HUMAN RESOURCES. HEALTH CARE FINANCING ADMINISTRATION. 1994. *Our Nation's Health Care Programs.*

———. DEPARTMENT OF HEALTH AND HUMAN RESOURCES. HEALTH CARE FINANCING ADMINISTRATION. 1995. *Your Medicare Handbook.*

———. DEPARTMENT OF HEALTH AND HUMAN RESOURCES. HEALTH CARE FINANCING ADMINISTRATION. OPERATIONS AND OVERSIGHT TEAM. 1995. *Medicare Managed Care Program Update.*

———. HEALTH CARE FINANCING ADMINISTRATION. NATIONAL COMMITTEE FOR QUALITY ASSURANCE. 1993. *Standards for Accreditation.*

———. HEALTH CARE FINANCING ADMINISTRATION. OFFICE OF ACTUARY. 1995–96. Personal communication.

UPTON, Hon. S. JULY 1991. *Your Health and the Public Health, A Statement of Government Health Policy.* New Zealand Ministry of Health.

VAN DE VEN, W. P. M. M., and F. T. SCHUT. 1994. Should catastrophic risks be included in a regulated competitive health insurance market? *Soc-Sci-Med.* 30(10): 1459–1472.

VAN DER ZEE, J., and J. B. F. HUTTEN. 1995. *Primary Health Care—The Case of the Netherlands.* Netherlands Institute for Primary Health Care.

WANKE, M. I., L. D. SAUNDERS, R. W. PONG, and W. J. B. CHURCH. 1995. *Building a Stronger Foundations: A Framework for Planning and Evaluating Community-Based Health Services in Canada.* Canadian Federal/Provincial/Territorial Deputy Ministers of Health.

WORLD HEALTH ORGANIZATION: ALMA ALTA. 1978. *Primary Health Care. A Joint Report by the Director General of the World Health Organization and the Executive Director of the United Nations Children's Fund.*

Issues for Canadian Pharmaceutical Policy

STEVEN G. MORGAN, M.A.

Doctorate Student in Health Economics
University of British Columbia

SUMMARY

The purpose of this paper is to identify broad directions for pharmaceutical policy in Canada based on the structure and dynamics of the pharmaceutical industry. The analysis here brings to light some of the economic and political incentives and constraints faced by major players in this industry. The role of key players and the impact of policy initiatives are discussed with such a framework in mind.

This paper does not *attempt to resolve any specific policy questions. Due to the breadth of topics covered, as well as time and space constraints, each topic receives brief attention. Some conclusions are drawn throughout the text based on the author's evaluation of the evidence presented. The paper concludes with recommendations for future policy research.*

The methodology used in this paper was, primarily, a literature search. Modern literature on pharmaceutical issues was sought through databases including OVID Health, EconLit, CBC, and catalogues at the University of British Columbia. Materials were also drawn from the author's private collection of literature. Data used for this paper come from the Canadian Institute for Health Information, the OECD, the Patented Medicine Prices Review Board, Statistics Canada, and citations from other studies.

This paper was written under the supervision of Professor Robert Evans. His guidance and comments are gratefully acknowledged. Comments and criticisms of an earlier draft were also received from members of the "Striking a

Balance" and "Evidence-Based Decision Making" working groups of the National Forum on Health. These, too, are gratefully acknowledged. The opinions expressed in this paper, as well as all errors and omissions, remain solely the author's.

TABLE OF CONTENTS

Introduction 681

    The Therapeutic Revolution 681

    Public Concern 682

The Steady Rise of Pharmaceutical Expenditures 683

    Past Analyses of the Industry 684

    Factors Contributing to Expenditure Growth 686

The Economics and Politics of the Pharmaceutical Industry 688

    Consumers 688

    Manufacturers 690

        The Canadian Industry 691

        Recouping Investment 691

        Profitability 693

    Doctors 694

    Pharmacists 695

    Government 696

    Achieving Cost Control 698

Industry Trends and Corporate Strategies 699

    Lobbying for Intellectual Property 699

    Locating Research and Development 700

    The Research Agenda 701

    Pharmaceutical Competition 703

    Generic Drugs 704

    A New Era of Competition 705

    Switching from Rx to OTC 705

Strategies for Managing Benefits 707

    Strategies Aimed at Consumers 707

Cost Sharing 707

Prescription Limits 708

Improving Compliance 709

Strategies Aimed at Pharmacists 710

Incentives for Efficient Retailing 710

Drug Cost Reimbursement 711

Strategies Aimed at Physicians 712

Physician Education and Training 712

Strategies Aimed at Manufacturers 713

Patent Policy 713

Price Controls 717

Restrictions on Advertising 722

Systemic Strategies 724

Universal Drug Insurance 724

Global Budgets 729

On-Line Pharmaceutical Information Systems 729

Conclusion 730

Bibliography 732

LIST OF FIGURES

Figure 1   Real expenditures on pharmaceuticals in Canada 683

Figure 2   Real pharmaceutical expenditures per capita
for selected OECD countries 685

Figure 3   Pharmaceutical and general price indexes for Canada 720

LIST OF TABLES

Table 1   New drug categorization in Canada 703

Table 2   Public pharmaceutical insurance coverage
in OECD countries 725

INTRODUCTION

The international pharmaceutical industry has shown spectacular growth and scientific achievement over the past half century. Driven by technological progress, changing disease patterns and the evolution of health care systems, pharmaceuticals have risen steadily in importance to the delivery of health care in developed and developing countries. Pharmaceuticals are used to control the onset and progress of disease, to relieve pain and the symptoms of sickness, to facilitate surgical procedures and recovery, and to eradicate illness. Drugs are used today for the treatment of many medical conditions that, in the past, were either untreatable or treatable only with more costly medical interventions, such as surgery.

The Therapeutic Revolution

Although the practice of pharmacology and therapeutics has roots in the teachings of the Greek physician Galen, for whom one of the pharmaceutical industry's most prestigious awards is named, the modern pharmaceutical industry is relatively young. The research-based pharmaceutical industry as we know it today originated during the "therapeutic revolution" of the 1930s and 1940s (Reekie and Weber 1979). During the early twentieth century, scientists started building an understanding of the basic mechanisms of disease and pharmacology. Scientists of the time were seeking the "magic bullet," a drug that would search out and attack diseased cells without harming healthy body tissue. This led to the discovery of several important medicines, including penicillin (1928), sulphanilamide (1935) and strep-tomycin (1943) (Reekie and Weber 1979). Over the years that followed, pharmaceutical discoveries grew at an exponential rate.

The health and economic effects of these early discoveries are practically beyond quantification. It would be impossible, for example, to place a value on the drastically reduced rate of death from pneumonia, tuberculosis, diphtheria, and measles brought about by antibiotic medicines in the 1940s and 1950s. Pharmaceutical innovation during these decades revolutionized modern medicine while providing a solid economic foundation upon which the research-based multinational pharmaceutical industry is built.

The rate of discovery slowed somewhat during the 1960s and 1970s; however, the role of pharmaceuticals in health care grew steadily. The availability of drugs increased as pharmaceutical manufacturers expanded distribution and marketing efforts, driven by the clinical and financial success of early discoveries. Meanwhile, corporations and governments intensified research efforts in the hopes of discovering the next breakthrough drug. Eventually, as the body of basic scientific knowledge grew, new discoveries emerged. Many "blockbuster drugs" were discovered and launched in the world market during the 1980s (Redwood 1993). Among these were treatments for cardiovascular conditions and gastrointestinal problems that eliminated the need for costly surgical interventions. Some of these products remain among the top-selling drugs worldwide.

Public Concern

These therapeutic achievements in the pharmaceutical industry did not come without cost. Parallel with the growth in scientific discoveries and use of new medicines came concern over the price of drugs, as well as their safety and efficacy (RCHS 1964; Cooper 1966; Comanor 1986). Rigorous analysis of the prices, profits, and practices of pharmaceutical manufacturers began with U.S. Senate Committee hearings in the 1950s, and continues around the world today.

This provokes the question: What is it about the pharmaceutical industry that leads to such critical investigation? To improve our understanding of why pharmaceutical manufacturers have come under such scrutiny, we must review the performance of the pharmaceutical industry more generally. Although pharmaceutical manufacturers—and policies that target them—are of central importance, they do not act alone. The pharmaceutical industry is made up of several key players including manufacturers, physicians, pharmacists, benefits providers (public and private), government regulators, and of course, consumers. Each of these players interacts with others in the process that brings a drug from an idea to a product consumed by patients seeking improved health.

Among the "market imperfections" that make the pharmaceutical industry unique are the following:
- drugs are "inputs" for health care, not "consumer goods";
- the pharmaceutical manufacturing industry is highly research intensive;
- significant economies of scale exist in the discovery and production of drugs;
- manufacturers are granted legally protected monopolies over their discoveries;
- diagnosing the indications for, and understanding the effects of, pharmaceuticals often requires significant medical and pharmacological knowledge;
- the choice of drug therapy is often made by a health professional, not the consumer;
- when a drug is needed, its purchase can seldom be deferred; and
- a significant portion of the population does not consider price when making drug purchases because public or private insurance covers the cost.

The analysis of the pharmaceutical industry in this paper tries to account for its uniqueness. In particular, this paper highlights the economic incentives, behaviours and interactions of key stakeholders, including consumers, manufacturers, physicians, pharmacists, and the government. Within this context, selected pharmaceutical policies directed at various players in the industry are discussed. This paper focuses largely on the market for and use of prescription drugs. Attention is paid to nonprescription products insofar as they relate to the recent trend of "switching" prescription-only products to nonprescription status.

THE STEADY RISE OF PHARMACEUTICAL EXPENDITURES

Pharmaceuticals account for one of the biggest components of health care expenditure in Canada. Canadians spend nearly as much on drugs as they do on physicians' services. By 1994, the total expenditure on drugs outside hospitals in Canada was approximately $9.17 billion, or 12 percent of all expenditures on health care (CIHI 1996; figure 1). Spending on physicians' services was $10.32 billion during that year. The growth of expenditure on pharmaceuticals has outpaced other components of health care expenditure in Canada for many years. Between 1975 and 1994, the average annual growth rate for drug expenditures in Canada was approximately 12 percent. In recent years, however, this growth rate has slowed to approximately 4 percent, due largely to much slower growth in public expenditures.

Figure 1

Real expenditures on pharmaceuticals in Canada

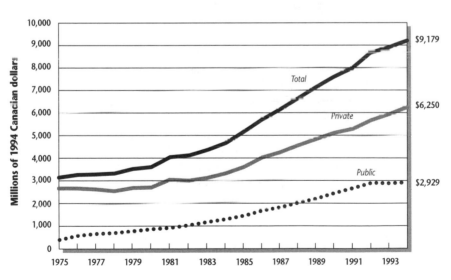

Source: CIHI 1996, deflated using Consumer Price Index (Stats Canada Label: P490000).

The total expenditure on pharmaceuticals may be broken down on two major lines. The first division is based on the product, dividing the market into prescription and nonprescription medicines. Prescription drugs have accounted for a remarkably stable 70 percent of Canadians' total expenditures on drugs for the past 20 years. The second division of pharmaceutical expenditure is between public and private expenditure. Public drug plans in Canada—predominantly covering the elderly and social assistance recipients—evolved during the late 1960s and 1970s, through to the mid-1980s. During this period, public expenditures on drugs grew substantially, outpacing private expenditures as illustrated in figure 1. As a result, public expenditures accounted for an increasing share of total expenditures on drugs between 1975 and 1985. Since 1985, public expenditure has accounted for about 30 percent of the total. The vast majority of public expenditure goes to prescription drugs (CIHI [1996] does not list *any* public expenditure on nonprescription drugs).

Steady growth in pharmaceutical expenditures is not peculiar to Canada. Many developed countries have experienced increases in real per capita spending on pharmaceuticals. Figure 2 shows this trend for Canada, Germany, France, the United States, Italy, the United Kingdom, Australia, and Sweden . For most of these countries, the upward trend in real pharmaceutical expenditures has been largely unabated. There are, however, a few exceptions: in Germany, for example, expenditures have *declined* since 1993,[1] similarly for Italy.[2] But these countries are in the minority. For the most part, developed countries have been unable to control expenditures due to increases in pharmaceutical prices, sales, or both.

Past Analyses of the Industry

Concern over the cost of drugs goes back several decades. The modern analysis of the pharmaceutical industry began in 1959 with the Kefauver Committee inquiries. The Kefauver Committee (a U.S. Senate Subcommittee) reported that drug costs were immense and that profits were high because excessive monopoly power had been granted to pharmaceutical manufacturers. The Kefauver findings had implications for Canada because many of the multinational manufacturers that dominated the Canadian market were based in the United States. The profitability of American

---

1. The dramatic decline in Germany is partially attributed to changes in physicians' prescribing patterns resulting from the introduction of an annual global budget for pharmaceuticals first implemented in 1993 (Munnich and Sullivan 1994).
2. Italian pharmaceutical expenditures have recently declined due to substantial increases in patient copayments for insured drugs (Mapelli 1995).

Figure 2

Real pharmaceutical expenditures per capita for selected OECD countries

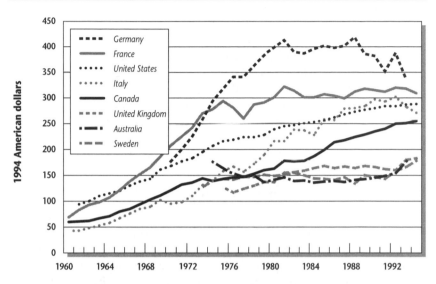

Source: OECD Health Data, monetary conversions with PPPs deflated using U.S. GDP deflator.

companies was, in part, due to operations in foreign markets such as Canada. Around the same time that the Kefauver Committee completed its hearings, Canadian policymakers were also investigating claims of excessive drug prices (RCHS 1964). These investigations, which culminated in the Harley Report of 1967, concluded that patent protection gave foreign-owned drug companies too much market power in Canada (RCHS 1964; also see Gorecki and Henderson 1981).

The early criticisms were not just that prices and profits were too high. The Kefauver Committee and others thought that much pharmaceutical research and development was mere "manipulation" of molecules to "innovate around" pioneering firms' patents by creating new products therapeutically similar to existing ones, thus yielding little increase in societal benefit (Cooper 1966; Walker 1971; Reekie and Weber 1979; Comanor 1986). Furthermore, analysts in Canada, the United States, and the United Kingdom were concerned that marketing, not science, was beginning to drive the use of new medicines in the 1960s. The Royal Commission on Health Services (1964) reported that pharmaceutical manufacturers spent an average of 29 percent of total sales on medical promotions, detailing, and direct selling in Canada during 1960; the same companies spent an average of 3.9 percent of total sales on Canadian research and development. In 1962, expenditure on promotional activities by manufacturers in the United Kingdom—home to many multinational pharmaceutical companies—outweighed expenditure on R&D for the first time (Cooper 1966). Even today, marketing expenditures exceed R&D expenditures on a global basis (Ballance 1996; Drake and Uhlman 1993).

Over the four decades that followed these early criticisms, the pharmaceutical industry has survived numerous academic analyses and public investigations, and remains largely unscathed. Although the industry has undergone significant technological and structural change, the critical issues from a policy perspective remain the same: real expenditure on drugs increases steadily from year to year; marketing plays a central role in drug use, potentially encouraging misuse and overuse of many drugs; and as discussed below, pharmaceutical profits remain extraordinarily high.

Factors Contributing to Expenditure Growth

The persistence of these issues has much to do with the economics and politics of the pharmaceutical industry. Every dollar of expenditure on pharmaceuticals is a dollar of income to stakeholders in the industry. There is, therefore, $9 billion of income at stake in the Canadian pharmaceutical industry, including both the prescription and nonprescription segments. Policy directed at reducing expenditures will directly affect these incomes.[3]

On the demand side, the steady rise in expenditure leads one to ask: Why? The aging of the population is often blamed for increasing expenditures on drugs and other health services; yet, upon review, evidence does not support this claim. The rapid growth of expenditure on drugs for the elderly has more to do with "modifiable factors," such as steady increases in the number of drugs doctors prescribe per elderly person, than with the inevitable aging of the population (Anderson and Lavis 1994). This finding

---

3. That this industry is so highly regulated—where barriers to competition exist through patents, marketing, professional associations, and licenses—makes this "expenditure equals income" relationship more interesting. In a perfectly competitive environment, "market forces" distribute resources such that the marginal value of expenditure (the price consumers are willing to pay for a good) is equal to the marginal value of income (the cost of producing the good). In industries with barriers to entry, the resulting markets no longer ensure this equality. The distribution of resources in imperfectly competitive markets will be effected, in part, by the market power of participating firms and the elasticity of demand (the sensitivity of demand to changes in price). It is likely that the distribution of expenditures and incomes in the pharmaceutical industry will be as profoundly influenced by government regulation as the anonymous forces of economic competition.

is consistent with other research on the perceived "crisis" in health care delivery and finance caused by the aging of the population. Demographic changes have contributed only slightly to rising costs of elderly patient care. Cost inflation that has occurred is almost entirely due to higher age-specific per capita utilization of services (Barer, Evans, and Hertzman 1995). Research in the pharmaceutical field indicates that overall pharmaceutical expenditure inflation has resulted from three principal factors: increased per capita utilization of drugs, the use of more costly new drugs instead of older ones, and escalating prices of existing drugs. Canadian evidence suggests that the most important determinant of increased expenditure is the substitution of new drugs for older drugs to treat the same condition (Castonguay et al. 1996; PMPRB 1996b; Crop Conseil 1995; Chiles 1995).

It is disconcerting that, although recent literature has warned against heavy reliance on new, expensive technologies, this has been true for decades. Reviews of Canadian drug costs show that an average of 75 of the 200 top-selling drugs in Canada from 1991 to 1994 had been on the market for only four years or fewer (PMPRB 1996b), and that the cost per insurance claim for new products is more than twice that of older drugs (Chiles 1995). Findings were very similar for the analysis of drug expenditures in the United States during 1960—44 percent of all sales that year were for products introduced over the previous five years (Comanor 1986). International evidence also suggests that new drugs account for most expenditure increases over time across countries (Denig and Haaijer-Ruskamp 1995).

The mere evolution of technology is not sufficient to explain the increased expenditure on drugs. Nor is it necessarily bad that new products make up a majority of sales in an industry. A larger portion of automobile sales, for example, are for models that have been introduced within a few years. But new technology, especially therapeutic improvements to existing pharmaceuticals, ought not to command utilization. Therapeutic improvements are often marketed at substantial cost. Costs and benefits of new technologies must be weighed against already established, or other new, technologies.

The increased use of newer drugs results from judgments made, for the most part, by physicians who act (ideally) on behalf of their patients and, perhaps, society.[4] Consumers enter this decision process only by paying for

---

4. Perhaps physicians should consider the interests of society as well as the interest of the individual patient. For example, efforts to reduce the use of broad-spectrum antibiotics are motivated by the undesirable effects of their excessive use on large populations, rather than on any single patient. Similarly, promoting "rational prescribing," by encouraging physicians to consider whether drugs are economical, is in the interest of those who could benefit from treatment made affordable with resources saved and by those who pay for drugs—in many cases, taxpayers.

the drugs, and in many cases this is done by a third-party payer. Doctors make judgments on patients' behalves based on their medical expertise and information available to them. In the case of pharmacotherapeutics, a great deal of the information available to practicing physicians is provided by the pharmaceutical companies (Anderson and Lexchin 1996). The quality of this information has been brought under question because it is provided for the dual purposes of informing physicians about alternative drug treatments and for selling the companies' products. Because physicians decide not just *whether* to prescribe, but *what* to prescribe, *how much* and *how often*, the information that they receive (and use) is crucial. If doctors make judgments without full information about the safety, efficacy, side effects, and cost of drugs (or if doctors ignore components of this information), the impact on drug utilization, health outcomes, and total costs could be enormous. This may be the reason that past pharmaceutical policies, which typically targeted patients and pharmacists, have failed to promote rational drug use and control costs. If we do not alter prescribing patterns through improved information and incentives for physicians, pharmaceutical expenditures will continue to rise and inappropriate drug use will remain.

THE ECONOMICS AND POLITICS OF THE PHARMACEUTICAL INDUSTRY

The pharmaceutical industry is composed of many agents: patients, doctors, pharmacists, governments, benefits providers, and manufacturers. Each has a different set of objectives and constraints: financial, professional, and legal. Agents in this industry pursue their objectives while interacting with others in a process that takes a drug from an idea to a product consumed by a patient. From a societal perspective, the overriding purpose of this process is to deliver one component of health care to patients where appropriate. This overriding purpose is subject to an interpretation that is bound to vary considerably according to an agent's role in the process. A physician seeking the best treatment for a patient might not consider price to be a component of the "appropriateness" of care, but a benefits provider or government official allocating scarce resources would. What follows is a description of major players in the industry: consumers, manufacturers, physicians, pharmacists, and governments.

Consumers

The relationship between consumers in the pharmaceutical industry and manufacturers and retailers is unique. The role of pharmaceuticals in health care provision, the regulation of drug distribution and consumption, and the various forms of drug insurance place constraints on, or alter the incentives of, consumers. Pharmaceutical consumers are, in many ways, unlike consumers in any other market.

The first striking dissimilarity between consumers of drugs and those of typical commodities is the nature of what is ultimately being demanded. Consumers in this industry do not demand the product in and of itself. Instead, consumers seek the positive health outcomes believed to be associated with health care. Pharmaceutical consumption is one component of health care, and is interrelated with many other components (physicians' and pharmacists' services in particular). Because drugs are inputs into health care, involving complicated chemical and physiological processes, the use of drugs includes a certain degree of uncertainty.

The uncertainty associated with pharmaceutical use is one reason that drug production, distribution, and consumption are strictly regulated. To aid in the determination of appropriate use of pharmaceuticals, consumers are often required to seek the advice of health care professionals before purchasing drugs. Restrictions on the sale of drugs—requiring a physician's prescription for many products, and limiting the sale of prescription and nonprescription drugs to pharmacists' retail outlets—are intended to ensure that consumers receive proper medical consultation about pharmaceutical therapies. As such, the sovereignty of consumers is partially abdicated to professionals who make many important decisions concerning consumers' pharmaceutical consumption.

Finally, the nature of drugs as inputs into health care places them very high on what might be described as a "hierarchy of consumer needs." If a drug is deemed medically necessary for the treatment of a serious illness, consumers may seldom defer its purchase. For this reason, the demand for pharmaceuticals may be highly inelastic (insensitive to price changes), making consumers vulnerable to catastrophic drug costs if prices and prescribing practices are not kept in check. When financial constraints are severe enough to bar a consumer from obtaining a drug, the delivery of appropriate medical care may be impeded.

Given that many new drugs are replacing insured medical services in Canada, moving toward pharmacotherapeutic treatment regimes may place a serious financial burden on consumers. Due to financial constraints faced by selected populations, this burden may create inequitable access to medical care. In order to relieve some of this financial pressure, provincial governments across Canada have insured those at greatest risk of incurring high drug costs (e.g., the elderly) and those with the fewest means to pay for drugs (e.g., social assistance recipients). Additionally, a significant portion of the population is insured through publicly subsidized, extended health coverage offered by many employers and unions. It is believed that insurance coverage adds to the inelasticity of pharmaceutical demand because many consumers are not responsible for the price of the drugs they consume (Egan, Higinbotham, and Weston 1982; Caves, Whinston, and Hurwitz 1991; Grabowski and

Vernon 1992; Scherer 1993; Coulson and Stuart 1995). Combined with the transfer of decision-making authority to professionals, this may remove consumers from the most important decisions concerning the choice of alternative treatments—leaving them with the responsibility to comply with prescribed regimes (discussed below).

Manufacturers

The pharmaceutical manufacturing industry is truly global in scope. With significant research costs to recoup, manufacturers seek to increase sales volumes by marketing their products internationally. Worldwide pharmaceutical markets are dominated by multinational manufacturers based in the United States, the United Kingdom, Germany, France, Switzerland, and Japan (Ballance 1996; Redwood 1993; Eden 1989).

Economies of scale in the two most costly production phases—R&D and fine chemical manufacturing—give significant advantages to large firms. These economies of scale make it most efficient for manufacturers to concentrate R&D and fine chemical production at company headquarters (Taggart 1991; Eden 1989), so little research other than clinical testing is done outside a multinational's home country, or at most one or two of its major markets (e.g., the United States; Ballance 1996). Most research done in "host markets" is regulatory testing required for marketing approval. The primary corporate activities in host markets are final production (the combining and packaging of ingredients) and marketing and sales activities (Ballance 1996; Eden 1989).

In 1995, the estimated worldwide pharmaceutical sales at factory-gate prices was $340 billion (PMPRB 1996a). Although no firm holds more than an 8 percent share of the global market, the industry is highly concentrated in individual classes of therapies (Moore 1996; Ballance 1996). In any particular drug class, there may be only a few competitors, with the leading firm controlling more than 50 percent of the market (Drake and Uhlman 1993). Recently, major players in the industry have merged or formed partnerships to gain synergies and economies of scale and scope in their research and marketing activities (Moore 1996; Anderson et al. 1995). The top 10 pharmaceutical manufacturers account for approximately 40 percent of the global market (PMPRB 1996a), and some analysts speculate that further mergers involving these firms are forthcoming.[5]

---

5. The speculated merger of Glaxo Wellcome PLC and Pfizer Inc. has been denied by company officials (*Financial Post Daily*, March 27, 1996, p. 9). However, major multinationals Sandoz AG and Ciba-Geigy recently merged in a U.S.$62-billion deal, making it the second-largest firm in the industry. Leading the industry is Glaxo Wellcome PLC, formed last year in a U.S.$41-billion takeover (*Financial Post Daily*, March 8, 1996, p. 5).

The Canadian Industry

Canada represents only about 2 percent of the world market for pharmaceuticals and is headquarters to no major multinational manufacturers (PMPRB 1996a; Eden 1989). The drug-manufacturing industry in Canada consists of large, multiproduct, research-oriented firms that are almost entirely foreign owned; generic drug manufacturers, dominated by two Canadian firms (Apotex and Novopharm); and smaller firms competing in niche markets, such as nonprescription drug segments. Canada also has several small research-oriented "biotechnology boutiques" (Crop Conseil 1995). Statistics Canada data indicate that factory-gate sales were $6 billion in 1995. The top 10 companies in Canada—two of which are Canadian-owned generic drug manufacturers—accounted for approximately 46 percent of Canadian drug sales in 1995 (PMPRB 1996a).

Recouping Investment

Typically, a new drug begins as a promising discovery in the field or laboratory resulting from deliberate search or happy accident. (Fortune, however, favours the prepared.) A very large number of such promising prospects are winnowed out during research and testing, and most fall by the wayside. By the time a drug comes to the market, it already represents a heavy investment, not only in its own development, but also in prospects that failed and in the years of clinical trials and research necessary to obtain regulatory approval for sale. The average research expenditure necessary for an American-based multinational manufacturer to bring a product to market is estimated at U.S.$200 million (Moore 1996).

To recoup the massive, fixed costs of investment, two things must happen: first, the product must sell for more than it cost to produce and, second, enough of the drug must be sold to recoup the investment. Unless the first requirement is satisfied, the second will never be reached. If a product is not priced at a premium over production costs, fixed costs cannot be recouped. Even when the product is marketed at a premium, corporate profitability depends on large-volume sales. Drug manufacturers are not charities, nor are they in public service. They are private, for-profit corporations in a competitive business, responsible to their shareholders for achieving the highest possible return on equity—profit. When a drug sells for more than it costs, the more you sell, the greater your profits. So both commercial survival and responsibility to shareholders demand that the product be marketed at all costs. Evidence of this has existed for decades, and continues to emerge today.[6]

To allow innovators to recoup their investment, countries grant temporary monopolies through patents. From the time a product is approved for sale until its patent expires, the patentholding firm has no direct competition. This allows firms approximately 10 to 15 years of monopoly before competitors can bid the price down. During this period, the patent-holder will charge the highest price the market will bear at the targeted sales level. This occurs not only in the country where the drug was discovered, but in every country where the manufacturer can patent and market it. There is no reason why the resulting margin of revenue over production costs should bear any relation to development costs; the drug may generate substantial monopoly profits in every country in which it is sold.

In defence of these profit margins, it has been noted that many drugs that enter the market do not fully recoup the costs of investment. However, successful products offset the losses from less-successful ones (Grabowski and Vernon 1990). This partly explains why the industry is dominated by massive, multinational companies: larger firms have a strategic advantage in financing and operating many simultaneous research projects. Recent evidence of economies of both scale and scope in research and development indicates that pursuing several projects at once both increases the odds of success and diffuses the risk of failure (Henderson and Cockburn 1996). Similarly, large companies, with their armies of sales representatives and established distribution channels, enjoy economies of scale in marketing and distribution as well. The pharmaceutical industry has managed to maintain extraordinarily high average profits for decades by managing many concurrent research projects and balancing the blockbuster drugs against the losers through aggressive marketing worldwide.

---

6. Financial incentives can cause companies to cover up unfavourable clinical trials, continue marketing ineffective drugs, and bribe government officials (Bero and Rennie 1996; Rosenberg 1996; Drake and Uhlman 1993). Most recently, evidence has accumulated to cast doubt on the safety of calcium channel blockers, a very common treatment for hypertension (*The Vancouver Sun*, Tues, May 28, 1996, B1). In the face of mounting clinical evidence that these products lead to increased rates of heart attack, relative to traditional treatments for hypertension, officials from Bayer Inc., the manufacturer of the best-selling calcium channel blocker in Canada, play down the risk. They continue to promote their product, suggesting that concerns with the short-acting form of the drug do not apply to the one-a-day version.

Profitability

In 24 of the 32 years between 1960 and 1991, pharmaceuticals held first or second rank on *Fortune* magazine's annual tabulation of industrial average return on shareholders' equity. In this period, the pharmaceutical industry's average return was 18.4 percent, compared to an average of 11.9 percent for the top 500 industrials (Scherer 1993). In the 1995 "*Fortune 500*" edition, drugmakers won the "triple crown": pharmaceuticals were ranked number one in return on revenues (16.4 percent), return on assets (12.7 percent), and return on equity (31.2 percent), with returns greater than three times the median for all 500 industries in each category (*Fortune*, May 15, 1995).

It is sometimes argued that extraordinary profits are needed to compensate for the risks of investment in research-intensive industries. Yet, even when the riskiness of investment is accounted for,[7] pharmaceuticals are, on average, very profitable.[8] Market power appears to be a basic characteristic of the pharmaceutical industry (Comanor 1986, 1182–1186).

Many question whether this profitability is justified. Profits per se are not indicative of unwarranted market power. For example, few people question the nature of competition in the cosmetics industry, which also ranks very high in profitability.

> To be sure, every business is certainly entitled to a *reasonable profit* as a reward to its investors and a guarantee of long-term stability. But the difficulty is judging a reasonable profit level. When, if ever, do profits become "unreasonable"? (Spinello 1992, 618)

---

7. The defence of high profits as a "risk premium" is inadequate. First, the consistent profitability of the pharmaceutical industry is not indicative of high risks. Second, the large size of manufacturers allows them to spread the risk associated with individual research projects by engaging in many projects simultaneously. Finally, it has been shown that the outliers in the industry earn unusually *high* rates of return, not *low* rates (Scherer 1993).

8. For nearly 30 years, academic literature in economics has focused on the question of how to calculate the profits of this industry appropriately (Comanor 1986). This cottage industry for economists proved little that was not already known. When calculating rates of economic rent (profit) for pharmaceutical firms, R&D and marketing expenditures should be capitalized as investment expenditures over time rather than as current outlays. Here, *depreciated values* of capital assets created by past and current outlays are included in the denominator, while only *current depreciation* on expenditures is subtracted from the numerator. Because both numerator and denominator are larger, these "economic rates of return" (versus accounting rates) for pharmaceuticals are still in excess of average returns by two standard deviations (Comanor 1986).

This question is difficult to answer when the industry in question produces goods that have a major impact on basic well-being: e.g., food, housing, or health care. The profitability of pharmaceutical manufacturers comes under scrutiny because drugs are inputs into health care, resulting in inelastic demand and the high social costs of financial barriers to access, and because governments grant firms significant market power through intellectual property protection. Evidence seems to suggest that, if any industry could be deemed excessively profitable, it would have to be the pharmaceutical industry. No other industry is so consistently profitable, and few others have as much legally protected market power.

Doctors

Physicians are among the most important figures in the pharmaceutical industry. Because they are presumed to have superior knowledge of diagnosis and medical intervention, physicians have been given the role of prescriber. As prescriber, the physician decides, on the consumer's behalf, which therapy would be best.

Few people think of physicians as entrepreneurs, but every practitioner in private practice operates a small business. Like all entrepreneurs, physicians make money from selling something; in this case, a service. Physicians paid on a fee-for-service basis have a financial incentive to see as many patients as possible in a working day, constrained only by the need to satisfy both themselves and their customers that a standard of professional care was met.

> Physician reimbursement policy is an important factor in shaping practice patterns. The time spent with patients and the type of services delivered are influenced by the method of payment (salary versus fee-for-service) and the fee schedule. Services with low economic return are performed with lower than expected frequency, the reverse being true for services with better economic returns. In keeping with these general observations, shorter patient contact times have been observed among fee-for-service physicians than salaried physicians. Shorter patient contact times and drug prescribing have been found to be strongly correlated in the two studies in which this was investigated (Tamblyn and Perreault 1995, 18).

Therefore, in the fee-for-service setting, a prescription is a convenient way to terminate patient visits (Soumerai, McLaughlin, and Avron 1989). Unfortunately, physicians do not have enough time to keep up with the clinical literature on drug safety and efficacy, or enough formal training in pharmacology (Anderson and Lexchin 1996). Drug companies attempt to fill this gap, albeit to their advantage. Because physicians want to provide the best possible care, manufacturers market the benefits of their drugs and downplay the risks. Currently accepted marketing practices in Canada (discussed below) appear to blur the distinction between education and persuasion (Lexchin 1989, 1993b, 1994). Cost is hardly mentioned in advertising that targets physicians because doctors do not pay for the drugs they prescribe and many patients have insurance that covers prescription drugs. Therefore, to remain on the leading edge of technology, doctors often prescribe the newest, most expensive drugs, without clinical evidence that they are superior to existing or alternative courses of treatment (Castonguay et al. 1996).

Pharmacists

In Canada, only a licensed pharmacist may sell a prescription medicine. This law has its roots in the days when a pharmacist compounded the drug prescribed by the doctor. Today, prescription drugs are manufactured in their dosage form and, as a result, pharmacists seldom compound prescriptions. Still, each time a prescription drug is dispensed, the pharmacists receives a dispensing (or professional) fee, in addition to retailing margins on the ingredient cost of the drug. Moreover, pharmacists lobby for the scheduling rules that require nonprescription drugs to be sold in pharmacies, or be available only from a pharmacist's dispensary.

The rationale for granting pharmacists a monopoly on retailing of both prescription drugs and many nonprescription drugs is that these products are not safe for sale without the professional consultation of a pharmacist. This monopoly over drug retailing has resulted in significant profits. Statistics Canada's most recent financial performance indicators show that "Drugs, Patented Medicines and Toiletries Retailing" has been one of the most profitable industries in Canada throughout the 1990s—with median rates of return on capital of more than twice the national average (Statistics Canada 1996).[9]

Trouble begins when the financial incentives of the pharmacist as retailer conflict with his professional role. Evidence of the overuse of drugs in Canada (Tamblyn and Perreault 1995), indicates that pharmacists should be refusing some potential sales of both prescription and nonprescription drugs, but sacrificing sales would reduce profits. The strong resistance to the removal of tobacco products from pharmacies in Canada shows that business interests sometimes outweigh professional obligations.

---

9. In 1994, drug retailers with annual revenues of more than $5 million had a median rate of return on capital employed of 16.8 percent, compared with a median rate of 7.7 percent for all similarly sized nonfinancial firms in Canada. According to these data, larger drug retailers held second place in profitability from 1988 to 1994. The return for drug retailers with annual revenues below $5 million was 11.5 percent, compared with a median rate of 5 percent for all similarly sized nonfinancial firms in Canada.

It has long been acknowledged that the pharmacist is the best-trained professional in the area of pharmacology, and that their pharmacological skills are grossly underused (Evans and Williamson 1978; Salmon 1996). The experience of hospital pharmacists indicates that a more effective application of pharmacists' expertise could help doctors prescribe more appropriately, and eventually improve quality of care and reduce costs. It is thus advocated that pharmacists be paid for "cognitive services," including patient counselling and monitoring, to promote more rational drug therapy. (Pay dispensers more to pay pharmaceutical manufacturers less.) But, although it is plausible in principle, this argument has been around for at least 25 years and shows few signs of being translated into reality because of the structural realities of the industry.

Community pharmacy lacks the structure necessary to make pharmacists "team members" in providing patient care. Community pharmacists have no access to diagnoses or medical records, so they can offer little therapeutic advice. The recent Community Pharmacist Intervention Study showed that Canadian retail pharmacists make approximately 1.2 interventions per 100 prescriptions filled (Poston, Kennedy, and Waruszynski 1995). In this study, checking for information missing from a prescription, such as dosage strength or quantity, was included as an intervention. Therapeutic problems such as incorrect dosage, drug duplication, and contraindication accounted for only 36.9 percent of reported interventions. According to these results, therapeutic interventions, used to justify the pharmacists' monopoly on drug retail and dispensing fees, occur fewer than five times out of every 1,000 prescriptions dispensed. Such a low rate of therapeutic intervention indicates either that the need for pharmacists' prescription-monitoring role is slight (e.g., due to a high level of appropriate prescribing) or that retail pharmacists in Canada are not (for whatever reason) fulfilling that role.

Improvements in information technology, such as on-line pharmaceutical records and prescriptions, will further erode the professional role of the retail pharmacist. Yet, even with adequate information, pharmacists have little incentive to question physicians about their prescriptions. Physicians who feel threatened could steer many patients away from a pharmacist who challenges them. Again, the professional duties of the pharmacist could conflict with business.

Government

Government also plays a major role in the pharmaceutical industry, both as a regulator and as a provider of drug benefits. Regulation is probably the government's most important task in this industry. Government agencies determine the rules of conduct in many ways, affecting the overall performance of the industry from both a health and safety perspective and an economic one.

Product safety regulation is critical to the pharmaceutical industry. With their obvious potency and the uncertainty of health outcomes, products must be scientifically proven safe and effective when used as indicated for the treatment of specified conditions. The Drugs Directorate of Health Canada is responsible for reviewing the clinical trials data submitted by manufacturers before their products can be marketed in Canada. Packaging, advertising, and scheduling are also responsibilities of the Drugs Directorate.[10]

The government also sets the terms of intellectual property protection in Canada. The Commissioner of Patents at Industry Canada is responsible for the laws and regulations under the Patent Act. By determining the length of Canadian patents, the type of patents to be granted (product, process, or use), the terms of permissible (and perhaps compulsory) licensing, as well as other related regulations, the federal government effectively defines the competitive environment.

Market power conferred by patents should be closely monitored to establish whether the patent system achieves the desired result at an acceptable cost. The federal government tracks some of the effects of pharmaceutical patents through the Patented Medicine Prices Review Board (PMPRB), which regulates the (factory-gate) prices of all patented medicines and monitors the research activities of patentholding drug manufacturers. Through their purchasing activities, provincial governments are also stakeholders in the monitoring and curtailing of patented (as well as nonpatented) drug costs.

Both federal and provincial governments play a major role as providers of pharmaceutical benefits. By offering drug benefits, governments relieve some of the financial burden of the pharmaceutical component of health care, and improve access to care. As major payers for drugs, governments can also use cost-cutting strategies not available to consumers. Governments can monitor drug use patterns, negotiate drug prices and volume discounts, and evaluate therapeutic alternatives to advise health professionals about optimal treatment regimes. As the importance of pharmaceutical benefits management increases, Canadian data indicate that managers of public drug plans are controlling costs more carefully than managers of private plans (figure 1). Unfortunately, managers of public drug plans have to balance the desire to control costs against the countervailing political influence of the pharmaceutical industry.

---

10. Provinces are also involved in drug scheduling. If Health Canada permits a product to be sold without a prescription, provincial authorities may schedule the product more strictly; for example, require that it be available only from a pharmacist's dispensary, or that it be available in that province only on prescription.

Finally, the government also has a significant indirect effect on the pharmaceutical industry through the regulation and organization of the health care system. By setting budgets and establishing remuneration mechanisms, the government influences the financial incentives of major players in this industry, including hospitals and physicians. The provincial health ministries can, for example, encourage greater use of medicines in outpatient care by increasing hospitals' financial incentives to schedule day surgeries. Moreover, remuneration mechanisms for physicians' services may influence incentives to prescribe drugs (Tamblyn and Perreault 1995).

Achieving Cost Control

Each major stakeholder in the pharmaceutical market has a vested interest in controlling the evolution of a cost containment strategy. Every dollar cut from expenditure in this sector is a dollar of income lost to a stakeholder. Effective solutions will not come voluntarily. The prolonged status quo, despite decades of calls for reform, indicates how hard it is to effect change. International experience is very similar. No country has managed substantial pharmaceutical cost reduction through cooperation, nor should we have expected such.

The Netherlands is a case in point. In 1988, the Dutch government proposed a reference-based pricing system to control high drug costs (Rigter 1994). In response, 10 industry associations, representing insurers, wholesalers, pharmacists, physicians and manufacturers, promised self-regulation through an "all-parties treaty." By 1990, it was clear that nothing was done— prices continued to rise. In 1991, the government stepped in with the Medicines Reimbursement System, followed in 1993 by further controls that signalled a radical shift from the Dutch government's traditional cooperative style.

A similar situation arose in Germany when the Health Insurance Cost Containment Act of 1977—which introduced revenue-based global budgets into the Statutory Health Insurance System—left to the organs of "self-administration" measures for a prescription review process with financial sanctions to discourage excessive prescribing. "The decentralised system of self-administration, which functions well as long as none of the involved parties stands to suffer a loss, never succeeded in implementing these measures." (Munnich and Sullivan 1994, 24). After 15 years of waiting for self-administration, the government enacted legislation in 1993 that preempted the ineffective voluntary process by introducing pharmaceutical budget constraints at the federal level. Though this legislation has been fiercely criticized (Schoffski 1996), it made an immediate and substantial impact on prescribing patterns. In fact, the strength of the industry's reaction to this (or any *effective*) legislation is testament to the fact that it caused real change, because altering prescribing patterns alters the distribution of incomes.

Some people argue that the difficulty of achieving cost control indicates that this is not a legitimate goal. According to this reasoning, escalation in pharmaceutical spending indicates growing demand for high-quality health care. Pharmaceutical expenditure is therefore defended on the basis that it saves money in other health care sectors where unmet needs would otherwise spill over. Consistent with this argument is the call for greater efficiency, but not less funding, in the pharmaceutical sector. Restructuring inputs to improve quality of care *and maintain (or increase) the level of expenditure* does not meet as much resistance as effective expenditure control because stakeholder incomes do not fall—except, of course, the incomes of consumers and taxpayers.

Another reform advocated by many stakeholders is simply to bring in more money from sources other than the government—usually patients. This shifts costs to avoid expenditure control. (It is little wonder that such policies are advocated by those whose incomes are affected by expenditure control.) According to this logic, more money means better care. However, if the current system involves overuse or misuse of costly medicine, it does not follow that bringing in more money—at the expense of consumers and taxpayers—will improve the performance of this health care component.

If pharmaceutical policy is to be truly effective in terms of expenditure control, some stakeholders must lose income. Trade-offs are inevitable, and "cooperative" solutions will produce little improvement.

INDUSTRY TRENDS AND CORPORATE STRATEGIES

Several trends and corporate strategies in the pharmaceutical industry shape the policy environment. Since the pharmaceutical industry is global, and multinational companies do most of the manufacturing and research, decisions made by these companies echo around the world. Selected trends and strategies in this multinational industry are discussed in this section.

Lobbying for Intellectual Property

One of the oldest questions in the literature on the pharmaceutical industry is balancing R&D incentives against the availability of low-cost drugs. Developed countries attempt to answer this question by giving innovating firms intellectual property rights, usually through patents. By granting a temporary monopoly on a new product, a patent allows the manufacturer to charge high prices because competitors cannot enter the market. Patent protection may also permit pharmaceutical manufacturers to make profits beyond those in other industries.

In light of the evidence of high pharmaceutical profits, few can dispute that intellectual property rights permit pharmaceutical manufacturers to recoup their investments, and more. Multinational pharmaceutical companies are not satisfied, however. They argue that not enough is being done to protect the rights of innovating firms *worldwide*. Since 1985, multinationals have warned governments in developed and developing countries that, without increased intellectual property protection, they will reduce innovation.

To extend their influence, multinational drug companies lobby in trade-related negotiations around the globe. For example, during the mid-1980s, U.S. President Ronald Reagan appointed Ed Pratt to chair the U.S. Business Roundtable, a top private sector advisory panel on Canada-U.S. free trade. Ed Pratt, president of Pfizer Inc., a U.S.-based multinational pharmaceutical manufacturer, wasted no time in bringing drug patents to the forefront of the Canada-U.S. free trade negotiations.

The U.S.-based multinationals that Ed Pratt represented particularly disliked Canada's long-standing compulsory drug patent licensing provision.[11] Due to intense pressure from the U.S. government, itself under pressure from U.S.-based drug companies, the Canadian government passed legislation that eliminated most of the scope of compulsory licensing in 1987, and completely removed this provision in 1993 (Lexchin 1993a; Gherson 1991; Eden 1989). Similar lobbies have taken place in the NAFTA negotiations and in the GATT negotiations, especially the Uruguay Round. With hundreds of billions of dollars at stake, multinationals pulled out all the stops to secure more advantageous patents through these trade negotiations.

Locating Research and Development

For countries like Canada with small pharmaceutical markets, the net benefit of increasing patent protection is not entirely obvious. One celebrated benefit, improved health through innovation, is not significant in a small market. Decisions concerning the scale, scope, and location of R&D are made by foreign multinationals according to a global research agenda. Greater profitability in a small country will *not* significantly affect the *scale* of research and, thus, discoveries. Profitability may, however, have some impact on the *location* of research.

One of the key locational determinants of R&D expenditure is the "strategic importance" of a firm's presence in the target country (Taggart 1991). One strategic consideration is negotiating with the target country's government. In this way, pharmaceutical companies use R&D expenditure as an international bargaining chip. To reward Canada for improving its patent protection in 1987, for example, multinational companies promised to increase R&D conducted in Canada.

---

11. Compulsory licensing allowed any manufacturer to sell a patented drug before its patent expiry, subject to a 4 percent royalty paid to the patentholder.

Even the location of R&D and production activities *within* a country is strategic. Because the pharmaceutical industry is highly regulated and profitability depends on government policy, firms have incentive to locate where they have the most political influence, a practice permitted by the fact that final production, clinical research, and marketing activities can be placed anywhere. When deciding whether to implement Bills C-22 and C-91, the federal Progressive Conservative government was well aware that multinational pharmaceutical companies were concentrated in key ridings in Quebec and Ontario (Lexchin 1993a).[12]

The Research Agenda

Given the R&D incentives, one should be aware of the incentives that come with various policies. Private sector firms conduct research to exploit profitable markets. The research agenda of a private sector firm will reflect that interest.

> There is little incentive for a commercial concern to pursue knowledge for its own sake. Only if knowledge can, somehow, be product or process linked and so provide extra revenue or reduce costs will a firm conduct research to gain that knowledge. As a consequence most industrial research (in any industry) is either applied research, rather than basic research, or development. Industrial research and development tends to build on the basic advances or discoveries made elsewhere (Reekie and Weber 1979, 11).

Faced with huge up-front investments and uncertain markets, the drug industry has several strategies to limit its risk. One is to focus research on known markets; that is, markets developed by the competition. By following a competitor's discoveries and by "innovating around their patent" (discovering nearly identical molecules with similar therapeutic effects), companies can gain market share. This 'me-too' style of research has been as heavily criticized by analysts in recent years as it was in the 1950s and 1960s, when it was referred to as "molecule manipulation" (RCHS 1964; Cooper 1966; Slatter 1977; Eastman 1985; Drake and Uhlman 1993).

Some argue that the development of me-too drugs is "necessary for companies to survive the long intervals between major discoveries" (Redwood 1993, 75). From a societal perspective, this opens the question of whether the valuable human resources used to innovate around patents should be applied elsewhere. Competing directly with a pioneering company's product

---

12. In Canada, Ontario and Quebec evenly split approximately 90 percent of annual R&D expenditures by patentholding firms from 1987 to 1994 (PMPRB 1989–1996).

through generic competition—under compulsory licensing and subject to suitable royalties, for example—would also produce revenue for firms that are between major discoveries, with much less duplicative research. This would eliminate the expense of molecule manipulation and the clinical trials necessary to get around the pioneers' patent (Eastman 1985).

However, corporations might *prefer* developing and marketing me-too products because me-too drugs earn significant margins over production costs; generic products earn smaller profits. As mentioned above, me-too products are similar to *but different from* the pioneering product; as such, they allow the manufacturers to sell their benefits, and justify the price. The only benefit of a generic product is the lower price.

Another research incentive in the pharmaceutical industry is to develop products that will have a stable and predictable market in the future. Strategic R&D investment requires the identification of a therapeutic need that cannot be exhausted easily. Therefore, the industry tends to innovate in "second-stage" therapies, especially symptomatic relief and maintenance products. Straight cures, such as the antibiotic that eliminates the *Helicobacter* bacteria that causes some recurring ulcers, can yield large margins but limited sales. Maintenance therapies, on the other hand, can generate the repeated, long-term sales that are crucial to commercial success.

These conditions produce both over- and underinvestment in R&D. Generally, like any other investment, research has both costs and benefits. These must be kept in balance, not just from the perspective of the private enterprise that steers the research, but also from the perspective of society. The presumption that more research is always better is based on a limited set of interests. Although policies to contain drug costs and drug manufacturer profits tend to reduce incentives to develop new drugs, society will not necessarily be worse off.

Although some new products offer significant therapeutic improvements ("breakthroughs"), most new drugs brought to market through the research efforts of drug companies do not. Table 1 categorizes new drugs marketed for human use in Canada from 1988 to 1995. Of the 581 new drugs, only 41 (7 percent) were breakthroughs: "the first product to treat effectively a particular illness or which provides substantial improvement over existing drug products" (PMPRB 1996a, 17). Two hundred and seventy-seven (47 percent) of the drugs introduced to the Canadian market during those years offered moderate, little, or no improvement over existing drugs. The remaining 248 new drugs were line extensions, usually a known drug in a new strength (PMPRB 1996a).[13]

If the current innovation and marketing trends are producing over- and inappropriate use of existing drugs, and the vast majority of new drugs

---

13. Fifteen products were unclassified.

Table 1

New drug categorization in Canada

Category	1988	1989	1990	1991	1992	1993	1994	1995
Line extension	15	35	26	51	23	35	29	34
Breakthrough	1	4	3	5	15	8	3	2
Moderate or no improvement	19	29	30	38	50	34	32	45
Not categorized	–	–	15	–	–	–	–	–
Total	35	68	74	94	88	77	64	81

Source: PMPRB Annual Reports 1991–1996.

coming onto the market offer neither significant (or any) therapeutic advantages nor significant cost savings, perhaps it is time to redirect the trend. It seems illogical to continue overusing increasingly expensive drugs simply to give the industry the incentive and wherewithal to develop still more expensive drugs for us to overuse. Usage and payments for new pharmaceuticals should provide sufficient incentive for the development of innovative products that offer improvements over current treatments.

Pharmaceutical Competition

When a new product is ready to be launched, enormous efforts go into marketing. Millions of dollars are spent to establish brand recognition among physicians and, in some cases, to establish the merits of a new class of therapies. Price is very important; instead of cost-plus pricing, the industry uses "market" pricing, which means that drug prices vary from region to region and country to country, and over time (Drake and Uhlman 1993; USGAO 1992; Caves, Whinston, and Hurwitz 1991; Comanor 1986; Egan, Higinbotham, and Weston 1982; Slatter 1977; RCHS 1964).

One pricing strategy, sometimes called "cream skimming," involves introducing the product at a high price to indicate quality and gain premiums from extremely brand-loyal prescribers (Drake and Uhlman 1993; Caves, Whinston, and Hurwitz 1991; Egan, Higinbotham, and Weston 1982, ch. 4; Slatter 1977). At the end of the introductory period, the price is lowered to increase market penetration. Finally, when the product is established, the price may rise over time, eventually losing some market share to new products.

New products often come on the market as me-too competitors— similar chemical compounds with similar therapeutic profiles. In the past, there was remarkably little price competition between brands with similar therapeutic effect. Instead, the industry competed fiercely on the basis of product differentiation through marketing and detailing (Comanor 1986; Egan, Higinbotham, and Weston 1982; Slatter 1977). The strategy with new products was often to exaggerate therapeutic differences, minimize potential disadvantages, and charge a high enough price to indicate that claims of superiority should be taken seriously. Until recently, this strategy worked.

A most spectacularly successful application of this strategy is ranitidine, the H_2 receptor blocker developed by Glaxo to compete with SmithKline's cimetidine. Under the trade name of Tagamet, cimetidine was, for a time, the world's largest-selling drug in dollars earned from sales. Glaxo developed ranitidine as a substitute; it produced fewer side effects in a minority of patients. On the strength of this advantage, Glaxo was able to sell ranitidine, under the trade name Zantac, as the better drug. Zantac duly replaced Tagamet as the world's largest-selling drug, earning U.S.$3.6 billion in 1994 alone (Moore 1996).

A manufacturer facing loss of market share to potential entrants may protect some of that share by applying for approval to market its product in modified dosage forms. This strategy usually involves "newer," long-acting or extended-release versions of the original product. The new dosage forms are protected by new patents, extending market protection for the branded firm. These therapeutic upgrades can achieve a significant sales advantage while maintaining its price-cost margin. As shown in table 1, line extensions account for almost 50 percent of new drugs entering the Canadian market since 1988.

Both these forms of product competition have been noted by commentators since the 1960s (RCHS 1964; Comanor 1986). Pharmaceutical companies' ability to compete through product differentiation permits them to avoid costly price competition. Product competition conducted through a cycle of product introduction and obsolescence has impeded the development of standardization of products, which is conducive to price competition.

Generic Drugs

Standardization does, eventually, enter the market with generic products. Either by way of licensing, or upon patent expiry, the generic equivalents of a branded product enter the market and subject the brand manufacturer to the fiercest competition of all—price competition.

An early paradox of generic competition was that, upon appearance of a generic competitor, brand manufacturers did not reduce their prices—in some cases the brand firm's price increased (Comanor 1986; Grabowski and Vernon 1992; Scherer 1993). A "segmented market" model has been used to describe this phenomenon. In this model, the market is made up of paying consumers, who are price sensitive, and insured consumers, who are not price sensitive. It is believed that, during the 1980s, a significant portion of the market was not price sensitive, so brand manufacturers were able to maintain sales at premium prices (Caves, Whinston, and Hurwitz 1991; Grabowski and Vernon 1992; Scherer 1993).

More recently, however, both private and public benefits providers have become increasingly cost conscious, and now have many techniques to promote more economical medicines, often generics. In response, brand manufacturers adopted an "if you can't beat 'em, join 'em" strategy. Rather than cut the prices of their brand-name products, brand manufacturers launch pseudogeneric copies of their own drugs.

For the brand manufacturer, this has two advantages (Anderson et al. 1995). First, by selling its own generic version, the manufacturer gains sales in the generic segment of its own market while retaining the premium prices for the branded version of the drug. Second, a brand manufacturer that launches a generic copy before patents have expired fills the generic inventory pipeline before competition can enter. The disadvantage of the brand manufacturer's participation in the generic market is that it lends credibility to generic manufacturers' claims of equivalence.

With the recent merger of small pseudogeneric firms into AltiMed, a giant generic drug manufacturer owned by three multinational drug companies (Pharmacia & Upjohn Inc., Hoffman-La Roche Ltd., and Glaxo Wellcome Inc.), pseudogenerics have established a significant presence in Canada. The generic drug manufacturers Apotex and Novopharm are asking the federal Bureau of Competition to block the creation of AltiMed because it will have an unfair advantage in Canada's generic drug industry (*Financial Post*, March 16/18, 1996, 1–2).

A New Era of Competition

Because benefits providers manage the prescription process, companies have fewer chances to charge premium prices for me-too products that offer little therapeutic improvement. Recently, in the United Kingdom and the United States, new products were introduced into therapeutic classes at significant discounts, indicating that manufacturers believe price competition will secure market share because *some* payers are no longer willing to pay extra for drugs that offer no real advantages (Bosanquet and Zammit-Lucia 1995).

Switching from Rx to OTC

For a growing number of branded prescription drugs, there is a new form of relief from profits lost to generic competition: the prescription to over-the-counter (Rx-to-OTC) switch. Branded prescription drugs face substantial losses in market share upon the arrival of generic copies. To extend a product's profitable life, prescription drug manufacturers can apply to have their product approved for sale over the counter.

If a product is approved for OTC sale, the manufacturer can effectively block competition from generic drugs through massive expenditure on marketing (Anderson et al. 1995). Generic drugs, which can be sold at low prices largely because almost nothing is spent on marketing them, are not as established in the OTC segment of the industry. Because many consumers are not aware that branded and generic products with identical ingredients are therapeutically equivalent, purchasers in the OTC segment are brand conscious. By establishing loyalty in customers who do not appear to shop by price, brand manufacturers may continue to charge premium prices for years after patent expiry.[14]

Rx-to-OTC switches are motivated almost solely by the manufacturer's desire to avoid generic competitors and thus to maintain high sales volumes at prices in excess of production costs (*Scrip Magazine*, Dec. 1993). Competition in this market may, however, come from other brand manufacturers marketing copies of the drug under different names—if the patent has expired. The patentholding firm still has a significant advantage here. If the patentholder gains approval for OTC sales before patent expiry, it can launch the OTC product before competitors can enter the market. This tactic is crucial to achieving and maintaining market share in many OTC categories (Anderson et al. 1995).

Increasing product sales is one reason why pharmacists also gain from Rx-to-OTC switches. Not only do they sell more product, they also get a higher retail margin on OTC drugs than on prescription drugs. This is a manufacturers' selling point for encouraging cooperation from pharmacists (Harrison 1994).

Although the Rx-to-OTC switch has tremendous implications for some products, the extent of this phenomenon should be limited by the number of eligible drugs. At Health Canada, the Drugs Directorate requires a detailed risk-benefit analysis for all switch applicants. Before a prescription product can be made available over the counter, it must be low in toxicity and intended for treating minor conditions that consumers can diagnose easily for themselves.[15] However, many fear that manufacturers will market watered-down versions of potent prescription medicines to maintain market share at high OTC prices, with little benefit to the consumer. The Drugs Directorate will be responsible for carefully assessing the overall impact of allowing

---

14. By establishing brand loyalty, the copyright on the brand name prevents direct imitation —remember, consumers do not often consider ingredients when buying medicines. For protecting OTC market share, trademarks and copyrights supplant expiring patents.

15. The requirement that OTC drugs be safe and effective for the treatment of self-diagnosable minor ailments contradicts the claims of pharmacists who insist that these products are not safe if sold outside a pharmacy.

more products to be sold without prescription in Canada and, where appropriate, to "hold the line" against intense pressures from manufactures who stand to gain from selling directly to consumers.

STRATEGIES FOR MANAGING BENEFITS

The remainder of this paper assesses several strategies used by drug benefits providers to control costs and improve drug utilization. The title of this section of the paper is "Strategies for Managing Benefits" because cost control seems too narrow a definition for optimal pharmaceutical policy. Pharmaceutical policy can improve the efficiency of drug use in Canada and, as a result, lower costs.

Strategies Aimed at Consumers

Cost Sharing

Faced with relentlessly escalating pharmaceutical costs, provincial governments and other benefits providers strive to control their liabilities. The simplest response is cost sharing with patients. Every provincial drug benefit plan in Canada now uses some form of cost sharing (Crop Conseil 1995).

Cost sharing is preferred by those who believe that increasing the cost to patients will make them consider whether the drug is necessary, thus reducing the use of marginally effective drugs. This rationale assumes that consumers know enough to weigh the costs and benefits of drug therapies, which is not likely.

> The whole *raison d'être* of the prescribing function of the physician is a social judgment that consumers/patients are inadequately informed to make their own utilization decisions—attempting to modify those decisions by incentives aimed at the consumer would seem inconsistent, to say the least (Evans and Williamson 1978, 53).

Furthermore, even if consumers had the medical knowledge to choose cost-effective drugs, few cost-sharing plans are designed to improve efficiency. For example, a fixed copayment gives the consumer only one choice—consume or not. Consumers with a fixed copayment plan have no incentive to ask for the most cost-effective drug because their copayment is independent of the choice of drug. Nor are such consumers encouraged to buy from a competitively priced retailer because their copayment is independent of where the drug is purchased. Thus, fixed copayments are merely aggregate usage-curbing tools that provide no incentive for efficiency at either the prescribing level or the dispensing level (Evans and Williamson 1978; Morgan 1994).

Copayments are widely used, however. More provinces employ fixed copayments than coinsurance on drug purchases (Crop Conseil 1995). Surprisingly, very little has been done to measure the effect of copayments on costs and health outcomes. The research that exists—conducted on Medicaid plans in the United States (Soumerai et al. 1993)—indicates that consumers respond to copayments of as little as 50 cents per prescription. Furthermore, usage declines the most with maintenance drugs for chronic conditions (e.g., diuretics), whereas copayments have minimal effect on usage of analgesics and sedatives.

The behavioural changes revealed by the copayment studies indicate that consumers do not always respond to copayments as policymakers might wish. People are more willing to give up medicines that do not produce predictable, immediate changes in health status. This indicates that patients and prescribers use different decision criteria. If consumer behaviour is indicative of a predictable choice model, then the usage effect of copayments on various drugs can be calculated, and drug plans managed accordingly.

This notion gives rise to a coinsurance philosophy like that adopted in France. Product reimbursement under such a system is guided by two considerations: the type of product and the disease (Huttin and Avorn 1996). These two factors influence the assignment of reimbursement levels for each drug. For example, a preventive therapy for a life-threatening illness may be reimbursed fully if consumers can be expected to abandon it if they must pay for it. The model can be extended further to produce coinsurance levels for specific populations based on income, age, and health status. Although theoretically interesting, such a coinsurance system may be administratively cumbersome.[16]

Prescription Limits

Another method of containing the cost of pharmaceutical benefits is to assign a monthly prescription limit per beneficiary. The limited evidence on prescription limits comes from a New Hampshire experiment where Medicaid recipients were limited to three prescriptions per month. This limit was replaced with a one-dollar copayment a year later (Soumerai et al. 1993). In this study, the number of prescriptions per beneficiary declined significantly. The largest proportional reduction in use was in drugs that were deemed ineffective. However, the use of drugs deemed essential (e.g., insulin) declined significantly; in fact, the volume of essential drug use was

---

16. This sort of coinsurance system acts like a modified version of Ramsey pricing. In such a system, products with the least elastic demand are taxed the most, with slight modifications to reflect judgements of "medical necessity." Choosing which drugs to insure would be administratively difficult.

so large that most of the $0.4 million saved by limiting prescriptions came from reducing use of essential drugs. A follow-up study associated the reduced use of drugs with a significant increase in nursing home admissions relative to a control group in New Jersey (Soumerai et al. 1993). The net financial savings were nil and people ended up in nursing homes prematurely; clearly, the real cost of the program was borne by those the Medicaid system was supposed to protect. This form of cost containment is, perhaps, the least desirable because of the perverse impact it can have on the health of vulnerable populations.

Improving Compliance

Once a doctor issues a prescription for a drug that he has decided a patient requires, the patient's behaviour is crucial if the drug's potential is to be realized. Patient compliance involves not only the purchase of drugs deemed necessary—deterred by copayment on prescription drugs—but also the appropriate administration of the drug. In a recent survey of the literature on noncompliance with prescription medicines in Canada, Coambs and associates (1995) revealed that approximately 50 percent of patients do not comply with their prescribed drug regimes. This raises costs substantially and may reduce quality of health care.

The most frequent noncompliance behaviour is neglecting to fill prescriptions or to consume drugs purchased. Approximately 33 percent of consumers exhibit these behaviours (Coambs et al. 1995). The remainder of noncompliant patients do not take their medication as directed—altering the timing and dosage of the therapy, ceasing therapy prematurely, or combining prescription drugs with nonprescription drugs or alcohol when contraindicated

Care should be taken when assessing patient compliance not to blame the consumer. It would be misleading to suggest that noncompliance is solely the fault of patients. Decisions made by a patient are based on their understanding of the information that they have available to them. This understanding hinges on the relationship between patients and medical professionals—most often doctors. Complete insurance coverage may reduce the rate of failure to fill prescriptions. The remainder of noncompliance behaviours, however, must be reduced in other ways. Coambs and associates (1995) suggest that health education may improve the rate of compliance. Providing written information to reinforce verbal instructions, for example, has been found to improve patients' understanding of their disease and the requirements of their medication (Coambs et al. 1995). Improving relationships between physicians and patients may also lead to better prescribing and compliance; physicians and patients often have different impressions of the nature of illnesses and the drugs used to treat them (Coambs et al. 1995; Tamblyn and Perreault 1995).

It has also been found that convenient dosage forms and delivery systems can improve compliance. Reduced dosage frequency, new formulations such as transdermal patches, and user-friendly packaging have all improved compliance with specific treatments (Coambs et al. 1995). Trade-offs, however, must be balanced when advocating modified dosage forms of drugs; new dosage forms come at premium prices. Compliance may decline if consumers cannot pay for the "new and improved" forms of a drug. Furthermore, there is evidence that some patients are less convinced of the value of extended-release drugs than doctors are (Denig and Haaijer-Ruskamp 1995).

Strategies Aimed at Pharmacists

Incentives for Efficient Retailing

Unlike drugs, whose purpose, characteristics, and even name may be unknown to the patient, the services pharmacists offer are standardized. Therefore, consumers who patronize competing retailers can compare the quality of their pharmacists' services. In systems that set pharmacists' fees competitively and apply coinsurance (*not* a fixed copayment) to only this part of the drug cost, pharmacists are encouraged to compete on service and price (Evans and Williamson 1978; Morgan 1994). Consumers willing to pay higher dispensing fees for increased professional service can patronize pharmacies that offer it. For any retail margin on the ingredient cost of a drug,[17] pharmacists will have incentives to provide services in the most efficient manner—allowing pharmacists to counsel patients and technicians to label packages.

Only British Columbia and Manitoba currently have competitively set dispensing fees for purchases covered by provincial drug benefit plans. In both provinces, the consumers are responsible for a portion of the dispensing

---

17. To a large extent, the pharmacist's margin on ingredient sales determines the number of pharmacists in practice. Competition in services and dispensing fees will cause pharmacists to use their time so that the marginal cost of increasing services equals the marginal benefits of offering them. Because the total payment to the pharmacist is the sum of both the dispensing fee and the ingredient costs, high margins on ingredients result in lower dispensing fees, higher levels of service, and more retailers, all other things being equal. Low margins induce pharmacists to reduce service levels, raise dispensing fees, or leave the market (Morgan 1994).

fee through coinsurance, with annual consumer contribution limits.[18] Dispensing fees in these provinces range dramatically (from $1 in some B.C. pharmacies to over $10 in provinces such as Alberta and Nova Scotia), which is consistent with the theory that different retailers offer different levels of service. Moreover, B.C. and Manitoba have some of the lowest average dispensing fees in Canada (Crop Conseil 1995).

Drug Cost Reimbursement

In addition to the dispensing fee, pharmacists derive income from the retail margin on the cost of the drug. Different systems of reimbursement of drug costs are applied in different provinces. These range from auction-style standing offer contracts to the audit-oriented actual acquisition cost arrangement.

Reimbursement systems have two objectives. First, when a prescription may be filled from a range of interchangeable, competing products, reimbursement should reward the pharmacist for selecting the lowest-cost product. This should be a chemically equivalent generic version of a branded product. Recently, however, B.C. has broadened the definition of interchangeability by grouping selected products that have similar therapeutic effects but are not necessarily chemically equivalent.

The second objective of a reimbursement system is to ensure that the lowest possible price is paid for any product, regardless of interchangeability. Of course, this objective must be balanced against the pharmacist's reward— a suitable retailing margin.

The most common form of drug price reimbursement in Canada is the Best Available Price (BAP) model; variants are used in all provinces except Saskatchewan (Grootendorst et al. 1996; Crop Conseil 1995). In this system, the government publishes a formulary listing the BAP price per unit of each drug. This price is meant to reflect the lowest price for the drug, accounting for volume purchases and retailing margins. Among a group of interchangeable products, as defined by the formulary, the province pays the lowest BAP in the group. This encourages pharmacists to select the lowest-cost drug, while earning the spread between the BAP paid by the government and the wholesale cost of the drug dispensed. This form of reimbursement seems to control costs more effectively than acquisition cost reimbursement does (Grootendorst et al. 1996; Gorecki 1992).

---

18. The limit varies slightly from province to province. Consumers insured by Pharmacare in B.C. pay 100 percent of the dispensing fee, up to an annual maximum of $200. Manitoba drug benefit recipients pay all drug costs up to an annual limit of $129 and 30 percent of costs thereafter. One might expect more competition in dispensing fees in B.C., where they are a more significant portion of the consumer's annual contribution to drug costs. Evidence shows that the fees charged in B.C. are lower than fees in Manitoba (Crop Conseil 1995).

Strategies Aimed at Physicians

Physician Education and Training

Even with perfectly efficient retailing and price systems, current prescribing patterns would still create inefficiencies. Evidence suggests that over-prescribing, underprescribing, inappropriate prescribing, and inefficient prescribing all exist in Canada (Anderson and Lexchin 1996; Tamblyn and Perreault 1995).

A factor contributing to excessive and inappropriate prescribing is the physician's heavy reliance on commercial sources of information about the costs and benefits of drugs. Evidence shows that doctors who are high-volume prescribers rank commercial sources of information most highly (Denig and Haaijer-Ruskamp 1995). Moreover, few doctors in practice can find enough time to keep up-to-date on pharmacotherapy developments (Anderson and Lexchin 1996).

Several strategies have been employed to address this problem. Programs have been implemented to educate doctors about the appropriate use of certain drugs and the costs of various treatments. Methods include news-letters, educational conferences, physician report cards, teleconferences, seminars, and individual educational visits (Anderson and Lexchin 1996; Denig and Haaijer-Ruskamp 1995). The results of these programs are mixed. However, evidence suggests that the most effective educational programs are multidimensional, and include individual visits from specially trained pharmacists or physicians. These visits, called counter detailing or academic detailing, were found to be cost-effective education (Anderson and Lexchin 1996). Not only do these programs save money, they do so by improving quality of care.

Some researchers question the effectiveness of large-scale physician education programs (Tamblyn and Perreault 1995). To date, individual education programs have been very limited in scope. Most programs address treatment alternatives for only one condition (e.g., hypertension), or focus on the appropriate use of one class of drugs (e.g., NSAIDs). Although individually successful, when nonindustry efforts to educate doctors escalate, doctors could be overwhelmed.

The ultimate solution to improving prescribing patterns will probably involve stricter regulation of pharmaceutical marketing practices, increased professional information and decision support for physicians, and new incentives for physicians to prescribe appropriately and cost-effectively.

Strategies Aimed at Manufacturers

Patent Policy

Canada is unique in its attempts to control the price of drugs. Instead of regulating pharmaceutical prices, profits or both, as other developed countries have, Canada promoted competition from generic drugs through compulsory licensing of patented medicines.[19] This law has been a focal point for discussion of Canadian pharmaceutical policy for decades. It remains contentious as the amendments that removed the compulsory licensing provision from the Canadian Patent Act—contained in Bill C-91 1993—come up for review in 1997.

Compulsory licensing for drug patents has been a part of the Canadian Patent Act since 1923. The original compulsory licensing provision—section 41(3) of the Canadian Patent Act—permitted firms to apply for a license to manufacture and sell a patented drug before the expiry of its 17-year patent. Innovating firms could not legally block these licenses (hence, compulsory). Because a compulsory license would diminish the value of a patent, the Commissioner of Patents was responsible for setting licensing terms, such as royalties paid by the licensee, to provide the innovator with "due reward."

In its early stages, this provision of the Canadian Patent Act allowed the sale of patented drugs under compulsory license, provided that all manufacturing was done in Canada. The Commissioner of Patents had hoped that many firms would compete for market shares of the same drug, thereby lowering prices. However, the manufacturing of active pharmaceutical ingredients was (and remains) extremely capital intensive. Returns to scale made the production of fine chemicals unprofitable in markets as small as Canada. Thus, since few active chemical ingredients were produced in Canada, the early compulsory licensing program was ineffective; only 22 compulsory licenses were granted between 1923 and 1969 (Lexchin 1993a, 148).

During the early 1960s, many Canadians were concerned about the high cost of patented medicines. This prompted the government to amend the compulsory licensing provision in 1969 (Gorecki and Henderson 1981).

---

19. Canada's regulatory approval process for generic drugs was also designed to facilitate competition. Generic drug manufacturers need only prove that their drugs are bioequivalent to the innovator's drug. This shortens the regulatory approval process for generic drug manufacturers, compared with their innovative counterparts, by eliminating the need to repeat expensive, time-consuming clinical trials. Upon receipt of regulatory approval certifying equivalency, a generic drug manufacturer may then market the product as a low-cost alternative to a branded drug.

With the addition of section 41(4), the Canadian Patent Act permitted any firm to import patented drugs, including the active ingredients, for sale under compulsory license subject to a 4 percent royalty fee.

With permission to import ingredients for sale before patent expiry, marketing generic copies of brand-name drugs became a viable business. Many Canadian companies began to sell generic drugs under compulsory license shortly after the 1969 amendments were passed. Between 1969 and 1982, more than 290 compulsory licenses were issued in Canada, many of them for best-selling drugs—21 of the top 50 in January of 1983 (Gorecki 1987, 60).

Over the years that followed the 1969 amendments to the Canadian Patent Act, in conjunction with the growth of provincial drug benefit programs, provincial governments created incentives for pharmacists to dispense the least-costly drug in an interchangeable class. Provincial substitution schemes would usually result in the use of a generic drug when such was available. Together with the addition of section 41(4) of the Canadian Patent Act, these measures made compulsory licensing indisputably successful at reducing the costs of Canadian pharmaceuticals (Eastman 1985).

In the early 1980s, the federal government established the Commission of Inquiry on the Pharmaceutical Industry to review the industry's performance. It found that compulsory licensing had successfully reduced the costs of pharmaceuticals to varying degrees, depending on province and drug class, without seriously harming the profitability of pharmaceutical manufacturers (Eastman 1985). Eastman found that, for the five years preceding his review, the weighted average of research spending, promotional expenditure, and profits for 55 leading firms in Canada were approximately as follows:

R&D:	4.5 percent of sales
Profits:	15.0 percent of sales
Promotions:	21.0 percent of sales

More recent data show that the pharmaceutical industry had a return on equity among the top 20 industries in Canada from 1972 to 1987— holding first, second, or third position from 1983 to 1987 (Lexchin 1993a).

In his report, Eastman stressed that Canada is a small market for pharmaceuticals, and home to none of the major multinationals. He recognized that patent protection in Canada would have little or no effect on the global scale and scope of R&D. Compulsory licensing, therefore, would not affect the rate of new product development.

In some ways this was unfortunate. Eastman thought that reducing the incentive for redundant research was one of the greatest benefits of compulsory licensing, besides cost savings. The competition under compulsory licensing, with suitable royalty payments, would supplant competition based on me-too research. Rather than trying to innovate around a competitor's patent protection, other firms could enter pioneers' markets directly. Unfortunately, compulsory licensing would have to be applied globally for it to affect research incentives.

In conclusion, Eastman recommended maintaining compulsory licensing with only minor changes. Notably, Eastman recommended a waiting period of *up to four years* before granting compulsory licenses, and increasing royalty fees from 4 to 14 percent. In 1987, the government introduced Bill C-22, which would create similar provisions. Amendments to the Canadian Patent Act in Bill C-22 gave patentholding firms a seven-year period of exclusive market protection, commencing upon the patentholder's receipt of the Notice of Compliance (NOC).[20] Market exclusivity could be extended to 10 years if the generic drug manufacturer's active ingredients were not made in Canada. In 1987, Canadian patents were extended from 17 to 20 years. Since the time required to obtain an NOC was approximately seven to 10 years after patent approval, pharmaceutical patents subsequent to 1987 permitted compulsory licensing only during the last few years of a patent.

In 1992, the government created even greater barriers to entry by introducing Bill C-91, which once again changed the structure of the Canadian patent for pharmaceuticals. Rather than offering a period of market exclusivity followed by a period of generic competition under compulsory license, as provided in Bill C-22, Bill C-91 eliminated compulsory licensing entirely. When Bill C-91 was brought into effect in 1993, it retroactively eliminated compulsory licenses granted subsequent to December 20, 1991. Following the enactment of Bill C-91, patentholders would effectively receive 10 to 13 years of exclusive market protection with a single patent—depending on the time taken to obtain an NOC.[21]

Bill C-91 also contained regulations that link the Canadian Patent Act to the Food and Drugs Act. These provisions allow a patentholder to block the issue of an NOC for drugs that are alleged (by the patentholder) to

---

20. The Notice of Compliance is the final stamp of regulatory approval from the Drugs Directorate of Health Canada. The process for obtaining an NOC is very long, involving years of clinical trials, submission of volumes of data, and a lengthy review by the Drugs Directorate.

21. The effective patent protection for drugs in Canada may be extended further by laws permitting a company to file many patents for one product. A single product may have patents covering its chemical compound, its manufacturing process, and its therapeutic use. Generic competition may not enter until the expiry of the last relevant patent. Thus, if patents for therapeutic uses are applied for after the patent on the chemical entity, the patentee can enjoy more than 20 years of protection, or more than 10 to 13 years of exclusive market protection.

violate existing patents. Although competitors may still produce a patented drug for the purposes of clinical testing and production engineering, stockpiling of patented drugs—necessary for product launch—is impracticable until the NOC is issued. This delays generic competition by up to 30 months more, and has resulted in more than 90 court challenges since 1993 (Anderson et al. 1995; *Report on Business*, May 20, 1996, B1). The new legislation also prohibited the export of drugs that are still under patent in Canada. Since Canadian patents often expire after patents for the same product expire in other countries, this can seriously affect the global competitiveness of Canadian generic drug manufacturers. It has been suggested that these additional regulatory provisions to the Patent Act have caused major generic drug manufacturers to divert investment from Canada to countries such as the United States and Mexico (Anderson et al. 1995).

A celebrated justification for longer patent protection in Canada is that it will encourage research into new drugs and, consequently, more new medicines for Canadians. This would then lead to improved treatments for Canadians and, thus, improved health. However, as stressed by Eastman (1985), the pharmaceutical industry is global, and Canada is a minor player with relatively little R&D activity.[22] Decisions concerning the scale, scope, and location of R&D are made at the multinationals' headquarters according to global research agendas (Taggart 1991; Eden 1989). Commercially viable discoveries made by such companies are patented and marketed world-wide, regardless of the country of origin. Furthermore, multinationals are unlikely to restrict the entry of new products to Canada because innovation occurred elsewhere. Therefore, the availability of new drugs in Canada is independent of the level of research done in Canada. For these reasons, the improvement in health by way of pharmaceutical innovation cannot be considered a substantial benefit of abolishing Canada's compulsory licensing.

The government has argued that removing the compulsory licensing provision made the Canadian pharmaceutical industry more competitive in the global market (Government News Release, NR-10770\92-21). Officials argue that firms will now invest more in Canada, creating jobs in the industry, which is located predominantly in Ontario and Quebec.

---

22. For decades before Bill C-22 and Bill C-91, multinational firms invested less in R&D as a percentage of sales in Canada than in their host countries (RCHS 1964; Eastman 1985). Moreover, very little research conducted in Canada was basic, innovative R&D. Figures for 1994 indicate that patentholding firms in Canada still spend only 11 percent of sales on R&D (PMPRB, 1995)—far below an estimated 18 percent spent on average in the United States, the United Kingdom, Sweden, Switzerland, France, Germany, or Italy (Potashnik 1995). Furthermore, basic research accounts for only 2.3 percent of sales in Canada; the remainder of Canadian research is predominantly regulatory clinical trials.

Indeed, as of 1991, pharmaceutical manufacturers met their promise to spend 10 percent of sales on R&D (Lexchin 1993a), but they have failed to create as many jobs as promised. Initially, multinational firms were to create "3000 scientific and research-related jobs" as a reward for Bill C-22 (Lexchin 1993a, 152). Lexchin (1993a) showed that, up to 1990, only about 150 jobs were created annually—far short of the more than 300 jobs per year needed to meet initial promises. More recent Statistics Canada data show that the total number of persons engaged in pharmaceutical R&D rose by approximately 1,300 person-years (from 900 to 2,231) between 1987 and 1993 (Statistics Canada 1987–1995).

Not only does the industry appear to be far below targeted employment growth, the jobs that have been created have come at a substantial cost. Extending longer patent protection is a decision made by the federal government which, in effect, bribes multinational firms to locate more R&D in Canada. The cost of "creating" related jobs is borne by the provincial governments and individual consumers. (In spite of the fact that the federal government played down its "costs", Bill C-22 provided $100 million in cash compensation to the provinces. This indicates that the federal government expected that public pharmaceutical benefits would rise significantly. It offered no compensation for cash-paying or privately insured consumers.) The questions that remain for the 1997 review of Bill C-91 are: How much did this amendment truly cost Canadians?; is this cost justified?; who bears this cost?; and who benefits from it?

Price Controls

Many believe that pharmaceutical costs can be controlled by controlling the price of drugs. Although this assumption ignores the importance of drug utilization, many countries employ price controls regulated by their national governments. Countries that use product-by-product price control include Australia, Belgium, Luxembourg, France, Greece, Italy, Portugal, and Spain (Gross et al. 1996; Federal/Provincial Task Force 1992).

Price controls are employed by governments as an attempt to counter some of the market power of pharmaceutical manufacturers. It is, however, questionable whether price controls have been successful in many countries. The trouble arises when regulatory bodies are subject to conflicting pressures from pharmaceutical manufacturers and from those who pay for their products. Governments who regulate prices are subject to intense pressure from manufacturers to allow "adequate" markups on drugs to reward their research and development. With the economic interests of domestic pharmaceutical sectors at stake in negotiations with multinational pharmaceutical companies, few governments are willing to apply intense countervailing pressure on these companies.

In most cases (except Australia, for example), the agency responsible for regulating pharmaceutical prices is not directly responsible for the cost of drugs purchased. Even when governments do pay for significant portions of drug costs, the price regulation is typically independent of the pharmaceutical insuring agency (as is the case in Canada). Thus, the cost of allowable price increases is off-loaded, in part or entirely, onto others. This is true of most forms of price regulation: negotiators independent of the market transaction are, in effect, bargaining with other people's money.

To justify allowable prices for new drugs, many countries use international price comparisons to determine what is a "reasonable" price. In Canada, regulations of the Patented Medicine Prices Review Board stipulate that introductory (factory-gate) prices of "breakthrough" drugs may not exceed the median of the prices of the drug in seven foreign markets: France, Germany, Italy, Switzerland, Sweden, the United Kingdom, and the United States. Due to the fact that multinational pharmaceutical companies exercise considerable market power *worldwide,* meeting the pricing standards of foreign markets creates a false sense of price control. Because of the politics of the industry, few regulators have demanded lower domestic prices than those abroad, leaving providers of drug benefits (private and public) to seek their own price discounts.

Canada is a case in point. Canada imposes factory-gate price controls on individual products through the Patented Medicine Prices Review Board (the Review Board). The Review Board, however, has quasi-judicial authority only over patented medicines; this excludes all nonpatented drugs, generic drugs marketed under compulsory license, and (until recently) products for which the patent has been dedicated.[23] In total, the Review Board has regulated about 3 percent of all pharmaceutical products, which represents about 40 percent of all sales by dollar volume (indicative of the prominent role played by new, patented drugs) (PMPRB 1995,1996a). The principal mandate of the Review Board is to ensure that factory-gate prices of patented medicines in Canada are not "excessive." The Review Board applies different standards for determining maximum allowable introductory prices, depending on the drug's classification (table 1).[24] The Review Board limits price increases of existing drugs to changes in the consumer price index for

---

23. To dedicate a patent is to abdicate the property rights conferred by it before expiry. Since, until recently, the Review Board did not monitor the price of drugs with dedicated patents, nor the research activity of their manufacturers, some companies dedicate their patents to avoid regulation.

24. The geometric price/quantity rules for establishing "nonexcessive" introductory prices used by the Review Board are unique to Canada. Anis and Wen (1996) argue that they are potentially subject to "gaming," but may nonetheless limit introductory prices of new drugs.

Canada.[25] Recently, the Review Board has reported estimates showing significant reductions in the rate of increase of factory-gate prices of patented drugs, compared to what might have occurred if Bills C-22 and C-91 had eliminated compulsory licensing without introducing price regulations.

Before the Review Board came into existence, Canada used competitive forces—through compulsory licensing of drug patents—to control prices (Lexchin 1993a). Because private competition is not subject to the political influence of multinational companies, this policy drove average prices down by introducing low-cost alternatives to branded drugs. On the other hand, the Review Board was established as a political compromise during the removal of the compulsory licensing. The very purpose of the legislation that removed the compulsory licensing provision was to raise the cost of drugs in Canada—thereby increasing the profits of patentholding firms and, supposedly, creating incentive for innovation. These conflicting interests were, therefore, apparent from the very formation of Canada's Review Board.

The Review Board originally reported to the Minister of Consumer and Corporate Affairs Canada, Industry Canada, making it potentially vulnerable—during, for example, the process of developing its guidelines and standards in consultation with industry stakeholders—to the political influence of multinational drug companies. It was never apparent that a price regulator under Industry Canada was the best guardian of health care consumers' (and payers') interests. Later, with the passage of Bill C-91, the Review Board was moved under the jurisdiction of the federal Minister of Health, who bears a closer (although imperfect) relationship to the payers for drugs. This shift is indicative of a change in the federal government's priorities concerning drug price regulation.

The potential efficacy of the Review Board has been more limited than it might have been, since its mandate is to review only the factory-gate price of patented medicines. Retail prices, which include retailer and wholesaler markups, and prices of nonpatented drugs are not regulated by the Review Board. As shown in figure 3, the consumer price index for all pharmaceuticals has outpaced the Review Board's index of regulated factory-gate prices.[26]

---

25. That the Patent Act requires the Review Board to use the CPI to limit factory-gate prices is intriguing. Other factory-gate indices exist, such as the Industrial Product Price Index (IPPI) which has remained below the CPI in most years since 1987.

26. Controversy over inherent biases in pharmaceutical price indexes is acknowledged. For a discussion of the difficulty constructing an accurate index of drug prices, the interested reader should see Bernt, Griliches, and Rosett (1993) and Griliches and Cockburn (1994). For present purposes, the consumer and industrial indexes are used to show differences between consumer and factory prices.

Figure 3

Pharmaceutical and general price indexes for Canada

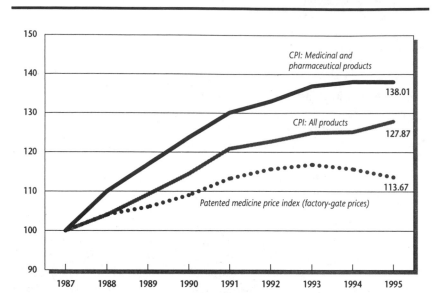

CPI: Medicinal and pharmaceutical products
138.01

CPI: All products
127.87

113.67

Patented medicine price index (factory-gate prices)

Sources: Statistics Canada (Labels: P490000, P800202), PMPRB (1996).

This evidence suggests that, although the Review Board may be limiting the growth in factory-gate prices of patented drugs, it has limited impact on the overall price of medicines in Canada.

One factor that diminished the control of the Review Board was patent dedication. Many patentholding firms have opted to dedicate their patents to avoid the Review Board. From 1969 to 1987, only two pharmaceutical patents were dedicated in Canada, whereas, from 1987 to 1994, more than 400 pharmaceutical patents were dedicated (Elgie 1995). This indicates that, for some products, the Review Board is a credible threat to price gouging. However, prior to 1995, once a product's patent was dedicated, the Review Board had no jurisdiction over its price, and payers were left to control the price of these products.[27] To counter this trend, the Review Board's jurisdiction has now been extended to include products with dedicated patents (Elgie 1995; PMPRB 1996a)—also indicative of a more aggressive stance on price regulation at the federal level.

---

27. For products with few competitors within their therapeutic class, this move could be highly profitable. Provided that a firm does not believe that generic competitors are ready to enter the market quickly, one route to high prices seems to be patent dedication.

It may be argued that most control of retail drug prices in Canada comes from the efforts of provincial drug benefits providers. Ministries of health in provinces across Canada have long insured segments of the population against the cost of prescription (and limited nonprescription) drugs in the ambulatory setting. Managers of benefits for these programs have developed various generic substitution laws, drug price reimbursement schemes (discussed above), formularies, and other mechanisms to control the cost of drugs provided under their plans. In effect, these government agencies use their concentrated buying power (monopsony power) to partially countervail the monopoly power of patentholding drug companies. In fact, provincial drug benefits providers are often stricter price regulators than the Review Board: just because the Review Board has not found a drugs price to be "excessive" does not mean that provinces will accept that drug into their formularies without further price concessions. The effect of the Ontario Drug Benefit formulary, for example, has been recognized by domestic and foreign researchers alike. Both Gross et al. (1996) and the USGAO (1992) found evidence consistent with the view that the ODB formulary was complimentary to the Review Board's regulations, contributing to the containment of retail drug prices.

If price regulation is going to be a more effective component of pharmaceutical policy, it must be integrated and complete. An integrated price regulator recognizes that the price of drugs is only one component of expenditure, the other being utilization, and that drugs are just one of many inputs into health care. An integrated regulator should *not* be independent of the market transaction. Ideally, a regulator would negotiate as a buyer of pharmaceutical products, with the objective of purchasing the most cost-effective pharmaceuticals subject to the real financial constraints of the system. Price regulation should also be complete, covering all products and all consumers. Gaps in the jurisdiction of a regulator will produce financial incentive to market the least-regulated products, not the most effective. Finally, given the global nature of the industry, with the widespread experience of expenditure escalation, domestic regulators must be willing to make honest appraisals regarding the trade-off between lower costs for pharmaceuticals and the multinational industry's location of R&D activities in Canada. Recent changes in the jurisdiction and powers of the Review Board indicate that Canada is moving toward greater price control. To be more effective, however, Canada's price regulator should regulate the (average) *retail* price of *all* pharmaceutical products, employ stricter standards for introductory prices and year-over-year price changes, and bear a closer relationship with the payers for pharmaceuticals, such as the provincial ministries of health.

Restrictions on Advertising

Drug companies spend between 15 and 20 percent of total sales on marketing and promotional activities in Canada, the United States, and elsewhere (Lexchin 1994; Drake and Uhlman 1993; Eastman 1985). Based on Canadian factory-gate sales of $6 billion, this implies that approximately $900 million was spent on pharmaceutical marketing in Canada in 1995.

Pharmaceutical manufacturers are noted for employing unique and sometimes controversial forms of marketing (Bleidt 1992a). For prescription drugmakers, marketing efforts do not typically target the consumer. Instead, companies target the much smaller and easily identifiable audience of physicians, the only licensed prescribers of their products. Most marketing expenditures go to sales representatives, or detailers (Lexchin 1989).

Expenditure on marketing is not wasted. Multinational drug manufacturers, who pour billions into these efforts every year, must know that their marketing programs result in more prescribing and, thus, sales (Lexchin 1989, 1994; Bleidt 1992b). From a business perspective, advertising and promotional activities are essential for profitability and survival. It has been argued that marketing is a cornerstone of private enterprise, including the pharmaceutical industry. Marketing is said to increase social welfare by bringing together individuals and groups for voluntary transactions that would not otherwise occur (Bleidt 1992b). There are, however, reasons why the generation of social welfare by *some forms* of advertising in the pharmaceutical industry is not obvious.

> In the real world of pharmaceutical promotion and medication use, the main assumptions of the social exchange perspective [on advertising] may not be valid. Patients often do not act rationally in making decisions to use medications. Consumers involved in self-care and self-medication usually are not aware of all treatment options in choosing their therapy. Prescribers of drug therapies, dominated by the Western biomedical approach to medicine, rarely know or discuss alternative healing models and nontraditional forms of therapy. Access to sufficient amounts of high-quality, objective drug information is limited or controlled by the drug producers (Montagne 1992, 197).

Pharmaceutical promotion in Canada is controlled by two codes of practice: the voluntary code of the Pharmaceutical Manufacturers' Association of Canada (PMAC), and the code of the Pharmaceutical Advertising Advisory Board (PAAB). Although in place since 1966, the PMAC guidelines have limited effect because they are optional and vague (Lexchin 1994). The PAAB was formed in 1975, partly in response to criticisms of marketing behaviour covered by the PMAC's "Principals and Code of Marketing Practice." The PAAB is not a government agency; it is made up of representatives of the PMAC, the Canadian Drug Manufacturers

Association (CDMA) (generic manufacturers), medical and pharmacy associations, consumers' associations, and Health Canada. The PAAB code of marketing practices covers both the print media and, since 1993, the electronic media.

Despite these codes of practice, concerns about the advertising and promotion of drugs in Canada still exist. Ideally, the promotional activities of drug companies would lead to better prescribing and self-medication practices by informing physicians and consumers about drugs and giving them complete, unbiased information concerning all benefits and risks of these therapies when compared with alternative treatments. This effect is seldom achieved through current marketing practices in Canada and elsewhere. Take, for example, print media targeting prescribing physicians. Drug companies spend millions of dollars on advertising in Canadian medical and pharmacy journals each year (Lexchin 1994). The image and text content of these full-page, glossy advertisements associates brand names with therapeutic benefits that sometimes exceed the clinical benefits of the advertised drug (Lexchin 1994; Wivell and O'Fallan 1992).

> Prescribing information usually does not accompany an ad, but is placed toward the end of the journal, a practice that is allowed by the [PAAB] code. In [a] 1991 survey [of 111 advertisements in professional journals] ... prescribing information was adjacent to the advertisement only 18 percent of the time. Following the editorial copy, the *Canadian Medical Association Journal* invariably contains 30 or so consecutive pages of small-print prescribing information for multiple drugs advertised elsewhere in the journal. Grouping the prescribing information in such a manner and using six-point or seven-point type size leads to doctors just skipping over these pages (Lexchin 1994, 94).

Does this practice improve prescribing or increase it? Moreover, although drug companies claim that detailers are educators who disseminate important information to doctors, detailers' principal function is to get doctors to prescribe their companies' products. Joel Lexchin (1993b, and 1989) has shown that, in Canada and elsewhere, the profit motives of manufacturers outweigh educational considerations when physicians contact pharmaceutical companies through detailers and company-sponsored seminars. Society could be paying a high price in overprescribing as a result of manufacturers misinforming, underinforming, or confusing physicians with questionable marketing.

Some may argue that this problem could be solved by limiting expenditure for marketing pharmaceuticals. Indeed, some promotional techniques should be limited or prohibited. However, this applies to specific activities that yield little more than brand loyalty, and do not improve physicians' scientific knowledge of alternative therapies. Limiting advertising expenditure may reduce problems, but will not eliminate them. Manufacturers will still have financial incentives to engage most vigorously in the activities that increase sales most, not necessarily the activities that improve prescribing most. Detailers concentrate their promotional activities on doctors who prescribe the most frequently, which indicates the incentive in this type of marketing (Comanor 1986; Lexchin 1989).

To ensure that marketing *improves* prescribing and self-medication in Canada, the government should make codes of conduct much stricter, with severe penalties for violations. Lexchin (1994) argued that a powerful, independent body could take more control over marketing practices. He suggests that government regulatory agencies are too easily influenced by major stakeholders and program administrators. Furthermore, Lexchin concludes that "…it is not possible to adequately regulate promotion through voluntary control, whether exercised by the industry or an outside body" (100).

Establishing an independent body with legislative authority to control advertising and promotion may improve prescribing in Canada. To ensure that doctors receive high-quality information about alternative drug treatments, therapeutics initiatives such as the one established in B.C. could provide practicing physicians with scientific information, assembled and evaluated by medical and pharmacy professionals. This could be achieved through newsletters and academic detailing. The desired result is to shift the basis of prescribing in Canada to medical and pharmacological science and away from marketing.

Systemic Strategies

Universal Drug Insurance

Pharmaceuticals have traditionally been left outside universal public health coverage in Canada, but they are a significant input to formal health care, the cost of which has grown faster than the cost of universally insured components of health care. Many developed countries offer universal or near-universal public pharmaceutical insurance, albeit with significant copayments in most cases. Table 2 shows estimated percentages of the populations covered by public prescription drug insurance, the percentage of payments covered by these government drug plans, and public pharmaceutical expenditures as a percentage of total expenditures in 22 OECD countries. As can be seen from this table, although Canada offers universal public health insurance, Canada has less public pharmaceutical coverage than most OECD countries. Fewer Canadians are covered by public drug plans, those covered pay more out-of-pocket and, as a result, the public share of total pharmaceutical expenditures is lower in Canada than in most other OECD countries.

Table 2

Public pharmaceutical insurance coverage in OECD countries

Country	Percentage of population covered by public plans	Percentage of beneficiaries costs covered by public plans	Public share of national pharmaceutical expenditures
Netherlands	100	91.2	91.2
United Kingdom	100	90	64.3
Luxembourg	100	84	–
Greece	100	74	–
Sweden	100	70.8	70.8
Iceland	100	68	66.1
Italy	100	65	41.0
Portugal	100	65	62.5
New-Zealand	100	64	–
Norway	100	58	–
Australia	100	47	–
Finland	100	45	45.6
Denmark	100	45	51.1
Switzerland	99.5	48	–
Spain	99.3	75	–
Austria	99	49	64.3
France	98	54	61.0
Belgium	94	50	45.3
Germany	92.2	48	–
Ireland	40	61	–
Canada	21 (44*)	33	31.9
United States	12	25	12.7

Source: OECD Health Care Data, 1996.

*Revised figure using other sources (Crop Conseil 1995). (OECD figures for Canadian public drug plan terms are believed to be low due to deductibles, copayments, and the inclusion of OTC products. Terms of specific plans covering the elderly and those on social assistance are much higher.)

Universal drug coverage was first proposed by the 1964 Hall Commission, but was not included in the Medical Care Act of 1968. Twenty years ago, Evans and Williamson (1978) investigated the merits of a universal Pharmacare program in Canada; however, until quite recently, little attention was paid to this idea. Today's high drug costs have encouraged some provinces to consider universal insurance as a way to ensure access to drugs while expanding government cost containment initiatives.

Because reliance upon the pharmaceutical component of health care has risen steadily since the introduction of universal health coverage in Canada, some question whether access to "needed" pharmacotherapy differs from access to nondrug treatments. In the absence of cross-subsidies created by the public pharmaceutical insurance, the people most likely to incur costs (the elderly, for example) may not be able to afford either drugs or insurance coverage. Testament to this is the fact that all provincial governments have insurance programs for people at greatest risk of high drug costs and people least able to pay.

The existing system of drug coverage for selected populations may seem to reduce the need for public insurance. Yet, because pharmaceutical costs are increasing steadily, nearly 50 percent of Canadians have chosen some kind of private drug insurance (Crop Conseil 1995), indicating that consumers think insurance benefits are worth the administration costs. However, there are significant inequities in the distribution of pharmaceutical insurance coverage. A survey conducted in 1995 indicated that nearly 75 percent of Canadians with more than $60,000 in annual income had some form of private drug coverage. Private coverage decreased proportionately with income: 68 percent of families with incomes between $40,000 and $59,000 had some private drug coverage, 35 percent of those with annual incomes between $20,000 and $39,999 had coverage, and only 7 percent of those with less than $20,000 in annual income had coverage (CROP survey cited in Crop Conseil 1995).

Although some statistics may report that public coverage in Canada is rising quickly, much of the growth is due to the implementation of universal provincial drug plans with very high deductibles. These "catastrophic drug cost" insurance programs are doubtlessly beneficial to Canadians with high-cost pharmacotherapeutic needs. Nevertheless, reporting that all residents of provinces with these plans are covered by public insurance may overstate the impact of these programs. Lexchin (1996) found that although the implementation of public pharmaceutical insurance plans since the 1960s has reduced the out-of-pocket drug costs for low-income Canadians, higher-income groups still have lower out-of-pocket drug expenses per capita, largely due to lower needs and private insurance. Out-of-pocket drug costs per capita as a percentage of total household expenditures for low-income groups is seven times that of high-income families (Lexchin 1996).

These findings indicate that pharmaceutical insurance in Canada is increasingly like health insurance in the United States, where middle- to low-income people fall through the cracks between the public and private insurance systems. A universal pharmaceutical insurance system would remove these inequities.

In addition to equity considerations, a universal, publicly funded pharmaceutical insurance system will improve the efficiency of the pharmaceutical component of the health care sector. This was deemed a necessary objective in Quebec's recent proposal for universal drug insurance (Castonguay et al. 1996). Lower administrative costs is an obvious benefit of a universal public plan. Many firms offer pharmaceutical coverage through group and individual plans, and the administration costs of this system could be drastically reduced by having consolidated drug plans administered by the provinces rather than small plans administered by small companies. Although the Castonguay report on insurance options for Quebec (Castonguay et al. 1996) recommended mixing private and public administration to preserve private sector jobs, this option proved too costly. In a wholly public system, the government estimates that administration costs would account for 3.7 percent of total program expenses, nearly half the private insurers' estimate for administration costs (*Globe and Mail,* June 11, 1996, B6). Furthermore, the cost of Canada's current private insurance system is already a public burden because employers can write off expenditures on health benefits made on behalf of their employees (tax expenditure subsidies). The real cost of the current system is, therefore, often underestimated.

Financing for universal public drug insurance would probably come, in part, from general tax revenues. This could result in a progressive financing arrangement, which may be desirable. Some may advocate the use of earmarked taxes or Pharmacare premiums. These financing systems, although appealing in principle, would needlessly increase the cost of revenue collection relative to tax financing.

Some argue that the public burden of a universal system could be reduced by cost sharing and deductibles. Castonguay and associates (1996) advocate a system of coinsurance, deductibles, and yearly contribution limits much like the Manitoba system (Crop Conseil 1995). All individuals whose benefits exceeded their deductible, which could vary according to age or income, would be covered for a portion of their drug expenses. Such consumers would be responsible for 25 percent of drug costs until their annual contribution limit was met. Thereafter, they would be fully insured. In addition to lowering the total public cost of the system, Castonguay and associates note that coinsurance encourages consumers to seek generic alternatives and to "question in more detail the merits of the simultaneous consumption of several drugs" (55). As mentioned above, the assumptions underlying the efficiency incentive of cost sharing on drugs do not necessarily hold: most often—and for good reason—the decision maker is the health professional, not the consumer. Moreover, building a system with deductibles that are too high may not prevent consumers from seeking supplementary private insurance, thus forsaking the basic goal of administrative efficiency.

The necessary assumptions for the efficiency argument supporting cost sharing may, however, hold for the choice of retail outlet. Consumers can make informed decisions about where to purchase drugs by weighing the dispensing fee against their desired level of service and convenience. Furthermore, given that dispensing fees accounted for an estimated 25 percent of privately funded drug costs in Canada in 1994 (GHM 1995), 100 percent coinsurance on this portion of total costs would have the desired effect on program expenses and would probably improve efficiency in the retail sector (Evans and Williamson 1978; Morgan 1994).

That is, consumers would be responsible for 25 percent of existing program expenses and, as a result of the forces of competition, the long-run cost to consumers may decline relative to what is paid in dispensing fees today. The government would be left to increase the efficiency—lower prices and improve prescribing—of the ingredient portion of retail pharmaceutical costs.

Although the public share of costs can be expected to rise when universal coverage begins, the overall system costs could decline significantly over time. A single payer for ingredient costs will have enormous buying power, will be able to track drug usage, and can coordinate cost containment efforts. Evidence of the superior benefits management of large buyers comes from recent experience. Economies of scale result from increased bargaining power, reduced administration costs, and efficiencies in services such as mail-order pharmacy. The major benefits managers in the United States—Medco, Diversified Pharmaceutical, and PCS—covered more than 30 million, 13 million, and 50 million consumers respectively in 1994 (*Wall Street Journal*, July 12, 1995, A3). Large pharmaceutical benefits managers like these are credited with slowing the growth of U.S. drug expenditure (Levit et al. 1994). In Canada, provinces have recently been more successful than the private sector in slowing the growth of public expenditure (figure 1).

By expanding coverage to the whole population, further efficiencies may be achieved in the public management of pharmaceutical benefits. To attain significant savings, program administrators must be proactive on benefits management. As with Lexchin's (1994) concerns regarding the regulation of advertisement, the effectiveness of government administration could be influenced by stakeholders and party politics, and by the ideology of program administrators.[28] If an independent body cannot be established to run a public system at arm's length from provincial ministries of health,

---

28. Take, for example, the Pharmacare program in B.C. Since Michael Corbeil became the executive director of Pharmacare, initiatives on drug cost reimbursement and reference-based pricing have been swiftly implemented (e.g., see Grootendorst et al. 1996), indicating a willingness to endure a legal and political backlash from industry. Corbeil's administration recently won a precedent-setting court case regarding reference-based pricing, leading the way for other provinces (*Globe and Mail*, June 4, 1996, A6).

current administrators will need encouragement to continue representing the interests of patients and payers vigorously.

Global Budgets

A benefits management technique that a single payer for pharmaceuticals could apply is a global budgeting scheme. Like the current global budgets for physicians' services, a global pharmaceutical budget would stipulate the maximum allowable expenditure on pharmaceuticals for each province. Physicians, who are in charge of prescribing, would be responsible for ensuring that this budget was not exceeded. Tying the pharmaceutical budget in each province to the physicians' budgets would encourage doctors to allocate expenditure for drugs and other health care inputs as efficiently as possible.

Germany has used this system since 1993. The German program included a threat to reduce physicians' incomes by a maximum of 2 percent if drug expenditure exceeded the limit. In January 1993, the first month of the program, prescribing declined by 26.5 percent, compared with January 1992. When Munnich and Sullivan (1994) reviewed the German program, they found that, in 15 of the 16 months between January 1993 and April 1994, expenditure on pharmaceuticals remained below limits. Some have criticized this program on the grounds that patients with high drug costs may have been referred to hospitals where drugs are paid for through other budgets (Schoffski 1996). If implemented in Canada, a mixed global budgeting system would need mechanisms to prevent off-loading of costly drug therapies to hospitals.

On-Line Pharmaceutical Information Systems

If physicians are to choose the most effective and economical therapies available, they must have new information sources. For example, the United Kingdom recently experimented with Prodigy, a computerized information system for physicians (*Lancet*, April 27, 1996; editorial). Prodigy contained information collected by a panel of medical professionals and pharmacists from clinical trial data originating with sources such as the Cochrane Collaboration. Prodigy provided treatment options for specific diagnoses based on the patient's history, and several drug choices listed by generic name, with the best available price. In Canada, a universal system of health and pharmaceutical coverage would provide the ideal databases for such a program.

The database and networking technologies necessary to implement such a computerized information system exist in some provinces today. Linked or linkable medical and pharmaceutical databases are now available for administrative and research purposes in all provinces in Canada (Anis et al. 1996). An office-based computer system would be the most costly stage of program implementation that remains.

If such a system is to work successfully in Canada, it must be designed in cooperation with medical professionals. Physicians' input should be sought throughout the design and implementation phases so the system meets their needs and is user friendly. The system will not succeed if practicing physicians do not like it. However, input from the pharmaceutical industry should be sought with caution; U.S. manufacturers already use computerized networks to monitor physicians' prescribing patterns and promote their products (Wivell and O'Fallon 1992). As with the regulation of marketing practices, on-line information systems should exist to facilitate prescribing by improving accepted medical and pharmacological knowledge, not to advance the marketing objectives of manufacturers.

CONCLUSION

A paper of this type does not readily lend itself to conclusions. The purpose of this paper was to lay out several issues facing pharmaceutical policymakers in Canada, not to resolve any specific issues. Consequently, the conclusions of this paper come in the form of recommendations for future research and evaluation.

It would be easy to advise governments to investigate more thoroughly each topic discussed in this paper; they are all fascinating from economic, social, and political standpoints. The following points concern areas where the government could make the greatest impact on the structure and conduct of the pharmaceutical component of Canada's health care system.

- Evidence discussed above indicates that prescribing in Canada is based substantially on commercial information. Prescribing patterns and marketing practices raise concerns about the quality of information physicians receive. The government should investigate ways to restructure the regulation of pharmaceutical marketing practices. Combined with increased professional information support for practicing physicians, this can improve health care significantly, and reduce costs substantially.
- The Canadian government will probably be unable to revive compulsory licensing. From an international political standpoint, this unique feature of Canadian pharmaceutical policy appears to be dead; therefore, policymakers should investigate ways to increase the use of generic drugs upon patent expiry and forestall development of costly me-too products through pharmacist reimbursement incentives and reference-based pricing systems.
- Given the upcoming review of Bill C-91, federal and provincial ministries of health, consumer groups, and private drug benefits providers should seek a detailed review of its regulatory provisions. Although the removal of compulsory licensing will not, unfortunately, be reversed, other regu-

lations that prevent immediate access to generic drugs upon the expiry of a single patent could be revoked.

- Finally, Canada should be moving toward universal drug insurance. This may improve access to care while reducing the total cost of the pharmaceutical component of Canada's health care system. The study of the appropriate implementation of such policies is encouraged. Attention should be paid to reducing barriers to needed care, managing benefits, and integrating pharmaceuticals with other components of health care. Particular caution should be taken when consumers are made responsible for drug costs (as opposed to dispensing fees) on the assumption that such arrangements lead to efficient product selection. The impact of new financial incentives (e.g., global budgeting) and remuneration mechanisms (e.g., capitation) for physicians should also be investigated in this regard.

It is hoped that this paper has brought to light some of the economic incentives and constraints that have shaped the pharmaceutical industry and have, in some cases, impeded policy change.

Steven G. Morgan *is a doctoral student at the University of British Columbia, specializing in health economics and industrial organization. He holds degrees from the University of Western Ontario and Queen's University. His primary area of research interest is pharmaceutical policy, in which he has conducted research for private and public agencies including the Queen's Health Policy Research Unit, and the Centre for Health Services and Policy Research UBC.*

BIBLIOGRAPHY

ANDERSON, G. M., and J. N. LAVIS. 1994. *Prescription Drug Use in the Elderly: Expenditures and Patterns of Use Under Ontario and British Columbia Provincial Drug Benefit Programs.* Queen's-University of Ottawa Press.

ANDERSON, G. M., and J. LEXCHIN. 1996. Strategies for improving prescribing practice. *Canadian Medical Association Journal* 154(7): 1013–1017.

ANDERSON, M., C. BOLTON, J. GORDON, S. MORGAN, and B. PAZDERKA. 1995. *Competition and the Pharmaceutical Value Chain: Competitive Issues in the Over-the-Counter and Generic Drug Segments of the Canadian Pharmaceutical Industry.* (A study commissioned by Industry Canada.) Queen's Health Policy: Queen's University, Kingston.

ANIS, A. H., and Q. WEN. 1996. *Price Regulation of Pharmaceuticals in Canada.* Working Paper. Centre for Health Services and Policy Research. University of British Columbia.

ANIS, A. H., G. CARRUTHERS, A. CARTER, and J. KIERULF. 1996. Variability in prescription drug utilization: Issues of research. *Canadian Medical Association Journal* 154(5): 635–640.

BALLANCE, R. H. 1996. Market and industry structure. In *Contested Ground: Public Purpose and Private Interest in the Regulation of Prescription Drugs,* ed. P. DAVIS. New York (NY): Oxford University Press.

BARER, M. L., R. G. EVANS, and C. HERTZMAN. 1995. Avalanche or glacier?: Health care and the demographic rhetoric. *Canadian Journal on Aging* 14(2): 193–224.

BERNDT, E. R., Z. GRILICHES, and J. G. ROSETT. 1993. Auditing the Producer Price Index: Micro evidence from prescription pharmaceutical preparations. *Journal of Business and Economic Statistics* 11(2): 251–264.

BERO, L .A., and D. R. DRUMMOND. 1996. Influences on the quality of published drug studies. *International Journal of Technology Assessment in Health Care* 12(2): 209–237.

BERO, L. A., and D. RENNIE. 1996. Influences on the quality of published drug studies. *International Journal of Technology Assessment in Health Care* (12(2): 209–237.

BLEIDT, B. 1992a. Recent issues and concerns about pharmaceutical industry promotional efforts. *Journal of Drug Issues* 22(2): 407–415.

_____. 1992b. Marketing activities: The keystone of capitalism—Increasing the availability of prescription drugs through pharmaceutical promotion. *Journal of Drug Issues* 22(2): 277–293.

BOSANQUET, N., and J. ZAMMIT-LUCIA. 1995. The effect of competition on drug prices. *Pharmaco-Economics* 8(6): 473–478.

Canadian Institute for Health Information (CIHI). 1996. *CANADIAN HEALTH EXPENDITURES.* Tables and figures made available on request.

CASTONGUAY, C., L. BORGEAT, L. CHAMPIGNY-ROBILLARD, D. LECLERC, and Y. MORIN. 1996. *Drug Insurance: Possible Approaches.* Report of the Committee of Experts on Drug Insurance. Bibliothèque nationale du Québec.

CAVES, R. E., M. D. WHINSTON, and M. A. HURWITZ. 1991. Patent expiration, entry, and competition in the U.S. pharmaceutical industry. *Brookings Papers: Microeconomics.* 1–66.

CHILES, V. 1995. Drug claims costs: A green shield Canada study. *Canadian Pharmaceutical Journal,* November: 37–43.

COAMBS, R. B., P. JENSEN, M. HAO HER, B. S. FERGUSON, J. L. JARRY, J. S. WONG, and R. V. ABRAHAMSOHN. 1995. *Review of the Literature on the Prevalence, Consequences, and Health Costs of Noncompliance and Inappropriate Use of Prescription Medication in Canada.* Prepared for the Pharmaceutical Manufacturers Association of Canada. University of Toronto Press.

COMANOR, W. S. 1986. The political economy of the pharmaceutical industry. *Journal of Economic Literature* 24(3): 1178–1217.

COOPER, M. H. 1966. *Prices and Profits in the Pharmaceutical Industry.* London: Pergamon Press.

COULSON, N. E., and B. C. STUART. 1995. Insurance choice and the demand for prescription drugs. *Southern Economic Journal* 61(4): 1146–1157.

CROP CONSEIL. 1995. *Drug Benefit Programs in Canada.*

DARBOURNE, A. 1993. OTC switching—pricing in a profitable market. *Scrip Magazine*, December: 14–16.

DENIG, P., and F. M. HAAIJER-RUSKAMP. 1995. Do physicians take costs into account when making prescribing decisions? *PharmacoEconomics* 8(4): 282–290.

DRAKE, D., and M. UHLMAN. 1993. *Making Medicine, Making Money.* Kansas (OK): Universal Press Syndicate.

EASTMAN, H.C. 1985. Report of the Commission of Inquiry on the Pharmaceutical Industry. Ottawa (ON): Supply and Services Canada.

EDEN, L. 1989. *Compulsory Licensing and Canadian Pharmaceutical Policy. International Business in Canada: Strategies for Management.* Ed. A. RUGHMAN. Scarborough: Prentice-Hall.

EGAN, J. W., H. N. HIGINBOTHAM, and J. F. WESTON. 1982. *Economics of the Pharmaceutical Industry.* New York (NY): Praeger.

ELGIE, R. G. 1995. Paper presented at C-PIC 1995. Canada's Pharmaceutical Industry Conference, Toronto.

EVANS, R. G. 1995. Manufacturing consensus, marketing truth: Guidelines for economic evaluation. *Annals of Internal Medicine* 123(1): 59–60.

EVANS, R. G., and M. F. WILLIAMSON. 1978. *Extending Canadian Health Insurance: Options for Pharmacare and Denticare.* Ontario Economic Council. Toronto (ON): University of Toronto Press.

FEDERAL/PROVINCIAL TASK FORCE. 1995. International models to influence pharmaceutical prices. Unpublished report to the Conference of Deputy Ministers of Health.

GHERSON, G. 1991. Patent protection issue heats up again despite success of Bill C-22. *Canadian Medical Association Journal* 145(2): 141–144.

GORECKI, P. 1984. Changing Canada's Drug Patent Law: The Minister's proposals. *Canadian Public Policy* 10: 77–80.

_____. 1987. Barriers to entry in the Canadian pharmaceutical industry: Comments, clarification and extensions. *Journal of Health Economics* 6: 59–72.

_____. 1992. *Controlling Drug Expenditures in Canada: The Ontario Experience.* Ottawa (ON): Economic Council of Canada.

GORECKI, P.K., and I. HENDERSON. 1981. Compulsory patent licensing of drugs in Canada: A comment of the debate. *Canadian Public Policy* 7(4): 559–568.

GRABOWSKI, H. G., and J. M. VERNON. 1992. Brand loyalty, entry, and price competition in pharmaceuticals after the 1984 Drug Act. *Journal of Law and Economics* 35(2): 331–350.

GRILICHES, Z., and I. COCKBURN. 1994. Generics and new goods in pharmaceutical price indexes. *American Economic Review* 84(5): 1213–1232.

GROOTENDORST, P., L. GOLDSMITH, J. HURLEY, B. O'BRIEN, and L. DOLOVICH. 1996. Financial incentives to dispense low cost drugs: A case study of British Columbia Pharmacare. Report submitted to Health System and Policy Division, Health Canada.

GROSS, D. J., J. KILE, J. RASTHER, and C. THOMAS. 1996. Prices for prescription drugs: The roles of market forces and government regulation. In *Contested Ground: Public Purpose and Private Interest in the Regulation of Prescription Drugs*, ed. P. DAVIS. New York (NY): Oxford University Press.

GROUP HEALTHCARE MANAGEMENT (GHM). 1995. Specific factors driving costs. Special report. *Group Healthcare Management* 3(11).

HARRISON, P. 1994. Rx to OTC: How will the switches impact pharmacies? *Pharmacy Practice* 10(4): 45–49.

HENDERSON, R., and I. COCKBURN. 1996. Scale, scope, and spillovers: The determinants of research productivity in drug discovery. *Rand Journal of Economics* 27(1): 32–59.

HOLBROOK, A. M., S. M. MCLEOD, P. FISHER, and M. A. LEVINE. 1996. Developing a Canadian prescribing practices network. *Canadian Medical Association Journal* 154(9): 1325–1331.

HUTTIN, C., and J. AVORN. 1996. Drug expenditures for hypertension: An empirical test of a disease-economic model in a French population. Paper presented at the Inaugural Conference of the International Health Economics Association, Vancouver, Canada.

KAITIN, K. 1996. Pharmaceutical innovation in a changing environment. In *Contested Ground: Public Purpose and Private Interest in the Regulation of Prescription Drugs*, ed. P. DAVIS. New York (NY): Oxford University Press.

KENNEDY, W., D. REINHARZ, M. PROULX., and A. CONTANDRIOPOULOS. 1995. *Selected National Drug Programs: Description and Review of Performance.*

LA PUMA, J. 1995. Physician rewards for postmarketing surveillance (seeding studies) in the U.S. *PharmacoEconomics* 7(3): 187–190.

LEVIT, K. R., C. A. COWAN, H. C. LAZENBY, P. A. McDONNELL, A. L. SENSENIG, J. M. STILLER, and D. K. WON. 1994. National health spending trends, 1960–1993. *Health Affairs* 13(5): 14–31.

LEXCHIN, J. 1989. Doctors and detailers: Therapeutic education or pharmaceutical promotion? *International Journal of Health Services* 19(4): 663–679.

_____. 1993a. Pharmaceuticals, patents, and politics. *International Journal of Health Services* 23(1): 147–160.

_____. 1993b. Interaction between physicians and the pharmaceutical industry: What does the literature say? *Canadian Medical Association Journal* 149(10): 1401–1407.

_____. 1994. Canadian marketing codes: How well are they controlling pharmaceutical promotion? *International Journal of Health Services* 24(1): 91–104.

_____. 1996. Income class and pharmaceutical expenditures in Canada: 1964–1990. *Canadian Journal of Public Health* 87(1): 46–50.

MAPELLI, V. 1995. Cost containment measures in the Italian healthcare system. *Pharmacoeconomics* 8(2): 85–90.

MONTAGNE, M. 1992. Drug advertising and promotion: An introduction. *Journal of Drug Issues* 22(2): 195–203.

MOORE, J. 1996. The pharmaceutical industry. Background paper for the National Health Policy Forum: Washington (DC).

MORGAN, S. G. 1994. Government drug plans and their side effects: An application of models of differentiated competition. Unpublished Master's essay. Department of Economics, Queen's University, Kingston, Ontario.

MUNNICH, F. E., and K. SULLIVAN. 1994. The impact of recent legislative change in Germany. *PharmacoEconomics* 6(1)suppl.: 22–27.

PATENTED MEDICINE PRICES REVIEW BOARD (PMPRB). 1989. *First Annual Report.* Supply and Services Canada.

_____. 1990. *Second Annual Report.* Supply and Services Canada.

_____. 1991. *Third Annual Report: For the Year Ended December 31, 1990.* Supply and Services Canada.

_____. 1992. *Fourth Annual Report: For the Year Ended December 31, 1991.* Supply and Services Canada.

_____. 1994. *Sixth Annual Report: For the Year Ended December 31, 1993.* Supply and Services Canada.

_____. 1995. *Seventh Annual Report: For the Year Ended December 31, 1994.* Supply and Services Canada.

_____. 1996a. *Eighth Annual Report: For the Year Ended December 31, 1995.* Supply and Services Canada.

_____. 1996b. *The Top 200 Selling Patented Drug Products in Canada (1994).* Supply and Services Canada.

POSTON, J., R. KENNEDY, and B. WARUSZYNSKI. 1995. Initial Results from the Community Pharmacist Intervention Study. *CPJ* Dec./Jan.: 18–25.

POTASHNIK, T. M. 1995. Patent expiration, generic competition and brand loyalty in the B.C pharmaceutical industry. Unpublished Master's thesis. Department of Economics, University of Victoria, Victoria, British Columbia.

REDWOOD, H. 1993. New drugs in the world market: Incentives and impediments to innovation. *The American Enterprise* 4(4): 72–80.

REEKIE, W. D., and M .H. WEBER. 1979. Profits, politics and drugs. London: Macmillan Press.

RIGTER, H. 1994. Recent public policies in the Netherlands to control pharmaceutical pricing and reimbursement. *PharmacoEconomics* 6(1)suppl.: 15–21.

ROSENBERG, S. A. 1996. Secrecy in medical research. *The New England Journal of Medicine* 334(6): 392–394.

ROYAL COMMISSION ON HEALTH SERVICES (RCHS). 1964. *Provision, Distribution, and Cost of Drugs in Canada.* Department of Health and Welfare. Supply and Services Canada.

SALMON, J.W. 1996. The professional and corporate context: Trends in the United States. In *Contested Ground: Public Purpose and Private Interest in the Regulation of Prescription Drugs*, ed. P. DAVIS. New York (NY): Oxford University Press.

SANTELL, J. P. 1996. Projecting future drug expenditures—1996. *American Journal of Health System Pharmacy* 53(15): 139–150.

SCHERER, F. M. 1993. Pricing. profits, and technological progress in the pharmaceutical industry. *Journal of Economic Perspectives* 7(3): 97–115.

SCHOFFSKI, O. 1996. Consequences of implementing a drug budget for office-based physicians in Germany. *Pharmacoeconomics* 10(suppl. 2): 37–47.

SLATTER, S. 1977. Competition and marketing strategies in the pharmaceutical industry. London: Croom Helm.

SOUMERAI, S. B., T. J. MCLAUGHLIN, and J. AVRON. 1989. Improving drug prescribing in primary care: A critical analysis of the experimental literature. *The Milbank Quarterly* 67: 268–317.

SOUMERAI, S. B., D. ROSS-DEGNAN, E. E. FORTESS, and J. ABELSON. 1993. A critical analysis of studies of state drug reimbursement policies: Research in need of discipline. *The Milbank Quarterly* 71(2): 217–252.

SPINELLO, R. A. 1992. Ethics, pricing, and the pharmaceutical industry. *Journal of Business Ethics* 11: 617–626.

STATISTICS CANADA. 1980–1996. Industrial Product Price Index (IPPI), Series D692601, D693877, and D693869.

STATISTICS CANADA. 1996. *Financial Performance Indicators for Canadian Business.* News Release: Industrial Organization and Finance Division.

STATISTICS CANADA. Various years. Industrial Research and Development Statistics. Cat. No. 88–202. Ottawa (ON).

TAGGART, J.H. 1991. Determinants of the foreign R&D locational decision in the pharmaceutical industry. *R&D Management* 21(3): 229–240.

TAMBLYN, R., and R. PERRFAULT. 1995. *Methods to Encourage the Sensible Use of Prescription Medication in the Elderly.* Position Paper. National Forum on Health. Ottawa (ON).

UNITED STATES GENERAL ACCOUNTING OFFICE (USGAO). 1992. *Prescription Drugs: Companies Typically Charge More in the United States than in Canada.* Report to the Chairman, House of Representatives: Washington.

WALKER, H. D. 1971. *Market Power and Price Levels in the Ethical Drug Industry.* Bloomington (IN): Indiana University Press.

WERTHEIMER, A., W. M. DICKSON, B. A. BRIESACHER. 1996. Pharmacy in the Western world health care system. In *Contested Ground: Public Purpose and Private Interest in the Regulation of Prescription Drugs*, ed. P. DAVIS. New York (NY): Oxford University Press.

WIVELL, M. K., and D. A. O'FALLON. 1992. Drug overpromotion: When is a warning not a warning? *Trial* 82(11): 21–27

Series
Canada Health Action: Building on the Legacy
Papers Commissioned by the National Forum on Health

Volume 1
Determinants of Health
Children and Youth

Jane Bertrand
Enriching the Preschool Experiences of Children

Paul D. Steinhauer
Developing Resiliency in Children from Disadvantaged Populations

David A. Wolfe
Prevention of Child Abuse and Neglect

Christopher Bagley and Wilfreda E. Thurston
Decreasing Child Sexual Abuse

Barbara A. Morrongiello
Preventing Unintentional Injuries among Children

Benjamin H. Gottlieb
Strategies to Promote the Optimal Development of Canada's Youth

Paul Anisef
Making the Transition from School to Employment

Pamela C. Fralick and Brian Hyndman
Youth, Substance Abuse and the Determinants of Health

Gaston Godin and Francine Michaud
STD and AIDS Prevention among Young People

Tullio Caputo and Katharine Kelly
Improving the Health of Street/Homeless Youth

Series
Canada Health Action: Building on the Legacy
Papers Commissioned by the National Forum on Health

Volume 2
Determinants of Health

Adults and Seniors

William R. Avison
The Health Consequences of Unemployment

Mary J. Breen
Promoting Literacy, Improving Health

Neena L. Chappell
Maintaining and Enhancing Independence and Well-Being in Old Age

Sandra O'Brien Cousins
Promoting Active Living and Healthy Eating among Older Canadians

Victor W. Marshall and Philippa J. Clarke
Facilitating the Transition from Employment to Retirement

Dr. Robyn Tamblyn and Dr. Robert Perreault
Encouraging the Wise Use of Prescription Medication by Older Adults

Daphne Nahmiash
Preventing, Reducing and Stopping the Abuse and Neglect of Older Canadian Adults in Canadian Communities

Volume 3
Determinants of Health
Settings and Issues

Susan A. McDaniel
Toward Healthy Families

Kathryn J. Bennett and David R. Offord
Schools, Mental Health and Life Quality

Michael F. D. Polanyi, Joan Eakin, John W. Frank, Harry S. Shannon and Terrence Sullivan
Creating Healthier Work Environments: A Critical Review of the Health Impacts of Workplace Change

Kimberly A. Scott
Balance as a Method to Promote Healthy Indigenous Communities

Pierre Hamel
Community Solidarity and Local Development: A New Perspective for Building Sociopolitical Compromise

Joseph Zayed and Luc Lefebvre
Environmental Health: From Concept to Reality

Marlies Sudermann and Peter G. Jaffe
Preventing Violence: School- and Community-Based Strategies

Ronald J. Dyck, Brian L. Mishara and Jennifer White
Suicide in Children, Adolescents and Seniors: Key Findings and Policy Implications

John Lord and Peggy Hutchison
Living with a Disability in Canada: Toward Autonomy and Integration

Benjamin H. Gottlieb
Protecting and Promoting the Well-Being of Family Caregivers

Peter A. Singer and Douglas K. Martin
Improving Dying in Canada

Terrence Sullivan, Okuri Uneke, John Lavis, Doug Hyatt and John O'Grady
Labour Adjustment Policy and Health: Considerations for a Changing World

Lars Osberg
Economic Policy Variables and Population Health

Series
Canada Health Action: Building on the Legacy
Papers Commissioned by the National Forum on Health

Volume 4
Striking a Balance
Health Care Systems in Canada and Elsewhere

Geoffroy Scott
International Comparison of the Hospital Sector

Astrid Brousselle
Controlling Health Expenditures: What Matters

Wendy Kennedy
Managing Pharmaceutical Expenditures: How Canada Compares

Centre for International Statistics
Health Spending and Health Status: An International Comparison

Damien Contandriopoulos
How Canada's Health Care System Compares with that of Other Countries: An Overview

Delphine Arweiler
International Comparisons of Health Expenditures

Marc-André Fournier
The Impact of Health Care Infrastructures and Human Resources on Health Expenditures

Ellen Leibovich, Howard Bergman and François Béland
Health Care Expenditures and the Aging Population in Canada

Raisa Deber and Bill Swan
Puzzling Issues in Health Care Financing

Terrence Sullivan
Commentary on Health Care Expenditures, Social Spending and Health Status

Allan M. Maslove
National Goals and the Federal Role in Health Care

Raiser Deber, Lutchmie Narine, Pat Baranek et al.
The Public-Private Mix in Health Care

John Marriott and Ann L. Mable
Integrated Models: International Trends and Implications for Canada

Steven G. Morgan
Issues for Canadian Pharmaceutical Policy

Series
Canada Health Action: Building on the Legacy
Papers Commissioned by the National Forum on Health

Volume 5
Making Decisions

Evidence and Information

Joan E. Tranmer, Susan Squires, Kevin Brazil, Jacquelyn Gerlach,
John Johnson, Dianne Muisiner, Bill Swan, Ruth Wilson
  Factors that Influence Evidence-Based Decision Making

Paul Fisher, Marcus J. Hollander, Thomas MacKenzie, Peter Kleinstiver,
Irina Sladecek, Gail Peterson
  Decision Support Tools in Health Care

Charlyn Black
  Building a National Health Information Network

Robert Butcher
  Foundations for Evidence-Based Decision Making

Carol Kushner and Michael Rachlis
  Consumer Involvement in Health Policy Development

Frank L. Graves and Patrick Beauchamp (EKOS Research Associates Inc.);
David Herle (Earnscliffe Research and Communications)
  Research on Canadian Values in Relation to Health and the Health Care System

Thérèse Leroux, Sonia Le Bris, Bartha Maria Knoppers, with
the collaboration of Louis-Nicolas Fortin and Julie Montreuil
  *The Feasibility of a National Canadian Advisory Committee on Ethics:
  Points to Consider*